Noninvasive Molecular Markers in Gynecologic Cancers

Noninvasive Molecular Markers in Gynecologic Cancers

Edited by
Debmalya Barh
Mehmet Gunduz

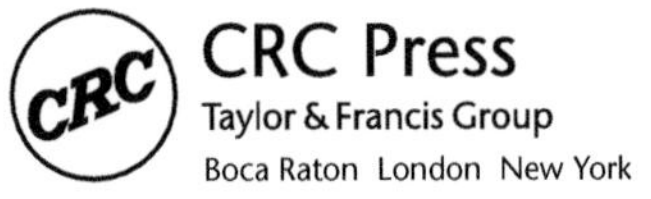

CRC Press is an imprint of the
Taylor & Francis Group, an **informa** business

First published in paperback 2024
First published in hardback 2020

Published 2015
by CRC Press
2385 NW Executive Center Drive, Suite 320, Boca Raton FL 33431

and by CRC Press
4 Park Square, Milton Park, Abingdon, Oxon, OX14 4RN

CRC Press is an imprint of Taylor & Francis Group, LLC

Publisher's Note
The publisher has gone to great lengths to ensure the quality of this reprint but points out that some imperfections in the original copies may be apparent.

ISBN 13: 978-1-4665-6938-6 (hbk)
ISBN 13: 978-1-138-74950-4 (pbk)
ISBN 13: 978-0-429-25427-7; 978-1-351-22883-1 (ebk)

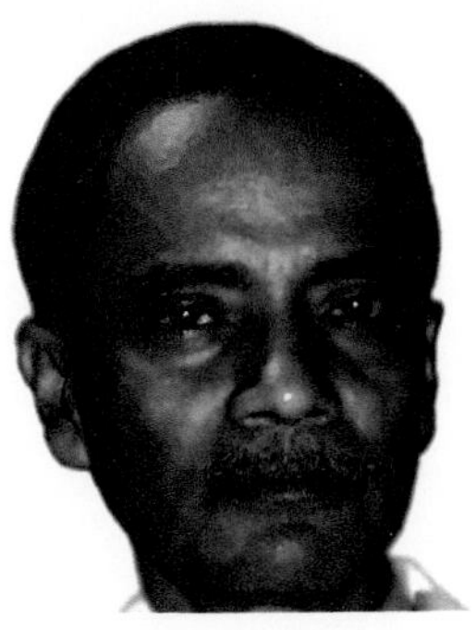

Dedicated to Deb's Maternal Uncle, Dr. S. Samanta, MBBS, DTMH,

a brave fighter against Non-Hodgkin's Lymphoma at 65 years.

Contents

Section VI Vaginal and Vulvar Cancers

Foreword

Gynecologic cancers are major causes of death in women worldwide. In practice, screening and early diagnosis provides an opportunity for better treatment and management and, thus, improves the prognosis and survivability. This book covers all the subsections of gynecologic cancers with the focus on noninvasive biomarkers. Biomarker identification and its critical usage for the early detection of cancer have accelerated in recent years, and the clinical use of noninvasive biomarkers seems to be especially promising. Thus, the topic has a wide appeal to basic scientists, clinical researchers, and physicians (especially from oncology and gynecology).

This *Noninvasive Molecular Markers in Gynecologic Cancers* book by Dr. Barh and Dr. Gunduz is a timely and valuable contribution to the field of gynecologic oncology. Chapters in this book cover all gynecological cancer types (ovarian, cervical, uterine, vaginal, fallopian tube, and vulvar cancers), from different perspectives. For readers' benefit, the book has also included breast cancer. After giving general information about the disease, identified biomarkers are presented in each chapter. The general information in each chapter about disease epidemiology, clinical features, diagnosis, treatment and prognosis will educate non-clinical readers about these particular cancers. The biomarker part of each chapter comprises the results of considerable amounts of research studies along with used, upcoming, and novel non-invasive molecular markers from various classes. Therefore, this book is a useful guideline for clinical researchers and basic scientists to have the overall idea of the non-invasive markers in various gynecologic cancers to be used clinically and also help us to find new and novel ones.

I certainly find this book fascinating and intellectually stimulating and I believe that there are a lot of scientific people and clinicians who will have the similar feelings about the book. I would like to thank all authors and editors for their all efforts to develop this highly useful book.

Dr. Haldun Guner, MD
Professor of Gynecology and Obstetrics,
Faculty of Medicine, Gazi University, Ankara, Turkey

Preface

Cancers that affect women's reproductive organs are collectively referred to as gynecologic cancers and are named according to the part of the body that is affected. Ovarian, cervical, uterine, vaginal, and vulvar cancers are the five main cancers that constitute the group. However, fallopian tube cancer, which is very rare, can also be included in this group. According to various reports, cervical cancer is the second most common cancer in women after breast cancer, and cumulatively both these cancers contribute over 40% of cancer-specific deaths in women worldwide, whereas ovarian and uterine cancers cause 10%–15% of all cancer-associated deaths. From this, we can conclude that gynecologic cancers along with breast cancer contribute to more than 50% of all cancer-associated deaths in women.

Early detection is critical for any given cancer. With the advent of the latest omics technologies, molecular markers in combination with conventional diagnostic and screening methods are emerging as next-generation early diagnostic and prognostic strategies that can allow early-stage diagnosis, resulting in more effective treatment and patient care and, in turn, increased rate of survival. The current trend in diagnosis is slowly shifting from invasive (tissue biopsy based) to minimally invasive or noninvasive (blood, serum, urine, and saliva) methods to avoid complications related to biopsy and other associated patient discomforts. Furthermore, obtaining samples noninvasively is easy and less time consuming. Moreover, molecular markers obtained noninvasively that are currently in use or under development show better sensitivity and specificity as compared to conventional markers obtained through biopsy.

Although there are several books available on various aspects of gynecologic cancers, none have documented the noninvasive molecular biomarkers that are under development or precisely used for screening, early diagnosis, prognosis, and/or therapy for cancers in female reproductive organs. This book, *Noninvasive Molecular Markers in Gynecologic Cancers,* is the first of its kind to fill this gap and to provide a ready-made resource that not only provides information on noninvasive molecular diagnostic biomarkers for gynecological cancers but also accounts for the epidemiology, clinical features, conventional diagnosis, treatment, and prognosis for these cancers. Each of these cancer types has unique signs and symptoms, risk factors, and molecular profile, and therefore requires different prevention strategies. A common factor in all of these cancers is risk, which increases with age and in some cases is associated with genetic predisposition or heritability. Different features of each cancer are explained in detail in dedicated chapters, where general information, epidemiology, clinical features, and biomarkers are given. Breast cancer is also included in the spectrum of cancers specific to women to make this book more complete and beneficial to the target audience: clinicians, oncologists, gynecologists, pathologists, radiologists, medical students, and researchers in biomarkers and targeted drug discovery.

Before the in-depth molecular investigation of gynecologic cancers, etiopathogenesis and clinics of these cancers should be known. To make the book more user-friendly, the 18 chapters are organized into six sections. In Section I, general topics are discussed. In Chapter 1, Dr. Kaygusuz and colleagues present an overview of gynecologic cancer in a compact but comprehensive way. In Chapter 2, Dr. Oznur's group gives a detailed account on early cytogenetic markers for gynecologic cancers.

Section II deals with breast cancer and includes Chapters 3 through 6. In this section, breast cancer biomarkers are investigated from different aspects. In Chapter 3, early molecular biomarkers in breast cancer are presented by Dr. Kaul-Ghanekar et al. Dr. Calomarde's group has specifically described clinical and molecular diagnostic and prognostic markers for invasive breast cancer in Chapter 4. Dr. Yılmaz and colleagues, in Chapter 5, have provided details on biomarkers in familial breast cancer. In the last chapter in this section, Chapter 6, Dr. Hasan's group summarizes the epigenetics of breast cancer and the influence of nutrients for methylation on this cancer.

In Section III, Chapters 7 through 9 deal with cervical cancer. Dr. Kaul-Ghanekar et al. provide a detailed account from the epidemiology to molecular markers of cervical cancer. In Chapter 8, Dr. Serrano's group presents the possible use of HPV, p16, Ki-67, and E6/E7 markers in cervical cancer. In Chapter 9, Dr. Kunos et al. summarize the biomarkers of nucleotide metabolism in cervical cancer.

In Section IV, Chapters 10 through 13, ovarian cancer is investigated from various aspects. In Chapter 10, Dr. O'Toole's group comprehensively presents various noninvasive early biomarkers in ovarian cancer. Dr. Oznur et al. have discussed biomarkers for ovarian endometrioid carcinoma in Chapter 11. In Chapters 12 and 13, two important biomarkers (CA125 and He4) in ovarian cancer are discussed by Dr. Bouanene et al. and Dr. Abehsera et al., respectively.

Section V, Chapters 14 through 16, discusses uterine and fallopian tube cancers. In Chapter 14, Dr. Nas and colleagues present molecular biomarkers for endometrial cancer, and in Chapter 15, Dr. Buery and Dr. Gunduz summarize biomarkers in uterine mesenchymal tumors. Chapter 16 by Dr. Peitsidis gives a detailed account on various aspects of fallopian tube carcinoma, including noninvasive early markers.

Finally, in Section VI, Dr. Ocak et al. and Dr. Iacoponi et al. describe noninvasive early markers associated with vaginal (Chapter 17) and vulvar (Chapter 18) cancer, respectively.

Leading international experts have authored these topics and each chapter is organized with a uniform structure: outline, abstract, detailed information for each title under outline, future perspectives, and references. A sufficient number of illustrations are included to support each topic. This basic structure makes understanding the topics easier. Almost all of the knowledge about all gynecological cancers and their biomarkers has been covered in this book.

We do hope this book will be a useful resource and a reliable and valuable reference on gynecological cancers that will help physicians manage early detection of any given gynecologic cancer and will motivate further research to find more noninvasive biomarkers. We also highly appreciate our readers' valuable comments on further improvements to the contents.

Debmalya Barh, MSc, MTech, MPhil, PhD, PGDM
Mehmet Gunduz, MD, PhD
Editors

Editors

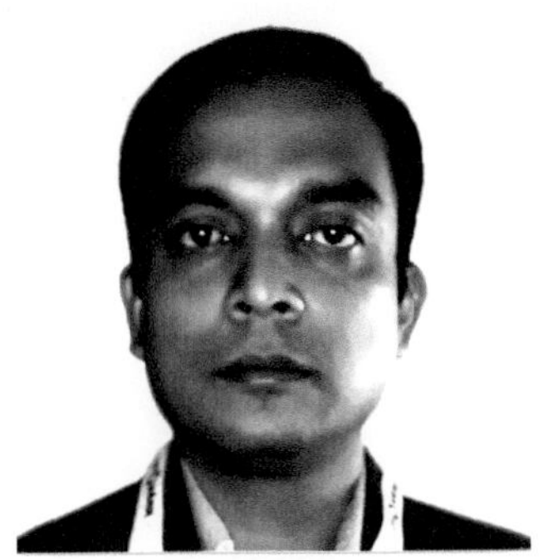

Debmalya Barh, MSc, MTech, MPhil, PhD, PGDM, is the founder of the Institute of Integrative Omics and Applied Biotechnology (IIOAB), India, a first-of-its-kind virtual global platform for multidisciplinary research and advocacy. He is a biotechnologist and active researcher in integrative *omics*-based biomarkers, targeted drug discovery, and personalized medicine for cancers and various complex diseases. He works with nearly 400 esteemed researchers from around 35–40 countries and has more than 125 high-impact international publications and several book chapters and conference presentations. He is a globally branded editor for cutting-edge *omics*-related reference books published by top-ranked international publishers. His cancer related books include *Cancer Biomarkers: Minimal and Noninvasive Early Diagnosis and Prognosis* by Taylor & Francis Group/CRC Press, *Omics Approaches in Breast Cancer: Towards Next-Generation Diagnosis, Prognosis and Therapy* and *Omics for Personalized Medicine* by Springer, among others. Due to his dedicated contribution to the field of applied biomedical and biological sciences and unique research strategies, he was recognized by *Who's Who in the World* in 2010 and was listed in the *Limca Book of Records*, the Indian equivalent to the *Guinness Book of World Records*, in 2014.

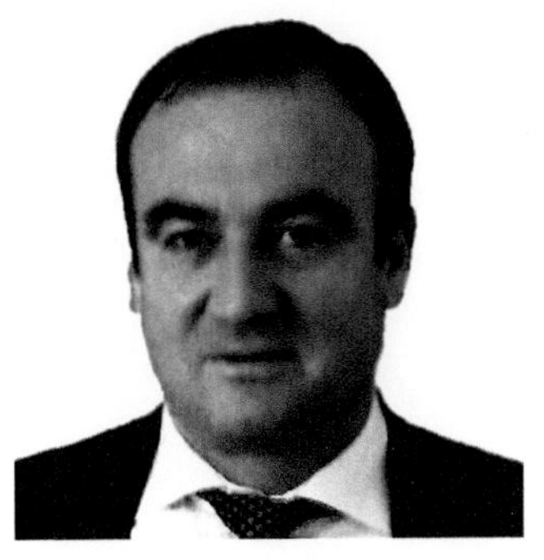

Mehmet Gunduz, MD, PhD, is the professor and head of the Department of Medical Genetics and Otolaryngology, Faculty of Medicine, Turgut Özal University, Ankara, Turkey. Dr. Gunduz graduated from the Medical School Hacettepe University, Ankara, Turkey, with the fourth highest rank in 1990. He completed his residency in otolaryngology, head and neck surgery, at the same university. He earned his PhD in medical genetics from Okayama University and Wakayama Medical University, Japan, and is a medical practitioner board-certified by both the Turkish and Japanese certification authorities. From 2003 to 2004, he worked as a visiting scientist at MD Anderson Cancer Center, Houston, Texas. Dr. Gunduz was one of the pioneers in identifying ING family tumor suppressors and has several publications on various cancer-related molecular markers, including breast cancer. He has more than 170 international publications and 3500 citations, several book chapters, and over 200 presentations in national and international conferences.

Contributors

Daniel Abehsera, MD, PhD
Gynecologic Oncology Unit
La Paz University Hospital
Madrid, Spain

Muradiye Acar, PhD
Faculty of Medicine
Department of Medical Genetics
Turgut Özal University
Ankara, Turkey

Eugen Ancuta, MSc, MD, PhD
Research Department
"Cuza-Voda" Obstetrics and Gynecology Clinical Hospital
Iasi, Romania

Debmalya Barh, MSc, MTech, MPhil, PhD
Centre for Genomics and Applied Gene Technology
Institute of Integrative Omics and Applied Biotechnology
Purba Medinipur, West Bengal, India

and

InterpretOmics India Pvt. Ltd.
Bangalore, Karnataka, India

Jemni Ben Chibani, PhD
Faculty of Pharmacy
Laboratory of Biochemistry and Molecular Biology
Monastir, Tunisia

Houda Bouanene, PhD
Faculty of Pharmacy
Laboratory of Biochemistry and Molecular Biology
Monastir, Tunisia

Dolores J. Cahill, PhD
Conway Institute of Biomedical and Biomolecular Research
University College Dublin
Dublin, Ireland

Maria C. Calomarde, MD
Gynecologic Oncology Unit
La Paz University Hospital
Madrid, Spain

Amit S. Choudhari, MSc
Interactive Research School for Health Affairs
Bharati Vidyapeeth University
Pune, Maharashtra, India

Marcos Cuerva, MD, PhD
Gynecologic Oncology Unit
La Paz University Hospital
Madrid, Spain

Serap Dede, MS
Faculty of Medicine
Department of Medical Genetics
Turgut Özal University
Ankara, Turkey

Javier De Santiago, MD, PhD
Gynecologic Oncology Unit
La Paz University Hospital
Madrid, Spain

María-Dolores Diestro, MD, PhD
Gynecologic Oncology Unit
La Paz University Hospital
Madrid, Spain

Gina Ferris, BA
Department of Radiation Oncology
Case Western Reserve University
Cleveland, Ohio

Mar Gil, MD
Gynecologic Oncology Unit
La Paz University Hospital
Madrid, Spain

Esra Gunduz, DMD, PhD
Faculty of Medicine
Department of Medical Genetics
Turgut Özal University
Ankara, Turkey

Mehmet Gunduz, MD, PhD
Faculty of Medicine
Department of Medical Genetics
Turgut Özal University
Ankara, Turkey

Tarique N. Hasan, MSc
R&D Center
Bharathiar University
Coimbatore, Tamil Nadu, India

Omer Faruk Hatipoglu, PhD
Faculty of Medicine
Department of Medical Genetics
Turgut Özal University
Ankara, Turkey

Alicia Hernández, MD, PhD
Gynecologic Oncology Unit
La Paz University Hospital
Madrid, Spain

Sara Iacoponi, MD, PhD
Gynecologic Oncology Unit
La Paz University Hospital
Madrid, Spain

Carlos Iglesias, MD
Gynecologic Oncology Unit
La Paz University Hospital
Madrid, Spain

Hasan Kafali, MD
Faculty of Medicine
Department of Obstetrics and Gynecology
Gazi University
Ankara, Turkey

Ruchika Kaul-Ghanekar, MSc, PhD
Interactive Research School for Health Affairs
Bharati Vidyapeeth University
Pune, Maharashtra, India

Ikbal Kaygusuz, MD
Faculty of Medicine
Department of Obstetrics and Gynecology
Turgut Özal University
Ankara, Turkey

Aydin Kosus, MD
Faculty of Medicine
Department of Obstetrics and Gynecology
Turgut Özal University
Ankara, Turkey

Charles A. Kunos, MD, PhD
Jean B and Milton Cooper Cancer Center
Summa Health System
Akron, Ohio

Ream Langhe, MB CHB, MSc
Department of Obstetrics and Gynaecology
Trinity Centre
and
Department of Histopathology
Trinity College Dublin
and
Sir Patrick Duns Research Laboratory
Central Pathology Laboratory
St. James's Hospital
and
Coombe Womens and Infants University Hospital
Dublin, Ireland

B. Leena Grace, PhD
Department of Biotechnology
Selvam Arts and Science College
Pappinayakkanpatti, Tamil Nadu, India

Lance Liotta, MD, PhD
Center for Applied Proteomics and Molecular Medicine
George Mason University
Manassas, Virginia

Adolfo Loayza, MD, PhD
Gynecologic Oncology Unit
La Paz University Hospital
Madrid, Spain

Cara Martin, MSc, PhD
Department of Histopathology
Trinity College Dublin
and
Sir Patrick Duns Research Laboratory
Central Pathology Laboratory
St. James's Hospital
and
Coombe Womens and Infants University Hospital
Dublin, Ireland

Lynda McEvoy, PhD
Department of Obstetrics and Gynaecology
Trinity Centre
and
Department of Histopathology
Trinity College Dublin
and
Sir Patrick Duns Research Laboratory
Central Pathology Laboratory
St. James's Hospital
and
Coombe Womens and Infants University Hospital
Dublin, Ireland

Serap Memik, MS
Faculty of Medicine
Department of Medical Genetics
Turgut Özal University
Ankara, Turkey

Elisa Moreno-Palacios, MD
Gynecologic Oncology Unit
La Paz University Hospital
Madrid, Spain

Catherine A. Moroski-Erkul, MS
Faculty of Medicine
Department of Medical Genetics
Turgut Özal University
Ankara, Turkey

Anjana Munshi, PhD
Department of Molecular Biology
Centre for Human Genetics
School of Health Sciences
Central University of Punjab
Bathinda, Punjab, India

Mairead Murphy, PhD
Department of Histopathology
Trinity College Dublin
and
Sir Patrick Duns Research Laboratory
Central Pathology Laboratory
St. James's Hospital
and
Coombe Womens and Infants University Hospital
and
Conway Institute of Biomedical and Biomolecular Research
University College Dublin
Dublin, Ireland

Gokhan Nas, MS
Faculty of Medicine
Department of Medical Genetics
Turgut Özal University
Ankara, Turkey

Zeynep Ocak, MD
Faculty of Medicine
Department of Medical Genetics
Turgut Özal University
Ankara, Turkey

John J. O'Leary, MD, MB, BCh, BAO, BSc, MSc, DPhil
Department of Histopathology
Trinity College Dublin
and
Sir Patrick Duns Research Laboratory
Central Pathology Laboratory
St. James's Hospital
and
Coombe Womens and Infants University Hospital
Dublin, Ireland

Sharon A. O'Toole, MSc, PhD
Department of Obstetrics and Gynaecology
Trinity Centre
and
Department of Histopathology
Trinity College Dublin
and
Sir Patrick Duns Research Laboratory
Central Pathology Laboratory
St. James's Hospital
and
Coombe Womens and Infants University Hospital
Dublin, Ireland

Murat Oznur, MD, PhD
Faculty of Medicine
Department of Medical Genetics
Turgut Özal University
Ankara, Turkey

Savita Pandita, MSc
Interactive Research School for Health Affairs
Bharati Vidyapeeth University
Pune, Maharashtra, India

Panagiotis Peitsidis, MSc, PhD
Department of Obstetrics and Gynecology
Helenas Venizelou Hospital
Athens, Greece

Emmanuel Petricoin, PhD
Center for Applied Proteomics and Molecular Medicine
George Mason University
Manassas, Virginia

Prerna Raina, MSc
Interactive Research School for Health Affairs
Bharati Vidyapeeth University
Pune, Maharashtra, India

Rosario Rivera Buery, DMD, PhD
Graduate School (Dentistry)
University of the East
Manila, Philippines

and

School of Dentistry
Centro Escolar University
Makati, Philippines

María Serrano, MD
Gynecologic Oncology Unit
La Paz University Hospital
Madrid, Spain

Gowhar Shafi, PhD
Department of Molecular Biology
Institute of Genetics and Hospital for Genetic Diseases
Begumpet, Hyderabad, India

and

Unit of Computational Medicine
Department of Medicine
Center for Molecular Medicine
Karolinska Institute
Stockholm, Sweden

Orla Sheils, MA, PhD
Department of Histopathology
Trinity College Dublin
and
Sir Patrick Duns Research Laboratory
Central Pathology Laboratory
St. James's Hospital
and
Coombe Womens and Infants University Hospital
Dublin, Ireland

Lauren Shunkwiler, BA
Department of Radiation Oncology
Case Western Reserve University
Cleveland, Ohio

Cathy Spillane, PhD
Department of Histopathology
Trinity College Dublin
and
Sir Patrick Duns Research Laboratory
Central Pathology Laboratory
St. James's Hospital
and
Coombe Womens and Infants University Hospital
Dublin, Ireland

Snehal Suryavanshi, MSc
Interactive Research School for Health Affairs
Bharati Vidyapeeth University
Pune, Maharashtra, India

Jesper Tegner, PhD
Unit of Computational Medicine
Department of Medicine
Center for Molecular Medicine
Karolinska Institute
Stockholm, Sweden

Tugce Yasar, MS
Faculty of Medicine
Department of Medical Genetics
Turgut Özal University
Ankara, Turkey

Burak Yılmaz, MS
Faculty of Medicine
Department of Medical Genetics
Turgut Özal University
Ankara, Turkey

Ignacio Zapardiel, MD, PhD
Gynecologic Oncology Unit
La Paz University Hospital
Madrid, Spain

Section I

General

1

Overview of Gynecologic Cancers

Ikbal Kaygusuz, MD, Aydin Kosus, MD, and Hasan Kafali, MD

CONTENTS

ABSTRACT Gynecologic cancers are an important cause of morbidity and mortality in women. Each gynecologic cancer is unique, with different signs and symptoms, different risk factors, and different prevention strategies. All women are at risk for gynecologic cancers, and risk increases with age. Uterine cancer is the most common gynecologic malignancy in developed countries. The majority of women with uterine cancer are diagnosed at an early stage because of early signs as uterine bleeding in a postmenopausal woman. Ovarian cancer is the leading cause of mortality among the gynecological malignancies, since the majority of ovarian cancers are diagnosed at an advanced stage. Cervical cancer screening and prevention programs have markedly decreased the incidence of the disease, and cervical cancer is the third most common cancer diagnosis and cause of death among gynecologic cancers in developed countries. Among all three of these reproductive-system cancers, early detection is crucial. But detection can be very difficult, especially in the early stages. Malignant tumors of the vulva, vagina, and fallopian tube are uncommon. There are several ways to treat gynecologic cancer. The treatment depends on the type of cancer and how far it has spread. If gynecologic cancers are discovered at an early stage, surgery can be curative. Radiotherapy or chemotherapy may be given postoperatively. A multidisciplinary approach to the treatment of gynecologic cancers is necessary.

1.1 Introduction

Gynecologic cancers include malignancies of the female genital tract involving the vulva, vagina, cervix, uterus, fallopian tubes, or ovaries. Gynecologic cancers are an important cause of morbidity and mortality in women. Therefore, it is important to determine their incidence and risk factors, investigate their causes, develop new methods for screening and diagnosis, predict about the survival of patients, and determine the appropriate strategies for the prevention and treatment of gynecological cancers. In the last two decades, considerable gains have been made in the detection and treatment of these cancers. When detected in early stages, most gynecologic cancers have a good cure rate.

This chapter focuses on the epidemiology, risk factors, clinical features, diagnosis, screening, prevention, mode of spread, staging, treatment, and prognosis of gynecologic cancers one by one. All women are at risk for gynecologic cancers, and risk increases with age.

1.2 Vulvar Cancer

1.2.1 Vulvar Squamous Cell Carcinoma

1.2.1.1 Epidemiology and Risk Factors

Malignant tumors of the vulva are uncommon, representing 5% of malignancies of the female genital tract [1]. Vulvar cancer is the fourth most common gynecologic cancer (following cancer of the uterine corpus, ovary, and cervix) [1]. It is encountered most frequently in postmenopausal women. The mean age at diagnosis is 65 [2]. Approximately 90% of vulvar malignancies are squamous cell carcinomas (SCCs); other histologies include melanoma, Bartholin's gland adenocarcinoma, sarcoma, Paget's disease, or basal cell carcinoma [3]. Risk factors for vulvar cancer include smoking, vulvar dystrophy (e.g., lichen sclerosus), vulvar or cervical intraepithelial neoplasia, human papillomavirus (HPV) infection, immunodeficiency syndromes, a prior history of cervical cancer, and northern European ancestry [4].

Recent studies suggest two different etiologic types of vulvar cancer. One type is seen mainly in younger patients, is related to mucosal HPV infection and smoking, and is commonly associated with vulvar intraepithelial neoplasia. Its prognosis is good. The second type is related to chronic inflammatory (vulvar dystrophy) or autoimmune processes. It is seen mainly in elderly women [5]. HPV has been shown to be responsible for 60% of vulvar cancers [6]. Specifically, HPV 16 and 33 are the predominant subtypes accounting for 55.5% of all HPV-related vulvar cancers [7]. The presence of the cervix does not appear to be necessary for oncogenic HPV to infect the genital tract. The prevalence of oncogenic HPV subtypes in the vagina is similar in women who have and have not undergone hysterectomy [8].

1.2.1.2 Clinical Features

Most patients are asymptomatic at the time of diagnosis. If symptoms exist, vulvar pruritus, a lump, and a mass are the most common findings. Pruritus is especially prevalent when there is an underlying vulvar dystrophy (e.g., lichen sclerosus or squamous cell hyperplasia). Less frequent symptoms include a vulvar bleeding or ulcerative lesion, discharge, pain, and dysuria. Occasionally, a large metastatic mass in the groin may be the initial symptom [9].

The lesions may be arisen, ulcerated, pigmented, or warty in appearance. Most lesions occur on the labia majora; the labia minora, perineum, clitoris, and mons are less frequently involved. Lesions are multifocal in 5% of cases. A synchronous second malignancy, most commonly cervical neoplasia, is found in up to 22% of patients with a vulvar malignancy [10].

1.2.1.3 Diagnosis

A careful inspection of the vulva is performed based upon vulvar complaints or during a routine pelvic examination. Vulvar cancer is a histologic diagnosis based upon a vulvar biopsy. The biopsy should be taken from the center of the lesion. If multiple abnormal areas are present, then multiple biopsies should be taken to *map* all potential sites of vulvar pathology. If a lesion is not grossly evident, but there is clinical suspicion of vulvar neoplasia, a 5% acetic acid solution application and colposcopic examination should be performed. Acetowhite areas with abnormal vascular patterns should be biopsied.

1.2.1.3.1 *Differential Diagnosis*

Differential diagnosis includes epidermal inclusion cysts, lentigos, disorders of Bartholin's gland, acrochordons, seborrheic keratoses, hidradenomas, lichen sclerosus and other dermatoses, and condyloma acuminata. If one of these disorders is initially suspected but does not respond to appropriate treatment, biopsy should be performed.

1.2.1.4 Mode of Spread

Vulvar carcinoma spread by the following modes:

- Direct extension to adjacent structures (e.g., vagina, urethra, clitoris, anus).
- Lymphatic embolization to regional inguinal and femoral lymph nodes. Lymphatic metastases can occur early in the course of disease, even in patients with small lesions. Ten percent of T1 tumors have lymph node metastases at diagnosis [11]. Most vulvar cancers spread firstly to the groin (inguinal–femoral) lymph nodes, which explains why these nodes are sampled as part of staging. Lesions that are on one side of the vulva generally spread only to the ipsilateral groin nodes. Lymphatic drainage from the clitoris, anterior labia minora, and perineum is bilateral.
- Hematogenous spread to distant sites, including the lungs, liver, and bone. It occurs late in the course of the disease and is rare in the absence of lymph node metastases.

1.2.1.5 Staging

Vulvar cancer is staged using surgical–pathologic staging system based upon findings from the biopsy of the vulvar lesion(s) and the inguinofemoral lymph nodes (Table 1.1) [12]. The prognostic importance of the lymph node status is significant, yet the accuracy of the clinical assessment of the lymph nodes is limited, so clinical staging is inadequate. Staging and primary surgical treatment are typically performed as a single procedure consisting of radical resection of the tumor and inguinofemoral lymphadenectomy (LND). Sentinel lymph node biopsy (SLNB) appears to be a promising approach but remains investigational.

TABLE 1.1

Staging Vulvar Cancer (FIGO)[a]

FIGO Stages	Definition
IA	Lesions 2 cm or less in size, confined to the vulva or perineum and with stromal invasion 1.0 mm or less[b]
IB	Lesions more than 2 cm in size or any size with stromal invasion more than 1.0 mm, confined to the vulva or perineum
II	Tumor of any size with extension to adjacent perineal structures (lower/distal one-third of the urethra, lower/distal one-third of the vagina, anal involvement)
IIIA	One or two regional lymph nodes
IIIB	Three or more lymph node metastases
IIIC	Lymph node metastasis with extracapsular spread
IVA	Tumor of any size with extension to any of the following: upper/proximal two-thirds of the urethra, upper/proximal two-thirds of the vagina, bladder mucosa, rectal mucosa, or fixed to pelvic bone and fixed or ulcerated regional lymph node metastasis
IVB	Distant metastasis (including pelvic lymph node metastasis)

Source: Data from American Joint Committee on Cancer, Corpus uteri, in: *AJCC Cancer Staging Manual*, 7th edn., Springer, New York, 2010.

[a] This staging classification does not apply to vulvar malignant melanoma.

[b] The depth of invasion is defined as the measurement of the tumor from the epithelial–stromal junction of the adjacent most superficial dermal papilla to the deepest point of invasion.

1.2.1.6 Treatment

1.2.1.6.1 Early-Stage Disease: Stages I and II

Traditional radical vulvectomy with en bloc inguinofemoral LND results in significant morbidity [13]. A more conservative approach has been used for the primary lesion. Depending upon the size and location of the lesion, this may necessitate radical local excision or partial radical vulvectomy. Women with stage IA disease with no clinically palpable groin nodes do not require inguinofemoral LND [14]. Women with stage IB disease that is unilateral and is not located in the anterior portion of the labia minora may undergo unilateral rather than bilateral inguinofemoral LND. All other patients require bilateral LND [15].

In general, primary surgical treatment for women with all stages of vulvar cancer is the most conservative technique that results in a ≥1 cm tumor-free margin. Primary radiation therapy (RT) is generally avoided for the management of early-stage vulvar cancers because of associated morbidity. If the patient is not fit enough to tolerate surgery, RT will be the preferred mode of therapy. In women with stage I or II disease with margins <1 cm after excision, reexcision rather than RT is suggested [16].

1.2.1.6.2 Advanced Disease: Stages III and IV

The standard management for patients with advanced vulvar cancer involving the proximal urethra, anus, or rectovaginal septum requires standard radical vulvectomy with en bloc bilateral inguinofemoral LND with partial removal of any involved structures or pelvic exenteration. Postoperative RT to the vulva for patients with high risk of local recurrence is suggested [16]. For patients with two or more positive inguinal lymph node, adjuvant pelvic RT is recommended [17]. Chemoradiation rather than vulvectomy is suggested for patients who would require an ostomy as a result of bowel or bladder resection and for patients with disease that is fixed to the bone [18].

Chemotherapy, RT, and surgery are options for management of regional recurrences and metastatic disease. Local perineal recurrences can be treated successfully by reexcision.

1.2.1.7 Prognosis

The presence of inguinofemoral node metastases is the most important prognostic factor for survival in patients with vulvar cancer [19]. Patients with negative lymph nodes have a 5-year survival rate of approximately 90%, which falls to approximately 50% for patients with positive lymph nodes [20]. Other prognostic factors include stage (which encompasses size and depth of invasion), capillary lymphatic space invasion, and older age [21].

1.2.2 Other Histologic Types

1.2.2.1 Melanoma

Melanoma is the second most common vulvar cancer histology, accounting for approximately 5%–10% of primary vulvar neoplasms [22]. It occurs predominantly in postmenopausal white women, at a median age of 68 years [22]. The initial symptoms are generally vulvar lesions, pruritus, or bleeding.

Vulvar melanoma is usually a pigmented lesion, but amelanotic lesions also occur. Most arise de novo on the clitoris or labia minora but can also develop within preexisting junctional or compound nevi [23]; thus, any nevus on the vulva should be removed. The International Federation of Gynecology and Obstetrics (FIGO) staging of vulvar cancer does not apply well to melanomas, which are usually smaller lesions and tend to metastasize early. Table 1.2 shows seventh (2010) tumor, node, metastasis (TNM) staging system for cutaneous melanoma. The prognosis correlates with the depth of penetration into the dermis. Lesions with less than 1 mm of invasion may be treated with radical local excision alone [24]. With more invasive lesions,

TABLE 1.2

Seventh (2010) TNM Staging System for Cutaneous Melanoma

Primary Tumor (T)	
TX	Primary tumor cannot be assessed (e.g., curettaged or severely regressed primary)
T0	No evidence of primary tumor
Tis	Melanoma in situ
T1	≤1.0 mm
	Without ulceration and mitoses $<1/\text{mm}^2$
	With ulceration or mitoses $\geq 1/\text{mm}^2$
T2	1.01–2.0 mm
	Without ulceration
	With ulceration
T3	2.01–4.0 mm
	Without ulceration
	With ulceration
T4	>4.0 mm
	Without ulceration
	With ulceration
Regional Lymph Nodes (N)	
NX	Patients in whom the regional nodes cannot be assessed (e.g., previously removed for another reason)
N0	No regional metastases detected
N1	One lymph node
	Micrometastases[a]
	Macrometastases[b]
N2	Two or three lymph nodes
	Micrometastases[a]
	Macrometastases[b]
	In-transit met(s)/satellite(s) without metastatic lymph nodes
N3	Four or more metastatic lymph nodes, matted lymph nodes, or in-transit met(s)/satellite(s) with metastatic lymph node(s)
Distant Metastasis (M)	
M0	No detectable evidence of distant metastases
M1a	Metastases to the skin, subcutaneous, or distant lymph node, normal serum LDH
M1b	Lung metastases, normal LDH
M1c	Metastasis to other visceral metastases with a normal LDH or any distant metastases and an elevated LDH

Source: Data from American Joint Committee on Cancer, Corpus uteri, in: *AJCC Cancer Staging Manual*, 7th edn., Springer, New York, 2010.

[a] Micrometastases are diagnosed after SLNB and completion LND (if performed).

[b] Macrometastases are defined as clinically detectable lymph node metastases confirmed by therapeutic LND or when any lymph node metastasis exhibits gross extracapsular extension.

en bloc resection of the primary tumor and regional groin nodes has traditionally been recommended [25]. The overall 5-year survival rate for vulvar melanomas is approximately 30% [23].

1.2.2.2 Verrucous Carcinoma

Verrucous carcinoma is a variant of squamous cell cancer that has distinctive features. It has a cauliflower-like appearance. The lesion grows slowly and rarely metastasizes to lymph nodes, but it may be locally destructive [26].

1.2.2.3 Basal Cell Carcinoma

Two percent of vulvar cancers are basal cell cancers, and 2% of basal cell cancers occur on the vulva [27]. They usually affect postmenopausal Caucasian women and may be locally invasive, however, usually nonmetastasizing [28]. They are often asymptomatic, but pruritus, bleeding, or pain may occur. Basal cell carcinomas are associated with a high incidence of antecedent or concomitant malignancy elsewhere in the body [28]. Thus, a thorough search for other primary malignancies should be performed.

1.2.2.4 Sarcoma

Soft tissue sarcomas (including leiomyosarcomas, rhabdomyosarcomas, liposarcomas, angiosarcomas, neurofibrosarcomas, fibrous histiocytomas, and epithelioid sarcomas) constitute 1%–2% of vulvar malignancies. The prognosis is generally poor [29].

1.2.2.5 Extramammary Paget's Disease

Extramammary Paget's disease, an intraepithelial adenocarcinoma, accounts for less than 1% of all vulvar malignancies [30]. Most patients are in their 60s and 70s and Caucasian. Pruritus is the most common symptom, present in 70% of patients. Vulvar Paget's disease is similar in appearance to Paget's disease of the breast. The lesion has an eczematoid appearance. It is usually multifocal and may occur anywhere on the vulva, mons, perineum/perineal area, or inner thigh. Extramammary Paget's disease and basal cell carcinomas are associated with a high incidence of antecedent or concomitant malignancy elsewhere in the body. Assessment for synchronous neoplasms is suggested.

1.2.2.6 Bartholin's Gland Adenocarcinoma

Although a rare malignancy, most primary adenocarcinomas of the vulva occur in the Bartholin's gland. The median age at diagnosis of Bartholin's gland cancer is 57 [31]. Bartholin's gland tumors are usually solid and infiltrate deep into the vulva. Enlargement of the Bartholin's gland in a postmenopausal woman is worrisome for malignancy, since benign inflammatory disease usually does not occur in this age group. The gland should be biopsied in older (over 40 years of age) women with a mass in this location, even if the lesion appears cystic or abscessed. Metastatic disease is common in cancers of Bartholin's gland because of the rich vascular and lymphatic network in this area.

1.3 Vaginal Cancer

1.3.1 Incidence and Risk Factors

Primary cancer of the vagina is a relatively uncommon tumor, represents only 1%–2% of malignant neoplasms of the female genital tract [1]. The majority of vaginal malignancies are metastatic, often arising from the endometrium, cervix, and vulva by direct extension and the ovary, breast, rectum, and kidney by lymphatic or hematogenous spread [32].

In general, vaginal cancers are associated with the same risk factors as in cervical cancers: multiple lifetime sexual partners, early age at first intercourse, and being current smoker [4]. Most cases of vaginal cancer appear to be related to HPV infection, just as with cervical cancer [33]. Thirty percent of women with vaginal cancer have a history of cervical cancer treated at least 5 years earlier [34]. Some lesions may occur after irradiation for cervical cancer.

1.3.2 Clinical Features

Painless vaginal bleeding, either postmenopausal or postcoital, and watery, blood-tinged, or malodorous discharge are the most common symptoms. With more advanced tumors, vaginal mass, urinary symptoms (e.g., frequency, dysuria, hematuria), gastrointestinal complaints (e.g., tenesmus, constipation, melena), and pelvic pain may occur [35]. However, as many as 20% of women are asymptomatic at the time of diagnosis [36]. These vaginal cancers may be detected as a result of cytologic screening for cervical cancer. Most of primary vaginal carcinomas occur in the posterior wall of the upper one-third of the vagina.

1.3.3 Diagnosis

The diagnosis of vaginal carcinoma can be difficult. The lesion may be missed on initial examination if it is small and situated in the lower two-thirds of the vagina. It is important to rotate the speculum to obtain a careful view. On physical examination, ulcerative, exophytic, and infiltrative growth patterns may be seen. Twenty percent of vaginal tumors are detected incidentally as a result of cytologic screening for cervical cancer by Papanicolaou (Pap) smear [36]. Definitive diagnosis is accomplished by biopsy of the suspected lesion. Colposcopy is valuable in evaluating patients with abnormal cytologic results, and it should be performed with acetic acid followed by Lugol's iodine stain to cervix and vagina.

1.3.4 Epidemiology and Pathology

1.3.4.1 Squamous Cell Carcinoma

SCCs are the most common form of vaginal cancer, occurring in 80%–90% of cases. The mean age at diagnosis is approximately 60 years, although the disease is seen occasionally in women in their 20s and 30s [37].

Verrucous carcinoma is an uncommon variant of vaginal SCC that is well differentiated and has low malignant potential [38]. It usually presents as a large, warty, fungating mass that is locally aggressive but rarely metastasizes.

1.3.4.2 Adenocarcinoma

Adenocarcinomas of the vagina occur in 9% of the vaginal cancers. Adenocarcinomas may arise in areas of vaginal adenosis, Wolffian rest elements, periurethral glands, and foci of endometriosis. Clear-cell variants of adenocarcinoma occur in women exposed in utero to diethylstilbestrol (DES) [39]. Grossly, clear-cell carcinomas of the vagina usually present as polypoid masses, most often on the anterior wall of the vagina. The median age at diagnosis is 19 years [40]. Approximately 70% of patients are stage I at the time of diagnosis and have good outcomes with primary radiation, surgery, or both [41]. On the other hand, adenocarcinomas that occur in non-DES-exposed women tend to have a poorer outcome [42].

1.3.4.3 Sarcoma

Leiomyosarcomas, endometrial stromal sarcomas (ESSs), malignant mixed Müllerian tumors, and rhabdomyosarcomas are the major types of primary vaginal sarcomas. The most common of these is the embryonal rhabdomyosarcoma (sarcoma botryoides), a highly malignant tumor that occurs in the vagina during infancy and early childhood (mean age 3 years) [43].

1.3.4.4 Melanoma

Melanoma of the vagina is rare [44] and extremely lethal. These malignancies occur at a mean age of approximately 60 years. They occur most frequently on the distal one-third of the anterior vaginal wall. The presenting symptom is most commonly vaginal bleeding. Importantly, they are often nonpigmented.

1.3.5 Mode of Spread

Vaginal cancer spreads most often by direct extension into the pelvic soft tissues and adjacent organs. The lymphatic drainage of the upper vagina is to the pelvic nodes and then to the para-aortic nodes. The distal one-third of the vagina drains primarily to the inguinofemoral nodes. Hematogenous spread to the lungs, liver, or bone may occur as a late phenomenon.

1.3.6 Staging

The FIGO staging for vaginal cancer is clinical and based upon findings from physical and pelvic examination, cystoscopy, proctoscopy, and chest and skeletal radiography (Table 1.3) [12].

1.3.7 Treatment

RT is the main method of treatment for vaginal cancer [45]. Surgery is limited to high selective cases. Women with stage I disease in the upper vagina that are less than 2 cm in diameter may be treated with either surgery or intracavitary RT. The surgical approach requires a radical hysterectomy, upper vaginectomy, and bilateral pelvic LND. Women with stage IV lesions with rectovaginal or vesicovaginal fistula and central pelvic recurrence after RT are candidates for pelvic exenteration [45].

TABLE 1.3

Staging Vaginal Cancer (FIGO)

FIGO Stages	Definition
I	Tumor confined to vagina.
II	Tumor invades paravaginal tissues but not to pelvic wall.
III	Tumor extends to pelvic wall. Pelvic or inguinal lymph node metastasis.
IVA	Tumor invades mucosa of the bladder or rectum and/or extends beyond the true pelvis (bullous edema is not sufficient evidence to classify a tumor as T4).
IVB	Distant metastasis.

Source: Data from American Joint Committee on Cancer, Corpus uteri, in: *AJCC Cancer Staging Manual*, 7th edn., Springer, New York, 2010.

RT is the treatment of choice for all patients except those described previously. Small superficial lesions may be treated with brachytherapy alone. Patients with stage I lesions that are greater than 2 cm in diameter and all patients with stages II–IV disease should be treated with external beam radiation with or without intracavitary or interstitial brachytherapy [46]. For stage II disease, neoadjuvant chemotherapy followed by radical surgery may be a promising alternative to RT [47].

1.3.7.1 Treatment-Related Complications

Rectovaginal or vesicovaginal fistulas, radiation cystitis or proctitis, rectal and vaginal strictures, and, rarely, vaginal necrosis will develop in 15% of patients treated for vaginal cancer. Radiation-induced premature menopause is another problem in women under 40 years of age. Oophoropexy may be performed to reduce the toxicity of radiation exposure in selected cases.

1.3.8 Prognosis

Stage is the most important variable to affect the prognosis. The overall 5-year survival rate for patients with vaginal cancer is 42% [45]. These lower rates may reflect the higher proportion of vaginal tumors initially diagnosed at an advanced stage and the potential for treatment complications that prevents aggressive therapy.

1.4 Cervical Cancer

1.4.1 Epidemiology and Risk Factors

Worldwide, approximately 500,000 new cases of cervical cancer (~1 case per minute) are diagnosed, and 275,000 deaths from cervical cancer occur annually, making it the second most common female cancer. More than 80% of all cervical cancers occur in women in developing countries [48]. Cervical cancer screening and prevention programs have markedly decreased the incidence of the disease, and cervical cancer is the third most common cancer diagnosis and cause of death among gynecologic cancers in developed countries [1]. The lifetime risk of developing cervical cancer is 0.76% [49], and its incidence and mortality are higher in nonwhite than in white women.

The mean age at diagnosis of cervical cancer is 47 years, and the distribution of cases is bimodal, with peaks at 35–39 and 60–64 years of age [48].

There are numerous risk factors for cervical cancer, but 99.7% of cervical cancers are attributed to infection with HPV, and about 70% of them are caused by types 16 and 18 [50]. While HPV is a necessary cause of cervical cancer, other cofactors are necessary for progression from cervical HPV infection to cancer. These cofactors include long-term use of hormonal contraceptives; high parity; tobacco smoking (especially SCC); coinfection with human immunodeficiency virus, herpes simplex virus type 2, and *Chlamydia trachomatis*; immunosuppression; certain dietary deficiencies; and genetic and immunological host factors [51]. Multiple sexual partners, early onset of sexual activity, a high-risk sexual partner, low socioeconomic status, and early age at first birth are also associated with an increased risk of cervical cancer. These are also likely due to exposure to HPV through sexual intercourse [52]. Cervical cancer is less common in sexual partners of circumcised males [53]. Genital tract HPV infection is extremely common, but results in cervical cancer in only a small proportion of infected women. It has been estimated that 75%–80% of sexually active adults will acquire genital tract HPV before the age of 50 [54]. When HPV infection persists, the time from initial infection to development of high-grade cervical intraepithelial neoplasia and, finally, invasive cancer takes an average of 15 years [55].

1.4.2 Histopathology

The two major histologic types of cervical cancer are SCC (69%) and adenocarcinoma (25%). Adenosquamous tumors exhibit both glandular and squamous differentiation. They may be associated with a poorer outcome than squamous cell cancers or adenocarcinomas [56]. Neuroendocrine or small-cell carcinomas, rhabdomyosarcoma, primary cervical lymphoma, and cervical sarcoma can originate in the cervix in women but are infrequent [57].

1.4.3 Clinical Features

Early cervical cancer is frequently asymptomatic. Irregular or heavy vaginal bleeding and postcoital bleeding are the most common symptoms [57]. Watery, mucoid, or purulent and malodorous vaginal discharge is another nonspecific finding and may be mistaken for vaginitis or cervicitis. Pelvic or lower back pain, which may radiate along the posterior side of the lower extremities, and bowel or urinary symptoms are uncommon and suggest advanced disease.

1.4.4 Diagnosis

The diagnosis of cervical cancer is established by biopsy. Symptomatic women without a visible lesion and those who have only abnormal cervical cytology should undergo colposcopy with directed biopsy and, if necessary, diagnostic conization [57].

Cervical cancer usually originates at the transformation zone. The lesion may manifest as superficial ulceration, exophytic tumor in the exocervix, or infiltration of the endocervix. Endophytic tumors can result in an enlarged, indurated cervix whose surface is smooth, referred to as a *barrel-shaped cervix*. Among cervical adenocarcinomas, approximately one-half are exophytic, others diffusely enlarge or ulcerate the cervix, and about 15% have no visible lesion because the carcinoma is within the endocervical canal [57].

A thorough pelvic examination including rectovaginal examination with assessment of tumor size and vaginal or parametrial involvement is required for staging cervical cancer. Other suspicious physical examination findings are palpable groin or supraclavicular lymph nodes.

1.4.4.1 Cervical Cytology

Cervical cytology is the principal method for cervical cancer screening. Cytology should also be performed for women with suspected cervical cancer [58].

HPV testing is used in combination with cervical cytology for cervical cancer screening and helps to determine which women with abnormal cytology results require further evaluation. However, it does not play a role in the diagnosis of malignancy in women with symptoms or a visible lesion suggestive of cervical cancer [58].

1.4.4.2 Cervical Biopsy and Colposcopy

Cervical biopsy may be performed as part of an initial evaluation or along with a full staging procedure. When obvious lesion is present, a cervical biopsy is usually sufficient for diagnosis. If gross disease is not present, a colposcopic examination with cervical biopsies and endocervical curettage is warranted. Colposcopic findings that suggest invasion are abnormal blood vessels, irregular surface contour with loss of surface epithelium, and color tone change. If the diagnosis cannot be established conclusively with colposcopy and directed biopsies, cervical conization may be necessary [59].

1.4.4.3 Differential Diagnosis

The differential diagnosis of cervical cancer includes other conditions that result in irregular or heavy vaginal bleeding, vaginal discharge, or visible cervical lesions as cervicitis, nabothian cysts, mesonephric cysts, cervical ectropion, ulcers associated with sexually transmitted infections, reactive glandular changes from inflammation, and endometriosis.

1.4.5 Screening and Prevention

The rate of cervical cancer has declined significantly in settings in which cervical cancer screening is employed. Widespread cytologic screening efforts include conventional Papanicolaou tests and, in developed, high-resource countries, liquid-based cytology (LBC). LBC improves the transfer of cells onto slides, yields more homogeneous cell samples, and is better suited for automated screening devices than conventional smears [58].

The discovery of a strong causal association between HPV infection and cervical cancer changed perspectives about cervical cancer prevention by introducing HPV DNA and RNA testing and spurring the development of prophylactic vaccines [54,55].

1.4.6 Mode of Spread

Cervical cancer can spread by direct extension or by lymphatic or hematogenous dissemination. Direct extension may involve the uterine corpus, vagina, parametria, peritoneal cavity, bladder, or rectum. Cervical cancer extends to pelvic and para-aortic lymph nodes by lymphatic spread, and it may extend to the lungs, liver, and bone by hematogenous spread.

1.4.7 Staging

Cervical cancer is a clinically staged disease [60]. The diagnosis of cervical cancer is made based upon histologic evaluation of a cervical biopsy. After histologic confirmation, the extent of disease is determined by the FIGO staging system that is largely based upon physical examination (pelvic examination with speculum, bimanual and rectovaginal examination, palpation of groin and supraclavicular lymph nodes, examination of the right upper quadrant), cervical biopsy (colposcopy with directed cervical biopsy, endocervical curettage, conization), and a limited number of endoscopic diagnostic procedures (hysteroscopy, cystoscopy, proctoscopy) and imaging studies (intravenous pyelogram [IVP], plain chest radiograph, and radiograph of the skeleton) (Table 1.4) [59,60].

The use of imaging studies to assess tumor size and local spread is controversial. If imaging is used, magnetic resonance imaging (MRI) is suggested rather than computed tomography (CT) or positron-emission tomography (PET). Cervical cancer may spread to the pelvic or para-aortic lymph nodes as well as more distal nodes. The presence of lymph node involvement does not alter the FIGO stage, but it is associated with a worse prognosis and impacts decisions regarding the RT field. Options for evaluating for lymph node metastases include lymph node dissection, imaging studies, or both [61]. Tumor stage is determined at the time of primary diagnosis of cervical cancer and is not changed because of subsequent findings, even upon recurrence [61].

TABLE 1.4

Staging Cervical Cancer (FIGO)

FIGO Stages	Definition
I	Cervical carcinoma confined to uterus (extension to corpus should be disregarded).
IA	Invasive carcinoma diagnosed only by microscopy. Stromal invasion with a maximum depth of 5.0 mm measured from the base of the epithelium and a horizontal spread of 7.0 mm or less. Vascular space involvement, venous or lymphatic, does not affect classification.
IA1	Measured stromal invasion 3.0 mm or less in depth and 7.0 mm or less in horizontal spread.
IA2	Measured stromal invasion more than 3.0 mm and not more than 5.0 mm in depth with a horizontal spread 7.0 mm or less.
IB	Clinically visible lesion confined to the cervix or microscopic lesion greater than IA2.
IB1	Clinically visible lesion 4.0 cm or less in the greatest dimension.
IB2	Clinically visible lesion more than 4.0 cm in the greatest dimension.
II	Cervical carcinoma invades beyond uterus but not to pelvic wall or to lower third of the vagina.
IIA	Tumor without parametrial invasion or involvement of the lower one-third of the vagina.
IIA1	Clinically visible lesion 4.0 cm or less in the greatest dimension with involvement of less than the upper two-thirds of the vagina.
IIA2	Clinically visible lesion more than 4.0 cm in the greatest dimension with involvement of less than the upper two-thirds of the vagina.
IIB	Tumor with parametrial invasion.
III	Tumor extends to pelvic wall and/or involves lower third of the vagina and/or causes hydronephrosis or nonfunctioning kidney.
IIIA	Tumor involves lower third of the vagina, no extension to pelvic wall.
IIIB	Tumor extends to pelvic wall and/or causes hydronephrosis or nonfunctioning kidney.
IVA	Tumor invades mucosa of the bladder or rectum and/or extends beyond true pelvis.

Source: Data from American Joint Committee on Cancer, Corpus uteri, in: *AJCC Cancer Staging Manual*, 7th edn., Springer, New York, 2010.

1.4.8 Treatment

Management of women with nonmetastatic invasive cervical SCC depends upon the FIGO stage of disease at diagnosis. Tumor size and local spread are important factors in planning cervical cancer treatment, particularly in determining which women are candidates for primary surgical treatment. RT can be used in all stages of disease, and the survival rates are similar both in RT and radical hysterectomy. There are advantages of the use of surgery instead of RT, particularly in younger women for whom conservation of the ovaries is important [59].

There are several options for the treatment of early-stage cervical cancer. Selected women with microscopic disease (stage IA1) may be treated with extrafascial hysterectomy, cone biopsy, or simple trachelectomy [62]. Women with a tumor that is confined to the cervix, uterus, and upper third of the vagina (stages IA2, IB1, IIA1) that is nonbulky (≤4 cm) are candidates for radical hysterectomy and bilateral pelvic LND. This surgery includes removal of the uterus and cervix, radical resection of the parametrial tissue and upper vagina, and complete pelvic LND. Obviously, the standard treatment does not allow future childbearing. Radical trachelectomy is a fertility-sparing surgical approach for the treatment of early invasive cervical cancer (for stage IA2 or small [≤2 cm] IB1) and may be performed either abdominally, vaginally, laparoscopically, or robotically [63].

There have recently been great strides in the treatment of cervical carcinoma, including adjuvant chemoradiation in patients discovered to have high risk for recurrence. For women who undergo hysterectomy, the presence of positive or close resection margins, positive lymph nodes, or microscopic parametrial involvement indicates a high risk for recurrence. Postoperative cisplatin-based concomitant chemoradiotherapy is recommended rather than adjuvant RT alone for these women. For women who are at intermediate risk of recurrence (large tumor size, deep cervical stromal invasion to the middle or deep one-third, or lymphovascular space invasion), adjuvant RT after hysterectomy is recommended. Adding concomitant chemotherapy to adjuvant RT is not universally accepted but will be treatment options [64].

Women with a clinically visible cervical cancer measuring ≥4 cm (stage IB2) alone or with involvement of less than the upper two-thirds of the vagina (stage IIA2) are generally treated with chemoradiation. Generally, it is prudent not to operate on lesions that are larger than 4 cm in diameter because these patients will require postoperative RT. They have a higher local failure rate and worse survival than those with smaller volume disease. Primary chemoradiotherapy, neoadjuvant chemotherapy, and primary surgery with adjuvant treatment are management options, but cisplatin-based primary chemoradiation has shown superior results. If the patients have acute or chronic pelvic inflammatory disease, an undiagnosed coexistent pelvic mass, or anatomic alterations that make optimal RT difficult, primary surgery is preferred [65]. If the patients have an initially large cervical lesion (>7 cm), lower uterine segment involvement, or a high posttreatment residual tumor volume, simple hysterectomy following completion of chemoradiation is suggested.

Women with stages IIB, III, and IVA cervical cancer have traditionally been treated with RT. Primary chemoradiation has been shown to be superior to RT alone, and cisplatin-based chemoradiation is now the preferred treatment strategy for these patients [66]. Women with widely metastatic disease (e.g., carcinomatosis or lung metastases) (stage IVB) are typically treated with full-dose chemotherapy alone. Palliative RT may be used to reduce vaginal bleeding or pain. Control of symptoms with the least morbidity is of primary concern in this patient population [67]. In women with a local recurrence or isolated metastatic disease, surgical resection is suggested if they are appropriate candidates [68].

1.4.9 Prognosis

Prognosis is related directly to clinical stage. With higher-stage disease, the frequency of nodal metastasis increases, and the 5-year survival rate diminishes. While stage I lesions have a 5-year survival rate of approximately 85%–90%, it falls to approximately 10%–15% for patients with stage IV lesions [59].

1.5 Uterine Cancer

1.5.1 Endometrial Cancer

1.5.1.1 Epidemiology

Uterine cancer is the most common gynecologic malignancy in developed countries and is the second most common in developing countries (cervical cancer is more common) [48]. Women have a 2.6% lifetime risk of developing uterine cancer, which accounts for 6% of all cancers in women [1]. The median age at diagnosis of uterine cancer is 61 years; 75% of cases occur in postmenopausal women. It is higher in whites [69]. The majority of women with uterine cancer are diagnosed at an early stage; distribution of stage at diagnosis is confined to primary site (68%), is spread to regional organs and lymph nodes (20%), and has distant metastases (8%) [70].

1.5.1.2 Histopathology and Risk Factors

The endometrium is the most common site of uterine cancer, and adenocarcinoma of the endometrium is the most common type. Among endometrial carcinomas, there are two histologic categories. Type I endometrioid carcinoma makes up more than 80% of all endometrial cancer cases, has a favorable prognosis [71], and is thought to be due to an excess of endogenous or exogenous estrogens, whose effect is inadequately antagonized by gestagens (or not at all). Endometrial hyperplasia is its histologic precursor [72]. Unopposed estrogen replacement therapy and the use of the partial estrogen agonist tamoxifen are the most common sources of exogenous estrogen [73], whereas endogenous sources such as obesity, chronic anovulation, early menarche (late menopause), cirrhosis, and estrogen-secreting tumors are also associated with the development of endometrial carcinoma [74].

Ten to twenty percent of endometrial carcinomas are of type II, which are histologically characterized as nonendometrioid histology: serous, clear cell, mucinous, squamous, transitional cell, mesonephric, and undifferentiated. These tumors are often high grade, have a poor prognosis, and are not clearly associated with estrogen stimulation. These cancers characteristically arise from atrophic endometrial tissue by way of a preliminary stage. The only known risk factors are age and prior irradiation of the uterus (e.g., for the treatment of cervical cancer) [75].

The disease is rare before the age of 40, and <20% occur before menopause [69]. Around 2%–5% of endometrial carcinomas have a hereditary basis, with Lynch syndrome, which is associated with germ line mutations to DNA mismatch repair genes and likely to develop the disease at a young age [76]. Nulliparity, diabetes mellitus, and hypertension are the other associated factors. Advanced maternal age at last birth, breast-feeding, the use of estrogen–progestin oral contraceptives (OCs), and tobacco use decrease the risk of endometrial carcinoma [77,78].

1.5.1.3 Clinical Features

Uterine bleeding in a postmenopausal woman is the main presenting sign of endometrial carcinoma. Occasionally, women with no abnormal uterine bleeding present with abnormal findings on cervical cytology. Pre- or perimenopausal women with acyclical bleeding should also undergo thorough diagnostic evaluation, particularly if they have risk factors for endometrial carcinoma [79].

1.5.1.4 Diagnosis

Women with abnormal bleeding should undergo firstly gynecological examination to localize the source of bleeding and determine its physical extent and transvaginal ultrasonography for evaluation of the endometrium and adnexa. Endometrial sampling is the gold standard for evaluation for endometrial neoplasia. For postmenopausal women, transvaginal ultrasound evaluation of endometrial thickness may be used as an initial study to evaluate for endometrial neoplasia in selected women, as an alternative to endometrial sampling. For these women, it is reasonable to defer endometrial sampling if the endometrial thickness is <4 mm. Sonography is not a valid alternative to endometrial sampling in premenopausal women. In contrast, no reliable cutoff has been reported in pre- or perimenopausal women as well as in postmenopausal women taking hormone replacement therapy or tamoxifen [80].

Endometrial carcinoma is a histologic diagnosis made based upon the results of evaluation of an endometrial biopsy, endometrial curettage, or hysterectomy specimen. Pelvic or abdominal imaging to assess myometrial invasion or cervical involvement is unnecessary if surgical staging is planned.

1.5.1.5 Screening

Routine screening for endometrial carcinoma is not suggested. The exception to this is women with Lynch syndrome who have a lifetime risk of endometrial cancer of 27%–71%, compared with 3% in the general population. Strategies for screening and prevention of endometrial cancer in these women with Lynch syndrome include endometrial sampling and risk-reducing hysterectomy [81].

1.5.1.6 Staging

Endometrial carcinoma is surgically staged according to the joint 2010 FIGO classification system (Table 1.5) [12,82]. In the 2010 classification system, the definition of stage I was changed to include only two substages: IA (tumor is limited to the endometrium or invades less than one-half of the myometrium) and IB (tumor invades one-half or more of the myometrium). In stage II, the subgroups were removed, and the definition was changed as "Tumor invades stromal connective tissue of the cervix but does not extend beyond the uterus."

1.5.1.7 Treatment

1.5.1.7.1 Surgery

Total extrafascial hysterectomy with bilateral salpingo-oophorectomy (BSO) with pelvic and para-aortic lymph node dissection is the standard staging procedure for endometrial

TABLE 1.5
Staging Uterine Carcinoma (FIGO)

FIGO Stages	Definition
I	Tumor confined to corpus uteri.
IA	Tumor is limited to endometrium or invades less than one-half of the myometrium.
IB	Tumor invades one-half or more of the myometrium.
II	Tumor invades stromal connective tissue of the cervix but does not extend beyond uterus.
IIIA	Tumor involves serosa and/or adnexa (direct extension or metastasis).
IIIB	Vaginal involvement (direct extension or metastasis) or parametrial involvement.
IIIC1	Regional lymph node metastasis to pelvic lymph nodes.
IIIC2	Regional lymph node metastasis to para-aortic lymph nodes, with or without positive pelvic lymph nodes.
IVA	Tumor invades bladder mucosa and/or bowel mucosa (bullous edema is not sufficient to classify a tumor as T4).
IVB	Distant metastasis. (It includes metastasis to inguinal lymph nodes; intraperitoneal disease; and the lung, liver, and bone. It excludes metastasis to para-aortic lymph nodes, the vagina, pelvic serosa, and adnexa.)

Source: Data from American Joint Committee on Cancer, Corpus uteri, in: *AJCC Cancer Staging Manual*, 7th edn., Springer, New York, 2010.

carcinoma [83]. The status of both the pelvic and para-aortic lymph nodes should be assessed intraoperatively in all patients. Cytoreduction often is performed when metastases are evident.

1.5.1.7.2 Adjuvant Therapy

Decisions about adjuvant therapy for endometrial carcinoma are based upon the risk of persistent or recurrent disease.

Women with low-grade (grade 1 or 2) endometrioid cancer confined to the endometrium (a subset of stage IA disease) and cancer that is not a high-risk histologic type (e.g., clear cell, serous, or carcinosarcoma) are classified as having low-risk endometrial cancer. Because their prognosis following surgery is excellent, no adjuvant treatment is required [84]. Women with low-risk endometrial carcinoma who wish to preserve fertility may be candidates for treatment with progestin therapy [85].

Women with intermediate-risk endometrial cancer have an increased risk of locoregional recurrence. Many patients undergo adjuvant treatment to reduce recurrence risk in the pelvis. Features of intermediate-risk disease include myometrial invasion (a subset of stage IA or stage IB) or occult cervical stromal invasion (stage II). Additional adverse prognostic factors are outer one-third myometrial invasion, grade 2 or 3 disease, and lymphovascular invasion. RT is recommended for the women with intermediate risk. In view of the toxicity of external teletherapy, vaginal brachytherapy seems to be a reasonable compromise, as vaginal recurrence rates, the occurrence of distant metastases, disease-free survival, and overall survival are similar but brachytherapy has significantly fewer adverse effects [86].

Women with high-risk disease have a high rate of recurrence and low survival rate without postoperative therapy. The features that identify women with endometrial cancer at high risk are serous or clear-cell adenocarcinoma of any stage, stage III or IV disease, regardless of histology or grade. They should receive adjuvant chemotherapy [87]. RT may also play a role in the treatment of this population to reduce the risk of local recurrence. According to lymph node involvement, options for RT include vaginal vault irradiation, external pelvic irradiation, extended field (pelvic and para-aortic) irradiation, and whole abdomen irradiation.

Endometrial carcinoma in women who initially present with extensive pelvic involvement or intra-abdominal disease is classified as advanced endometrial cancer. For them, treatment is individualized. Surgical cytoreduction reduces pelvic symptoms and improves the patient's quality of life by temporarily decreasing abdominal discomfort and ascites. If women are not amenable to surgical cytoreduction, medical treatment is recommended [88,89].

Some patients have regional and distant metastases that, though occasionally responsive to standard hormone therapy, are rarely curable. The most common hormonal treatment has been progestational agents, which produce good antitumor responses in as many as 15%–30% of patients. Responses to hormones are correlated with the presence and level of hormone receptors and the degree of tumor differentiation [90]. In the presence of a relative contraindication to high-dose progestin therapy, tamoxifen is recommended.

1.5.1.8 Prognosis

The prognosis of endometrial carcinoma is determined primarily by disease stage and histology (included both grade and histologic subtype). Fortunately, most women with endometrial carcinoma have a favorable prognosis, since the majority have endometrioid histology and present with early-stage disease. In general, the rate of 5-year survival for stage I disease is approximately 80%–90%, for stage II is 70%–80%, and for stages III and IV is 20%–60% [91]. Five-year survival rate of serous or clear-cell adenocarcinomas is less than 50%, even for patients with stage 1 disease.

1.5.1.9 Posttreatment Surveillance

The majority of recurrences of endometrial carcinoma occur within 3 years after treatment (68%–100%) [91]. The most common sites of recurrent disease are the vaginal vault, pelvis, abdomen, and lungs [92]. The risk of local, but not distant, recurrence is lower in patients who have received RT. Posttreatment surveillance for women with endometrial carcinoma consists mainly of monitoring for symptoms and physical examination every 3–6 months for 2 years, then every 6 months or annually. Signs or symptoms suggestive of recurrence include vaginal bleeding, abdominal or pelvic pain, persistent cough, and unexplained weight loss. It is important to take a vault Pap smear every 6 months for 2 years, then annually. Patients with a family history suggestive of Lynch syndrome should take genetic counseling [92].

1.5.2 Uterine Sarcoma

Uterine sarcomas, which include ESS, leiomyosarcoma, and undifferentiated endometrial sarcoma, arise from the myometrium or from connective tissue elements within the endometrium. Compared with the more common endometrial carcinomas, uterine sarcomas behave more aggressively and are associated with a poorer prognosis.

1.5.2.1 Epidemiology and Risk Factors

Uterine sarcomas are rare, accounting for 3%–8% of all uterine malignancies [93]. The mean age at diagnosis is approximately 60 years. Black women have a higher incidence of leiomyosarcomas. There is an increased incidence of uterine sarcoma after pelvic radiation, but this association appears to be stronger for carcinosarcoma, which is no longer classified as a sarcoma [94]. Long-term use of tamoxifen (5 years or more) may be associated with an increased risk of developing uterine sarcoma [95]. There are few data regarding genetic determinants of uterine sarcoma. Hereditary leiomyomatosis and renal cell carcinoma (HLRCC) syndrome and childhood retinoblastoma have been associated with an increased risk of uterine sarcoma.

1.5.2.2 Classification

Uterine sarcomas are classified as nonepithelial or mixed epithelial–nonepithelial tumors (Table 1.6). The three most common types are all nonepithelial: ESS, leiomyosarcoma, and undifferentiated endometrial sarcoma [96]. Uterine carcinosarcoma, also known as malignant mixed Müllerian tumor, is now regarded as a variant of endometrial carcinoma rather than a pure sarcoma. The sarcomatous component is the result of the metaplastic or dedifferentiated change of the epithelial component [97].

Uterine sarcomas are referred to as homologous or heterologous. The majority are homologous (i.e., arise from native uterine tissue), including endometrium (ESS), muscle (leiomyosarcoma), and sarcomas of nonspecific supporting tissue (e.g., connective tissue, blood vessels, lymphatics). In contrast, heterologous tumors contain elements with nonnative differentiation (e.g., skeletal muscle, cartilage, bone).

1.5.2.2.1 Endometrial Stromal Sarcomas

Endometrial stromal tumors can be either benign (endometrial stromal nodules) or malignant (ESS), but are generally indolent. ESSs are low-grade, well-differentiated tumors. ESS is usually disseminated throughout the myometrium (appearance is similar to adenomyosis) and may invade the serosa; less commonly, it occurs as a solitary intramural nodule [98]. These tumors were previously referred to as low-grade ESS.

TABLE 1.6

Classification of Uterine Sarcomas

Nonepithelial Tumors
Endometrial stromal tumors
Stromal nodule (benign)
ESS
Undifferentiated endometrial sarcoma
Smooth muscle tumors of uncertain malignant potential
Leiomyosarcoma
Epithelioid
Myxoid
Mixed endometrial stromal and smooth muscle tumors
Other soft tissue tumors
Homologous
Heterologous
Mixed Epithelial–Nonepithelial Tumors
Adenosarcoma
Homologous
Heterologous
With high-grade stromal overgrowth

Note: Modified from the Gynecologic Oncology Group classification of uterine sarcoma.

1.5.2.2.2 Undifferentiated Endometrial Sarcoma

Undifferentiated endometrial sarcomas are aggressive tumors that lack specific differentiation. They are also characterized by significant cellular atypia and mitotic activity [98]. Undifferentiated endometrial sarcomas can grow to large sizes. These tumors were previously referred to as high-grade ESS.

1.5.2.2.3 Leiomyosarcoma

Leiomyosarcomas are characterized by prominent cellular atypia, abundant mitoses (≥10 per 10 high-power fields), and areas of coagulative tumor cell necrosis. These three features are called the Stanford criteria in which the presence of two of the three features indicated a risk of metastatic spread of >10% [99]. Leiomyosarcomas appear grossly as a large (>10 cm) yellow or tan solitary mass with soft, fleshy cut surfaces exhibiting areas of hemorrhage and necrosis [99]. The mass may bulge into the uterine cavity, but the epicenter is in the myometrium.

1.5.2.2.4 Mixed Endometrial Stromal and Smooth Muscle Tumor

These tumors, also referred to as stromomyomas, are defined as having at least 30% each of endometrial stromal and smooth muscle components [100].

1.5.2.2.5 Adenosarcoma

Adenosarcoma of the uterus is a rare mixed tumor in which a benign epithelial component is mixed with a malignant stromal (i.e., sarcomatous) element. They generally have low malignant potential and a good prognosis [101].

1.5.2.3 Clinical Features

Uterine sarcomas typically present with vaginal bleeding, pelvic pressure symptoms (e.g., pressure, urinary frequency, constipation), enlarged uterus, or abdominal distension. The amount of bleeding varies and may be accompanied by a foul-smelling vaginal discharge [96]. On pelvic examination, the uterus is often enlarged, but may be normal in size. It is not possible to reliably distinguish between a leiomyoma and a leiomyosarcoma by history or physical examination. Rapid growth of a uterine mass is a sign of a potential uterine sarcoma [102], but the data do not support an increased risk of malignancy in such patients.

1.5.2.4 Diagnosis

The diagnosis of uterine sarcoma is based upon histologic examination. Uterine sarcomas are most commonly diagnosed following myomectomy or hysterectomy. Endometrial sampling will yield the correct diagnosis in some, but not all, patients [103]. Data regarding diagnostic accuracy of serum markers, biopsy, or imaging are limited for these rare tumors.

1.5.2.5 Staging

Uterine sarcomas are staged surgically. Previously, all uterine sarcomas were staged according to the criteria for uterine carcinomas. Now, uterine leiomyosarcomas and ESSs and adenosarcoma are staged using a FIGO staging system for uterine sarcoma (Table 1.7) [104]. The histologic type and stage of the uterine sarcoma are the most important prognostic factors [105].

TABLE 1.7

Staging Uterine Sarcoma (FIGO)

FIGO Stages	Definition
Leiomyosarcoma and ESS	
I	Tumor limited to the uterus.
IA	Tumor 5 cm or less in the greatest dimension.
IB	Tumor more than 5 cm.
II	Tumor extends beyond the uterus, within the pelvis.
IIA	Tumor involves adnexa.
IIB	Tumor involves other pelvic tissues.
III	Tumor infiltrates abdominal tissues.
IIIA	One site.
IIIB	More than one site.
IIIC	Regional lymph node metastasis.
IVA	Tumor invades the bladder or rectum.
IVB	Distant metastasis (excluding adnexa, pelvic, and abdominal tissues).
Adenosarcoma	
I	Tumor limited to the uterus.
IA	Tumor limited to the endometrium/endocervix.
IB	Tumor invades to less than half of the myometrium.
IC	Tumor invades more than half of the myometrium.
II	Tumor extends beyond the uterus, within the pelvis.
IIA	Tumor involves adnexa.
IIB	Tumor involves other pelvic tissues.
III	Tumor involves abdominal tissues.
IIIA	One site.
IIIB	More than one site.
IIIC	Regional lymph node metastasis.
IVA	Tumor invades the bladder or rectum.
IVB	Distant metastasis (excluding adnexa, pelvic, and abdominal tissues).

Source: Data from American Joint Committee on Cancer, Corpus uteri, in: *AJCC Cancer Staging Manual*, 7th edn., Springer, New York, 2010.

1.5.2.6 Treatment

Total abdominal hysterectomy (TAH) is the standard procedure, and BSO should also be performed in all patients except premenopausal women with leiomyosarcoma [105]. Extirpative surgery alone is potentially curative; there are no additional benefits from more radical surgery.

Although there is no clear improvement in survival by the addition of postoperative pelvic RT in women undergoing surgery for uterine sarcoma, a reduction in local recurrence has been demonstrated in many studies [106]. But there is no consensus as to the indications for or optimal type of adjuvant therapy for any histologic subtype. Most endometrial stromal tumors (ESS) express steroid hormone receptors; hormonal therapy (with progestins, gonadotropin-releasing hormone analogs, and aromatase inhibitors) is the cornerstone of adjuvant therapy for ESS [107]. Observation alone is also an option for women with completely resected disease. Leiomyosarcoma and undifferentiated endometrial sarcoma are associated with high rates of extra-abdominal recurrence. Despite the absence of definitive data from randomized controlled trials, adjuvant chemotherapy (gemcitabine plus docetaxel) is commonly recommended for women with resected stages I through IVA disease. Adjuvant RT is a reasonable option for patients at high risk for local recurrence [108].

1.6 Ovarian Cancer

1.6.1 Epidemiology

Ovarian cancer is the second most common gynecologic malignancy in developed countries and the third most common gynecologic malignancy in developing countries [109]. It is the leading cause of mortality among the gynecological malignancies and the fifth leading cause of all cancer-related deaths since the majority of ovarian cancers are diagnosed at an advanced stage [109]. More than 90% of ovarian malignancies develop from epithelial ovarian cancer (EOC) [110]. It is higher in whites and usually diagnosed in the sixth decade of life [111].

Ovarian germ cell tumors (OGCTs) arise most frequently in the second and third decades and represent 70% of ovarian neoplasms in this age group [112]. They account for 3%–5% of ovarian cancers [113]. Malignant ovarian sex cord–stromal neoplasms are rare, comprising only 1.2% of all primary ovarian cancers. They are more frequent in black women and the average age at diagnosis is 50 years. These tumors occur with equal frequency among pre- and postmenopausal women [111].

1.6.2 Classification

In general, ovarian tumors are divided as epithelial and nonepithelial. Histologic classification of ovarian tumors according to World Health Organization (WHO) is shown in Table 1.8 [114].

1.6.2.1 Epithelial Ovarian Cancer

EOC is developed from epithelial cells that cover the ovarian surface [115]. It can be grouped into predominant histologic types as follows: serous cystadenocarcinoma (75%), mucinous cystadenocarcinoma (10%), endometrioid carcinoma (10%), undifferentiated carcinoma, clear-cell carcinoma, and Brenner's tumor. *Serous carcinoma,* the most common histologic subtype of EOC, is regarded as closely related to fallopian tube and primary peritoneal serous carcinoma, based upon similarities in histology and clinical behavior. Some experts have proposed that these carcinomas all originate in the fallopian tubes. Serous carcinoma is often associated with concentric rings of calcification known as psammoma bodies. On gross examination, serous carcinoma has an irregular and multilocular appearance. It is the most common bilateral EOC [116]. *Mucinous cystadenocarcinoma* may resemble intestinal or endocervical epithelium. They tend to remain confined to the ovaries longer than serous carcinomas and are the largest epithelial ovarian neoplasms, measuring 20 cm or more in diameter. They are usually unilateral. A clinical picture of pseudomyxoma peritonei may be present [117]. *Endometrioid tumors* closely resemble the components of endometrial cancer and arise in association with primary endometrial cancer in about 20% of patients [118]. They occasionally arise from foci of endometriosis [119]. Their survival is better than serous adenocarcinoma [118]. *Clear-cell carcinomas* of the ovary resemble glycogen-filled vaginal rests. They have also been called mesonephroid carcinomas because their histologic features include *clear cells,* similar to those seen in renal cell carcinomas. They occur in association with endometriosis. Rarely, they may be associated with humorally mediated hypercalcemia [120]. *Brenner tumors* are the fibroadenomatosis proliferation of the ovary. Fewer than 2% of these tumors are malignant. About 10% of them occur in conjunction with a mucinous cystadenocarcinoma or dermoid cyst in the same or opposite

TABLE 1.8

WHO Histologic Classification of Ovarian Tumors

1. Surface epithelial–stromal tumors
   - 1.1 Serous tumors: benign, borderline, malignant
   - 1.2 Mucinous tumors, endocervical like and intestinal type: benign, borderline, malignant
   - 1.3 Endometrioid tumors: benign, borderline, malignant, epithelial–stromal, and stromal
   - 1.4 Clear-cell tumors: benign, borderline, malignant
   - 1.5 Transitional cell tumors: Brenner tumor, Brenner tumor of borderline malignancy, malignant Brenner tumor, transitional cell carcinoma (non-Brenner type)
   - 1.6 Squamous cell tumors
   - 1.7 Mixed epithelial tumors (specify components): benign, borderline, malignant
   - 1.8 Undifferentiated carcinoma
2. Sex cord–stromal tumors
   - 2.1 Granulosa–stromal cell tumors: granulosa cell tumors, thecoma–fibroma group
   - 2.2 Sertoli–stromal cell tumors, androblastomas: well-differentiated, Sertoli–Leydig cell tumor of intermediate differentiation, Sertoli–Leydig cell tumor poorly differentiated (sarcomatoid), retiform
   - 2.3 Sex cord tumor with annular tubules
   - 2.4 Gynandroblastoma
   - 2.5 Unclassified
   - 2.6 Steroid (lipid) cell tumors: stromal luteoma, Leydig cell tumor, unclassified
3. Germ cell tumors
   - 3.1 Dysgerminoma: variant—with syncytiotrophoblast cells
   - 3.2 Yolk sac tumors (endodermal sinus tumors): polyvesicular vitelline tumor, hepatoid, glandular
   - 3.3 Embryonal carcinoma
   - 3.4 Polyembryoma
   - 3.5 Choriocarcinoma
   - 3.6 Teratomas: immature, mature, monodermal, mixed germ cell
4. Gonadoblastoma
5. Germ cell sex cord–stromal tumor of nongonadoblastoma type
6. Tumors of rete ovarii
7. Mesothelial tumors
8. Tumors of uncertain origin and miscellaneous tumors
9. Gestational trophoblastic diseases
10. Soft tissue tumors not specific to ovary
11. Malignant lymphomas, leukemias, and plasmacytomas
12. Unclassified tumors
13. Secondary (metastatic) tumors
14. Tumor-like lesions

WHO, World Health Organization.

ovary [121]. *Undifferentiated carcinoma* refers to tumors with no discernible histologic differentiation or only minor areas of differentiation.

1.6.2.2 Nonepithelial Cancer

Nonepithelial cancer of the ovary accounts for about 10% of all ovarian cancers. They include germ cell malignancies, sex cord–stromal tumors, metastatic carcinomas to the ovary, and a variety of extremely rare ovarian cancers (e.g., sarcomas, lipoid cell tumors). The ovary can also be involved by metastatic disease, especially from breast cancer or

Krukenberg's tumors (mucin-producing neoplastic signet ring cells involving the ovarian stroma) from the gastrointestinal tract [115].

1.6.2.2.1 Germ Cell Malignancies

Germ cell malignancies are derived from primordial germ cells of the ovary. They can be broadly divided into those that differentiate toward embryo-like neoplasms (teratomas and their subtypes and dysgerminomas) and those that differentiate primarily toward extraembryonic fetal-derived (endodermal sinus [yolk sac] tumors, nongestational choriocarcinomas) cell populations or a mixture of both [122]. *Teratomas* are the most common type of germ cell neoplasm. Most, but not all, teratomas are benign. Teratomas are divided into four categories: mature (cystic or solid, benign), immature (malignant), malignant due to a component of another somatic malignant neoplasm, and monodermal or highly specialized [123]. *Dysgerminoma* is the most common malignant ovarian germ cell neoplasm. Bilateral ovarian disease is more common than with any other ovarian germ cell neoplasm [113]. Dysgerminoma is the ovarian counterpart of testicular seminoma; histologically, it has a similar appearance. Dysgerminomas may develop within a gonadoblastoma, and if it is present, oophorectomy should be performed in these patients to prevent the development of gonadal neoplasia [124].

1.6.2.2.2 Ovarian Sex Cord–Stromal Neoplasms

Ovarian sex cord–stromal neoplasms develop from the cells surrounding the oocytes, including the cells that produce ovarian hormones. They are divided into several histologic subtypes, including fibromas, fibrothecomas, granulosa cell neoplasms, Sertoli or Sertoli–Leydig cell neoplasms, and gynandroblastoma [116]. *Granulosa cell tumors* are the most common type of malignant ovarian sex cord–stromal tumors [125]. They typically present as large masses; the mean diameter is 12 cm and often produces estrogen, and symptoms related to hyperestrogenism are common at diagnosis. There is a well-documented association between granulosa cell tumors and both endometrial hyperplasia (25%–50%) and adenocarcinoma (5%–10%) [126]. Clinically, the most useful serum marker for granulosa cell tumors is inhibin. They have a distinct histologic pattern: small groups of cells called Call–Exner bodies are the hallmark. Among sex cord–stromal tumors, *fibromas* are the most common histology, and they are benign solid tumors, usually unilateral that primarily occur in postmenopausal women and do not produce hormones [127]. The association of ovarian fibroma with ascites and/or pleural effusion is termed Meigs' syndrome [128]. Ovarian fibromas associated with basal cell cancers are called nevoid basal cell carcinoma syndrome or Gorlin's syndrome. *Sertoli-stromal cell tumors* often produce androgens, so the affected women will present with virilization.

1.6.3 Etiology

The cause of EOC remains poorly understood. Traditionally, two main hypotheses were proposed:

- Incessant ovulation—repeated ovulation results in minor trauma to the ovarian epithelium, causing an increased proliferation-associated DNA damage during the reproductive years, and subsequently appears to play a central role in tumorigenesis. Early menarche and late menopause have also been associated with an increased risk of ovarian cancer likely due to increased ovulation [129].

- Exposure to gonadotropins—81% of cases in postmenopausal women, over age 50; during this period, the level of gonadotropins is very high; thus, elevated follicle stimulating hormone and luteinizing hormone concentrations may be carcinogenic. This hypothesis is supported by the observation that experimentally induced ovarian tumors contain gonadotropin receptors [130].

As a result of epidemiological studies, risk factors have been identified [131]. The incidence of EOC increases with increasing age, early menarche or late menopause, infertility, nulligravidity, endometriosis, polycystic ovarian syndrome, and genetic factors. Ovulation induction for treatment of infertility does not appear to increase the risk for ovarian cancer. Endometriosis-associated EOC appears to develop in younger women and have a better prognosis than most cases of EOC. Clear-cell, endometrioid, and low-grade serous subtypes are most common in endometriosis-associated EOC.

1.6.3.1 Genetic Factors

It has been estimated that approximately 10% of ovarian tumors are hereditary and associated with highly penetrant, autosomal, dominant genetic predisposition. Three clinical manifestations of hereditary ovarian cancer have been identified: site-specific ovarian cancer, hereditary breast and/or ovarian cancer (HBOC), and hereditary nonpolyposis colorectal cancer (HNPCC) syndromes. The presence of known high-penetrance cancer susceptibility genes (i.e., *BRCA1*, *BRCA2*, *MLH1*, *MSH2*) is likely responsible for the increased risk [132]. While *BRCA1* mutation carriers have 35%–46% lifetime risk of ovarian cancer, *BRCA2* mutation carriers have 13%–23% [133]. *MLH1* and *MSH2* mutations are susceptibility genes of HNPCC and account for 10% of hereditary EOC. Hereditary ovarian cancers generally develop in women about 10 years earlier than sporadic disease. A part of ovarian cancers can also occur from epithelial rests in the normal peritoneum or the fimbriae of fallopian tubes. Prophylactic BSO (PBSO) in healthy mutation carriers, after their last birth, results in an 80% reduction in the risk of ovarian cancer [134]. However, even after PBSO, there is still a risk of approximately 4% of developing primary peritoneal cancer. Serous tubal epithelial carcinomas and tubal carcinomas with *TP53* mutations have been found in up to 80% of prophylactic salpingo-oophorectomy specimens from carriers of mutant *BRCA1* or *BRCA2* gene [135].

1.6.3.2 Environmental Factors

Current smoking or past smoking appears to increase the risk of mucinous ovarian cancer, but not other types of EOC [136]. The association between genital use of talcum powder (talc) and EOC is controversial [137].

1.6.3.3 Protective Factors

Risk is halved by the use of OCs for as long as 5 years before menopause, possibly related to reduced ovulation and treatment of transforming cells with progestational agents, and the duration of protection lasts for more than 30 years after the last use. A history of a full-term pregnancy and later age (>35 years old) at last pregnancy decrease the risk. One interesting theory to explain this protective effect is that pregnancy may induce shedding of premalignant ovarian cells. Alternatively, pregnancy may simply decrease the number of lifetime ovulations, thereby resulting in less capsular repair that when altered can result in a transforming event. Tubal ligation and hysterectomy have each been associated with a substantial reduction in risk of developing ovarian cancer, possibly through local disruption of ovarian blood supply. Also, tubal neoplasia is a precursor lesion for serous ovarian cancer. Presumably, by extending the duration of amenorrhea, breast-feeding has a protective effect [131].

1.6.4 Clinical Features

The symptoms associated with ovarian cancer are nonspecific and may also be caused by gastrointestinal, urologic, or other conditions. Possible symptoms are bloating, increased abdominal size, urinary urgency or frequency, difficulty in eating or feeling full, and abdominal or pelvic pain, meteorism, changes in bowel habits, and unexplained weight loss. As these complaints are fairly nonspecific, early diagnosis is difficult. In particular, ovarian cancer should be suspected when these symptoms coexist with other symptoms, occur almost daily, and are more severe than expected [138]. In advanced EOC, abdominal distention, nausea, anorexia, and early satiety are typically due to the presence of ascites and omental or bowel metastases; dyspnea is occasionally present due to a pleural effusion. Infrequently, women with EOC present initially with venous thromboembolism [139].

The finding of an adnexal mass on pelvic examination is a common presentation of ovarian cancer. An adnexal mass may be discovered due to symptoms of pelvic pain or pressure, or it may be found on a routine pelvic examination or an imaging study performed for another indication. A solid, irregular, fixed adnexal mass is suggestive of ovarian cancer, and if combined with an upper abdominal mass, ascites, or both, the diagnosis is almost certain.

In addition, sex cord–stromal neoplasms secrete estrogens or androgens, and germ cell malignancies often produce the beta subunit of human chorionic gonadotropin (hCG) that results in endocrine-dependent clinical signs (e.g., precocious puberty, abnormal uterine bleeding, endometrial hyperplasia, carcinoma, or virilization) or symptoms of pregnancy [140]. Ovarian germ cell malignancies usually grow rapidly. As a result, patients often present with sudden abdominal enlargement and pain. Pain is caused by rupture or torsion of the mass.

1.6.5 Diagnosis

1.6.5.1 Physical Examination

Women with symptoms suggestive of ovarian cancer should be evaluated with a physical examination, including an abdominal, pelvic, and rectovaginal examination as well as palpation of groin and supraclavicular lymph nodes. Findings suggestive of ovarian cancer include adnexal mass; abdominal ascites; a mass in the mid to left upper abdomen, which may represent an omental cake; pleural effusion; and groin or supraclavicular lymphadenopathy [141].

1.6.5.2 Pelvic and Abdominal Imaging

Of all imaging procedures used to diagnose ovarian cancer, transvaginal ultrasound is the most valuable in determining whether lesions are benign or malignant. It can help to assess for the presence of ascites and the extent of disease. CT or MRI may be used in particular cases, for example, for differential diagnosis between ovarian cancer and a primary gastrointestinal tumor [142]. Chest radiography is performed in most patients to evaluate for pleural effusion, pulmonary metastases, and mediastinal lymphadenopathy.

1.6.5.3 Laboratory Evaluation for Tumor Markers

CA 125 concentration used alone does not perform well for diagnosis or exclusion of EOC in premenopausal women [131]. Moreover, half of patients with stage I EOC have a normal CA 125 level. Nevertheless, a very high level is suggestive of EOC and a baseline value is useful in monitoring women who are subsequently diagnosed with EOC.

Some germ cell malignancies secrete hCG (embryonal cell carcinomas and ovarian choriocarcinomas, mixed germ cell tumors), alpha-fetoprotein (AFP) (endodermal sinus tumors, embryonal cell carcinomas and polyembryoma carcinomas, mixed germ cell tumors, and some immature teratomas), and lactate dehydrogenase (LDH) (dysgerminomas) [122,143,144], and sex cord–stromal neoplasms secrete inhibin, estrogen, and androgens [135]. The measurement of these diagnostic markers may play a role in the diagnosis.

However, even in the absence of an adnexal mass, if symptoms associated with ovarian cancer and/or abdominal distention or ascites are present and tumor markers associated with ovarian cancer are elevated, a *diagnostic laparoscopy* should be considered as part of the evaluation.

Women should undergo appropriate screening for breast and cervical cancers prior to surgical exploration. If abnormal uterine bleeding or a uterine mass is present, endometrial sampling should be performed preoperatively. Infrequently (~20% of women with advanced disease), the diagnosis is based upon tissue or fluid obtained via image-guided biopsy, paracentesis, or thoracentesis [145].

1.6.6 Screening

The goal of early detection of EOC is to improve prognosis by diagnosing the disease while it is confined to the ovary or when the disease volume is low. As yet, there is no approach that justifies a recommendation of general screening for ovarian cancer. Ultrasonography and CA 125 glycoprotein antigen, the most widely studied tumor marker for ovarian cancer screening, lack specificity and sensitivity for early-stage disease. Serum concentration of the CA 125 can be elevated in endometriosis; uterine leiomyoma; pelvic inflammatory disease; cirrhosis with or without ascites; cancers of the endometrium, breast, lung, and pancreas; and pleural or peritoneal fluid due to any cause. Moreover, CA 125 levels are elevated in approximately 1% of healthy women and fluctuate during the menstrual cycle [131]. Therefore, CA 125 is more useful in postmenopausal women. Screening with a single measurement of CA 125 alone, in either average- or high-risk women, is not recommended. The change in CA 125 levels over time appears to be a more promising screening method. Patients with a familial ovarian cancer syndrome, who have not undergone prophylactic oophorectomy, may benefit from surveillance with a combination of CA 125 and serial transvaginal ultrasound [132].

1.6.7 Mode of Spread

Ovarian cancer typically spreads through transcoelemic, lymphatic, and blood vessels by exfoliating cells that disseminate and implant throughout the peritoneal cavity. The distribution of intraperitoneal metastases tends to follow the circulatory path of peritoneal fluid, so metastases are commonly seen on the posterior cul-de-sac, paracolic gutters, right hemidiaphragm, liver capsule, and omentum. Lymphogenous dissemination takes place along the ovarian vascular bundles into the para-aortic lymph nodes and over the parametria into the pelvic lymph nodes. Blockage of diaphragmatic lymphatics prevents outflow of proteinaceous fluid from the peritoneal cavity, causing the accumulation of ascites fluid in advanced disease. Hematogenous metastases are not common, and parenchymal metastases to the liver and lungs are seen in only about 2% of patients at initial presentation [110].

In contrast to EOC, nodal involvement is more common with malignant OGCTs, and they have a somewhat greater predilection for hematogenous metastases to the liver and lung [146]. On the other hand, ovarian sex cord–stromal neoplasms may spread by local or regional extension, but nodal metastases are rare [147].

1.6.8 Staging

Over carcinoma is surgically staged according to the FIGO classification system (Table 1.9) [149]. The steps for surgical staging are summarized in Table 1.10.

TABLE 1.9

Staging Ovarian, Fallopian Tubal, Carcinoma (FIGO)

FIGO Stages	Definition
I	Tumor limited to ovaries (one or both) or fallopian tubes.
IA	Tumor limited to one ovary (capsule intact) or fallopian tubes no tumor on ovarian or fallopian tubes surface. No malignant cells in ascites or peritoneal washings.
IB	Tumor limited to both ovaries (capsules intact) or fallopian tubes, no tumor on ovarian or fallopian tubes surface. No malignant cells in ascites or peritoneal washings.
IC	Tumor limited to one or both ovaries or fallopian tubes, with any of the following:
IC1	Surgical spill.
IC2	Capsule ruptured before surgery or tumor on ovarian or fallopian tube surface.
IC3	Malignant cells in the ascites or peritoneal washings.
II	Tumor involves one or both ovaries or fallopian tubes with pelvic extension or peritoneal cancer.[a]
IIA	Extension and/or implants on uterus and/or tube(s) and/or ovaries.
IIB	Extension to implants on other pelvic tissues.
III	Tumor involves one or both ovaries or fallopian tubes, or peritoneal cancer, with cytologically or histologically confirmed spread to the peritoneum outside the pelvis and/or metastasis to the retroperitoneal lymph nodes.
IIIA	Positive retroperitoneal lymph nodes and/or microscopic peritoneal metastasis beyond the pelvis.
IIIA1	Positive retroperitoneal lymph nodes only (cytologically or histologically proven).
IIIA1(i)	Metastasis up to 10 mm in the greatest dimension.
IIIA1(ii)	Metastasis more than 10 mm in the greatest dimension.
IIIA2	Microscopic extrapelvic (above the pelvic brim) peritoneal involvement, with or without positive retroperitoneal lymph nodes.
IIIB	Macroscopic peritoneal metastasis beyond the pelvis 2 cm or less in the greatest dimension, with or without positive retroperitoneal lymph nodes.
IIIC	Peritoneal metastasis beyond the pelvis more than 2 cm in the greatest dimension (includes extension of tumor to capsule of liver and spleen without parenchymal involvement of either organ), with or without positive retroperitoneal lymph nodes.
IV	Distant metastasis (excludes peritoneal metastasis).
IVA	Pleural effusion with positive cytology.
IVB	Parenchymal metastases and metastases to extra-abdominal organs (including inguinal lymph nodes and lymph nodes outside the abdominal cavity).

Sources: Data from American Joint Committee on Cancer, Corpus uteri, in: *AJCC Cancer Staging Manual*, 7th edn., Springer, New York, 2010; Prat J., *Int. J. Gynaecol. Obstet*, 124, 1, 2014.

[a] Dense adhesions with histologically proven tumor cells justify upgrading to stage II.

TABLE 1.10

Steps in Staging Ovarian Cancer

1. Obtain any free fluid for cytologic evaluation.
2. If no free fluid is present, obtain washings by instilling and recovering 50–100 mL of saline. The fluid should irrigate the cul-de-sac, paracolic gutters, and area beneath each diaphragm.
3. Systematically explore all intra-abdominal organs and surfaces: the bowel, liver, gallbladder, diaphragms, mesentery, omentum, and the entire peritoneum should be visualized and palpated, as indicated.
4. Suspicious areas or adhesions should be biopsied. If there are no suspicious areas, multiple biopsies should be obtained from the peritoneum of the cul-de-sac, paracolic gutters, bladder, and intestinal mesentery.
5. The diaphragm should be biopsied or scraped for cytology. A laparoscope and biopsy instrument may be used.
6. The omentum should be resected from the transverse colon.
7. The retroperitoneum should be explored to evaluate pelvic nodes. Suspicious nodes should be removed and sent for frozen section examination. An ipsilateral dissection may be performed only for unilateral tumor.
8. The para-aortic nodes should be exposed and enlarged nodes removed. Nodes superior to the inferior mesenteric artery should also be resected. (Routine LND is not required for sex cord–stromal tumors.)
9. In the absence of suspicious nodes, pelvic and para-aortic nodes should still be sampled to exclude the possibility of microscopic stage III disease. (Routine lymph node sampling is not required for sex cord–stromal tumors.)
10. A total abdominal hysterectomy and BSO is performed. (Fertility-conserving surgery may be an option for some women.)

1.6.9 Treatment

The initial management of women with ovarian cancer is surgical. Surgery is performed in women with suspected ovarian cancer to obtain tissue to confirm the diagnosis, assess the extent of disease (staging), and attempt to remove as much of the gross tumor as possible, which is crucial for successful treatment.

Approximately 25% of patients present with tumor confined to the ovary (stage I) or tumor beyond the ovary but confined to the pelvis (stage II). For women with EOC confined to the ovary (IA or IB) and/or well-differentiated (grade 1) tumors, prognosis is excellent with survival of at least 90% following surgery total abdominal hysterectomy–bilateral salpingo-oophorectomy (TAH BSO) alone [149].

The other 75% of women with EOC present with tumor that has spread throughout the peritoneal cavity or involves para-aortic or inguinal lymph nodes (stage III) or tumor that has spread to more distant sites (stage IV) [150]. The standard of care for these patients is maximal surgical cytoreduction followed by platinum and taxane-based chemotherapy (carboplatin plus paclitaxel) [151].

Cytoreductive surgery is the cornerstone of therapy for ovarian cancer. There are several potential benefits of aggressive primary surgical management in women with EOC, particularly those with advanced disease: Optimal response to postoperative systemic chemotherapy is achieved in the setting of minimal disease burden that are well perfused and therefore mitotically active. Removal of bulky disease rapidly improves symptoms that are related to tumor burden. The other benefit is that ovarian neoplasms produce multiple cytokines, at least some of which are immunosuppressive (e.g., interleukin-10, vascular endothelial growth factor) [152,153]. Removal of tumor bulk may improve or restore host immune competence. Studies have consistently shown that the volume of residual disease remaining after cytoreductive surgery inversely correlates with survival. Patients with <1 cm of disease in any one location are considered to have optimally cytoreduced EOC. All other patients have suboptimally cytoreduced disease. A growing body of literature reports an association between cytoreduction to <1 mm or to no visible disease and improved response to chemotherapy, less platinum resistance, and improved survival [154,155].

For women with optimally cytoreduced EOC, a combination of intravenous plus intraperitoneal (IV/IP) chemotherapy rather than intravenous chemotherapy alone is recommended. Patients who are not good candidates for surgery due to the location and volume of disease involvement or medical comorbidities at the time of diagnosis may be considered for neoadjuvant chemotherapy [150]. If the initial surgical attempt at cytoreduction was not optimal and was not a maximal surgical effort, then chemotherapy and secondary surgical cytoreduction and repeated staging should be performed, and those with at least stable disease should proceed with an interval debulking surgery, followed by adjuvant chemotherapy, but survival is not as high as with optimal cytoreduction at primary surgery [156].

The treatment principles for all types of malignant *OGCT* include surgery for diagnosis and complete surgical staging, cytoreductive surgery if advanced disease is present, and adjuvant chemotherapy in most cases. Most women with OGCTs are young and wish to preserve future childbearing capacity. Unilateral salpingo-oophorectomy with preservation of the uterus and the contralateral ovary if these organs appear normal can be offered as a treatment option [157]. These tumors are highly chemotherapy sensitive. In adult women with completely resected stage I nondysgerminomatous ovarian germ cell malignancies, postoperative adjuvant platinum-based combination chemotherapy is recommended instead of cytoreductive surgery. In stage IA, dysgerminoma surgery followed by close surveillance is recommended rather than RT or adjuvant chemotherapy. And unilateral salpingo-oophorectomy alone is adequate treatment for stage IA grade 1 unruptured immature teratomas [158].

One notable difference between *sex cord–stromal* and other ovarian neoplasms is that lymph node metastases are rare [147]. Pelvic and para-aortic LND may result in lymphedema that impacts postoperative quality of life. Thus, for most women with malignant sex cord–stromal neoplasms, we suggest not performing pelvic and para-aortic LND. Nodes should be palpated, however, and LND is required for women with palpable nodal enlargement. For young women with stage I disease who desire for fertility preservation with a unilateral ovarian mass or avoid estrogen therapy, unilateral oophorectomy alone is appropriate.

1.6.10 Prognosis

Tumor stage, residual disease after initial surgery, histologic type, tumor grade, age, and general health are independent, significant parameters in the survival prognosis of patients with ovarian cancer. Mucinous tumors have a significantly worse prognosis than serous papillary and endometrial cancers and respond less favorably to conventional platinum-based combined chemotherapy. Both the risk of recurrence and the risk of a fatal outcome are more than twice as high [159].

1.7 Fallopian Tube Carcinoma

Primary carcinoma of the fallopian tube comprises 0.2% of cancers and diagnostically confused with ovarian carcinoma [160]. It is higher in whites, and the highest incidence is in women aged 70–79. The average age at diagnosis is 55–60 years [161]. Almost all cancers are of epithelial origin, most frequently of serous histology, but sarcomas and mixed tumors can occur [162].

1.7.1 Clinical Features

The classic triad of symptoms and signs associated with fallopian tube carcinoma is a prominent watery vaginal discharge, pelvic pain, and pelvic mass. However, this triad is noted in fewer than 15% of patients. In postmenopausal patients, the vaginal discharge may be yellow, watery, and similar to that seen with a urinary fistula. A fallopian tube cancer should be suspected in postmenopausal patients whose bleeding or abnormal cytologic findings are not explained by endometrial or endocervical curettage. In most patients, it is found incidentally in asymptomatic women at the time of TAH BSO [163].

1.7.2 Staging

Fallopian tube carcinoma is staged according to FIGO (Table 1.9) [161]. It is staged like ovarian cancer because the mode of dissemination is similar. Stage at diagnosis of primary fallopian tube carcinoma is fairly evenly distributed: localized (36%), regional (30%), and distant (32%) [160].

1.7.3 Treatment

Fallopian tube carcinoma is similar to ovarian cancer; thus, the treatment is essentially the same. TAH BSO should be done. Staging operation should be performed in patients whose disease appears to be confined to the pelvis. The retroperitoneal lymph nodes should be evaluated, and peritoneal cytologic studies and biopsies should be performed, along with an infracolic omentectomy. In patients with metastatic disease, cytoreductive surgery is appropriate. Postoperatively, combination chemotherapy is the same as for EOC [161,164].

1.7.4 Prognosis

The overall 5-year survival for patients with fallopian tube carcinoma is about 40%, and this number is higher than for patients with ovarian cancer and reflects the higher proportion of patients diagnosed with early-stage disease [161].

1.8 Conclusion and Future Direction

Gynecologic cancers are an important cause of morbidity and mortality in women. Among them, there is only a slight decrease in the incidence of cervical cancer in settings in which cervical cancer screening is employed. It is the third most common cancer diagnosis and cause of death among gynecologic cancers in the developed countries. Cervical cancer is highly preventable because only cervical cancer has a screening test—the Pap test. Furthermore, gynecologic cancers, caused by HPV infection (servix, vulva, and vagen), could be largely prevented by appropriate vaccination strategies. In countries that do not have screening and prevention programs, cervical cancer remains the second most common type of cancer and cancer-related deaths among all types of cancer in women. Dissemination of routine physical exams and screening in developing countries would reduce the rate of cervical cancer in developing countries and worldwide.

Early detection is an essential goal of all types of cancer. When cancer is found early, it is highly treatable and associated with long survival and good quality of life. Furthermore, mortality rates of cancers are decreased if they are detected at early stages. Although uterine cancer mortality rates are declining, because of early signs as uterine bleeding in a postmenopausal woman, additional effort is warranted to reduce the incidence and mortality of gynecologic cancer in the future, by education of public for warning signs, implementation of early detection programs, accurate surgical staging and the use of optimal therapeutic strategies.

Several evidence-based interventions are available to reduce the incidence, morbidity, and mortality from these cancers. But recent mortality data suggest that gynecologic cancer death rates are not decreasing. An area that can be expanded is inclusion of activities related to genomics, as inherited mutations increase risk for ovarian and uterine cancers in some individuals. Increased knowledge and understanding of this increased risk may lead to risk-reducing behaviors among individuals that may ultimately result in decreases in incidence.

References

1. Siegel R, Ward E, Brawley O, Jemal A. 2011. Cancer statistics, 2011: The impact of eliminating socioeconomic and racial disparities on premature cancer deaths. *CA Cancer J Clin* 61:212.
2. Messing MJ, Gallup DG. 1995. Carcinoma of the vulva in young women. *Obstet Gynecol* 86:51.
3. Dittmer C, Katalinic A, Mundhenke C, Thill M, Fischer D. 2011. Epidemiology of vulvar and vaginal cancer in Germany. *Arch Gynecol Obstet* 284(1):169–174.
4. Madsen BS, Jensen HL, van den Brule AJ et al. 2008. Risk factors for invasive squamous cell carcinoma of the vulva and vagina—Population-based case-control study in Denmark. *Int J Cancer* 122:2827.
5. de Koning MN, Quint WG, Pirog EC. 2008. Prevalence of mucosal and cutaneous human papillomaviruses in different histologic subtypes of vulvar carcinoma. *Mod Pathol* 21:334.
6. Monk BJ, Burger RA, Lin F et al. 1995. Prognostic significance of human papillomavirus DNA in vulvar carcinoma. *Obstet Gynecol* 85:709.
7. Insinga RP, Liaw KL, Johnson LG, Madeleine MM. 2008. A systematic review of the prevalence and attribution of human papillomavirus types among cervical, vaginal, and vulvar precancers and cancers in the United States. *Cancer Epidemiol Biomarkers Prev* 17:1611.
8. Castle PE, Schiffman M, Bratti MC et al. 2004. A population-based study of vaginal human papillomavirus infection in hysterectomized women. *J Infect Dis* 190:458.
9. Zacur H, Genadry R, Woodruff JD. 1980. The patient-at-risk for development of vulvar cancer. *Gynecol Oncol* 9:199.
10. Collins CG, Lee FY, Roman-Lopez JJ. 1971. Invasive carcinoma of the vulva with lymph node metastasis. *Am J Obstet Gynecol* 109:446.
11. Hacker NF, Nieberg RK, Berek JS et al. 1983. Superficially invasive vulvar cancer with nodal metastases. *Gynecol Oncol* 15:65.
12. Benedet JL, Bender H, Jones H 3rd et al. 2000. FIGO staging classifications and clinical practice guidelines in the management of gynecologic cancers. FIGO Committee on Gynecologic Oncology. *Int J Gynaecol Obstet* 70:209.
13. Stehman FB, Look KY. 2006. Carcinoma of the vulva. *Obstet Gynecol* 107:719.
14. Farias-Eisner R, Cirisano FD, Grouse D et al. 1994. Conservative and individualized surgery for early squamous carcinoma of the vulva: The treatment of choice for stage I and II (T1-2N0-1M0) disease. *Gynecol Oncol* 53:55.

15. Hacker NF, Berek JS, Lagasse LD et al. 1984. Individualization of treatment for stage I squamous cell vulvar carcinoma. *Obstet Gynecol* 63:155.
16. de Hullu JA, van der Zee AG. 2006. Surgery and radiotherapy in vulvar cancer. *Crit Rev Oncol Hematol* 60:38.
17. Kunos C, Simpkins F, Gibbons H et al. 2009. Radiation therapy compared with pelvic node resection for node-positive vulvar cancer: A randomized controlled trial. *Obstet Gynecol* 114:537.
18. Moore DH, Thomas GM, Montana GS et al. 1998. Preoperative chemoradiation for advanced vulvar cancer: A phase II study of the Gynecologic Oncology Group. *Int J Radiat Oncol Biol Phys* 42:79.
19. Maggino T, Landoni F, Sartori E et al. 2000. Patterns of recurrence in patients with squamous cell carcinoma of the vulva. A multicenter CTF study. *Cancer* 89:116.
20. Hacker NF. 2005. Vulvar cancer. In: *Practical Gynecologic Oncology*, 4th edn., Berek JS, Hacker NF (eds.), pp. 543–583. Philadelphia, PA: Lippincott, Williams & Wilkins.
21. Woolderink JM, de Bock GH, de Hullu JA et al. 2006. Patterns and frequency of recurrences of squamous cell carcinoma of the vulva. *Gynecol Oncol* 103:293.
22. Sugiyama VE, Chan JK, Shin JY et al. 2007. Vulvar melanoma: A multivariable analysis of 644 patients. *Obstet Gynecol* 110:296.
23. Podratz KC, Gaffey TA, Symmonds RE, Johansen KL, O'Brien PC. 1983. Melanoma of the vulva: An update. *Gynecol Oncol* 16(2):153–168.
24. Chung AF, Woodruff JM, Lewis JL Jr. 1975. Malignant melanoma of the vulva: A report of 44 cases. *Obstet Gynecol* 45(6):638–646.
25. Trimble EL, Lewis JL Jr, Williams LL et al. 1992. Management of vulvar melanoma. *Gynecol Oncol* 45(3):254–258.
26. Kabir N, Ara I, Ahmed A, Muhsin AU. 2007. Verrucous carcinoma of vulva. *Mymensingh Med J* 16(2 Suppl.):S53–S56.
27. de Giorgi V, Salvini C, Massi D et al. 2005. Vulvar basal cell carcinoma: Retrospective study and review of literature. *Gynecol Oncol* 97:192.
28. Benedet JL, Miller DM, Ehlen TG, Bertrand MA. 1997. Basal cell carcinoma of the vulva: Clinical features and treatment results in 28 patients. *Obstet Gynecol* 90:765.
29. Magné N, Pacaut C, Auberdiac P et al. 2011. Sarcoma of vulva, vagina and ovary. *Best Pract Res Clin Obstet Gynaecol* 25(6):797–801.
30. Parker LP, Parker JR, Bodurka-Bevers D et al. 2000. Paget's disease of the vulva: Pathology, pattern of involvement, and prognosis. *Gynecol Oncol* 77:183.
31. Copeland LJ, Sneige N, Gershenson DM et al. 1986. Bartholin gland carcinoma. *Obstet Gynecol* 67:794.
32. WAY S. 1951. Vaginal metastases of carcinoma of the body of the uterus. *J Obstet Gynaecol Br Emp* 58:558.
33. Daling JR, Madeleine MM, Schwartz SM et al. 2002. A population-based study of squamous cell vaginal cancer: HPV and cofactors. *Gynecol Oncol* 84:263.
34. Benedet JL. 1991. Vaginal malignancy. *Curr Opin Obstet Gynecol* 3(1):73–77.
35. Choo YC, Anderson DG. 1982. Neoplasms of the vagina following cervical carcinoma. *Gynecol Oncol* 14:125.
36. Gallup DG, Talledo OE, Shah KJ, Hayes C. 1987. Invasive squamous cell carcinoma of the vagina: A 14-year study. *Obstet Gynecol* 69:782.
37. Creasman WT, Phillips JL, Menck HR. 1998. The national cancer data base report on cancer of the vagina. *Cancer* 83:1033.
38. Isaacs JH. 1976. Verrucous carcinoma of the female genital tract. *Gynecol Oncol* 4:259.
39. Herbst AL, Ulfelder H, Poskanzer DC. 1971. Adenocarcinoma of the vagina. Association of maternal stilbestrol therapy with tumor appearance in young women. *N Engl J Med* 284:878.
40. Melnick S, Cole P, Anderson D, Herbst A. 1987. Rates and risks of diethylstilbestrol-related clear-cell adenocarcinoma of the vagina and cervix. An update. *N Engl J Med* 316:514.
41. Senekjian EK, Frey KW, Anderson D, Herbst AL. 1987. Local therapy in stage I clear cell adenocarcinoma of the vagina. *Cancer* 60:1319.

42. Frank SJ, Deavers MT, Jhingran A et al. 2007. Primary adenocarcinoma of the vagina not associated with diethylstilbestrol (DES) exposure. *Gynecol Oncol* 105:470.
43. Hilgers RD, Malkasian GD Jr, Soule EH. 1970. Embryonal rhabdomyosarcoma (botryoid type) of the vagina. A clinicopathologic review. *Am J Obstet Gynecol* 107:484.
44. DeMatos P, Tyler D, Seigler HF. 1998. Mucosal melanoma of the female genitalia: A clinicopathologic study of forty-three cases at Duke University Medical Center. *Surgery* 124:38.
45. Frank SJ, Jhingran A, Levenback C, Eifel PJ. 2005. Definitive radiation therapy for squamous cell carcinoma of the vagina. *Int J Radiat Oncol Biol Phys* 62:138.
46. Tewari KS, Cappuccini F, Puthawala AA et al. 2001. Primary invasive carcinoma of the vagina: Treatment with interstitial brachytherapy. *Cancer* 91:758.
47. Benedetti Panici P, Bellati F, Plotti F et al. 2008. Neoadjuvant chemotherapy followed by radical surgery in patients affected by vaginal carcinoma. *Gynecol Oncol* 111:307.
48. Jemal A, Bray F, Center MM et al. 2011. Global cancer statistics. *CA Cancer J Clin* 61:69.
49. Ries LAG, Melbert D, Krapcho M et al. 2007. *SEER Cancer Statistics Review, 1975–2004*. Bethesda, MD: National Cancer Institute.
50. Walboomers JM, Jacobs MV, Manos MM et al. 1999. Human papillomavirus is a necessary cause of invasive cervical cancer worldwide. *J Pathol* 189:12.
51. Munoz N, Castellsagué X, Berrington de González A, Gissmannet L. 2006. HPV in the etiology of human cancer. *Vaccine* 24:S1.
52. Berrington de González A, Green J, International Collaboration of Epidemiological Studies of Cervical Cancer. 2007. Comparison of risk factors for invasive squamous cell carcinoma and adenocarcinoma of the cervix: Collaborative reanalysis of individual data on 8,097 women with squamous cell carcinoma and 1,374 women with adenocarcinoma from 12 epidemiological studies. *Int J Cancer* 120:885.
53. Castellsagué X, Bosch FX, Muñoz N et al. 2002. Male circumcision, penile human papillomavirus infection, and cervical cancer in female partners. *N Engl J Med* 346:1105.
54. Manhart LE, Holmes KK, Koutsky LA et al. 2006. Human papillomavirus infection among sexually active young women in the United States: Implications for developing a vaccination strategy. *Sex Transm Dis* 33:502.
55. Society of Gynecologic Oncologists Education Resource Panel Writing group, Collins Y, Einstein MH et al. 2006. Cervical cancer prevention in the era of prophylactic vaccines: A preview for gynecologic oncologists. *Gynecol Oncol* 102:552.
56. Grisaru D, Covens A, Chapman B et al. 2001. Does histology influence prognosis in patients with early-stage cervical carcinoma? *Cancer* 92:2999.
57. DiSaia PJ, Creasman WT. (eds.) 2007. Invasive cervical cancer. In: *Clinical Gynecologic Oncology*, 7th edn., pp. 54–57. Philadelphia, PA: Mosby Elsevier.
58. Partridge EE, Abu-Rustum NR, Campos SM et al. 2010. Cervical cancer screening. *J Natl Compr Cancer Netw* 8:1358.
59. Bidus MA, Elkas JC. 2007. Cervical and Vaginal Cancer. In: *Berek & Novak's Gynecology*, 14th edn., Berek JS (ed.), pp. 1403–1444. Philadelphia, PA: Lippincott, Williams & Wilkins.
60. Pecorelli S, Zigliani L, Odicino F. 2009. Revised FIGO staging for carcinoma of the cervix. *Int J Gynaecol Obstet* 105:107.
61. Amendola MA, Hricak H, Mitchell DG et al. 2005. Utilization of diagnostic studies in the pretreatment evaluation of invasive cervical cancer in the United States: Results of intergroup protocol ACRIN 6651/GOG 183. *J Clin Oncol* 23:7454.
62. Bisseling KC, Bekkers RL, Rome RM, Quinn MA. 2007. Treatment of microinvasive adenocarcinoma of the uterine cervix: A retrospective study and review of the literature. *Gynecol Oncol* 107:424.
63. Mejia-Gomez J, Feigenberg T, Arbel-Alon S, Kogan L, Benshushan A. 2012. Radical trachelectomy: A fertility-sparing option for early invasive cervical cancer. *Isr Med Assoc J* 14(5):324–328.
64. Green J, Kirwan J, Tierney J et al. 2005. Concomitant chemotherapy and radiation therapy for cancer of the uterine cervix. *Cochrane Database Syst Rev* (3):CD002225.

65. Allen HH, Nisker JA, Anderson RJ. 1982. Primary surgical treatment in one hundred ninety-five cases of stage IB carcinoma of the cervix. *Am J Obstet Gynecol* 143:581.
66. Committee on Practice Bulletins-Gynecology. 2002. ACOG practice bulletin. Diagnosis and treatment of cervical carcinomas. *Obstet Gynecol* 99:855.
67. Hong JH, Tsai CS, Lai CH et al. 2004. Recurrent squamous cell carcinoma of cervix after definitive radiotherapy. *Int J Radiat Oncol Biol Phys* 60:249.
68. Lim MC, Lee HS, Seo SS et al. 2010. Pathologic diagnosis and resection of suspicious thoracic metastases in patients with cervical cancer through thoracotomy or video-assisted thoracic surgery. *Gynecol Oncol* 116:478.
69. Allard JE, Maxwell GL. 2009. Race disparities between black and white women in the incidence, treatment, and prognosis of endometrial cancer. *Cancer Control* 16:53.
70. Lewin SN, Herzog TJ, Barrena Medel NI et al. 2010. Comparative performance of the 2009 international Federation of gynecology and obstetrics' staging system for uterine corpus cancer. *Obstet Gynecol* 116:1141.
71. Bokhman JV. 1983. Two pathogenetic types of endometrial cancer. *Gynecol Oncol* 15:10–17.
72. Furness S, Roberts H, Marjoribanks J et al. 2009. Hormone therapy in postmenopausal women and risk of endometrial hyperplasia. *Cochrane Database Syst Rev* (2):CD000402.
73. Fisher B, Costantino JP, Wickerham DL et al. 1998. Tamoxifen for prevention of breast cancer: Report of the National Surgical Adjuvant Breast and Bowel Project P-1 Study. *J Natl Cancer Inst* 90:1371–1388.
74. Brinton LA, Berman ML, Mortel R et al. 1992. Reproductive, menstrual, and medical risk factors for endometrial cancer: Results from a case-control study. *Am J Obstet Gynecol* 167:1317–1325.
75. Felix AS, Weissfeld JL, Stone RA et al. 2010. Factors associated with Type I and Type II endometrial cancer. *Cancer Causes Control* 21:1851.
76. McMeekin DS, Alektiar KM, Sabbatini PJ et al. 2009. Corpus: Epithelial tumors. In: *Principles and Practice of Gynecologic Oncology*, Barakat RR, Markman M, Randall ME, (eds.), pp. 683–732. Philadelphia, PA: Lippincott.
77. Mueck AO, Seeger H, Rabe T. 2010. Hormonal contraception and risk of endometrial cancer: A systematic review. *Endocr Relat Cancer* 17:R263.
78. Zhou B, Yang L, Sun Q et al. 2008. Cigarette smoking and the risk of endometrial cancer: A meta-analysis. *Am J Med* 121:501.
79. Kimura T, Kamiura S, Yamamoto T et al. 2004. Abnormal uterine bleeding and prognosis of endometrial cancer. *Int J Gynaecol Obstet* 85:145.
80. Timmermans A, Opmeer BC, Khan KS et al. 2010. Endometrial thickness measurement for detecting endometrial cancer in women with postmenopausal bleeding: A systematic review and meta-analysis. *Obstet Gynecol* 116(1):160–167.
81. Tan MH, Mester JL, Ngeow J et al. 2012. Lifetime cancer risks in individuals with germline PTEN mutations. *Clin Cancer Res* 18:400.
82. American Joint Committee on Cancer. 2010. Corpus uteri. In: *AJCC Cancer Staging Manual*, 7th edn., Edge S, Byrd DR, Compton CC, Fritz AG, Greene FL, Trotti A (eds.), p. 403. New York: Springer.
83. Straughn JM Jr, Huh WK, Kelly FJ et al. 2002. Conservative management of stage I endometrial carcinoma after surgical staging. *Gynecol Oncol* 84:194.
84. Kong A, Johnson N, Kitchener HC, Lawrie TA. 2012. Adjuvant radiotherapy for stage I endometrial cancer. *Cochrane Database Syst Rev* 3:CD003916.
85. Martin-Hirsch PP, Bryant A, Keep SL et al. 2011. Adjuvant progestogens for endometrial cancer. *Cochrane Database Syst Rev* (6):CD001040.
86. Alektiar KM, Venkatraman E, Chi DS, Barakat RR. 2005. Intravaginal brachytherapy alone for intermediate-risk endometrial cancer. *Int J Radiat Oncol Biol Phys* 62:111.
87. Johnson N, Bryant A, Miles T et al. 2011. Adjuvant chemotherapy for endometrial cancer after hysterectomy. *Cochrane Database Syst Rev* (10):CD003175.
88. Lin LL, Grigsby PW, Powell MA, Mutch DG. 2005. Definitive radiotherapy in the management of isolated vaginal recurrences of endometrial cancer. *Int J Radiat Oncol Biol Phys* 63:500.

89. Khoury-Collado F, Einstein MH, Bochner BH et al. 2012. Pelvic exenteration with curative intent for recurrent uterine malignancies. *Gynecol Oncol* 124:42.
90. Lentz SS. 1994. Advanced and recurrent endometrial carcinoma: Hormonal therapy. *Semin Oncol* 21(1):100–106.
91. Fung-Kee-Fung M, Dodge J, Elit L et al. 2006. Follow-up after primary therapy for endometrial cancer: A systematic review. *Gynecol Oncol* 101:520.
92. Sartori E, Pasinetti B, Chiudinelli F et al. 2010. Surveillance procedures for patients treated for endometrial cancer: A review of the literature. *Int J Gynecol Cancer* 20:985.
93. Brooks SE, Zhan M, Cote T et al. 2004. Surveillance, epidemiology, and end results analysis of 2677 cases of uterine sarcoma 1989–1999. *Gynecol Oncol* 93:204–208.
94. Fang Z, Matsumoto S, Ae K et al. 2004. Postradiation soft tissue sarcoma: A multiinstitutional analysis of 14 cases in Japan. *J Orthop Sci* 9:242.
95. Wysowski DK, Honig SF, Beitz J. 2002. Uterine sarcoma associated with tamoxifen use. *N Engl J Med* 346:1832.
96. D'Angelo E, Prat J. 2010. Uterine sarcomas: A review. *Gynecol Oncol* 116:1319.
97. McCluggage WG. 2002. Uterine carcinosarcomas (malignant mixed Mullerian tumors) are metaplastic carcinomas. *Int J Gynecol Cancer* 12:687–690.
98. Moinfar F, Azodi M, Tavassoli FA. 2007. Uterine sarcomas. *Pathology* 39:55.
99. Bell SW, Kempson RL, Hendrickson MR. 1994. Problematic uterine smooth muscle neoplasms. A clinicopathologic study of 213 cases. *Am J Surg Pathol* 18:535.
100. Oliva E, Clement PB, Young RH, Scully RE. 1998. Mixed endometrial stromal and smooth muscle tumors of the uterus: A clinicopathologic study of 15 cases. *Am J Surg Pathol* 22:997.
101. Verschraegen CF, Vasuratna A, Edwards C et al. 1998. Clinicopathologic analysis of mullerian adenosarcoma: The M.D. Anderson Cancer Center experience. *Oncol Rep* 5:939.
102. Parker WH, Fu YS, Berek JS. 1994. Uterine sarcoma in patients operated on for presumed leiomyoma and rapidly growing leiomyoma. *Obstet Gynecol* 83:414.
103. Bansal N, Herzog TJ, Burke W et al. 2008. The utility of preoperative endometrial sampling for the detection of uterine sarcomas. *Gynecol Oncol* 110:43.
104. Prat J. 2009. FIGO staging for uterine sarcomas. *Int J Gynaecol Obstet* 104:177.
105. Gadducci A, Cosio S, Romanini A, Genazzani AR. 2008. The management of patients with uterine sarcoma: A debated clinical challenge. *Crit Rev Oncol Hematol* 65:129.
106. Vongtama V, Karlen JR, Piver SM et al. 1976. Treatment, results and prognostic factors in stage I and II sarcomas of the corpus uteri. *Am J Roentgenol* 126:139.
107. Amant F, De Knijf A, Van Calster B et al. 2007. Clinical study investigating the role of lymphadenectomy, surgical castration and adjuvant hormonal treatment in endometrial stromal sarcoma. *Br J Cancer* 97:1194.
108. Kanjeekal S, Chambers A, Fung MF, Verma S. 2005. Systemic therapy for advanced uterine sarcoma: A systematic review of the literature. *Gynecol Oncol* 97:624.
109. Siegel R, Naishadham D, Jemal A. 2012. Cancer statistics, 2012. *CA Cancer J Clin* 62:10.
110. Romero I, Bast RC Jr. 2012. Minireview: Human ovarian cancer: Biology, current management, and paths to personalizing therapy. *Endocrinology* 153(4):1593–1602.
111. Quirk JT, Natarajan N. 2005. Ovarian cancer incidence in the United States, 1992–1999. *Gynecol Oncol* 97:519.
112. Zalel Y, Piura B, Elchalal U et al. 1996. Diagnosis and management of malignant germ cell ovarian tumors in young females. *Int J Gynaecol Obstet* 55:1.
113. Smith HO, Berwick M, Verschraegen CF et al. 2006. Incidence and survival rates for female malignant germ cell tumors. *Obstet Gynecol* 107:1075–1085.
114. Scully R, Sobin L. 1999. *Histologic Typing of Ovarian Tumors*, World Health Organization (ed.), Vol. 9. Berlin, Germany: Springer-Verlag.
115. Lacey JV, Sherman ME. 2009. Ovarian neoplasia. In: *Robboy's Pathology of the Female Reproductive Tract*, 2nd edn., Robboy SL, Mutter GL, Prat J, Bentley RC, Russell P, Anderson MC (eds.), pp. 601–639. Oxford, U.K.: Churchill Livingstone Elsevier.

116. Scully RE, Young RH, Clement PB. 1998. Surface epithelial-stromal tumors. Serous tumors. In: *Atlas of Tumor Pathology. Tumors of the Ovary, Maldeveloped Gonads, Fallopian Tube, and Broad Ligament*, Scully RE, Young RH, Clement PB (eds.), pp. 51–79, Washington, DC: Armed Forces Institute of Pathology.
117. Scully RE, Young RH, Clement PB. 1998. Mucinous tumors and pseudomyxoma peritonei. In: *Atlas of Tumor Pathology. Tumors of the Ovary, Maldeveloped Gonads, Fallopian Tube, and Broad Ligament*, Scully RE, Young RH, Clement PB (eds.), pp. 81–105, Washington, DC: Armed Forces Institute of Pathology.
118. Scully RE, Young RH, Clement PB. 1998. Endometrioid tumors. In: *Tumors of the Ovary, Maldeveloped Gonads, Fallopian Tube, and Broad Ligament*, Scully RE, Young RH, Clement PB (eds.), p. 107. Washington, DC: Armed Forces Institute of Pathology.
119. McMeekin DS, Burger RA, Manetta A et al. 1995. Endometrioid adenocarcinoma of the ovary and its relationship to endometriosis. *Gynecol Oncol* 59:81.
120. Scully RE, Young RH, Clement PB. 1998. Clear cell tumors. In: *Tumors of the Ovary, Maldeveloped Gonads, Fallopian Tube, and Broad Ligament*, Scully RE, Young RH, Clement PB (eds.), Washington, DC: Armed Forces Institute of Pathology.
121. Scully RE, Young RH, Clement PB. 1998. Transitional and squamous cell tumors. In: *Tumors of the Ovary, Maldeveloped Gonads, Fallopian Tube, and Broad Ligament*, Scully RE, Young RH, Clement PB (eds.), Washington, DC: Armed Forces Institute of Pathology.
122. Talerman A. 1994. Germ cell tumours of the ovary. In: *Blaustein's Pathology of the Female Genital Tract*, Kurman RJ, (ed.), p. 849. Springer Verlag: New York.
123. Ayhan A, Bukulmez O, Genc C et al. 2000. Mature cystic teratomas of the ovary: Case series from one institution over 34 years. *Eur J Obstet Gynecol Reprod Biol* 88:153.
124. Krasna IH, Lee ML, Smilow P et al. 1992. Risk of malignancy in bilateral streak gonads: The role of the Y chromosome. *J Pediatr Surg* 27:1376.
125. Young RH. 2005. Sex cord-stromal tumors of the ovary and testis: Their similarities and differences with consideration of selected problems. *Mod Pathol* 18:81.
126. Adamian RT. 1991. Hyperplastic processes and endometrial cancer in patients with hormone-producing ovarian tumors. *Vopr Onkol* 37:48.
127. Chen VW, Ruiz B, Killeen JL et al. 2003. Pathology and classification of ovarian tumors. *Cancer* 97:2631.
128. Peparini N, Chirletti P. 2009. Ovarian malignancies with cytologically negative pleural and peritoneal effusions: Demons' or meigs' pseudo-syndromes? *Int J Surg Pathol* 17:396.
129. Purdie DM, Bain CJ, Siskind V, Webb PM, Green AC. 2003. Ovulation and risk of epithelial ovarian cancer. *Int J Cancer* 104:228–232.
130. Kammerman S, Demopoulos RI, Ross J. 1977. Gonadotropin receptors in experimentally induced ovarian tumors in mice. *Cancer Res* 37:2578.
131. Schorge JO, Modesitt SC, Coleman RL et al. 2010. SGO White Paper on ovarian cancer: Etiology, screening and surveillance. *Gynecol Oncol* 119(1):7–17.
132. Pennington KP, Swisher EM. 2012. Hereditary ovarian cancer: Beyond the usual suspects. *Gynecol Oncol* 124:347.
133. Chen S, Parmigiani G. 2007. Meta-analysis of BRCA1 and BRCA2 penetrance. *J Clin Oncol* 25:1329.
134. Rebbeck TR, Kauff ND, Domchek SM. 2009. Meta-analysis of risk reduction estimates associated with risk-reducing salpingo-oophorectomy in BRCA1 or BRCA2 mutation carriers. *J Natl Cancer Inst* 101(2):80–87.
135. Stuart GC, Kitchener H, Bacon M et al. 2011. Gynecologic Cancer InterGroup (GCIG) consensus statement on clinical trials in ovarian cancer: Report from the Fourth Ovarian Cancer Consensus Conference. *Int J Gynecol Cancer* 21:750–755.
136. Tworoger SS, Gertig DM, Gates MA et al. 2008. Caffeine, alcohol, smoking, and the risk of incident epithelial ovarian cancer. *Cancer* 112:1169.
137. Huncharek M, Geschwind JF, Kupelnick B. 2003. Perineal application of cosmetic talc and risk of invasive epithelial ovarian cancer: A meta-analysis of 11,933 subjects from sixteen observational studies. *Anticancer Res* 23:1955.

138. Olson SH, Mignone L, Nakraseive C, Caputo TA, Barakat RR, Harlap S. 2001. Symptoms of ovarian cancer. *Obstet Gynecol* 98(2):212–217.
139. Sørensen HT, Mellemkjaer L, Olsen JH, Baron JA. 2000. Prognosis of cancers associated with venous thromboembolism. *N Engl J Med* 343:1846.
140. Varras M, Vasilakaki T, Skafida E, Akrivis C. 2011. Clinical, ultrasonographic, computed tomography and histopathological manifestations of ovarian steroid cell tumour, not otherwise specified: Our experience of a rare case with female virilisation and review of the literature. *Gynecol Endocrinol* 27:412.
141. Goff BA, Muntz HG. 2005. Screening and early diagnosis of ovarian cancer. *Women's Health in Primary Care* 8:262.
142. Kinkel K, Lu Y, Mehdizade A et al. 2005. Indeterminate ovarian mass at US: Incremental value of second imaging test for characterization—Meta-analysis and Bayesian analysis. *Radiology* 236(1):85–94.
143. Talerman A, Haije WG, Baggerman L. 1978. Serum alphafetoprotein (AFP) in diagnosis and management of endodermal sinus (yolk sac) tumor and mixed germ cell tumor of the ovary. *Cancer* 41:272.
144. Schwartz PE, Morris JM. 1988. Serum lactic dehydrogenase: A tumor marker for dysgerminoma. *Obstet Gynecol* 72:511.
145. Goff BA, Mandel L, Muntz HG, Melancon CH. 2000. Ovarian carcinoma diagnosis. *Cancer* 89:2068.
146. Kumar S, Shah JP, Bryant CS et al. 2008. The prevalence and prognostic impact of lymph node metastasis in malignant germ cell tumors of the ovary. *Gynecol Oncol* 110:125.
147. Thrall MM, Paley P, Pizer E et al. 2011. Patterns of spread and recurrence of sex cord-stromal tumors of the ovary. *Gynecol Oncol* 122:242.
148. Heintz AP, Odicino F, Maisonneuve P et al. 2006. Carcinoma of the ovary. FIGO 26th Annual Report on the Results of Treatment in Gynecological Cancer. *Int J Gynaecol Obstet* 95(1):161–192.
149. Young RC, Walton LA, Ellenberg SS et al. 1990. Adjuvant therapy in stage I and stage II epithelial ovarian cancer. Results of two prospective randomized trials. *N Engl J Med* 322:1021.
150. Young RC, Decker DG, Wharton JT et al. 1983. Staging laparotomy in early ovarian cancer. *JAMA* 250:3072.
151. du Bois A, Quinn M, Thigpen T et al. 2005. 2004 consensus statements on the management of ovarian cancer: Final document of the Third International Gynecologic Cancer Intergroup Ovarian Cancer Consensus Conference (GCIG OCCC 2004). *Ann Oncol* 16(Suppl. 8):viii7.
152. Merogi AJ, Marrogi AJ, Ramesh R et al. 1997. Tumor-host interaction: Analysis of cytokines, growth factors, and tumor-infiltrating lymphocytes in ovarian carcinomas. *Hum Pathol* 28:321.
153. Santin AD, Hermonat PL, Ravaggi A et al. 1999. Secretion of vascular endothelial growth factor in ovarian cancer. *Eur J Gynaecol Oncol* 20:177.
154. Eisenkop SM, Spirtos NM, Lin WC. 2006. "Optimal" cytoreduction for advanced epithelial ovarian cancer: A commentary. *Gynecol Oncol* 103:329.
155. Eisenhauer EL, Abu-Rustum NR, Sonoda Y et al. 2008. The effect of maximal surgical cytoreduction on sensitivity to platinum-taxane chemotherapy and subsequent survival in patients with advanced ovarian cancer. *Gynecol Oncol* 108:276.
156. Bristow RE, Chi DS. 2006. Platinum-based neoadjuvant chemotherapy and interval surgical cytoreduction for advanced ovarian cancer: A meta-analysis. *Gynecol Oncol* 103:1070.
157. Low JJ, Perrin LC, Crandon AJ, Hacker NF. 2000. Conservative surgery to preserve ovarian function in patients with malignant ovarian germ cell tumors. A review of 74 cases. *Cancer* 89:391.
158. O'Connor DM, Norris HJ. 1994. The influence of grade on the outcome of stage I ovarian immature (malignant) teratomas and the reproducibility of grading. *Int J Gynecol Pathol* 13:283.
159. Teramukai S, Ochiai K, Tada H et al. 2007. PIEPOC: A new prognostic index for advanced epithelial ovarian cancer—Japan Multinational Trial Organization OC01-01. *J Clin Oncol* 25:3302.
160. Stewart SL, Wike JM, Foster SL, Michaud F. 2007. The incidence of primary fallopian tube cancer in the United States. *Gynecol Oncol* 107:392.

161. Heintz AP, Odicino F, Maisonneuve P et al. 2006. Carcinoma of the fallopian tube. FIGO 26th Annual Report on the Results of Treatment in Gynecological Cancer. *Int J Gynaecol Obstet* 95(1):145–160.
162. Salvador S, Gilks B, Köbel M et al. 2009. The fallopian tube: Primary site of most pelvic high-grade serous carcinomas. *Int J Gynecol Cancer* 19:58.
163. Berec JS, Natarajan S. 2007. Ovarian and fallopian tube cancer. In: *Berek & Novak's Gynecology*, 14th edn., Berek JS (ed.), pp. 1528–1529. Philadelphia, PA: Lippincott, Williams & Wilkins.
164. Podratz KC, Podczaski ES, Gaffey TA, O'Brien PC, Schray MF, Malkasian GD Jr. 1986. Primary carcinoma of the fallopian tube. *Am J Obstet Gynecol* 154(6):1319–1326.

2

Cytogenetic Early Markers in Gynecologic Cancers

Murat Oznur, MD, PhD, Serap Dede, MS, Debmalya Barh, MSc, MTech, MPhil, PhD, and Mehmet Gunduz, MD, PhD

CONTENTS

ABSTRACT The identification of the true chromosome complement in human cells followed by the investigation of abnormal chromosome constitution in malign tumor cells led cytogenetic analysis to be used for the diagnosis and management of many malignancies. A number of studies have identified clinical applications of cytogenetic analysis for different cancers. Cytogeneticists accompany clinicians in this struggle by using current and future diagnostic technologies. Conventional cytogenetic, fluorescence in situ hybridization (FISH), and array comparative genomic hybridization (CGH) tests are current diagnostic technologies that are useful for the management of malignancies and for the diagnosis as well as the prediction of cancers. The karyotypes of some tumors are very complex and unstable, which might be considered as useful markers for their diagnosis. There are an increasing number of researches evaluating these markers for specific tumors. Conventional cytogenetic analysis accompanied by molecular genetic tests might be the main course of diagnosing tumors in the near future. Among cancer diseases, gynecologic cancers rank as the second highest cause of mortality and morbidity in women after breast cancer. This chapter focuses on the novel biomarkers that are being used or proposed for use for early diagnosis of gynecologic cancers, including ovarian, endometrial, cervical, vulvar, and vaginal cancers. According to the suitability of tissue, the detection of suspicious genetic abnormalities and their role in the diagnosis and prognostic prediction of a variety of solid tumors are rising. As the knowledge of malignancies and of their abnormal genetic structure increases, the importance and significance of conventional cytogenetic techniques become more evident.

2.1 Introduction

2.1.1 Development of Cytogenetic Techniques

Theodor Boveri investigated the chromosome constitution of malignant tumors and found that there is an abnormal chromosome number and structure in malignant tumor cells. He emphasized that any event that leads to an abnormal chromosome constitution is an indication of malignant tumors (Sandberg 1979). Subsequently, cytogenetic analysis is required for the diagnosis and management of many malignancies. With the identification of the true chromosome complement in human cells by Tjio and Levan (1956), reports about abnormalities of chromosome number and subsequently chromosome structure have risen.

Encouraged by these studies, other new investigations have brought cytogenetic analysis into current procedures. The main steps in this process are as follows:

- The discovery of hypotonic solution pretreatment
- Using colchicines, which has been used for arresting cells in the metaphasic stage of the cell cycle, thus increasing the number of mitoses available for analysis
- Tjio and Levan's (1956) report about identifying 46 chromosomes in the human cell
- The discovery of phytohemagglutinin (PHA), which induces peripheral blood lymphocytes to divide
- Staining by Giemsa

Although the progression of cytogenetic abnormalities was observed in various cancers, it was difficult to link those abnormalities with different morphological subtypes of tumors. After the improvement in chromosome banding, chromosomes could clearly be distinguished from each other, and thus, their abnormalities could be termed as deletion, inversion, duplication, or balanced translocation.

After the description of the Philadelphia chromosome by Nowell and Hungerford, the clinical utility of cytogenetic methods evolved step by step. A number of studies have identified clinical applications of cytogenetic analysis in different cancers. The development of in situ hybridization (ISH) also contributed to these processes (Campbell 2011).

Studies in translocations helped the identification of genes and resulted in the development of ISH and advanced cytogenetic analysis. In the early studies of ISH, DNA fragments labeled by thymidine were used as probes (Harper and Saunders 1981). However, the difficulties in conducting ISH such as the necessity of performing most of the steps in total darkness and the required time for hybridization have caused certain failures of tests. These problems have been partially solved by the development of FISH. Moreover, FISH probes were developed to determine the presence or absence of extra copies of chromosomes, translocations, and deletions. In nondividing cells, the studies of FISH that used panels of probes to identify chromosome rearrangements have seen great success.

By the improvement of FISH methods, in which each chromosome can be painted with a different color, it is easy to detect complex karyotypes.

The usage of FISH tests has become a necessary step in developing CGH. In CGH, labeled with green and red fluorochromes, the DNA of the patient and the DNA of the normal control compete with each other on a slide containing normal chromosome preparations for hybridization. Then a computer reads each chromosome and evaluates the DNA, which has hybridized along the length of each chromosome, according to its label. If the DNA of the patient sample does not include gains or losses, a yellow sign appears on the computer. This is the sign of an equal mixture of green and red fluorescence, which represents the patient's DNA and the control's DNA hybridized to each chromosome. If there is any loss of the patient's DNA, which is labeled green, then the sign on the computer will be red, representing the extra amount of normal control DNA and vice versa. Arrays of bacterial artificial chromosomes (BACs) or oligonucleotide-dotted slides/chips by CGH applications improved cytogenetics in cancer research. Deletions or amplifications in kilobase sizes could be evaluated by array CGH while balanced translocations could not be detected (Campbell 2011).

In clinicians' struggle for their patients' well-being, cytogeneticists help by using current and future diagnostic technologies. Conventional cytogenetic, FISH, and array CGH tests are current diagnostic technologies that are useful for the management of malignancies and for diagnosis and prediction of cancers (Campbell 2011).

2.1.2 Cytogenetic Techniques in Solid Tumors

The study and evaluation of chromosomal abnormalities in various malignancies are valuable for the diagnosis and prognostic stratification. According to the suitability of the tissue, the detection of suspicious genetic abnormalities and their role in the diagnosis and prognosis of a variety of solid tumors is rising.

With the increasing knowledge of malignancies and their abnormal genetic structure, the importance and significance of conventional cytogenetic techniques become evident as these methods can seek and evaluate all chromosomes at once. Molecular cytogenetic techniques are also useful for diagnosis. They may have some limitations in assessing all chromosome abnormalities simultaneously when used alone, so they could be used as a complementary process of conventional cytogenetic techniques.

The karyotypes of some tumors are very complex and unstable, which might be considered as useful markers for their diagnosis. There are an increasing number of researches evaluating these markers for specific tumors. These researches encourage clinicians. Conventional cytogenetic techniques accompanied by molecular genetic techniques might become the main processes in the diagnosis of tumors in the near future (Campbell 2011).

2.2 Gynecologic Cancers

After heart diseases, cancer is the second disease that causes death in developed countries. Among cancer diseases, after breast cancer, gynecologic cancers are the second reason that causes mortality and morbidity in women. Although it differs from one country to another in the world, the prevalence of gynecologic cancers in Eastern countries is in the order of endometrial, ovarian, and cervical cancers (CCs) (Uçar and Bekar 2010).

2.2.1 Ovarian Cancer

Ovarian cancer in women generates 4% of all cancers and causes 6% of cancer deaths. It is predicted that there are 192,000 cases all over the world. The prevalence of ovarian cancer could change according to different geographic regions. Especially in European countries like Scandinavian countries, the United Kingdom, Canada, and North America, its incidence is higher. In the United States, the incidence is 16/100,000 women while in Japan it is 3/100,000. The variety of environment and lifestyle may be the reason for this diversity (Uçar and Bekar 2010).

Early detection of ovarian cancer is rare, and when it is detected, it has pelvic spread. It is mostly sporadic but has got familial cancer syndromes.

According to histological specifications, ovarian cancers are heterogeneous. In histological classification, *ovarian epithelial carcinomas* are the most common form of ovarian cancers. This subtype of cancer develops from the ovary's surface cells. The other subtypes are *serous*, *clear cell*, *endometrioid*, and *mucinous* forms.

While genetic aberrations of serous carcinomas develop first of all in K-RAS and BRAF and then in p53 pathways, the other subtypes show various alterations. Gene amplifications are frequently seen aberrations of many ovarian cancers, among which CCNE1 (which encodes Cyclin E1), ERBB2, AKT2, PIK3CA, and the MYC family member L-MYC are more often identified (Bunz 2008a,b,c).

2.2.1.1 Cytogenetic Findings of Ovarian Cancer

Micci et al. (2010) studied cytogenetic aberrations of a group consisting of 23 patients determined as borderline ovarian tumor cases (Table 2.1). The analysis was done by cell culturing, g-banding, and karyotyping steps of the conventional cytogenetic technique and by high-resolution CGH. Finally, they reported that the cases with an abnormal karyotype had simple chromosomal aberrations of trisomy 7 and 12 as the most common ones. They also reported the detection of a common breakpoint of 3q13. As a result of CGH analysis gains from chromosome arms 2q, 6q, 8q, 9p, and 13q and losses from 1p, 12q, 14q, 15q, 16p, 17p, 17q, 19p, 19q, and 22q were detected (Micci et al. 2010).

Grygalewicz et al. (2009) compared cytogenetic changes in primary (6/11) and relapsed (5/11) borderline tumors of the ovary at stages I and III by conventional trypsin and Giemsa produce G-banded chromosome (GTG) banding analysis and FISH. They detected genomic imbalances in both groups. They reported that they observed chromosomal aberrations in chromosomes 12, 7, 8, and 21 as gains and in X as loss in a primary ovarian group. Their study also revealed chromosomal aberrations in chromosomes 7 and 12 as gains and in chromosomes 1, 2, 4, 6, 9, 10, 16, 17, 20, and 22 as losses in the relapsed group (Grygalewicz et al. 2009).

Bruchim et al. (2009) studied 45 epithelial ovarian cancers by CGH. They reported that among the 45 cases, they observed gains of DNA copy number at 3q (51%), 8q (47%), 2q (33%), and 1q (31%) and losses at 19 (20%) and 22 (20%) followed by 5q (13%) regions as the most common ones. Besides these aberrations, gains at 1p (20%), 2p (4%), 5p (18%), 7q (18%), 19 (2%), and 20q (2%) were the other observed alterations (Bruchim et al. 2009).

Caserta et al. (2008) applied microarray comparative genomic hybridization (A-CGH) in their study as an alternative technique besides the routine cytogenetic investigations, FISH

TABLE 2.1

Summary of Cytogenetic Findings of Ovarian Cancer

Researcher	Technique	Findings
Micci et al. (2010)	Conventional cytogenetic CGH	Trisomy 7 and 12 as the most common Common breakpoint of 3q13 Gains: 2q, 6q, 8q, 9p, and 13q Losses: 1p, 12q, 14q, 15q, 16p, 17p, 17q, 19p, 19q, and 22q
Grygalewicz et al. (2009)	Conventional cytogenetic	Primary ovarian group Gains: 12, 7, 8, and 21 Loss: X
	FISH	Relapsed group Gains: 7 and 12 Losses: 1, 2, 4, 6, 9, 10, 16, 17, 20, and 22
Bruchim et al. (2009)	CGH	The most common ones Gains: 3q (51%), 8q (47%), 2q (33%), and 1q (31%) Losses: 19 (20%), 22 (20%), and 5q (13%)
Caserta et al. (2008)	A-CGH FISH	The most common findings Gains: 8q, 9q, and 12p Losses: 6q, 9p, 10q, 21q, and 22q
Panani and Roussos et al. (2006)	Conventional cytogenetic	Structural aberrations at regions 1p13, 1p36, 3p13-14, 3q21, 11p15, 11q23, 11q10, 17q24-25, and 19q13 Isochromosomes i(5p), i(17q), i(8q), and i(11q) Translocations t(1;11), t(3;19), t(3;17), t(7;11), and t(11;17)
Park et al. (2006)	SNP array Digital karyotyping FISH Quantitative real-time PCR	Amplicon at 19p13.12 region
Fishman et al. (2005)	CGH	Gains: 1q, 2p, 2q, 3q, 6q, 8q, and 12p Losses: 18q and X
Lin et al. (2005)	CGH	Remarkable gains: 14 (25%), 12 (14%), and 7p15-p21 (6%) Losses: 22q (31%), 1p33-p36 (6%), 16p13.1 (6%), and 16q (6%)
Sahin et al. (2004)	Conventional cytogenetic	The most common abnormalities in 1, 3, 6, 7, 8, 11, 21, 22, and X Complex karyotypes at later stages
Partheen et al. (2004)	CGH	The most common gains: 1q24-qter (39%), 2pter-p14 (31%), 2q21-q34 (31%), 3q13.3-qter (49%), 8q13-q21.2 (47%), 8q23-q24.2 (57%), and 12p (32%) Losses: 4q13-q26 (37%), 4q31.1-qter (37%), 5q12-q22 (43%), 8p (42%), 17pter-q21 (35%), and X (51%)

application, and classical CGH techniques for overcoming their own limitations. They studied a group of 10 ovarian carcinoma patients, 9 of whom were serous papillary cystadenocarcinoma (8 patients were grade III, and 1 was grade II) and the other one was endometrial carcinoma according to their histological analysis. Finally, they reported the most common findings of 6q (four cases with mosaic loss of 6q), 9p (four cases), 10q (three cases), 21q (three cases), and 22q (four cases) as deletional aberration of chromosomes and gains of 8q and 9q (occurring together in eight cases) and gain of 12p. They also reported that they had observed monosomy X (in two cases) and a microdeletion of 17p terminal (in two cases).

They detected that some cases showed a genomic profile with total or mosaic segmental gain on chromosomes 2p, 3q, 4q, 7q, and 13q (Caserta et al. 2008).

Panani et al. (2006) studied 15 cases of ovarian adenocarcinomas by conventional cytogenetic technique for investigating the presence of recurrent structural aberrations with common chromosomal breakpoints. They noted that previous cytogenetic studies had reported chromosomes 1, 3, 6, 7, 11, 12, 17, and 19 as being the most common chromosomal rearrangements. Additionally, CGH studies had reported that recurrent abnormalities including gains on 1p, 1q, 3q, 6p, 8q, 11q, 12p, 17q, 19p, 19q, and 20q and losses of 4q, 5q, 8p, 11p, 13q, 17p, and 18q are common in ovarian cancer. Contributing to these findings, they reported that they observed recurrent structural aberrations involving chromosomal regions 1p13, 1p36, 3p13-14, 3q21, 11p15, 11q23, 11q10, 17q24-25, and 19q13. They also reported the observation of isochromosomes i(5p), i(17q), i(8q), and i(11q) and translocations t(1;11), t(3;19), t(3;17), t(7;11), and t(11;17) (Panani and Roussos 2006).

Joon T. Park et al. (2006) studied the biopsies of 31 high-grade ovarian serous carcinomas using single nucleotide polymorphism (SNP) array to analyze genome-wide DNA copy number. As a result, they reported that they had identified an amplicon at the 19p13.12 region in 6 of 31 (19.5%) ovarian high-grade serous carcinomas. They also validated the result by digital karyotyping, quantitative real-time polymerase chain reaction (PCR), and dual-color FISH analysis (Park et al. 2006).

Fishman et al. (2005) studied the genetic abnormalities in the primary tumors of seven epithelial ovarian cancer patients that appeared to be stage III ovarian serous cancer by using CGH. They analyzed the cytogenetic changes in six of the seven primary tumors as complex karyotypic patterns. They reported that they had revealed chromosomal aberrations in six patients with certain repeated changes as amplification of 1q, 2p, 2q, 3q, 6q, 8q, and 12p and underrepresentation of 18q and X chromosomes (Fishman et al. 2005).

Lin et al. (2005) studied 36 ovarian cancer patients with stage I granulosa cell tumors (GCTs) that are ovarian sex cord stromal tumors of low-grade malignancy which may occasionally metastasized. They used CGH to detect the chromosomal imbalances. They reported that although they observed remarkable losses of 22q (31%), 1p33-p36 (6%), 16p13.1 (6%), and 16q (6%) and gains of chromosomes 14 (25%), 12 (14%), and 7p15-p21 (6%). There were also losses at chromosomes 9, 13, 15, 17, and 21 and gains at chromosomes 6, 8, 9, 10, 13, and 18, which they figured as an ideogram (Lin et al. 2005).

Sahin et al. (2004) studied 15 serous papillary adenocarcinoma samples at different stages by using conventional cytogenetic technique. They reported that they observed chromosomal abnormalities in chromosomes 1, 3, 6, 7, 8, 11, 21, 22, and X as the most common ones and complex karyotypes at later stages (Sahin et al. 2004).

Partheen et al. (2004) used CGH to determine chromosomal alterations in 98 patients with stage III serous papillary adenocarcinomas. They reported that they detected cytogenetic alterations on all chromosomes and noticed that some changes were recurrent and rather specific. They also reported that they observed aberrations of some of the chromosomes or parts of chromosomes most often involved in the regions of 1q24-qter (39%), 2pter-p14 (31%), 2q21-q34 (31%), 3q13.3-qter (49%), 8q13-q21.2 (47%), 8q23-q24.2 (57%), and 12p (32%) as gains and in the regions of 4q13-q26 (37%), 4q31.1-qter (37%), 5q12-q22 (43%), 8p (42%), 17pter-q21 (35%), and X (51%) as losses of genetic material. They declared and figured as an ideogram that besides these most common regions, they also detected aberrations at chromosomes 5p, 6p, 7q21-q31, 7q32-qter, 11q13-q23, 12q14-q22, 18q11.2-q21, 19q12-q13.2, 20p, and 20q as gain and 4p, 6q16-q24, 9qter-p21, 9q, 16q, and 18q21-qter as loss (Partheen et al. 2004).

2.2.2 Endometrial Cancer

Endometrial cancer is the most commonly seen gynecologic cancer in Western countries. While this cancer is frequently seen between the fifth and seventh decades, it is rare before the age of 40. As populations are getting older, the incidence of endometrial cancer is rising. The prevalence of endometrial cancer also changes among countries according to differences of their ethnicity and geographic region. It shows the importance of the environment and genetic effects on the development of cancer (Uçar and Bekar 2010).

The endometrium is the inner layer of the uterus that consists of cells of *epithelial* and *stromal origin*. Cancers can develop from both these cells, but predominantly endometrial cancers are carcinomas that develop from epithelial cells. Additionally, endometrial carcinomas can be classified as *endometrioid carcinoma, serous papillar carcinoma, clear cell carcinoma, adenosquamous carcinoma, mucinous carcinoma,* and *squamous carcinoma* according to their histologic specifications. Endometrioid carcinoma is the most common form of endometrial carcinomas and develops from its noninvasive form called complex atypical hyperplasia (CAH). The other form of endometrial carcinoma, serous papillar carcinoma, develops from endometrial intraepithelial carcinoma (EIC). These lesions are distinguishable by their clinical and molecular structures (Gordon and Ireland 2008, Bunz 2008).

Microsatellite instability, which represents DNA mismatch repair defects, could be exhibited in nearly a quarter of sporadic cancers. These defects could be seen in both endometrioid carcinoma and its precursor, CAH.

In endometrial cancers, the most common mutations are caused by the affected PIK3 pathway. Nearly half of endometrioid carcinomas have mutations in PTEN. In endometrioid carcinomas, the mutations of PIK3CA and PTEN coexist. Furthermore, K-RAS, P53, and CTNNB1 mutations are common in endometrioid carcinomas.

In comparison to endometrioid carcinomas, uterine serous carcinoma is less common. In this group, PTEN mutations are rare, microsatellite instability is uncommon, but P53 mutations occur in more than 90% of cases (Bunz 2008).

2.2.2.1 Cytogenetic Findings of Endometrial Cancer

Lee et al. (2012) studied endometrial stromal sarcoma (ESS) and reported a transforming 14-3-3 oncoprotein, which they identified through conventional cytogenetic and whole-transcriptome sequencing analysis (Table 2.2). They observed that this oncoprotein resulted from a t(10;17) genomic rearrangement, leading to fusion between 14-3-3ε (YWHAE) and either of two nearly identical FAM22 family members (FAM22A or FAM22B). To characterize the genetic basis of high-grade ESS, they performed prospective cytogenetic G-banding and FISH analyses, which identified a translocation, t(10;17)(q22;p13), as a recurrent and predominant aberration (Lee et al. 2012).

Amador-Ortiz et al. (2011) used an interphase FISH technique to evaluate the prevalence of the t(7;17)(p15;q21) and JAZF1-JJAZ1 gene fusion in a series of six cases (three cases arising from the ovary and three from the abdominopelvic cavity) of primary extrauterine ESS. They evoked the knowledge that although ESS is a primary tumor of the uterus, it is at the same time a primary tumor that originates from the ovaries, vagina, pelvic wall, omentum, and gastrointestinal tract and exhibits similar morphologic features to its uterine counterpart. They also demonstrated their findings as the presence of t(7;17)(p15;q21) and associated JAZF1-JJAZ1 fusion transcripts only in a subset of primary extrauterine ESS and its 17% prevalence (one of six cases). As the

TABLE 2.2

Summary of Cytogenetic Findings of Endometrial Cancer

Researcher	Technique	Findings
Lee et al. (2012)	Conventional cytogenetic FISH analyses Sequencing analysis	t(10;17)(q22;p13)
Amador-Ortiz et al. (2011)	Interphase FISH	t(7;17)(p15;q21)
Chiang and Oliva (2011)	REVIEW	Translocations involving partners on chromosome arms 6p, 7p, and 17q
Levan et al. (2006)	CGH	Gains: 1q25-q42 (30%) and 19pter-p13.1 (26%), 19q13.1-q13.3 (19%), 8q (8q21-q22 and 8q22-qter) (17%), 10q21-q23 (14%), and 10p (13%) Losses: 4q22-qter, 16q21-qter, and 18q21-qter (all 8%)
Muslumanoglu et al. (2005)	CGH	Gains: 8q (46.7%), 1q (33.3%), 3q26 (26.7%), and 4p (20.0%) Losses: 1p36-pter and 10q (33.3%), 9q and 14q (26.7%), 11q (20.0%)
Micci et al. (2004)	CGH	Type I endometrial carcinomas Gains: 1q and 8q Losses: Xp, 9p, 9q, 17p, 19p, and 19q Type II endometrial carcinomas Gains: 1q, 2p, 3q, 5p, 6p, 7p, 8q, 10q, and 20q Losses: Xq, 5q, and 17p

reported range is 33%–80% for uterine ESS, they associated this low prevalence to an indication of heterogeneity of ESS (Amador-Ortiz et al. 2011).

Chiang and Oliva (2011) reviewed the literature about endometrial stromal tumors. They analyzed cytogenetic findings of the publications of chromosomal aberrations and classified them into 35 chromosomal rearrangements of ESS. They showed that the rearrangements often include specific, recurrent translocations involving partners on chromosome arms 6p, 7p, and 17q. They emphasized that t(7;17)(p15;q21) and its variants have been found in 11 of 35 (31%) chromosomal rearrangements and suggested that this was a significant development in at least a subset of ESS. They pointed out a breakpoint on the short arm of chromosome 6 at the 6p21 locus, which recombines with partners on chromosome 7, in particular 7q34-7q11, 7p22, 7p21, 7p15, and 7q22. This breakpoint of 6p21 locus has also been rearranged with partners on chromosome 3 including 3p12 and 3q29. Besides these rearrangements, t(6;7)(q21;p15)/t(6;10;10)(p21;q22;p11)/add(6)(p21.3)/loss of 6p21.3-pter/t(X;17)(p11;q23), and t(10;17)(q22;p13) are some of the other aberrations (Chiang and Oliva 2011).

Levan et al. (2006) studied 98 patients with endometrioid adenocarcinomas to investigate their chromosomal alterations by using the CGH technique. They reported that they detected gain alteration at region 1q25-q42 as the most frequent one (30%). Besides this alteration, gains at 19pter-p13.1 (26%), 19q13.1-q13.3 (19%), 8q (8q21-q22 and 8q22-qter) (17%), 10q21-q23 (14%), and 10p (13%) were also reported. The common reported losses were found in the three regions 4q22-qter, 16q21-qter, and 18q21-qter, all of which were detected at 8% rates (Levan et al. 2006).

Muslumanoglu et al. (2005) studied paraffin-embedded tissue specimens from 15 cases of endometrial carcinoma, 32 cases of endometrial hyperplasia, and 20 cases of normal endometrial tissue by using the CGH technique. They aimed to evaluate the sequential genomic copy alterations related to the development of precursor lesions and endometrioid-type endometrial carcinomas. They reported that they observed aberrations as gains on 8q (46.7%), 1q (33.3%), 3q26 (26.7%), and 4p (20.0%) and losses on 1p36-pter and 10q (33.3%), 9q and 14q (26.7%), and 11q (20.0%). In conclusion, they commented that they observed different patterns of chromosomal aberrations in precursor lesions than in endometrial carcinomas, except for the loss of 1p36-pter. According to them, this is a suggestion of an early event in the development of carcinoma (Muslumanoglu et al. 2005).

Micci et al. (2004) studied 67 patients with endometrial carcinomas and 15 patients with carcinosarcomas by karyotyping and CGH. They reported that as chromosomal aberrations they observed gains from chromosome arms 1q and 8q and losses from Xp, 9p, 9q, 17p, 19p, and 19q in the type I endometrial carcinoma group, whereas the type II endometrial carcinomas of group showed a more complex imbalanced picture, with gains from chromosome arms 1q, 2p, 3q, 5p, 6p, 7p, 8q, 10q, and 20q and losses from Xq, 5q, and 17p. Their observations about the carcinosarcomas were gains of or from 1q, 5p, 8q, and 12q but losses from 9q. According to their comprehensive study, they also defined the aberration regions and reported that type I adenocarcinomas that were highly differentiated mostly showed gains from 1q24-q42 and 10p13-p15 with the only loss scored at 13q14-q34; those that were moderately differentiated showed gains from 1q32-q42, 7p13-p22, 7q11-q36, and 10q21-q26 as well as losses from Xp11, 9p12-p13, 9q11-q34, 17p13, 19p13, and 19q13; and those that were poorly differentiated showed gains from 1q25-q31, 2p16-p24, 2q23-q35, 3q26-q29, 6p12, 8q23-q24, and 20q13 but losses from Xp11-p22, Xq12-q13, and Xq23-q28; 5q14, 9p21, 9q13-q22, and 9q34, 17p12-p13, and 17q. They reported that besides these groups serous papillary carcinomas showed gains from 1q25-q41, 2p24-p25, 2q12-q13, 3q13-q26, 5p14-p15, 6p21-q12, 6q13, 7p21, 8q24, 18q12, 20p12-p13, and 20q12-q13 but losses from 17p13, whereas the clear-cell carcinomas showed gains from 3q22-q29, 7p11-p21, 8q11-q23, 10q25-q26, 16p13, and 20q13 but losses from 6q16-q23 (Micci et al. 2004).

2.2.3 Cervical Cancer

After breast cancer, CC is the second highest cancer diagnosed all over the world. This cancer causes 9% of cancer deaths in a year around the world. The prevalence of this cancer differs according to the country's development level. CC causes the death of women between 25 and 64 years. It has frequently been seen in underdeveloped countries (Uçar and Bekar 2010).

Squamous cell carcinomas (SCCs) are the most common form of CCs, which develop from the transition zone of the cervical epithelium called the squamocolumnar junction. They cause 80% of CCs. The other 20% are caused by *adenocarcinomas*, which develop from the endocervix, and are usually ulcerative and infiltrative (Fotra and Gupta 2011).

The underlying cause of CC differs from the other common cancers as it is an infection of the human papillomavirus (HPV). The other genetic aberrations, which trigger cervical tumorigenesis, are yet to be investigated. K-RAS mutations and P53 gene mutations in CCs rarely occur. Besides this, in cervical neoplasia, aberrations of the PIK3CA pathway are frequently seen (Bunz 2008).

2.2.3.1 Cytogenetic Findings of Cervical Cancer

Pinto et al. (2012) reviewed CC and its precursors. They detected the high prevalence of chromosome 3 alterations in SCCs. Although generally alterations of "3p loss," especially the loss of the whole short arm or breakage at 3p14.2 which harbor the most common chromosomal fragile site named the FHIT gene, were detected, the most characteristic

TABLE 2.3

Summary of Cytogenetic Findings of Cervical Cancer

Researcher	Technique	Findings
Pinto et al. (2012)	REVIEW	3p loss or breakage at 3p14.2 region.
		Gain at the segment between chromosome bands 3q24/25 and 3q28.
Fotra et al. (2011)	Conventional cytogenetic	Squamous cervical cancer Trisomy of chromosomes 3, 8, 11, 12, 13, 17, 18, 19, 20, and 22. Adenocarcinoma
		Monosomy of chromosome 3 and trisomy of chromosomes 1, 3, and 17.
Darroudi et al. (2010)	PCC	Gains at chromosomes 1, 3, 9, 14, 15, and 22.
	COBRA	Losses: 1, 2, 3, 8, 11, 14, 15, 18, and 22.
	FISH	They have not observed any aberration in chromosomes 5, 12, 16, and 21.
Wilting et al. (2009)	Array CGH	Gains: on chromosome **1** at regions [1p36.11-p35.2 (%21.7); 1p31.3-p21.1 (%26.1); 1q25.3-q32.1 (%23.9); 1q32.2-q44 (%23.9)], on chromosome **3** at regions [3p26.3-p26.1 (%21.7); 3p14.3-p14.2 (%21.7); 3q11.2-q29 (%26.1)], on chromosome **7** at region [7q31.1-q31.2 (%28.3)], and on chromosome **20** at regions [20p13-p11.21 (%26.1); 20q12 (%32.6)].
		Losses: on chromosome **4** at regions [4p16.3-p16.1 (%32.6); 4q31.21 (%21.7); 4q35.2 (%26.1)], on chromosome **11** at region [11q13.3 (%28.3)], on chromosome **16** at region [16q24.2-q24.3 (%21.7)], on chromosome **17** at regions [17p13.3 (%34.8); 17q25.3 (%41.3)], and on chromosome **19** at region [19p13.11-q12 (%32.6)].
Jancarkova et al. (2008)	Conventional cytogenetic	Amplifications 3q and 5p.
	CGH	Deletions 13q and isochromosome 5p.
Choi et al. (2007)	Array CGH	Gains: 1p36.33-1p36.32, 8q24.3, 16p13.3, 3q27.1, and 7p21.1.
		Losses: 2q12.1, 22q11.21, 3p14.2, 6q24.3, 7p15.2, and 11q25.

chromosomal abnormality identified in invasive CC was the gain of chromosome arm 3q. In this review, they reported that this identified chromosomal abnormality was detected in approximately 70% of CCs. They also noted that by CGH studies, the chromosomal alterations of 3q, or more specifically a gain at the segment between chromosome bands 3q24/25 and 3q28, were commonly identified, which had led to the hypothesis that this genetic aberration might play a pivotal role in the transition from preinvasive lesions to invasive CCs (Pinto et al. 2012) (Table 2.3).

Fotra and Gupta (2011) studied cytogenetic aberrations in CC. The study group consisted of 78 patients among whom 66 were confirmed as SCC and 12 were adenocarcinoma according to their histopathological specifications. They emphasized that the numerical chromosomal changes were more common (95%) than structural changes (5%). They reported trisomy 3, 8, 11, 12, 13, 17, 18, 19, 20, and 22 in SCC, as well as monosomy 3 and trisomy 1, 3, and 17 in adenocarcinoma as chromosomal aberrations. These results led them to consider the conventional cytogenetic analysis as a powerful tool and established technique that can provide a picture of the human genome at a glance (Fotra and Gupta 2011).

Darroudi et al. (2010) used a newly developed assay based on chemically induced premature chromosome condensation (PCC) and multicolor combined binary ratio labeling (COBRA) FISH techniques in order to investigate recurrent cytogenetic aberrations in primary CC at different stages of progression. They analyzed the cytogenetic profiles of 17 CC patients' biopsies, which were derived from SCCs (14/17) and from adenocarcinomas (3/17).

According to their assessments for the loss and gain of specific chromosomes at stages IB1, IIA, and IIB of CC, the most frequent numerical changes observed were in chromosomes 1, 3, 9, 14, 15, and X as gain and in chromosomes 1, 2, 3, 8, 11, 14, 15, 18, and 22 as loss. They reported that they did not observe any aberration in chromosomes 5, 12, 16, and 21 (Darroudi et al. 2010).

Wilting et al. (2009) studied 46 high-grade cervical intraepithelial neoplasia (CIN 2/3) lesions on biopsies using the array CGH technique. They reported that they observed frequent alterations including gains located at chromosome 1 [1p36.11-p35.2 (21.7%), 1p31.3-p21.1 (26.1%), 1q25.3-q32.1 (23.9%), 1q32.2-q44 (23.9%)], 3 [3p26.3-p26.1 (21.7%), 3p14.3-p14.2 (21.7%), 3q11.2-q29 (26.1%)], 7 [7q31.1-q31.2 (28.3%)], and 20 [20p13-p11.21 (26.1%), 20q12 (32.6%)] and losses located at chromosome 4 [4p16.3-p16.1 (32.6%), 4q31.21 (21.7%), 4q35.2 (26.1%)], 11 [11q13.3 (28.3%)], 16 [16q24.2-q24.3 (21.7%)], 17 [17p13.3 (34.8%), 17q25.3 (41.3%)] and 19 [19p13.11-q12 (32.6%)] (Wilting et al. 2009).

Jancarkova et al. (2008) studied 20 patients with CC. They reported that they applied both conventional (direct culture and a G-banding technique, the FISH technique with whole chromosome painting probes) and molecular techniques (the CGH method) for genetic testing. As a result, they reported that the most typical findings in cervical tumor cells that they observed were amplifications of 3q and 5p, and deletions of 13q and isochromosome 5p. They noted that some of the less frequent findings in their study were amplifications of chromosome 2 and deletions of chromosome 10, 11p, and 21q (Jancarkova et al. 2008).

Choi et al. (2007) studied 15 cases of CC to identify novel genomic regions of interest and provide highly dynamic range information on the correlation between SCC and its related gene expression patterns by a genome-wide array CGH. They reported that they observed chromosomal aberrations at regions 1p36.33-1p36.32, 8q24.3, 16p13.3, 3q27.1, and 7p21.1 as gains and at regions 2q12.1, 22q11.21, 3p14.2, 6q24.3, 7p15.2, and 11q25 as losses (Choi et al. 2007).

2.2.4 Vulvar Cancer

Vulvar cancer, which is rarely seen, comprises 5% of gynecologic cancers. Its incidence is predicted as 2/100,000 (Uçar and Bekar 2010).

2.2.4.1 Cytogenetic Findings of Vulvar Cancer

Ouyang et al. (2007) studied 21 cases of vulvar squamous cell carcinoma (VSCC) to identify genetic alterations by using the CGH technique. They reported that among multiple chromosomal aberrations that they observed, gains of chromosomes 3q, 8q, and 12q and losses of chromosomes 4p and 3p were the most common chromosomal alterations (Ouyang et al. 2007) (Table 2.4).

Yangling et al. (2007) studied patients of VSCC with HPV-positive and HPV-negative groups for the documentation of chromosomal gains and losses by using CGH. They reported that while the losses of 4p and 3p were seen in both HPV-positive and HPV-negative groups, gains of 3q and 12q were significantly more common in HPV-positive and gain of 8q was more common in HPV-negative groups. According to them, this indicates that one or more oncogenes, which are important in the development and progression of HPV-induced carcinomas, are located on 3q and 12q regions (Yangling et al. 2007).

Ouyang et al. (2006) studied 21 patients with VSCC to investigate chromosomal gains and losses by using CGH. As a result, they reported that they had observed gains on chromosomes 3q (43%), 8q (38%), 12q (33%), and 9p (19%) and losses of 4p (52%), 3p (43%), and 9p (10%).

TABLE 2.4
Summary of Cytogenetic Findings of Vulvar Cancer

Researcher	Technique	Findings
Ouyang et al. (2007)	CGH	Gains: 3q, 8q, and 12q. Losses: 4p and 3p.
Yangling et al. (2007)	CGH	Losses of 4p and 3p were in both HPV-positive and HPV-negative groups. Gains of 3q and 12q were significantly more common in HPV-positive groups. Gain of 8q was more common in HPV-negative groups.
Ouyang et al. (2006)	CGH	Gains: 3q (43%), 8q (38%), 12q (33%), and 9p (19%). Losses: 4p (52%), 3p (43%), and 9p (10%).

TABLE 2.5
Summary of Cytogenetic Findings of Vaginal Cancer

Researcher	Technique	Findings
Habermann et al. (2004)	CGH	Gains: 3q (69%) and 19p (50%), 5p (50%), 6q and 19q (44%), 1q and 17p (38%), 1p, 7p, 14, 16q, 18p, and 22 (31%), and 2p, 9q, 12, and 18q (25%). Losses: 13q, 8p, and 9p.

They also added that while comparing the groups, they observed gains of 3q (73%) and 12q (64%) significantly more commonly in HPV-positive VSCC group and gains on chromosome 8q (70%) more commonly in HPV-negative VSCC group (Ouyang et al. 2006).

2.2.5 Vaginal Cancer

Vaginal cancer is a gynecologic cancer that is rarely seen. Its incidence is 1/100,000. Ninety percent of this cancer is seen as an invasion or metastasis from cervical, endometrial, and vulvar cancers (Uçar and Bekar 2010).

2.2.5.1 Cytogenetic Findings of Vaginal Cancer

Habermann et al. (2004) studied 16 biopsies taken from patients with primary carcinomas of the vagina, which are rare tumors of all gynecologic malignancies. They established a pattern of genomic imbalances in vaginal SCCs by using the CGH technique. They reported that they observed chromosomal imbalances in all tumors and the most common DNA gains were mapped to chromosome arms 3q (69%) and 19p (50%), 5p (50%), 6q and 19q (44%), 1q and 17p (38%), 1p, 7p, 14, 16q, 18p, and 22 (31%), and 2p, 9q, 12, and 18q (25%). They have also observed chromosomal losses mapped to chromosome arms 13q, 8p, and 9p (Habermann et al. 2004) (Table 2.5).

2.3 Conclusion and Future Direction

Conventional cytogenetic, FISH, and array CGH tests are current diagnostic technologies, which are useful for the management of malignancies and for diagnosis and prediction of cancers. The karyotypes of some tumors are very complex and instable, which might be considered as useful markers for their diagnosis. There are increasing numbers of researches evaluating these markers for specific tumors.

By the increasing knowledge of malignancies and of their abnormal genetic structure, the importance and the significance of conventional cytogenetic become more evident. Molecular cytogenetic techniques are also useful for the diagnosis of cancer diseases, but when used alone, they have some limitations.

The studies of FISH, which has been used with panels of probes to identify chromosome rearrangements, have got great success. The improvement of FISH methods, which succeeded in painting each chromosome with a different color, has made it easy to detect complex karyotypes. The use of FISH tests has become a step for developing comparative genomic hybridization (CGH), which could evaluate deletions or amplifications in patients' genome.

Near-future conventional cytogenetic accompanied by molecular genetic applications might be the main part of the diagnosis of tumors.

References

Amador-Ortiz, C., A. A. Roma, P. C. Huettner, N. Becker, and J. D. Pfeifer. 2011. JAZF1 and JJAZ1 gene fusion in primary extrauterine endometrial stromal sarcoma. *Hum Pathol* 42 (7):939–946. doi: 10.1016/j.humpath.2010.11.001.

Bruchim, I., O. Israeli, S. M. Mahmud, A. Aviram-Goldring, S. Rienstein, E. Friedman, G. Ben-Baruch, and W. H. Gotlieb. 2009. Genetic alterations detected by comparative genomic hybridization and recurrence rate in epithelial ovarian carcinoma. *Cancer Genet Cytogenet* 190 (2):66–70. doi: 10.1016/j.cancergencyto.2008.11.013.

Bunz, F. 2008a. Genetic alternations in common cancers: Endometrial cancer. In *Principles of Cancer Genetics*, pp. 235–237. Springer Science.

Bunz, F. 2008b. Genetic Alternations in common cancers: Ovarian cancer. In *Principles of Cancer Genetics*, pp. 242–243. Springer Science.

Bunz, F. 2008c. Genetic Alternations in common cancers: Cancer of the uterine cervix. In *Principles of Cancer Genetics*, pp. 248–250. Springer Science.

Campbell, L. 2011. Evolution of cytogenetic methods in the study of cancer. In *Cancer Cytogenetics Methods and Protocols*, 2nd edn, Campell, L. (ed.), pp. 3–12. Springer–Humana Press.

Caserta, D., M. Benkhalifa, M. Baldi, F. Fiorentino, M. Qumsiyeh, and M. Moscarini. 2008. Genome profiling of ovarian adenocarcinomas using pangenomic BACs microarray comparative genomic hybridization. *Mol Cytogenet* 1:10. doi: 10.1186/1755-8166-1-10.

Chiang, S. and E. Oliva. 2011. Cytogenetic and molecular aberrations in endometrial stromal tumors. *Hum Pathol* 42 (5):609–617. doi: 10.1016/j.humpath.2010.12.005.

Choi, Y. W., S. M. Bae, Y. W. Kim, H. N. Lee, T. C. Park, D. Y. Ro, J. C. Shin, S. J. Shin, J. S. Seo, and W. S. Ahn. 2007. Gene expression profiles in squamous cell cervical carcinoma using array-based comparative genomic hybridization analysis. *Int J Gynecol Cancer* 17 (3):687–696. doi: 10.1111/j.1525-1438.2007.00834.x.

Darroudi, F., J. W. Bergs, V. Bezrookove, M. R. Buist, L. J. Stalpers, and N. A. Franken. 2010. PCC and COBRA-FISH a new tool to characterize primary cervical carcinomas: To assess hall-marks and stage specificity. *Cancer Lett* 287 (1):67–74. doi: 10.1016/j.canlet.2009.05.034.

Fishman, A., E. Shalom-Paz, M. Fejgin, E. Gaber, M. Altaras, and A. Amiel. 2005. Comparing the genetic changes detected in the primary and secondary tumor sites of ovarian cancer using comparative genomic hybridization. *Int J Gynecol Cancer* 15 (2):261–266. doi: 10.1111/j.1525-1438.2005.15213.x.

Fotra, R. and S. Gupta. 2011. Study of the cytogenetic and non-cytogenetic factors in cervical carcinoma in the Jammu region of J and K state. *J Cancer Res Ther* 7 (3):286–291. doi: 10.4103/0973-1482.87019.

Gordon, M. D. and K. Ireland. 2008. *Pathology of Endometrial Carcinoma. The Global Library of Women's Medicine*, doi: 10.3843/GLOWM.10238.

Grygalewicz, B., P. Sobiczewski, P. Krawczyk, R. Woroniecka, J. Rygier, A. Pastwinska, M. Bidzinski, and B. Pienkowska-Grela. 2009. Comparison of cytogenetic changes between primary and relapsed patients with borderline tumors of the ovary. *Cancer Genet Cytogenet* 195 (2):157–163. doi: 10.1016/j.cancergencyto.2009.07.005.

Habermann, J. K., K. Hellman, S. Freitag, K. Heselmeyer-Haddad, A.-C. Hellström, K. Shah, G. Auer, and T. Ried. 2004. A recurrent gain of chromosome arm 3q in primary squamous carcinoma of the vagina. *Cancer Genet Cytogenet* 148 (1):7–13. doi: 10.1016/s0165-4608(03)00245–0.

Harper, M. E. and G. F. Saunders. 1981. Localization of single copy DNA sequences of G-banded human chromosomes by in situ hybridization. *Chromosoma* 83 (3):431–439.

Jancarkova, N., M. Krkavcova, M. Janashia, P. Freitag, J. Duskova, and D. Cibula. 2008. Importance of chromosomal changes correlated to prognostic factors in ovarian and cervical malignant tumors. *Ceska Gynekol* 73 (2):79–86.

Lee, C. H., W. B. Ou, A. Marino-Enriquez, M. Zhu, M. Mayeda, Y. Wang, X. Guo et al. 2012. 14-3-3 fusion oncogenes in high-grade endometrial stromal sarcoma. *Proc Natl Acad Sci USA* 109 (3):929–934. doi: 10.1073/pnas.1115528109.

Levan, K., K. Partheen, L. Osterberg, K. Helou, and G. Horvath. 2006. Chromosomal alterations in 98 endometrioid adenocarcinomas analyzed with comparative genomic hybridization. *Cytogenet Genome Res* 115 (1):16–22. doi: 10.1159/000094796.

Lin, Y. S., H. L. Eng, Y. J. Jan, H. S. Lee, W. L. Ho, C. P. Liou, W. Y. Lee, and C. C. Tzeng. 2005. Molecular cytogenetics of ovarian granulosa cell tumors by comparative genomic hybridization. *Gynecol Oncol* 97 (1):68–73. doi: 10.1016/j.ygyno.2004.12.014.

Micci, F., L. Haugom, T. Ahlquist, H. K. Andersen, V. M. Abeler, B. Davidson, C. G. Trope, R. A. Lothe, and S. Heim. 2010. Genomic aberrations in borderline ovarian tumors. *J Transl Med* 8:21. doi: 10.1186/1479-5876-8-21.

Micci, F., M. R. Teixeira, L. Haugom, G. Kristensen, V. M. Abeler, and S. Heim. 2004. Genomic aberrations in carcinomas of the uterine corpus. *Genes Chromosomes Cancer* 40 (3):229–246. doi: 10.1002/gcc.20038.

Muslumanoglu, H. M., U. Oner, S. Ozalp, M. F. Acikalin, O. T. Yalcin, M. Ozdemir, and S. Artan. 2005. Genetic imbalances in endometrial hyperplasia and endometrioid carcinoma detected by comparative genomic hybridization. *Eur J Obstet Gynecol Reprod Biol* 120 (1):107–114. doi: 10.1016/j.ejogrb.2004.08.015.

Ouyang, L., S. L. Zhang, R. L. Chen, B. Li, and L. L. Chen. 2007. Chromosomal aberration in vulvar squamous cell carcinoma analyzed by comparative genomic hybridization. *Ai Zheng* 26 (6):572–575.

Ouyang, L., S. L. Zhang, and X. Wang. 2006. Genetic aberrations and human papillomavirus status in vulvar squamous cell carcinomas. *Zhonghua Fu Chan Ke Za Zhi* 41 (10):701–705.

Panani, A. D. and C. Roussos. 2006. Non-random structural chromosomal changes in ovarian cancer: i(5p) a novel recurrent abnormality. *Cancer Lett* 235 (1):130–135. doi: 10.1016/j.canlet.2005.04.010.

Park, J. T., M. Li, K. Nakayama, T.-L. Mao, B. Davidson, Z. Zhang, R. J. Kurman, C. G. Eberhart, I.-M. Shih, and T.-L. Wang. 2006. notch3 gene amplification in ovarian cancer. *Cancer Res* 66:6312–6318.

Partheen, K., K. Levan, L. Osterberg, K. Helou, and G. Horvath. 2004. Analysis of cytogenetic alterations in stage III serous ovarian adenocarcinoma reveals a heterogeneous group regarding survival, surgical outcome, and substage. *Genes Chromosomes Cancer* 40 (4):342–348. doi: 10.1002/gcc.20053.

Pinto, A. P., M. Degen, L. L. Villa, and E. S. Cibas. 2012. Immunomarkers in gynecologic cytology: The search for the ideal 'biomolecular Papanicolaou test'. *Acta Cytol* 56 (2):109–121. doi: 10.1159/000335065.

Sahin, I., Z. Yilmaz, and F. I. Sahin. 2004. Cytogenetic abnormalities in serous papillary adenocarcinoma of the ovary. *Eur J Gynaecol Oncol* 25 (5):585–586.

Sandberg A.A. 1979. Before 1956: Some historical background to the study of chromosomes in human cancer and leukemia. *Cancer Genet Cytogenet* 1:87–94.

Tjio J.H. and A. Levan. 1956. The chromosome number of man. *Hereditas*. 42:1–6.

Uçar, T. and M. Bekar. 2010. Türkiye'de ve Dünyada Jinekolojik Kanserler. Türk Jinekolojik Onkoloji Dergisi. *Haziran* 13 (3):55–60.

Wilting, S. M., R. D. Steenbergen, M. Tijssen, W. N. van Wieringen, T. J. Helmerhorst, F. J. van Kemenade, M. C. Bleeker et al. 2009. Chromosomal signatures of a subset of high-grade premalignant cervical lesions closely resemble invasive carcinomas. *Cancer Res* 69 (2):647–655. doi: 10.1158/0008-5472.CAN-08-2478.

Yangling, O., Z. Shulang, C. Rongli, L. Bo, C. Lili, and W. Xin. 2007. Genetic imbalance and human papillomavirus states in vulvar squamous cell carcinomas. *Eur J Gynaecol Oncol* 28 (6):442–446.

Section II

Breast Cancer

3

Early Biomarkers in Breast Cancer

Ruchika Kaul-Ghanekar, MSc, PhD, Snehal Suryavanshi, MSc, and Prerna Raina, MSc

CONTENTS

ABSTRACT Breast cancer is one of the leading causes of cancer deaths in women worldwide. However, over the past few decades, there has been a steady decline in mortality rates due to increasingly effective adjuvant medical treatments. Mammography screening programs have increased the diagnosis of early-stage breast cancer with better prognosis. Moreover, the discovery of specific prognostic and predictive biomarkers in the past few years have enormously helped in the early detection and treatment of breast cancer. With the advent of high-throughput technologies, more and more biomarkers based on either genomics or proteomics are being explored for early detection as well as better prognosis of breast cancer. This chapter focuses on the traditional as well as novel biomarkers that are being used or proposed to use for early prognosis, diagnosis, as well as treatment of the breast cancer to reduce morbidity as well as mortality.

3.1 Introduction

Breast cancer is the most commonly diagnosed cancer and the leading cause of death in women worldwide (National NCI program database, Jennifer et al., 2011; Patnaik et al., 2011). It accounts for about 23% (1.38 million) of the total cancer cases and 14% (458,400) of the total cancer-related deaths (Jemal et al., 2011). The incidence rates are higher in Western and Northern Europe, Australia, New Zealand, and North America; moderate in South America, the Caribbean, and Northern Africa; and lower in sub-Saharan Africa and Asia (Jemal et al., 2011). However, 60% of the breast cancer–related deaths have been found to occur in economically developing countries.

Breast cancer is a clinically heterogeneous disease with multifactorial etiology (Jensen et al., 2008). Age; hormonal, genetic, and environmental factors; molecular oncogenic aberrations in DNA repair; cell cycle control; and cell survival are some of the factors that may contribute toward the development of breast cancer (Perou et al., 2000; King et al., 2003; Nguyen et al., 2008; Norman et al., 2003). Increased lifetime exposure to endogenous or exogenous hormones has been recognized as one of the major risk factors in the development of the disease (Kurian et al., 2009; Crooke et al., 2011). Besides these, socioeconomic status (SES) has also been found to determine the risk of breast cancer. Unlike other cancers, the risk of breast cancer development has been shown to be positively associated with higher SES (Heck and Pamuk, 1997; Robert et al., 2004). The socioeconomic factors that affect the breast cancer risk include reproductive, lifestyle and behavioral factors that involve age, parity, age at first childbirth, body mass index (BMI), alcohol consumption, age at menarche, and hormonal imbalance (Adami et al., 2002; Braaten et al., 2004; Butt et al., 2012; Fabian and Kimler, 2001).

Breast cancer has been categorized into various major classes by different research groups based on molecular characterization such as gene expression profiling or immunohistochemical characteristics (Cakir et al., 2012). Some studies divide the breast cancer into five major classes: normal breast-like, luminal A, luminal B, basal-like, and human epidermal growth factor receptor 2 (HER2) positive (Perou et al., 2000; Sorlie et al., 2001). Other studies categorize it into three major classes: HER2+/ER+, ER–/HER2–, and HER2+ breast cancers based on ER/PR and Her2 expression (Onitilo et al., 2009; Zhang and Liu, 2008). Such type of heterogeneity in breast cancer subtypes poses a great challenge in the early detection of the disease, thereby inviting attention toward identification of more biomarkers that are differentially expressed during carcinogenesis. Even though routine mammography screening programs have led to an increase in early diagnosis of the breast cancer (Sakorafas et al., 2008; Wiechmann and Kuerer, 2008), but due to its suboptimal accuracy, discovery of more specific diagnostic markers is needed.

Biomarkers are powerful tools that would help in identification of high-risk subjects and timely regulation of the cancer (Weigel and Dowsett, 2010). The discovery of biomarkers has increased the early diagnosis, prognosis, and therapeutics of breast cancer. This chapter focuses on traditional and new biomarkers that are being used or have potential to be used for early detection of breast cancer that would help in the management of the disease.

3.1.1 Why Is It Important?

Breast cancer, reported dating back to 3000 BC, is the most threatening socioeconomic burden in the world that affects not only the patients but also their families (Donegan and Spratt, 1995; Jacques et al., 2010). Despite advanced diagnosis and therapeutics, management of breast cancer is a major clinical challenge due to its heterogeneity, complexity, and aggressiveness

(Harnett et al., 2009). The treatment strategies available are linked with enormous side effects (Wood et al., 2001). Besides this, inadequate access to the screening programs, social and cultural barriers, lack of awareness, financial problems, and certain taboos are some of the important barriers in the prognosis and diagnosis of the disease, particularly in developing and underdeveloped nations (Parsa et al., 2006). Contrarily, in the developed countries, such problems are rare because of the high SES as well as awareness of the advanced health-care system that includes screening and treatment modalities (Jemal et al., 2010). However, the limitations associated with the diagnosis and imaging of breast cancer have focused the global attention toward the use of biomarkers that would help in the early diagnosis of the disease, thereby leading to timely intervention strategies (Bhatt et al., 2010).

3.1.2 Epidemiology

Despite the availability of advanced diagnostics and therapeutic interventions, breast cancer remains a leading cause of cancer deaths worldwide in the women aged between 35 and 55 years (American Cancer Society, 2012). Table 3.1 elucidates the

TABLE 3.1

World Key Statistic of Breast Cancer

	Incidence			Mortality		
Regions	Cases (1000)	[a]ASR per (100,000)	[a]Cum. Risk (%) (Age 0–74)	Cases (1000)	[a]ASR per (100,000)	[a]Cum. Risk (%) (Age 0–74)
World	1383.5	39	4.1	458.4	12.5	1.3
More developed regions	692.2	66.4	7.1	189.5	15.3	1.7
Less developed regions	691.3	27.3	2.8	269	10.8	1.2
Eastern Africa	17.9	19.3	2.1	10	11.4	1.3
Middle Africa	8.3	21.3	2.1	4.7	13.1	1.4
Northern Africa	28	32.7	3.2	14.6	17.8	1.8
Southern Africa	9	38.1	4.2	4.5	19.3	2.1
Western Africa	29.4	31.8	3.4	16.3	19	2.1
Caribbean	9	39.1	4.3	3.4	14.2	1.6
Central America	17.5	26	2.8	6.5	9.6	1
South America	88.4	44.3	4.8	27.1	13.2	1.4
Northern America	205.5	76.7	8.4	45.6	14.8	1.6
Eastern Asia	240.3	25.3	2.6	61.7	6.3	0.7
South-Eastern Asia	87	31	3.2	36.8	13.4	1.4
South-Central Asia	173	24	2.5	82.6	12	1.3
Western Asia	28.5	32.5	3.4	12.3	14.3	1.5
Central and Eastern Europe	114.6	45.3	5	47.5	17	1.9
Northern Europe	69.5	84	9	18.3	17.8	1.9
Southern Europe	91.3	69	7.4	25.6	15.3	1.7
Western Europe	149.4	90	9.6	37.3	17.5	1.9
Australia/New Zealand	16.1	85.5	9.4	3.4	15.4	1.7
Melanesia	0.6	22.8	2.4	0.3	13.2	1.4
Micronesia/Polynesia	0.3	58	6.1	0.1	13.2	1.5
India	115	22.9	—	53	11.1	—

Source: The data have been gathered from GLOBOCAN 2008, http://globocan.iarc.fr.

[a] ASR, age-standardized rates; Cum. Risk, cumulative risk.

incidence and mortality of breast cancer, depicting a wide geographical distribution all over the world. Breast cancer is most frequent among women both in the developed and the developing regions with almost similar incidence rates; however, the mortality rates vary between 189.5×10^3 and 269×10^3 in more developed and underdeveloped regions, respectively (GLOBOCAN 2008). The rate of occurrence is on the rise in urban areas compared with the rural ones with widespread incidence in the women of higher SES (Hausauer et al., 2009). According to the recent reports, the mortality rate in females has been estimated to be around 130,000/year (Kohrmann et al., 2009). The chance that breast cancer would be responsible for a woman's death has been reported to be around 1 in 35 (about 3%) wherein the incidence of developing invasive breast cancer is approximately 1 in 9 (American Cancer Society, 2012). In the recent years, substantial progress has been made in understanding the genetics and molecular biology of the disease (Eroles et al., 2012). Various factors such as environmental, hormonal, dietary, lifestyle, and genetic factors, radiation as well as age, race, ethnicity, gender, and family history are considered to be involved in the development of the disease (Figure 3.1) (MacMahon, 2006).

All these factors may disturb the cellular signaling pathways, which results in altered molecular mechanisms leading to carcinogenesis (Nguyen et al., 2008; Marotta et al., 2011). Exposure to radiations and mutagenic agents (Ronckers et al., 2005), use of oral contraceptives, postmenopausal hormone therapy (PHT), hormone replacement therapy (HRT), and menopausal hormone therapy (MHT) are some of the reasons that may be responsible for the rise in breast cancer incidence rates (Norman et al., 2003). Alcohol consumption and cigarette smoking are some other lifestyle factors that may also increase the cancer risk (Chen et al., 2011). Obesity is also considered to be one of the main risk factors and is positively associated with postmenopausal women (Sinicrope and Dannenberg, 2011) as it may raise the estrogen levels. Besides the aforementioned factors, around 5%–10% of breast cancer cases have been attributed to genetic mutations (Stoppa-Lyonnet et al., 2009). For example, inherited mutations in *BRCA1* and *BRCA2* genes are the most common hereditary cause of breast cancer (Pijpe et al., 2012). Older age has also been linked to the cancer development wherein one out of eight invasive breast cancers are

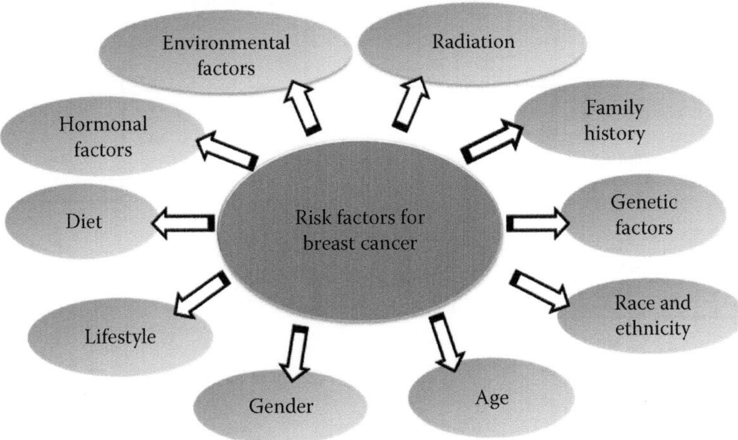

FIGURE 3.1
Risk factors for breast cancer development. Several factors are involved in breast cancer development that include environmental, hormonal, dietary, lifestyle and genetic factors, exposure to the ionizing radiation, as well as age, race, ethnicity, gender, and family history.

found in women younger than 45, while about two out of three invasive breast cancers are found in women around 55 years of age or older (Harrison et al., 2010). Breast cancer has been reported to be common in American-African women than in Asian, Hispanic, and Native American women (Chen et al., 2011). Incidences are more prevalent in women than men; especially, the women having a family history are at a greater risk (Metcalfe et al., 2010).

3.1.3 Types of Breast Cancer

Breast cancer may be invasive or noninvasive depending upon the type and the stage of the disease (Souzaki et al., 2011) (Figure 3.2). It has been divided into ductal carcinoma in situ (DCIS), invasive ductal carcinoma (IDC), noninvasive lobular carcinoma (lobular carcinoma in situ [LCIS]), and invasive lobular carcinoma (ILC) (Hanby and Hughes, 2008; Muggerud et al., 2010) (Figure 3.3). DCIS, representing around one in five cases, is the noninvasive type wherein the cancer cells are present inside the ducts and do not invade the surrounding breast tissue (Suryadevara et al., 2010). IDC starts in the milk duct of the breast wherein the cancer cells break all the way through the wall of the duct into the fatty tissue of the breast followed by metastasis to other parts of the body. These represent around 8 out of 10 cancer cases and are further divided into various subtypes such as adenocystic, adenosquamous, medullary, mucinous, papillary, micropapillary, tubular, and metaplastic carcinomas (Suryadevara et al., 2010). LCIS is not generally regarded as a true cancer wherein the cells remain confined to the lobules (Foster et al., 2004).

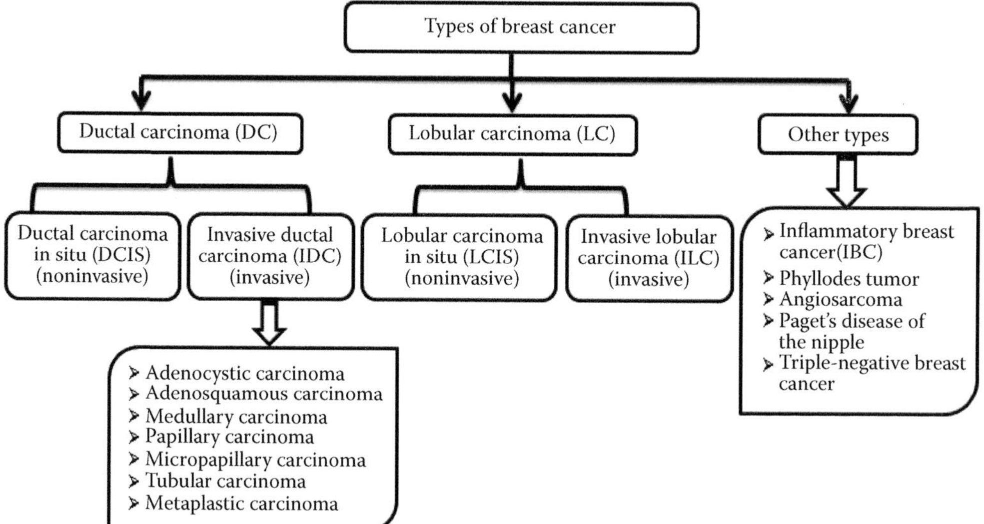

FIGURE 3.2
Types of breast cancer. Breast cancer is broadly classified into two types: ductal carcinoma (DC) and lobular carcinoma (LC). DC is divided into DCIS (noninvasive) and IDC, the latter being divided into adenocystic, adenosquamous, medullary, mucinous, papillary, micropapillary, tubular, and metaplastic carcinomas. LC is further grouped into noninvasive or LCIS and ILC. However, there are some other types that include IBC, phyllodes tumor, angiosarcoma, Paget's disease of the nipple, and triple-negative breast cancer.

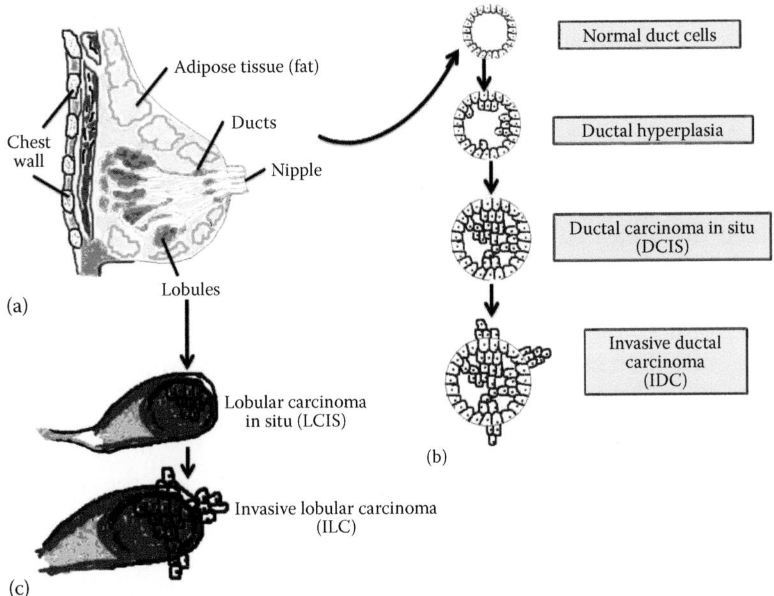

FIGURE 3.3
Anatomy of normal breast along with different types of breast cancer: (a) Anatomy of normal breast. Anatomy of breast showing ducts, lobules, nipple, adipose tissue, and chest wall. (b) Development of ductal carcinoma: Hyperplasia is a precancerous condition that describes an accumulation of abnormal cells in a normal breast duct and is associated with an increased risk of developing cancer. In atypical hyperplasia, cells keep dividing and become more abnormal, then the condition may be reclassified as noninvasive breast cancer (DCIS). When the abnormal cells tend to outgrow and start migrating to the nearby organs, the condition may be classified as IDC. (c) Development of lobular carcinoma: If the cells start proliferating abnormally and tend to accumulate inside the lobules but do not spread to the other tissues, the condition is known as LCIS. If LCIS cells tend to outgrow and metastasize to the nearby organs, then the condition is known as ILC.

ILC represents around 1 out of 10 invasive cases and starts in the milk-producing glands (lobules) wherein the cancer cells undergo metastasis (Suryadevara et al., 2010).

Besides these, there are additional types that include inflammatory breast cancer (IBC), phyllodes tumor, angiosarcoma, Paget's disease of the nipple, and triple-negative breast cancer (Dalberg et al., 2007; Glazebrook et al., 2008; Yang et al., 2009). IBC is the invasive form wherein the breast looks red and its skin becomes thick and pitted. Phyllodes tumor develops in the stroma of the breast and is usually benign that may become malignant only in rare cases (Kapali et al., 2010). Angiosarcoma, rarely found in the breast, usually occurs in cells that line the blood or lymph vessels (Desbiens et al., 2011). It can also be found in the patients with lymphedema that may be caused due to lymph node surgery or radiation therapy (Tahir et al., 2006). These cancers have the tendency to grow and metastasize rapidly. Paget's disease is the rarest form that arises from the breast ducts, affects the skin of the nipple and areola showing crusted, scaly and reddish appearance with areas of bleeding or oozing (Dalberg et al., 2007). In triple-negative breast cancer, the cells lack estrogen, progesterone, and HER2 receptors on their surfaces, and such cancers tend to grow and metastasize more quickly (Williams Jones and Carriyan, 2003; Roberti et al., 2012).

The staging of any cancer describes upon the extent of its spread in the body and helps in better prognosis and treatment, thereby increasing the chances of survival in the patients. Stages can be decided by the tumor size (less than 2 cm, between 2 and 5 cm, or more than 5 cm), lymph node involvement, as well as invasiveness or noninvasiveness of the tumor (Abeloff et al., 2008).

The American Joint Committee on Cancer (AJCC) has designated TNM system ("T" stands for tumor, "N" for node, and "M" for metastasis) for staging the cancer and has categorized the breast tumors into stages 0, I, IIA, IIB, IIIA, IIIB, and IV (Table 3.2) (Singletary et al., 2002). Stage 0 is noninvasive, whereas I–IV are the invasive stages of the breast cancer. In stage 0, the cancer has not spread to the lymph nodes or to the distant sites. Around 30% of the breast cancers are detected at the stage 0 with 99% of 5-year survival rate (Lee et al., 2007). It includes DCIS, LCIS, and Paget's disease of the nipple (Atoum et al., 2010). Stage I tumor is less than or equal to 2 cm in size and has not spread to the lymph nodes (N0) or distant sites (M0). Stage II is divided into IIA and IIB. The tumors that are less than 2 cm with micrometastases in axillary lymph nodes or tumors between 2 and 5 cm without axillary lymph node involvement are grouped into stage IIA. Tumors between 2 and 5 cm with micrometastases in one to three axillary lymph nodes or the tumors larger than 5 cm that do not grow into the chest wall or skin and have not spread to the lymph nodes are included in stage IIB. Stage III is also

TABLE 3.2

Breast Cancer Stages

Stage	TNM	Description	Five-Year Survival (%)
0	Tis N0 M0	No tumor in regional lymph nodes, no distant metastases.	99
I	T1 N0 M0	Tumor is less than or equal to 2 cm, no spread of tumor to regional lymph nodes, no distant metastases.	92
IIA	T0 N1 M0	Tumor is smaller than 2 cm with micrometastases in 1–3 axillary lymph nodes, no distant metastases.	82
	T1 N1 M0	Tumor is less than or equal to 2 cm, metastases to movable ipsilateral nodes, no distant metastases.	
	T2 N0 M0	Tumor is between 2 and 5 cm, no tumor is regional lymph nodes, no distant metastases.	
IIB	T2 N1 M0	Tumor is between 2 and 5 cm, metastases to movable ipsilateral nodes, no distant metastases.	65
	T3 N0 M0	Tumor is over 5 cm, no tumor is regional lymph nodes, no distant metastases.	
IIIA	T0 N2 M0	Tumor is less than or equal to 2 cm, metastases to 4–9 axillary lymph nodes, no distant metastases.	47
	T1 N2 M0	Tumor is between 2 and 5 cm, metastases to 4–9 axillary lymph nodes, no distant metastases.	
	T2 N2 M0	Tumor is over 5 cm, metastases to movable ipsilateral nodes, no distant metastases.	
	T3 N2 M0	Tumor is over 5 cm, metastases to 4–9 axillary lymph nodes, no distant metastases.	
IIIB	T4 Any N M0	Tumor of any size growing into the chest wall or skin, any nodal involvement, no distant metastases.	44
	Any T N3 M0	Any primary tumor involvement, metastases to more than 10 axillary lymph nodes, no distant metastases.	
IV	Any T Any N M1	Any primary tumor involvement, any nodal involvement, distant metastases.	14

divided into IIIA and IIIB. Stage IIIA, also called local spread of breast cancer, includes tumor of any size that has spread to four to nine axillary lymph nodes or to internal mammary nodes, as well as tumors larger than 5 cm with micrometastases in one to three axillary lymph nodes. Stage IIIB tumors are of any size (T0–T4) that extend to the chest wall or the skin with any member of lymph node involvement (N0–N4). Stage IV is the most aggressive stage wherein the tumor, irrespective of its size, has spread to other organs of the body with nodal involvement and is always associated with poor survival (Carey et al., 2005; Weigel and Dowsett, 2010).

3.1.4 Current Methods for Early Diagnosis, Prognosis, and Therapy

Detection of breast cancer at an early stage would not only help to cure the disease (by providing an opportunity for treatment) but would also improve the survival rate. Early detection has become easy with advances in screening techniques that include routine mammography programs and/or palpation (either self-examination or by physician or nurse practitioner), digital mammography, sonogram, thermography, transillumination, xeromammograpy, computed tomography (CT) scan, magnetic resonance imaging (MRI), biopsy as well as genetic testing (Lehtimaki et al., 2011; Vaughan, 2012). In the latter, detection of *BRCA1* and *BRCA2* gene mutations is recommended, usually for women having a strong family history of breast or ovarian cancer. It is also tested in women who have been detected earlier with DCIS or LCIS or whose biopsies have tested positive for precancerous lesions (Nelson et al., 2005; Palma et al., 2006; Mackay and Szecsei, 2010). Breast cancers detected by screening mammography have more favorable prognostic characteristics than cancers detected by other methods (McCann et al., 2002; Kobeissi et al., 2011). Despite the available screening facilities, diagnosis of the breast cancer remains inadequate due to the low sensitivity/specificity, relative complexity, and high cost-to-benefit ratio (Prasad and Houserkova, 2007; Heiko, 2009).

During the past few years, biomarkers have gained significant importance in the diagnosis of many diseases. Prognostic and predictive biomarkers such as ER, PR, HER2, p53, BRCA1/2, and many others are currently being used for the early diagnosis of breast cancer that would help in determining the risk of the disease (Cianfrocca and Goldstein, 2004). The biomarkers can be measured more quickly and have high sensitivity and specificity, thereby making them promising candidates for breast cancer detection. Table 3.3 enlists various imaging methods that are being used in the breast cancer detection along with their sensitivity, specificity, as well as advantages and disadvantages.

3.1.5 Test Providers and Popular Tests with Cost Involved

Mammogram and magnetic resonance imaging are the two commonly used tests for breast cancer screening (Lehman et al., 2005; Vaughan, 2012). These can be performed by clinicians (doctor or nurse). A mammogram is an x-ray of the breast that may help in finding tumors that are too small to be palpable (Kobeissi et al., 2012). It can detect DCIS as well as abnormal cells in the lining of a breast duct, which may become invasive in some women. The sensitivity of a mammogram depends on the size of the tumor as well as on the density of the breast tissue. The cost for mammography in developed countries such as the United States is around 150–200 USD, whereas in developing countries such as India, the cost is around 54 USD. MRI is more sensitive than mammography and may be used

TABLE 3.3

List of Imaging Tools along with Their Sensitivity, Specificity, as well as Advantages and Disadvantages

Imaging Tools	Sensitivity (%)	Specificity (%)	Advantages	Disadvantages	References
Screening mammography by x-ray	90	75	Mortality reduction, improved treatment of early disease, low cost, minimal discomfort.	Radiation risk and other risks; risk of false alarm.	Gotzsche et al. (2013)
Ultra sound by sound waves	89	78	Ultrasound pictures may show whether a lump is solid or filled with fluid; useful for detecting cancer in women at higher risk.	Associated with false positive and false negative results; not widely available or routinely used.	Kelly et al. (2010)
CT scan by computerized tomography	—	—	Best way to image internal mammary nodes and to evaluate the chest and axilla after mastectomy.	Radiation exposure in CT scan can accumulate and can increase the risk of developing cancer; risk of allergic reaction due to dye administration.	Boone et al. (2006)
PET scan by radioactive material	75	92.3	PET diagnoses disease even before the structural changes are visible, provides both an anatomical and functional view of the suspected cells.	It does not reliably detect tumors smaller than 5–10 mm.	Pennat et al. (2010)
MRI by magnetic fields	90	72	MRI is more sensitive, identifies the primary site of cancer in the breast, noninvasive, and usually a painless medical test.	False positive results; more expensive than mammography.	Houssami et al. (2014)

to detect lumps in the breast that may have been left behind even after surgery or radiation therapy. It helps to study breast lumps or enlarged lymph nodes suspected during a clinical breast exam or a breast self-exam as well as in presurgical planning of patients with detected breast cancer. The cost for MRI screening in developed countries such as the United States is around 1080 USD, whereas in developing countries such as India, the cost is around 216 USD.

The National Breast and Cervical Cancer Early Detection Program (NBCCEDP) and the Indiana Breast and Cervical Cancer Program (BCCP) are among the leading programs for the breast cancer prevention (Howard et al., 2010). The NBCCEDP is unique in being the first and the only national cancer screening program in the United States (American Cancer Society, 2012). It aims to provide access to breast cancer screening services to the underprivileged women; emphasizes on rescreening of women at recommended time intervals; and invests resources on rescreening (Eheman et al., 2006). The BCCP offers breast cancer screening, diagnostic testing, as well as treatment to women with nonprivileged or underprivileged status. It offers free treatment to the needy women and provides free services for breast cancer screening as well as diagnostic tests that include liquid-based cytology tests, clinical breast exams (CBEs), mammograms (screening and diagnostic), and diagnostic breast ultrasounds (BCCP website: www.healthoregon.org/bcc). At the National Cancer Institute (NCI), National Institutes of Health (NIH), the Early Detection Research Network (EDRN) is a program where biomarkers for early detection of cancer are identified and validated clinically (http://edrn.nci.nih.gov/).

3.2 Treatment Strategy, Targeted Therapy, Drug Targets, and Pharmacogenomics for Breast Cancer

3.2.1 Treatment Strategy

Treatment options for the breast cancer vary with the stage and the type, certain characteristics of the cancer cells, menopausal status, as well as the general health of the patient (Clarke and Fuller, 2006; Naeim et al., 2010). The currently available treatment options include surgery, radiation therapy, chemotherapy, hormone therapy, and targeted therapy.

In surgery, the affected part of the breast is removed. It involves various options such as lumpectomy, quadrantectomy, total or simple mastectomy, modified radical mastectomy, and sentinel lymph node biopsy (SLNB). In lumpectomy, only the breast lump is removed whereas quadrantectomy involves removal of one-quarter of the breast (Fisher et al., 2002). Both the surgical procedures are followed by chemotherapy and/or radiotherapy (Bassiouny et al., 2005). In total or simple mastectomy, the entire breast is removed along with other nearby tissues, whereas in modified radical mastectomy, the whole breast along with some lymph nodes is removed (Dooley et al., 2001). In SLNB, the sentinel lymph node is removed during the surgery whose presence is often associated with metastatic breast disease (Weaver, 2010).

Radiation therapy is also used to treat the cancer that has metastasized to the other parts of the body, for example, to the bones or brain. It uses high-energy x-rays to shrink the tumors as well as to kill the cancer cells. Radiation therapy can be used in the form of either external beam or brachytherapy. In the former, an external source of radiation is directed at the tumor site from outside the body, whereas in brachytherapy, the radiation source is placed inside or next to the area requiring the treatment (Fisher et al., 2002; Smith et al., 2012).

- Chemotherapy involves the use of drugs to damage or kill the cancer cells. It can be given either as an adjuvant or a neoadjuvant chemotherapy wherein the former is given to the patient after the surgery and the latter is given to the patient before the surgery. Adjuvant chemotherapy has been reported to reduce the risk of relapse and death (Fornier and Norton, 2005). Neoadjuvant chemotherapy may shrink the size of large tumors so that they are small enough to be removed with less extensive surgery (Schott and Hayes, 2012). Table 3.4 mentions various Food and Drug Administration (FDA)–approved drug combinations that are being given to the breast cancer patients.

Chemotherapy is usually associated with several side effects that include hair loss, mouth sores, loss of appetite or increased appetite, nausea and vomiting, low blood cell counts, neuropathy, cardiotoxicity, increased risk of leukemia, increased chances of infections,

TABLE 3.4
FDA-Approved Drug Combinations Used in Breast Cancer

Abbreviations	Commonly Used Drug Combinations
AC	Doxorubicin hydrochloride (adriamycin) + cyclophosphamide
AC-T	Doxorubicin hydrochloride + (adriamycin) cyclophosphamide + paclitaxel (taxol)
CAF	Cyclophosphamide + doxorubicin hydrochloride (adriamycin) + fluorouracil
CMF	Cyclophosphamide + methotrexate + fluorouracil
FEC	Fluorouracil + epirubicin hydrochloride + cyclophosphamide

Source: The data have been gathered from American Cancer Society (2012).

easy bruising or bleeding, as well as fatigue (Tchen et al., 2003; Hermelink et al., 2007; Lemieux et al., 2008; Azim et al., 2011). However, these side effects are outweighed by potential benefits of chemotherapy in terms of decreasing the mortality rates and increasing the patient survival. Chemotherapy kills both invasive and noninvasive cancer cells, thereby reducing the likelihood of recurrence or death after adjuvant therapy (Cianfrocca and Goldstein, 2004). It can shrink the large tumors to operable size and thus make surgery less invasive. Chemotherapy can also help in increasing the effectiveness of radiation therapy (Schott and Hayes, 2012).

Besides the mentioned treatments, hormone therapy is used to block the female hormones (estrogen and progesterone) that might promote the growth of any cancer cells that may have remained even after surgery (Lea et al., 2004). This may be done either by using drugs that block the action of hormones such as tamoxifen or an aromatase inhibitor or by surgical removal of hormone-making organs, such as the ovaries. Hormone therapy does not help patients having ER- and PR-negative tumors.

3.2.2 Targeted Therapy

Targeted therapy uses drugs to identify and attack specific markers on cancer cells. It may interfere with the molecules involved in the malignant cell signal transduction, cell invasion, metastasis, apoptosis, cell cycle, and angiogenesis (Suter and Marcum, 2007; Munagala et al., 2011). Targeted therapy mainly focuses on inhibition of HER2, estrogen, insulin-like growth factor, PARP, and PI3K/Akt/mTOR signaling pathways (Martelli et al., 2010; Sachdev, 2010; Higgins and Baselga, 2011; Nielsen, 2012). Some targeted therapies use the monoclonal antibodies that work like the natural antibodies synthesized by our immune system to target cancer cells (Bernard-Marty et al., 2006). These therapies are new and are sometimes called immune-targeted therapies.

The first molecular target for breast cancer treatment was the cellular receptor for the female sex hormone, estrogen (Hanstein et al., 2004; Suter and Marcum, 2007). The binding of estrogen to the estrogen receptor (ER) in cells activates the hormone–receptor complex, which in turn activates the genes involved in cell growth and proliferation (Lindberg et al., 2011). Interference with estrogen ability to stimulate the growth of breast cancer cells (ER-positive breast cancer cells) could serve as an effective treatment approach (Kumar and Kumar, 2008). Several drugs have been approved by the FDA for the treatment of ER-positive breast cancers. Drugs such as herceptin (trastuzumab) kill the breast cancer cells having high levels of HER2 protein, whereas tamoxifen and toremifene (Fareston®) bind to the ER and prevent estrogen binding (Verma et al., 2012). Another drug, fulvestrant (Faslodex®), binds to the ER and promotes its destruction, thereby reducing ER levels inside the cells (Lynn, 2004). In Table 3.5, the list of FDA-approved drugs for the treatment of breast cancer has been mentioned.

TABLE 3.5

List of FDA-Approved Drugs for the Treatment of Breast Cancer

FDA-Approved Drugs for Breast Cancer	Key Targets
Tamoxifen, raloxifene, toremifene, fulvestrant	Selective estrogen receptor modulators
Anastrozole, exemestane, letrozole	Aromatase inhibitors
Cetuximab, lapatinib, gefitinib, erlotinib	EGFR (HER1) inhibitors
Trastuzumab, pertuzumab, lapatinib	HER2 inhibitors
Rapamycin (also called sirolimus), temsirolimus, everolimus	mTOR inhibitors
Perifosine	Akt inhibitors

Source: The data have been gathered from American Cancer Society (2012).

3.2.3 Pharmacogenomics in Breast Cancer

The field of pharmacogenomics (PG) involves studying the influence of an individual's genetic variations on drug response (Yiannakopoulou, 2012). The efficacy and toxicity of drugs in an individual depend upon genetic polymorphisms in drug-metabolizing enzymes, transporters, receptors, and other drug targets (Wajapeyee and Somasundaram, 2004). This relatively new field combines pharmaceutical sciences with molecular biology, high-throughput biotechnology, and bioinformatics to develop effective, safe, and customized drug treatment regimens for a particular individual or patient population (Rofaiel et al., 2010; Wang, 2010).

Several factors such as genetics of an individual, environmental factors, diet, age, lifestyle, and state of health of a patient can influence an individual's response to medicines (Wajapeyee and Somasundaram, 2004). PG determines how genetic variations would influence the drug response in an individual and thus provides personalized therapy based on individual genetic variability (Evans, 2003). This in turn helps not only in maximizing the efficacy of the drug but also in reducing the drug-associated side effects. The advantages of PG include improved therapeutic index as well as dose regimen and selection of optimal drug (Ingle, 2008). For example, tamoxifen is an anticancer drug that is used for treating breast cancer patients having ER+ tumors. The pharmacological activity of tamoxifen depends on cytochrome P450 2D6 (CYP2D6) enzyme that converts tamoxifen to its active metabolite, endoxifen (Rofaiel et al., 2010). Patients with reduced CYP2D6 activity (owing to genetic polymorphisms in the cytochrome p450 gene) produce little endoxifen and, thus, get partial therapeutic benefit from tamoxifen (Holmes and Liticker, 2005). Thus, PG would help in selection of optimal drugs for the patients who are genetically resistant to the specific drugs.

The study of the PG of chemotherapy response mainly examines metabolizing enzymes such as cytochrome P450, UDP-glucuronosyltransferase (UGT), and drug transporters such as ATP-binding cassette (ABC) (Fajac et al., 2010). The field of PG offers personalized medicine compared with the traditional *one-drug-fits-all* approach. FDA (United States) has approved two commercially available pharmacogenomic tests that detect variations in the genes coding for enzymes involved in drug metabolism. These include cytochrome P450 CYP2C19 and CYP2D6 (Roche AmpliChip, http://www.roche.com/), and UDP-glucuronosyltransferase (Invader UGT1AI Molecular Assay; Third Wave Technologies, http://www.twt.com/) (Swen et al., 2007). However, the usage of these tests remains limited in routine clinical practice because of many challenges that may include analytic, ethical, and technological issues involved in generation and management of large drug response datasets (Williams-Jones and Carriyan, 2003; Bansal et al., 2005).

However, implementation of PG in routine clinical practice presents significant challenges. These include identifying candidate genes and pathways involved in variable drug response; correlating disease genes with drug response genes; describing drug response phenotypes; selection of clinically relevant tests that could also predict the outcome of drug treatment; cost-effective and wide availability of tests; and focusing on analytic, ethical, and technological issues involved in generation and management of large datasets (Williams-Jones and Carriyan, 2003; Roden et al., 2006; Swen et al., 2007). By overcoming such challenges and by generating strong scientific evidence, PG can help in safe and more effective usage of drugs through personalized therapy (Swen et al., 2007). Moreover, regulatory agencies should recommend the use of PG-based tests prior to drug prescriptions and pharma companies as well as patient groups should advocate the use of such tests, which would gear up its use in clinical practice (Swen et al., 2007).

3.3 Invasive and Noninvasive Biomarkers: Advantages and Disadvantages

A biomarker is a signature molecule used as an indicator of biological state that may be either secreted by a tumor in body fluids or it can be a specific response of the body to the presence of cancer (Falasca, 2012). Biomarkers include nucleic acids, proteins, sugars, lipids, small metabolites, cytogenetic and cytokinetic parameters, as well as whole tumor cells found in the body fluid whose expression may be altered in tumors (Bhatt et al., 2010). Some of the clincopathological features of the tumor that are routinely used as biomarkers include tumor size, histological type, cellular and nuclear characteristics, mitotic index, lymphovascular invasion, hormonal receptors, lymph node metastases, and axillary lymph node status (Sarkar et al., 2008). However, these parameters are not sufficient to predict the course of cancer (Weigel and Dowsett, 2010). Thus, massive efforts have been put together to identify and validate specific prognostic and predictive biomarkers of breast cancer that would reduce the mortality through early detection, risk stratification, prediction, and better prognosis (Weigel and Dowsett, 2010).

Depending upon sampling method, biomarkers could be either invasive or noninvasive (Song et al., 2012). Invasive biomarkers involve invasive surgical procedures that require penetration into body through incision or cut. For example, immunohistochemical analyses of ER, PR, HER2, Ki-67, and p53 require biopsy samples or tissue samples that could be obtained by surgery. Invasive biomarkers are specific, sensitive, and widely used for rapid and accurate diagnosis and prognosis of the disease. However, invasive surgical procedures are associated with anxiety, prolonged recovery time, and high follow-up costs that cause discomfort to the patients.

Noninvasive biomarkers are proteins, enzymes, hormones, tumor cells, or cell-free DNAs and nucleic acids produced and released either by tumor cells or by host cells and would be easily detected in the body fluids such as serum, nipple aspirate fluid (NAF), tear, urine, or saliva. Biomarkers that have been used clinically for breast cancer detection are mostly noninvasive (Beverly, 2009; Zhang et al., 2010). For example, development of novel methylation-based biomarkers (obtained noninvasively from patient) as well as serum microRNAs help in early detection of the disease. Noninvasive biomarkers are more sensitive, specific, and easily detectable than invasive biomarkers. They are more valuable in prognosis, diagnosis, and in making therapeutic decisions. They are associated with the less anxiety and discomfort to the patients (Madu and Lu, 2010; Misek and Kim, 2011a;

Robertson et al., 2011). However, limited availability of sufficient number of good quality samples for the evaluation of biomarkers is one of the drawbacks of noninvasive biomarkers (Richard, 2011). Both invasive and noninvasive biomarkers in panels may provide higher predictive potential, resulting in improved clinical outcomes (Zhu et al., 2011).

3.4 Different Invasive Biomarkers Currently Used and Under Development

3.4.1 Currently Used Invasive Biomarkers in Breast Cancer Detection

3.4.1.1 Estrogen Receptors (ERα, ERβ)

The steroid hormone, estrogen, plays a central role in the etiology of breast cancer (Baglietto et al., 2010). It mediates its biological effects through estrogen receptors (ER) that are expressed in around 70% of human breast cancers. ER is a ligand-inducible transcription factor that belongs to the nuclear receptor NR3B subfamily. It is the most powerful predictive and prognostic biomarker in breast cancer that provides the index for sensitivity to endocrine treatment (Giguere et al., 1988).

ER has two different isoforms, namely, ERα and ERβ, that are encoded on different chromosomes and act as hormone-dependent transcriptional regulators. ERα, located on chromosome 6q (Menasce et al., 1993), is a 66 kDa protein (Kong et al., 2003) while ERβ, located on chromosome 14q (Gosden et al., 1986), is a 59 kDa protein (Ogawa et al., 1998). ERα acts as a tumor promoter, whereas ERβ is a tumor suppressor. The presence of ERβ in breast tumors is associated with better prognosis and longer disease-free survival (Chen et al., 2008). ERα is an important functional modulator of the estrogen-signaling pathway and is more frequently expressed than ERβ. ERα expression is a useful clinical biomarker of breast tumor progression and thereby an effective therapeutic target. ERα-positive breast cancers have long been considered relatively resistant to traditional chemotherapeutic drugs (Allegra and Lippman, 1978). These are characterized by slow growth, high degree of differentiation, and increase in the relapse-free survival (Schiff et al., 2005). It has been reported that the patients with ER-positive tumors have a significantly higher response rate to antiestrogens such as tamoxifen than patients with ER-poor/ER-negative tumors.

3.4.1.2 Progesterone Receptor

The progesterone receptor (PR) is a member of the nuclear receptor superfamily, which specifically regulates the expression of target genes in response to the hormonal stimulus (Yin et al., 2012). PR exists in two isoforms, namely, PR-A (94 kDa protein) and PR-B (116 kDa protein) wherein the latter activates transcription of target genes and PR-A represses transcription of PR-B as well as few other nuclear receptors (Dressing and Lange, 2009; Pathiraja et al., 2011). Fu et al. (2010) showed that progesterone receptor enhances breast cancer cell motility and invasion through activation of focal adhesion kinase. The ratio of PR-A to PR-B expression controls the PR signaling, and any imbalance between the two isoforms may lead to alterations in PR signaling (Viale et al., 2007). Progesterone receptor is an important biomarker for predicting the outcome in breast cancer patients. Several clinical studies have reported ER-/PR-negative breast cancer patients at a high risk of mortality than ER-/PR-positive ones as the latter respond better to endocrine therapies (Varghese, 2007).

3.4.1.3 HER-2

HER-2/neu/c-ErbB-2 proto-oncogene is located in chromosome 17q12 and encodes for a 185 kDa transmembrane glycoprotein belonging to the epidermal growth factor receptor (EGFR) family (Ross et al., 2004). Other members of EGFR family include EGFR (HER-1 or erbB1), HER-2, HER-3 (erbB3), and HER-4 (erbB4). HER-2 is found to be amplified in about 10%–35% of human breast carcinomas and is considered as a key prognostic factor in early stages of the disease (Bofin et al., 2004). Amplification of HER-2/neu is an established predictive and prognostic factor in aggressive breast cancer. Studies have also reported that the overexpression of HER-2 may influence the sensitivity of breast carcinoma to chemotherapy (Yu and Zhang, 2008). Vijver et al. (1988) reported for the first time the overexpression of HER-2/neu oncogene in 189 samples of breast cancer patients by using immunohistochemistry. Berger et al. (1988) determined HER-2/neu protein overexpression associated with lymph node status and breast cancer tumor grade. Slamon et al. found that the overexpression of HER2/neu gene is associated with a more aggressive phenotype and poor prognosis (Slamon and Clark, 1988; Paik et al., 1990). The humanized monoclonal antibody trastuzumab has been reported to have high affinity for the extracellular domain of HER-2 and is, thus, used against human epidermal growth factor receptor-2 (HER2)–positive early breast cancer (Vogel et al., 2002). Recent prospective randomized trials of adjuvant trastuzumab therapies have demonstrated the reduced risk of recurrence and mortality in patients with HER-2-positive early-stage breast cancer (Simpson and Simth, 2005).

3.4.1.4 Ki-67

Proliferation is a key feature of the tumor progression, and it has a major impact on the risk of recurrence. Breast cancers expressing high levels of Ki-67, a nuclear marker of cell proliferation, are associated with worse outcomes (Miglietta et al., 2010). Studies have confirmed that Ki-67 is an important predictive and prognostic factor in early breast cancer. It is a nonhistone nuclear antigen, universally expressed in the cells during the proliferative phases of the cell cycle (mid G1, S, G2, and M phase) and is absent in G0 phase (Lopez et al., 1991). The prognostic and predictive value of Ki-67 is independent of age, nodal and hormonal status, as well as estrogen receptors and is thus associated with poor prognosis (Cheang et al., 2009). Patients having tumors overexpressing Ki-67 in more than 50% of the cells are at a high risk of developing the recurrent disease. Increased expression of Ki-67 in breast cancer is associated with poor prognosis and better response to chemotherapy (Jung et al., 2009; Jones et al., 2007). Many studies have shown that Ki-67 expression gets progressively increased from benign carcinoma to DCIS and to invasive breast cancer, thereby leading to worse clinical outcomes (Kim et al., 2011).

3.4.1.5 p53

p53 is a short-lived transcription factor located in 17 p13.1 chromosome that acts as a *guardian of the genome* and is also known as a master tumor suppressor protein (Wang et al., 2009a). Several studies have established the role of p53 in tumor suppression, regulation of genes involved in cell adhesion, cell cycle, apoptosis, control of genome stability, neuronal growth, angiogenesis, metastasis, oxidative stress, cell fate, and cytoskeleton organization (Qin et al., 2007; Stokłosa and Gołąb, 2005). Oxidative stress and exposure to mutagenic

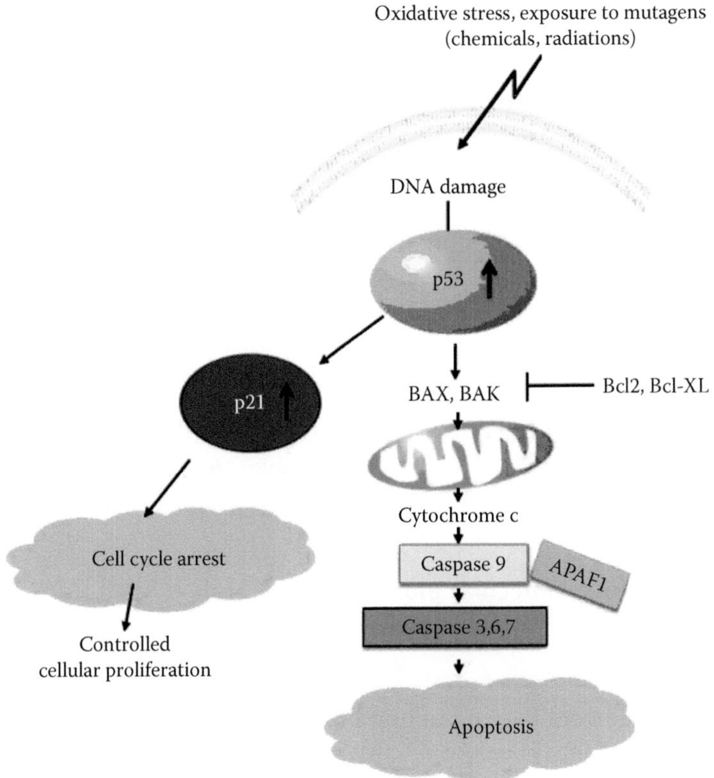

FIGURE 3.4
p53 signaling pathway. p53 plays an important role in regulation of cell proliferation and apoptosis. Oxidative stress as well as exposure to mutagens (chemicals, radiations) leads to DNA damage, resulting into the activation of tumor suppressor protein p53 that results into transcriptional activation of pro-apoptotic proteins BAX and BAK and repression of antiapoptotic Bcl2 and Bcl-XL proteins. BAX and BAK help in the activation of procaspase-9 by the release of cytochrome c from the mitochondria as well as the cleavage of caspase 9 into caspase 3, 6, and 7 resulting into the apoptosis. Activation of p53 also causes the transcriptional induction of p21 (a cell cycle regulator), which in turn inhibits CDK-cyclin activity and arrests the cell cycle leading to the regulation of cell proliferation.

agents involved in DNA damage result in the activation of p53 that in turn further activates p21 (a cell cycle regulator) and pro-apoptotic proteins, resulting in regulation of the cell proliferation and apoptosis (Figure 3.4).

p53 mutation has gained attention as a potential prognostic and predictive marker of breast cancer. It is estimated that almost one-third of breast cancers have altered p53, which is associated with more aggressive phenotype (Miller et al., 2005). Results by several groups have shown that p53 mutation status is a useful predictive marker that is linked with a two- to threefold increased risk of recurrence and death (Bull et al., 2004; Bourdon et al., 2011). Recent immunohistochemical studies suggest that p53 mutation is associated with several other adverse prognostic factors such as high tumor grade, high proliferation rate, and ER^-/PR^- status. Olivier et al. studied the prognostic value of mutant p53 gene in 1794 patients with breast cancer wherein they found that patients with mutated p53 have worse prognosis. They also found that p53 mutations were more frequent in aggressive tumors and node-positive cases and in women less than 60 years (Olivier et al., 2006). Gonzalez-Angulo et al. (2004) found the altered expression of p53 in majority of patients with inflammatory

TABLE 3.6
Role of Breast Cancer Invasive Biomarkers with Their Testing Methods

Proteins	Testing Methods	Role in Breast Cancer
ER	Immunohistochemistry	Stimulates proliferation of mammary cells; involved in cell division and DNA replication
PR	Immunohistochemistry	Involved in metastatic disease; predicting outcome in cancer patients
HER-2	Immunohistochemistry fluorescence in situ hybridization (FISH)	Strongly associated with increased disease recurrence; prognostic factor in early stages of the disease
Ki-67	Immunohistochemistry, antibody labeling	Prognosis and prediction of cellproliferation
p53	Antibody labeling	Potential prognostic and predictive biomarker of breast cancer involved in apoptosis, cell proliferation, and metastasis

breast cancer 2006. Thus, p53 is a useful biomarker for predicting prognosis and patient's response to therapy (Stoklosa and Golab, 2005). Table 3.6 enlists currently used invasive molecular biomarkers along with their regulatory role in breast cancer.

3.4.2 Different Invasive Molecular Biomarkers Currently under Development for This Cancer

3.4.2.1 SMAR1

Scaffold/matrix attachment region binding protein 1 (SMAR1) (Chattopadhoy, Genomics 2000) is a matrix-associated region (MAR)–binding protein, whose tumor suppressor function was first reported by Kaul et al. (2003). SMAR1 gene is located in 16q24.3 chromosome, and its expression has been reported to be downregulated in several breast cancer cell lines and tissues (Kaul et al., 2003; Singh et al., 2007). SMAR1 has been shown to regulate the cell proliferation by arresting the cells at G2/M phase through direct interaction and activation of tumor suppressor p53 (Kaul et al., 2003; Jalota et al., 2005). Rampalli et al. (2005) reported that SMAR1 represses cyclin D1 expression by recruiting HDAC1-mSin3A co-repressor complex at cyclin D1 promoter locus. Moreover, SMAR1 has been reported to downregulate the metastasis of breast cancer through TGF-β pathway (Singh et al., 2007). It has also been shown to regulate T-cell receptor beta enhancer activity through interaction with CDP/CUX, a positive regulator of cell cycle (Kaul-Ghanekar et al., 2004). Kamini Singh et al. (2007) performed SMAR1 expression analysis in 30 fibroadenoma benign cases and 30 malignant breast cancer patients including grades I, II, and III, wherein they found that SMAR1 is downregulated during the advanced stages and the decreased SMAR1 expression correlated with defective p53 subcellular localization. They et al. showed that SMAR1 inhibited TNF-α-induced induction of NF-κB, thereby suggesting that SMAR1-regulated tumorigenesis through modulation of NF-κB target genes (Singh et al., 2009). Kaul-Ghanekar et al. (2009) have shown by atomic force microscopy studies that SMAR1 expression correlated with cell surface smoothness in different cancer cell lines, in different grades of human breast cancer tissues as well as in mouse tumor sections. They found that human breast cancer tissues showing lower expression of SMAR1 exhibited increased surface roughness compared to the normal breast tissue. Based on their findings, the authors indicated that the tumor suppressor protein SMAR1 might be used as a phenotypic differentiation marker between cancerous and noncancerous cells (Kaul-Ghanekar et al., 2009). Figure 3.5 depicts the different molecular targets and pathways regulated by SMAR1.

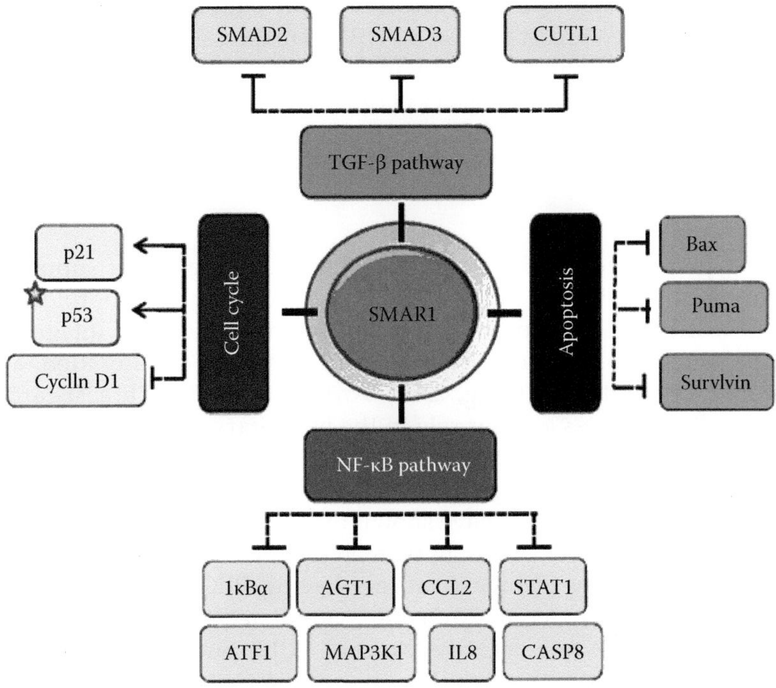

FIGURE 3.5
Different molecular targets and pathways regulated by SMAR1. The figure shows the role of SMAR1 in cell cycle regulation, apoptosis, as well as TGF-β and NF-κB signaling pathways. (From Malonia, S.K. et al., 2011.)

3.4.2.2 CDP/Cux

The CCAAT-displacement protein/cut homeobox (CDP/Cux) is an MARBP as well as a transcriptional activator that has been reported to regulate mammary-specific gene transcription as well as breast tumorigenesis (Zhu et al., 2004). It has been found to be overexpressed in breast cancer (Michl and Downward, 2005). Cux/CDP/CUTL1 is involved in higher-order chromatin organization and may be able to target certain regulatory loci to specific regions of the nucleus (Truscott et al., 2003). Cux is known to regulate transcription of developmental genes and plays an important role in cell proliferation and differentiation (Nepveu, 2001; Goulet et al., 2007). Studies have reported that CDP/Cux represses a large number of genes, particularly those expressed in precursor cells prior to terminal differentiation (Vadnais et al., 2012). Michl et al. (2005) have shown that increased expression of Cux enhances tumor metastasis Michl and Downward, 2005. In transgenic mice, both CDP/Cux isoforms, p75 and p110, were shown to cause malignancies in several organs and cell types including breast cancer (Cadieux et al., 2006).

3.4.2.3 SATB1

Special AT-rich sequence binding protein 1 (SATB1) is a genome organizer that regulates chromatin structure, histone modification, and nucleosomal positioning (Galande et al., 2007; Han et al., 2008; Fessing et al., 2011). It is one of the key proteins involved in the development and progression of breast cancer (Iorns et al., 2010; Hanker et al., 2011).

SATB1 expression is upregulated in aggressive rather than nonaggressive breast cancer cells. In highly aggressive breast cancer, SATB1 overexpression has been reported to be associated with metastasis, whereas its downregulation has been reported to overturn the metastatic and tumorigenic characteristics of cells. Several studies have reported SATB1 as a prognostic marker for breast cancer (Patani et al., 2009; Chen et al., 2011).

3.4.2.4 BRCA1

Breast cancer type 1 susceptibility protein (BRCA1) gene is a tumor suppressor located on 17q21 chromosome that encodes a 220 kDa nuclear phosphoprotein (Suter and Marcum, 2007). It plays an important role in regulating genome integrity, cell cycle checkpoint proteins, key mitotic or cell division steps, cell proliferation, apoptosis as well as chromatin remodeling (Deng, 2006). Around 5%–10% of breast carcinomas are hereditary, and BRCA1 plays a major role in the hereditary susceptibility for the cancer (Christopoulou and Spiliotis, 2006). Women with BRCA1 germline mutations have more than three times the risk of developing breast cancer (Christopoulou and Spiliotis, 2006; Mackay and Szecsei, 2010). Studies have shown that there is a cumulative lifetime risk of 50%–85% of developing breast cancer in women having a germline mutation in BRCA1 (King et al., 2003). Majority of breast cancers having BRCA1 mutations are estrogen receptor negative (ER^-) (Tung et al., 2010). BRCA1-mutated tumors occur at an early age and are ER, PR, and HER2/neu negative (Xu et al., 2012). Such tumors are poorly differentiated and have the worst prognosis (Bowman-Colin C et al., 2013).

3.4.2.5 BTG3/ANA/APRO4

BTG3/ANA/APRO4 is a member of the antiproliferative B-cell translocation gene (BTG)/transducer of ErbB2 (Tob) gene family (Matsuda et al., 2001). The BTG family of antiproliferative gene products has been shown to play a significant role in the negative control of the cell cycle (Ou et al., 2007). BTG3 is negative regulator of SRC tyrosine kinase, and it inhibits the activity of the E2F1 transcription factor (Yu et al., 2008). The latest reports show that BTG3 is a p53 target and provides evidence for its DNA damage response and explains its anticancer potential through inhibition of E2F1 transcription factor (Ou et al., 2007). Some reports suggest that promoter region of the BTG3 gene is hypermethylated in breast cancer, thereby implicating its potential as a possible biomarker (Yu et al., 2008).

3.4.2.6 Cyclin D1

Cyclin D1 gene, located on chromosome 11q13, has been reported to regulate G1-S phase during the cell cycle (Kim et al., 2009a; Saha et al., 2011). It activates cdk 4/6 and plays an important role in sequestering cdk inhibitors in the G1/S phase (Alao, 2007). Cyclin D1 has been found to promote cell proliferation and differentiation by shortening the G1/S transition in many human tumors including breast cancer (Colozza et al., 2005). It is a key factor amplified in 15% breast cancer patients and overexpressed at genetic and protein levels in over 50% of breast cancer cases (Ormandy et al., 2003; Zelivianski et al., 2010). Overexpression of cyclin D1 in both in situ ductal and lobular subtypes suggests its possible role as a biomarker in the early detection of breast cancer (Rennstam et al., 2001). Several studies have shown a strong positive correlation of cyclin D1 with ER and

TABLE 3.7

Different Invasive Biomarkers Having the Potential for Prognostic Markers

Protein	Role in Breast Cancer
SMAR1	Regulates the cell proliferation, cell cycle, chromatin modulator.
SATB1	Proliferation marker that regulates histone modification, nucleosomal positioning.
BRCA1	Regulates cell proliferation, apoptosis, chromatin remodeling.
BTG3/ANA/APRO4	It has antiproliferative activity; acts as chromatin modulator.
Cyclin D1	It is a proliferation marker and plays a regulatory role in cell cycle regulation.

PR expression levels, wherein overexpression in ER-positive breast cancer patients has been found to be associated with relapse-free survival (Tobin et al., 2011). Table 3.7 enlists various invasive molecular biomarkers that are currently under development and their regulatory role in breast cancer.

3.5 Different Noninvasive Biomarkers Currently Used and under Development

3.5.1 Noninvasive Biomarkers Currently Used in Breast Cancer

3.5.1.1 Nipple Aspirate Fluid or Ductal Lavage Fluid Biomarkers

Nipple aspiration is a noninvasive and low-cost procedure used for obtaining breast fluids from the duct openings of the nipple for the evaluation of abnormalities associated with breast cancer (Fabian et al., 2005). Nipple fluid may provide a better source of ductal epithelial cells, cell-free nucleic acids (DNA, RNA, miRNA), and proteins released from the tumors (Dooley et al., 2001; Suijkerbuijk et al., 2008). Breast fluid provides a rich and superior source of biomarkers for breast cancer because the proteins present are specifically released from the breast tissue (Li et al., 2005). In combination with high-throughput novel proteomic profiling technology, specific biomarkers of nipple fluid have been discovered and validated (He et al., 2007). Sauter et al. collected NAF from 177 subjects using a modified breast pump, and out of that samples from 144 subjects were analyzed to evaluate promising cellular biomarkers (epithelial cells obtained from NAF). They analyzed cytology by computerized image analysis of NAF epithelial cells and observed that DNA index as well as percentage of cells in G2/M phase or with hypertetraploidy increased with abnormal cytology that correlated with increased breast cancer risk. All these results suggest that biomarkers from NAF may prove useful either as an adjunct to currently accepted breast cancer screening methods or to evaluate response to chemopreventive agents (Sauter et al., 1997).

Zhao Y analyzed carcinoembryonic antigen (CEA) and prostate-specific antigen (PSA) in NAF samples from 44 women with newly diagnosed invasive breast cancers, 67 women with proliferative breast lesions (DCIS and LCIS as well as atypical ductal hyperplasia) and 277 controls without these lesions. They found elevated levels of nipple fluid CEAs in breast cancer patients compared to the healthy controls. However, nipple fluid PSAs levels were similar in breast cancer patients as well as healthy control women. Their results suggested that nipple fluid CEA could be a potent biomarker for early breast cancer detection (Zhao et al., 2001).

Pawlik et al. collected NAF samples from the breasts of 18 women with stage I or II unilateral invasive breast carcinoma and 4 healthy volunteers as well using a handheld suction cup. The samples were analyzed using isotope-coded affinity tag (ICAT) labeling, sodium dodecyl sulfate–polyacrylamide gel (SDS-PAGE), liquid chromatography and mass spectrometry (LC/MS) to quantify and identify differential expression of tumor-specific proteins in NAF. They identified around 353 peptides and found that 5 proteins were differentially expressed in the NAF samples from cancer patients compared to that from healthy controls. Alpha2 HS-glycoprotein (heavy:light (H:L) ratio 0.63) was down-regulated while lipophilin B (H:L ratio 1.42), beta-globin (H:L ratio 1.98), hemopexin (H:L ratio 1.73), and vitamin D–binding protein precursor (H:L ratio 1.82) were overexpressed in NAF from cancer patients. Thus, proteomic-based techniques could be used to find markers for diagnosis of breast cancer (Heianbo et al., 2011; Pawlik et al., 2006).

He et al. analyzed NAF samples from 76 different women, including 63 samples from noncancerous breasts and 38 samples from breasts with invasive cancer, by surface-enhanced laser desorption ionization coupled to time-of-flight mass spectrometry (SELDI-TOFMS) technique to identify protein biomarkers. A set of eight markers were identified, which include albumin, apolipoprotein A-I, apolipoprotein D, hemoglobin ß, hemoglobin α, lactotransferrin, prolactin-induced protein, and α-1-antitrypsin, which collectively gave 63% sensitivity, 89% specificity, and 76% accuracy for distinguishing cancerous cases from noncancerous one (He et al., 2007).

Aberrantly methylated genes found in breast epithelial cells of NAF can be used as promising candidates for the early detection of breast cancer (Krassenstein et al., 2004). Methylation markers in NAF can be detected by various techniques that include methylation-specific PCR (MSP), quantitative multiplex methylation-specific PCR (QM-MSP), and sodium bisulfite treatment-based nested quantitative assay (Suijkerbuijk et al., 2011). Krassenstein et al. analyzed methylation status of GSTP1 (glutathione S-transferase P), retinoic acid receptor beta (RARB), p16INK4a, p14 alternate reading frame ($p14^{ARF}$), ras association domain-containing protein 1A (RASSF1A), and death-associated protein kinase 1 (DAPK) from matched specimens of tumor and normal tissues as well NAF from 22 breast cancer patients. They found hypermethylation of one or more genes in 82% of NAF DNAs in breast cancer patients compared to the normal controls (Krassenstein et al., 2004). Besides these, methylation of cyclin D2, HIN1, RAR-b2, CCND2 (cyclin D2), cyclin-dependent kinase inhibitor 2A (CDKN2A), RARB, RASSF1, twist-related protein 1 (TWIST1), BRCA1/2, secretoglobin 3A1 (SCGB3A1), and adenomatous polyposis coli (APC) genes in NAF samples has been reported in other studies to predict the breast cancer risk (Lewis et al., 2005; Euhus et al., 2007; Locke et al., 2007).

3.5.1.2 Serum Biomarkers

3.5.1.2.1 MUC-1

Mucins are large glycoproteins with high carbohydrate content (50%–90% by weight) and are divided into seven structurally identifiable families (MUC1–MUC7) (Rose and Voynow, 2006). These are normally expressed at the apical surface of polarized epithelial cells of normal mammary glands. However, in cancer, transformation and disruption of polarity lead to their release into the bloodstream of patients.

The MUC1 gene product is a transmembrane glycoprotein that is frequently overexpressed in malignant glandular cell surfaces and leads to increased serum levels of MUC1 that could be measured as an important predictive marker of breast cancer (Rakha et al., 2005). It is a high-molecular-weight (250–1000 kDa) protein that can activate membrane receptors for growth factors, reduce E-cadherin-mediated cell adhesion, and diminish cell–cell and cell–extracellular matrix interactions, thereby promoting cell migration and invasion. It can also reduce the cellular apoptotic response to oxidative stress (Hudson et al., 2001; Costa et al., 2011). Detection of high levels of these mucins in breast cancer patients correlates with increasing tumor burden and poor prognosis (Mukhopadhyay et al., 2011). Members of the MUC1 family include CA15.3, BR27.29, mucin-like carcinoma-associated antigen (MCA), and CA549 that are the most commonly implicated serum tumor markers in breast cancer.

3.5.1.2.1.1 CA15-3 and CA 27.29 (aka BR 27.29) Cancer antigen 15-3 (CA15-3) is a mucin-like transmembrane glycoprotein with a molecular weight of 290 kDa that is shed from the tumor cells into the bloodstream (Nicolini et al., 2006). It is overexpressed in more than 90% of breast carcinomas and is used in the diagnosis, treatment, and clinical management of the disease (Senapati et al., 2006). It is a useful marker in evaluating recurrence of the disease as well as response to the treatment (Al-azawi et al., 2006). The potential uses of CA15-3 in clinical practice lead to improved diagnosis and cost effectiveness (Prabasheela and Arivazhagan, 2011). CA15-3 is the most sensitive test in detecting metastatic breast cancer (Kruit et al., 2010).

Cancer antigen 27.29 (CA27.29) is a soluble form of the glycoprotein MUC1 (Cen et al., 2008) and can be detected by the monoclonal antibody B27.29 (Treon et al., 2000). It is overexpressed in a variety of cancers including breast cancer (Handy, 2009). Elevated serum CA27.29 protein levels are highly associated with progression of breast cancer (Harris et al., 2007) and has been reported in approximately one-third of women with early stage (stage I or II) and two-thirds of women with late stage of breast cancer (stage III or IV) (Hussain et al., 2006). It is highly specific and sensitive in detecting metastatic disease (Duffy, 2006). The US FDA has approved CA27.29 as a biomarker for monitoring breast cancer (Kurian et al., 2008).

CA15-3 and CA27.29 are useful markers in monitoring the response to either endocrine or cytotoxic therapy. Both are well-characterized serum biomarkers that allow the detection of circulating MUC1 antigen in the peripheral blood. Several studies have reported CA15-3 and CA27.29 as the predictive markers for breast cancer detection (Kumpulainen et al., 2002; Molina et al., 2010). Keyhani et al. in their study have measured CA15-3 levels in 54 patients with benign lesions, 43 with malignant lesions, and 39 normal controls before and after mastectomy. They tried to find out the correlation between serum levels of CA15-3 and age, clinical stage, as well as the number of lymph nodes involved. They found elevated levels of CA15-3 in 10% of patients with stage I, 20% with stage II, 40% with stage III, and 75% with stage IV breast cancer (Keyhani et al., 2005).

3.5.1.2.1.2 MCA, MSA, and CA549 MCA is a macromolecular glycoprotein belonging to the heterogeneous family of mucins (Ogawa et al., 2000). It has a molecular weight of 35 kDa and has been tested for breast cancer detection although it is not widely used as a biomarker (Seregni et al., 2008).

Mammary serum antigen (MSA) is a mucin-like glycoprotein of molecular weight of 30 kDa (Stacker et al., 1988). It is defined by the antibody 3EL.2 and is an important biomarker in breast cancer detection (Smart et al., 1990; Nicolini et al., 2006).

Cancer antigen 549 (CA549) is an acidic glycoprotein of molecular weight of around 400–512 kDa (Chan et al., 1988). It is a serum antigen defined by the monoclonal antibody BC4E 549 and belongs to the polymorphic epithelium mucins (PEMs) (Dnistrian et al., 1991). Elevated levels of CA549 have been reported in serum of breast cancer patients by using sensitive immunoassays. However, these assays have high sensitivity and specificity for advanced breast cancer than the early-stage breast cancer (Malati, 2007).

Gion et al. evaluated serum levels of CA549, CA15.3, and MCA markers from 184 healthy women and 237 patients with primary breast cancer by using immunometric assay technique. All these three markers significantly associated with tumor size and lymph node status and thus could be effective indicators of the tumor (Gion et al., 1994).

Nicolini et al. evaluated MCA, CEA, CA15.3, and TPA markers in serum samples of 289 breast cancer patients aged between 27 and 80 years. In this study, they compared sensitivity and specificity of MCA with that of CEA, CA15.3, and TPA for early detection of relapse. Moreover, they compared the diagnostic accuracy and predictive value of the MCA–CA15.3 association to that of CEA–TPA–CA15.3 panel. MCA sensitivity was higher than that of CEA or TPA or CA15.3 while specificity of MCA was similar to TPA and lower than that of CEA and CA15.3. MCA–CA15.3 association showed higher sensitivity but lower specificity, accuracy, and positive predictive value than CEA–TPA–CA15.3 panel. These findings concluded that CEA–TPA–CA15.3 panel is more accurate than MCA–CA15.3 association and can detect early relapsed patients with limited metastatic disease, thereby suggesting more favorable prognosis (Nicolini et al., 2006).

Verring et al., in their study, analyzed serum levels of CA549, MCA, and CA15-3 from 56 healthy women, 63 primary breast cancer patients, and 232 breast cancer patients with different stages. They reported elevated serum levels of CA549, MCA, and CA15-3 markers in the patients with breast cancer, thereby suggesting them as good indicators for predicting the disease extent as well as prognosis (Verring et al., 2011).

3.5.1.2.2 Carcinoembryonic Antigen

Carcinoembryonic antigen (CEA) is a serum glycoprotein of 200 kDa and belongs to the immunoglobulin gene super family (Schumann et al., 2004). It is expressed in normal mucosal cells and is found to be overexpressed in a variety of malignancies including breast cancer (Park et al., 2008). It is detected in the serum of cancer patients by using radioimmunoassay or enzyme-linked immunosorbent assay and can also be determined by immunohistochemical analysis of biopsy samples (Lkeda et al., 1994). In breast tumors, CEA is more prevalent in ductal compared to the lobular carcinomas. Since it has been found in patients with DCIS, CEA could be used as an early marker of the tumorigenic process. High levels of CA15-3 and/or CEA in breast cancer patients are an indicative of metastatic disease (Molina et al., 2010). Recent reports suggest that CEA and CA15-3 are the markers used for early detection of recurrence of the disease (Ghasabeh and Keyhanian 2013).

3.5.1.2.3 Cytokeratins

Fragments of cytokeratins 8, 18, and 19 are proposed as serum markers for early-stage breast cancer (Giovanella et al., 2002; Olofsson et al., 2007; Cîmpean et al., 2008).

3.5.1.2.3.1 Cytokeratin 19 (CK-19)/CYFRA21-1 Cytokeratin 19 fragment (CK-19), also known as CYFRA21-1, is an acidic cytoplasmic protein that has been reported in the serum of cancer patients (Marrakchi et al., 2008; Kosacka and Jankowska, 2009). It is a member of the intermediate filament group of proteins with a molecular weight of 40 kDa and is the most widely studied biomarker in the early detection of breast cancer (Oremek et al., 2007; Chang et al., 2009). Serum CYFRA 21-1 levels have a prognostic and predictive value for detecting disease relapse as well as the treatment efficacy (Nakata et al., 2004; Xenidis et al., 2009; Saloustros et al., 2011). Stathopoulou et al. (2002) were the first to detect the presence of CK-19 mRNA in the peripheral blood of patients with stage I and II breast cancer before initiation of adjuvant therapy.

Xenidis et al. evaluated the clinical relevance of CK-19 mRNA-positive circulating tumor cells (CTCs) in a total of 437 patients who had received adjuvant chemotherapy for stage I to III cancer by using a quantitative real-time RT-PCR assay. CK-19 mRNA-positive CTCs were detected in 179 patients before chemotherapy (41.0%). Around 51% patients with CK-19 mRNA-positive disease turned negative after adjuvant chemotherapy and around 22% of patients with initial CK-19 mRNA-negative disease became positive. These findings suggest that the detection of CK-19 mRNA-positive CTCs in the blood after adjuvant chemotherapy is an independent risk factor indicating the presence of chemotherapy-resistant residual disease (Xenidis et al., 2009).

The prognostic value of CK-19 mRNA-positive CTCs has been found to be associated with the hormone receptor status (Saloustros et al., 2011). Ignatiadis et al. observed that detection of CK-19 mRNA-positive CTCs before adjuvant chemotherapy in early stages was related to the status of estrogen receptor and HER2. The poor clinical outcome was observed in patients with ER-negative, triple-negative, and HER-2-positive early stage (Ignatiadis et al., 2007). Gaforio et al. (2003) found that CK-19 mRNA-positive CTCs correlated with estrogen receptor status in a positive manner, thereby indicating poor clinical outcome (Lianidou and Markou, 2011).

3.5.1.2.3.2 TPA and TPS Tissue polypeptide antigen (TPA) is a circulating complex of polypeptide fragments of low-molecular-weight cytokeratins 8, 18, and 19 (Barak et al., 2004). These three cytokeratins are characteristic of internal epithelium and are widely distributed in normal tissues and in tumors derived from them. These fragments are shed into the bloodstream during necrosis and lysis of the carcinoma cells (Śliwowska et al., 2006). TPA has been reported as a marker of cell proliferation, and its elevated levels in serum have been found in a variety of cancers, including breast, lung, gastrointestinal, urological, and gynecological cancers (Sugita et al., 2002; Barak et al., 2004). It is used in the early diagnosis, treatment planning, as well as in the follow-up of breast cancer. It is known to be sensitive but nonspecific tumor marker; however, along with other serum markers, TPA helps in monitoring the disease (Malati, 2007).

Tissue polypeptide-specific antigen (TPS) is a specific epitope structure of a peptide in serum associated with human cytokeratin 18 (Gonzalez-Quintela et al., 2006). It is associated with the proliferative activity of breast tumors (Liska et al., 2007), and its presence indicates poor disease-free survival (Ahn et al., 2013).

Śliwowska et al. analyzed serum levels of CA15-3, TPA, and TPS in 90 female breast cancer patients at various stages of the disease. They found a positive association between percentage of women with increased levels of all the three markers and the advanced stage of the disease. Their results suggested that the serum levels of CA15-3, TPA, and TPS may be useful markers to establish the stage of the disease and would help in deciding the treatment options (Śliwowska et al., 2006).

3.5.1.2.4 Her-2

C-erbB-2/HER2/neu is the most frequently used and the best-known biomarker (Fritz et al., 2005) that is overexpressed in 20%–30% of patients with breast cancer (Fiszman and Jasnis, 2011). This oncoprotein is cell membrane bound, but its extracellular domain is shed into circulation; thus, it becomes a potent serum biomarker (Carney, 2007). Elevated c-erbB-2/HER2/neu protein levels have been found in the serum of patients with breast carcinoma and have been associated with poor clinical outcome (Lipton et al., 2002). It is a key biomarker that is useful to detect therapy response as well as recurrence in patients with diagnosed breast carcinoma (Misek et al., 2011b).

3.5.1.2.5 *Mammaglobin*

Mammaglobin is a member of the secretoglobin family, mapped onto the human chromosome 11q13, that is overexpressed in around 70%–80% of primary and metastatic breast cancer tissues (Bhargava et al., 2007; Rehman et al., 2010).

Zehentner et al. studied peripheral blood samples from 147 breast cancer patients and 50 healthy controls. The samples were tested for mammaglobin gene expression by a multigene real-time RT-PCR assay and for serum mammaglobin protein by a sandwich ELISA assay. Mammaglobin expression was detected in 61% of blood samples from women with confirmed breast cancer and was not found in 50 healthy controls. Circulating mammaglobin protein was detected in 70% of the samples of the breast cancer sera. The RT-PCR assay and the ELISA for mammaglobin produced a combined sensitivity of 84% and specificity of 97%, suggesting that these are valuable tools in diagnosis and prognosis of breast cancer (Zehentner et al., 2004).

Bernstein et al. performed an ELISA-based study to identify the expression of mammaglobin in sera from 56 healthy control and 26 metastatic breast cancer patients. The level of mammaglobin was significantly high in diseased group as compared to the healthy controls. Thus, mammaglobin protein is an important serum marker for breast cancer diagnosis (Bernstein et al., 2005).

Chen et al. investigated cytokeratin 19, human mammaglobin, and carcinoembryonic antigen-positive CTCs from peripheral blood of 50 patients with early-stage breast cancer. The study was carried before giving any systemic adjuvant therapy, and it suggested that cytokeratin 19, mammaglobin, and CEA markers have important predictive and prognostic value in detection of the disease (Chen et al., 2010). In Table 3.8, different serum biomarkers along with their structure and function have been mentioned that could be used in early detection.

3.5.1.2.6 *Autoantibody Biomarkers*

Serum and other body fluids of the cancer patients are rich sources of antigens, glycoproteins, CTCs, and autoantibodies that could be used as biomarkers for the early detection (Zhong et al., 2008). These autoantibodies are stable, highly specific, easily purified from serum and are readily detected with well-validated secondary reagents (Anderson et al., 2011). Detection of serum antibodies against tumor antigens may provide reliable serum markers for cancer diagnosis and prognosis (Macdonald et al., 2012). Chapman et al.

TABLE 3.8

Serum Biomarkers for Early Detection of Breast Cancer

Markers	Structure	Function	References
CA 15-3	Glycoprotein	Mucins	Chourb et al. (2011)
CA27.29	Glycoprotein	Mucins	Klee et al. (2004)
MCA	Glycoprotein	Mucins	Ogawa et al. (2000)
CA549	Glycoprotein	Mucins	Chan et al. (1988)
CEA	Glycoprotein	Cell–cell interaction	Bidard et al. (2012)
Cytokeratin 19	Protein	Cytokeratin	Molina et al. (2010)
TPA	Protein	Cytokeratin	Nolen et al. (2008)
TPS	Protein	Tumor-associated antigen	Duffy (2006)
HER-2 (shed form)	Protein	Cell proliferation	Carney (2007)
Mammaglobin	Immunoglobulin	Cell signaling	Bernstein et al. (2005)
RS/DJ-1	Protein	Circulating tumor antigen	Naour et al. (2001)

detected the presence of autoantibodies against the known tumor-associated proteins such as p53, c-myc, HER2, NY-ESO-1 (cancer-testis antigen), BRCA1, BRCA2, and MUC1 antigens from serum samples of 94 normal controls, 97 primary breast cancer patients, and 40 patients with DCIS by ELISA. Elevated levels of antibodies in serum samples against one or more of these tumor-associated antigens were observed in 64% of the primary breast cancer patient sera and 45% of patients with DCIS at a specificity of 85%. These findings concluded that autoantibody assays against a panel of antigens could be used as biomarkers in the detection and diagnosis of early breast cancer (Chapman et al., 2007).

3.5.1.2.7 Circulating Tumor Cells Biomarkers

CTCs are the key predictive markers in breast cancer (Bidard et al., 2012; Ramona and Massimo, 2011), and their detection is useful in prognosis, diagnosis, prediction of response to therapy, as well as treatment of primary or metastatic disease (Swaby and Cristofanilli, 2011). Wiedswang et al. (2004) observed that isolated tumor cells present in bone marrow from stage I and II breast cancer patients predict unfavorable clinical outcome. Similar findings were observed by Braun et al. (2005) wherein they analyzed bone marrow micrometastasis in breast cancer patients of stages I, II, and III, indicating reduced disease-free and overall survival. There are multiple approaches to detect CTCs in blood that include immunocytochemical methods, cell search system, and RT-qPCR (Auwera et al., 2010). Among these, multimarker qRT-PCR is one of the most sensitive and specific methods utilized for the molecular detection of circulating cancer cells in blood (Mario Giuliano et al., 2011; Rosa Nadal et al., 2012). Circulating tumor markers such as HER2/neu, p53 autoantibodies, cytokeratin-positive cells, autoantibodies to nucleophosmin (NPM), serum soluble vascular cell adhesion molecules such as intracellular adhesion molecule-1 (ICAM-1), vascular cell adhesion molecule-1 (VCAM-1), E-selectin, and CK-19 mRNA-positive cells are some of the interesting and mostly studied biomarkers that can predict progression-free and overall survival of the patients (Nicolini et al., 2006).

3.5.1.3 Tear Fluid Biomarkers

Tear fluid offers a potential noninvasive source of biomarkers (Mann and Tighe, 2007). It is composed of a complex mixture of mucins, glycoproteins, unglycosylated proteins, peptides, lipids, lysozyme, lactoferrin, secretory immunoglobulin A (sIgA), lipocalin, and lipophilin (Li, 2010). Tear biomolecules have been presumed to act as biomarkers for local eye diseases, autoimmune diseases (Sjogren's syndrome), ocular bacterial infections (trachoma), diabetes, as well as different cancers (Wu and Zhang, 2007; Lebrecht et al., 2009; Zhou et al., 2009; CsőszÉ et al., 2012; Kelly and Amy, 2011). The global interest is rising in using tear biomarkers for prognosis as well as diagnosis of breast cancer because the collection of tears is relatively simple, safe, noninvasive, inexpensive, and repetitive with minimal discomfort to the patients (Li, 2010; Böhm et al., 2012; Yong, 2010). However, tear fluid biomarkers have not been clinically assessed due to few hurdles such as low throughput, lack of automation potential, and the requirement of large sample volume. Another challenge is the need for highly sensitive and reliable techniques for the analysis of a small amount of tear samples to ensure reproducible and quantifiable results (Karns et al., 2011).

Lebrecht et al. had established protein biomarker profile from tear fluid samples of 50 breast cancer patients and 50 healthy women by using SELDI-TOFMS technique. They generated a panel of 20 tear biomarkers that differentiate the breast cancer patients from healthy controls with 70.94% accuracy and approximately 70% specificity and sensitivity.

The study suggested that the proteomic pattern of tear fluid may be useful in the diagnosis as well as high-throughput biomarker discovery (Lebrecht et al., 2009). The hurdles in tear fluid biomarker discovery highlight the need for standard sampling procedure as well as very sensitive techniques for detection.

3.5.1.4 Salivary Biomarkers

Over the past decade, considerable efforts have been expended to discover and validate the salivary biomarkers for the noninvasive detection of breast cancer by using transcriptomic and proteomic approaches (Al-Tarawneh et al., 2011). Several studies have been conducted to detect putative salivary biomarkers for early detection of breast cancer wherein the potential use of salivary proteins such as c-erbB-2, VEGF, EGF, and CEA has been implicated (Brooks et al., 2008; Zhang et al., 2010; Streckfus et al., 2012).

3.5.1.5 Heat Shock Protein

Heat shock proteins (HSPs) are a family of highly conserved proteins that play an important role in the regulation of apoptosis (Gupta and Knowlton, 2005). Desmetz et al. (2008) showed that heat shock protein 60 (HSP60) could be considered as a relevant tumor-associated antigen for early-stage ductal in situ breast carcinoma detection (Hamrita et al., 2010).

3.6 Genetic Biomarkers

Cancer involves deregulation of gene expression profiles and disruption of molecular networks (Bhatt et al., 2010). Various genetic alterations that have been found to be associated with cancer include nonrandom mutations and single-nucleotide polymorphisms (SNPs), insertions, deletions, and translocations/rearrangements within the regulatory region of the gene (Sadikovic et al., 2008). Copy number variations (CNV) as well as microsatellite instability (MSI) are also known to play a significant role in breast tumorigenesis (Sadikovic et al., 2008). Recent advances in high-throughput genomics as well as application of integrative approaches have resulted in the discovery of promising candidate biomarkers that would help in diagnosis and better prognosis of the disease (Hicks et al., 2011).

3.6.1 Genetic Variations

3.6.1.1 Mutations and SNPs in Breast Cancer

Genomic instability refers to an increased rate of genomic alteration that plays an important role in cancer development (Kwei et al., 2010). Germline mutations in several genes, due to an abnormal number of centrosomes, inefficient DNA repair, and unwanted telomere maintenance, confer high risk in developing breast cancer (Antoniou et al., 2008). Several genes have been shown to exhibit germline mutations in breast cancer that include TP53, core-binding factor subunit beta (CBFB), phosphatidylinositol-4,5-bisphosphate 3-kinase (PIK3CA), v-akt murine thymoma viral oncogene homolog 1 (AKT1), GATA3, mitogen-activated protein kinase kinase kinase 1 (MAP3K1), and v-erb-b2 erythroblastic leukemia viral oncogene homolog 2 (ERBB2) (Usary et al., 2004; Ralhan et al., 2007; Lim et al., 2009; Kancha et al., 2011; Banerji et al., 2012). Germline mutations in BRCA1 and BRCA2 genes have been linked to the development of hereditary breast cancers (Mote et al., 2004). Telomere dysfunction has also been regarded as one of the possible mechanisms responsible for genomic instability (Artandi and DePinho, 2000). It has been reported to play an imperative role in situ progression of breast cancer from ductal hyperplasia to DCIS (Chin et al., 2004).

Besides these mutations, SNPs have been reported as the primary cause of genetic disorders in humans and may be used as therapeutic markers in determining the individual's risk of developing breast cancer (Gobbi et al., 2006; Onay et al., 2006). SNPs refer to single-nucleotide variation in an individual's genome that may occur within the coding sequences of genes, noncoding regions of genes or in the intergenic regions (Onay et al., 2006; Schmid et al., 2012). SNPs are divided into normal and abnormal types wherein the former polymorphisms occur in the DNA sequence that does not alter the normal protein structure. In abnormal SNPs, polymorphisms occur in the DNA sequence that encodes for the structural or functional domains of the protein. Abnormal SNPs have been found to be involved in the development of breast cancer (Huang et al., 2010). Approximately 500,000 noncoding, 200,000 silent coding, and 200,000 replacement coding SNPs are likely to occur in the human genome (Halushka et al., 1999).

Onay et al. in their study have reported a cross talk among genes/SNPs from DNA repair, cell cycle, immune system, and cancer metabolism pathways. Recently, it has been shown that breast cancer–associated SNPs are enriched in the cistromes (set of cis-acting targets for a trans-acting factor) of forkhead box protein A1 (FOXA1), estrogen receptor 1 (ESR1), and the epigenome of histone H3 lysine 4 monomethylation (H3K4me1) (Cowper-SalLari et al., 2012). FOXA1 is highly correlated with $ER\alpha^+$ and PR^+ protein expressions as well as endocrine signaling in breast cancer (Badve et al., 2007; Albergaria et al., 2009). FOXA1 acts as a marker to identify $ER\alpha^+$ cancers that are resistant to endocrine therapy. In $ER\alpha^-$ breast cancer, the expression of FOXA1 is highly correlated with improved disease-free survival. Overexpression of neurogenic locus notch homolog protein 2 (NOTCH2) has been reported in the patients with rs11249433 SNP, which has been reported to promote the development of ER^+ luminal tumors (Fu et al., 2010). Table 3.9 enlists the different mutated genes, types of mutations involved, and their role in breast cancer.

3.6.1.2 Insertions, Deletions, and Translocations

Chromosome rearrangements such as translocations, inversions, and deletions have been frequently reported in breast cancer (Hanahan and Weinberg, 2000; Albertson et al., 2003). The aberrant function of the genes may result from naturally occurring DNA polymorphisms that include gene amplification or duplication, deletion or insertion in coding regions and splice sites, chromosomal translocation, as well as inversion (Futreal et al., 2004; Kolusayin and Orta, 2005). Such aberrations may lead to changes in genome copy number, chromosome structure, as well as epigenetic modifications that may have been reported to suppress the expression of tumor suppressor genes or activate the oncogenes leading to breast cancer development (Feinberg and Tycko, 2004; Mitelman et al., 2004; Ushijima, 2005). For example, BRCA1-deficient tumors have been reported to exhibit gross mutations (inversions, deletions) at the locus of tumor suppressor gene PTEN resulting into its dysfunction (Heikkinen et al., 2011).

TABLE 3.9

List of Mutated Genes, Type of Mutation, and Their Role in Breast Cancer

Mutated Genes	Full Form	Type of Cancer	Type of Mutation	Role in Breast Cancer
BRCA1 & BRCA2	Breast cancer type 1 susceptibility protein	Hereditary breast cancer	Somatic/point mutations	• Uncontrolled cell proliferation.
CBFB	Core-binding factor subunit beta	ER-positive breast cancer	Recurrent mutations	• Involved in metastasis.
TP53	Tumor protein 53	Node-positive breast cancer	Somatic mutations	• Controls cell fate in response to DNA damage. • It has a specific role in blocking homologous recombination between divergent sequences.
PIK3CA	Phosphatidylinositol-4,5-bisphosphate 3-kinase	ER-positive breast cancer	Hot spot mutations	• Activate the phosphatidylinositol-3-kinase (PI3K) pathway.
AKT1	V-akt murine thymoma viral oncogene homolog	ER-positive breast cancer	Somatic mutations	
GATA3	Trans-acting T-cell-specific transcription factor	ER-positive breast cancer	Somatic mutations	• Involved in metastasis, aggressive tumor development. • Deletion of GATA3 in the mammary epithelium is also involved in morphogenesis and differentiation of luminal epithelial cells.
MAP3K1	Mitogen-activated protein kinase kinase kinase 1	ER-positive breast cancer and luminal type breast cancer	Somatic mutations	• MAP3K1 encodes serine/threonine protein kinases that play a major role in activation of JUN signaling pathway.
ERBB2	v-erb-b2 erythroblastic leukemia viral oncogene homolog 2	Her2-enriched and luminal B subtypes, typically have ERBB2 amplification	Point mutations	• ErbB2 overexpression leads to increased chemoresistance. • It is also associated with increased metastasis.
MAGI3-AKT3 fusion gene	Membrane-associated guanylate kinase-3-v-akt murine thymoma viral oncogene homolog 3	Triple-negative breast cancer	Somatic mutations	• MAGI3–AKT3 translocation and deletion result in loss of function of a tumor suppressor gene PTEN and activation of an oncogene AKT3.

3.6.1.3 Copy Number Variations

Several studies have demonstrated the role of DNA CNV in normal development and disease (Krepischi et al., 2012). CNV deletions have been reported in almost 30% of genes involved in breast cancer development that include BRCA1, BRCA2, adenomatous polyposis coli (APC), SMAD4, tumor protein p53 (TP53), as well as mismatch repair genes human mutL homolog 1 (hMLH1) and human mutS homolog 2 (hMSH2) (Krepischi et al., 2012).

3.6.1.4 Microsatellite Instability

Microsatellites/short tandem repeats (STRs) are simple sequence repeats of 2–6 base pairs in the human genome (Turnpenny and Ellard, 2005). These are genetic markers having biological functions, according to their location, such as affecting protein coding (in coding regions) or regulating gene expression (in regulatory regions) (Gemayel et al., 2010; Lacroix-Triki et al., 2010). They are involved in genetic mapping, forensic analysis, and bone marrow engraftment monitoring. MSI results from defects in DNA mismatch repair, leading to mutations at simple sequence repeats (microsatellites) (Siah et al., 2000). The reported incidence of MSI in breast cancers is 5%–30% (Lee et al., 2001; Kamat et al., 2012). Microsatellites in the estrogen receptor (ESR1, ESR2) and androgen receptor (AR) genes have been hypothesized to be predisposing factors for breast cancer. Over the past decade, various studies have been conducted to test the relationship between these three microsatellites and breast cancer risk in men and women (Zheng et al., 2012).

MSI, a type of genetic instability involving frequent errors during the replication of short nucleotide repeats, is mostly due to a defective DNA mismatch repair gene such as hMSH2, hMLH1, hPMS2, and hMSH6 (Anghel et al., 2006; Lin et al., 2007; Stacey et al., 2010; Huo et al., 2012). Two MSI phenotypes have been described in cancer that include MSI-high (MSI-H) cancers, resulting from defective mismatch repair; and MSI-low (MSI-L) tumors, having lower levels of MSI but are not associated with defective mismatch repair (Cavazzana-Calvo et al., 1999; Cox et al., 2006a). Murata et al. in their study have investigated the MSI, protein expression of hMSH2 and hMLH1, as well as genetic and epigenetic modifications of these genes in sporadic breast tumors. They revealed the association of MSI with reduced expression of hMLH1 and hMSH2 genes in the patients with sporadic breast tumors. They have also shown that the tumors with MSI contain both genetic and epigenetic modifications of these mismatch repair genes (Murata et al., 2002; Fonseca et al., 2005). MSI has been reported in a number of breast cancer–related genes such as BAT25, BAT-26, BAT-40, D17S250, D5S346, D2S123, D18S55, D18S58, mutation frequency decline-28 (MFD-28), mutation frequency decline-41 (MFD-41), and tumor protein p53ALU repeat polymorphism (TP53ALU) (Fonseca et al., 2005; Lee et al., 2001; Kamat et al., 2012; Luqmani and Mathew, 2004). MSI, thus, plays a chief role in the genomic instability and tumorigenesis in sporadic breast cancer and can serve as a therapeutic target in future.

3.7 Epigenetic Biomarkers

Epigenetics refers to the study of heritable changes in gene expression with no change in the gene sequence (Sadikovic et al., 2008). DNA methylation, histone tail modifications, posttranslational modifications, as well as alterations in microRNA expression profiles are the most important epigenetic changes associated with the cancer (Veeck and Esteller, 2010).

3.7.1 Methylation Biomarkers in Breast Cancer

DNA methylation plays an important role in chromatin organization, silencing of transposable elements, X-chromosome inactivation, tissue-specific expression, and genetic imprinting (Miranda and Jones, 2007). Methylation has been reported as one of the imperative factors in tumor development and thus may serve as a valuable biomarker in breast cancer early detection (Kornegoor et al., 2012). During the process of tumorigenesis, hypermethylation at tumor suppressor genes leads to silencing of transcription, cancer initiation, as well as progression (Brook et al., 2009). It has been found that around 600–10,000 genes show aberrant methylation in a single tumor (Ushijima and Asada, 2010). Within these genes, some are important in cancer development whereas some code for important microRNAs (Costello et al., 2000; Momparler, 2003; Jones, Baylin, 2007; Esteller, 2008; Novak et al., 2009). Moreover, not only the malignant cells but the surrounding tissue also shows defective methylation pattern (Yan et al., 2006).

3.7.1.1 Methylation Markers in Nipple Fluid

Nipple aspiration is a noninvasive procedure, and the aspirate fluid is known to contain breast epithelial cells (Fabian et al., 2005). Methylation of *GSTP1*, RARB, CDKN2A/p16INK4a, p14^{ARF}, RASSF1A, and DAPK genes has been reported in breast cancer by a number of studies (Suijkerbuijik et al., 2010). Genes such as CDKN2A, CCND2, APC, SCGB3A1, RASSF1, TWIST, or RARB have been shown to be associated with the history of breast cancer (Suijkerbuijik et al., 2010).

3.7.1.2 Methylation Markers in Blood

Methylation has been found to be rarely detectable in serum or plasma of healthy individuals than that of the patients with breast cancer. Matuschek et al., in their study, collected serum samples from 85 breast cancer patients and 22 healthy controls and analyzed the methylation status of APC, RASSF1A, ESR1, CDKN2A/p16, and GSTP1 genes. They observed the hypermethylation of APC, RASSF1A, GSTP1, and ESR1 in 29%, 26%, 18%, and 38% of breast cancer patients, respectively. On the other hand, hypermethylation of ESR1 and RASSF1A, APC, and GSTP1 was found to be around 23%, 9%, and 6% in healthy controls, respectively. They also found a strong correlation between the hypermethylation of GSTP1 and ESR1 with Her2/neu status of cancer patients (Matuschek et al., 2010).

Sebova et al. analyzed the DNA methylation levels of RASSF1A and CDH1 genes in blood samples collected from 92 breast cancer patients and 50 healthy controls. They observed methylation of RASSF1A in 82.6% and CDH1 in 21.7% of breast cancer patients. However, no methylation of these genes was found in healthy controls. A positive correlation was observed between the elevated levels of RASSF1A methylation with the tumor size, lymph node status, as well as TNM stage. Thus, RASSF1A and CDH1 genes could be useful methylation markers for breast cancer detection (Sebova et al., 2011).

Radpour et al. investigated the methylation profiles of cancer-related genes APC, bridging integrator 1 (BIN1) (bridging integrator 1), bone morphogenetic protein 6 (BMP6), BRCA1, CST6 (cystatin E/M), ESR-b, GSTP1, p14/ARF, p16/CDKN2A, p21/CDKN1A, PTEN, and TIMP3 in the axillary lymph node metastasis in breast cancer. They reported a higher rate of methylation of genes APC, BMP6, BRCA1, and p16 genes in the lymph node metastasis than in the normal tissue, thereby suggesting them to be useful for screening metastasis (Radpour et al., 2011). In Table 3.10, the methylation markers found in the blood of breast cancer patients have been enlisted.

TABLE 3.10

Methylation Markers in Blood, Their Chromosomal Location, and Their Role

Methylation Markers	Full Forms	Chromosome Location	Role	References
CDKN2A/ p16Ink4A	Cyclin-dependent kinase inhibitor 2A	9p21	Acts as a tumor suppressor; negative regulator of cyclin-dependent kinases and p14(ARF1); an activator of TP53	Aravidis et al. (2012)
CDH1	Cadherin-1	16q22.1	Acts as a tumor suppressor gene; plays an important role in cell adhesion, thus may keep cancer cells from metastasizing	Pecina-Slaus (2003)
RASSF1	Ras association domain-containing protein 1	3p21.31	Acts as a tumor suppressor	Suijkerbuijk et al. (2011), Voyatzi et al. (2010)
APC	Adenomatous polyposis coli	5q21	Acts as a tumor suppressor; plays an important role in cell attachment and signaling	Aoki and Taketo (2007)
DAPK1	Death-associated protein kinase 1	9q21.33	Acts as a tumor suppressor gene; plays an important role in cell growth, apoptosis	Suijkerbuijk et al. (2011)
RARβ	Retinoic acid receptor beta	3p24	Steroid receptor; antiproliferative	Piperi et al. (2010), Voyatzi et al. (2010)
MGMT	O-6-methylguanine-DNA methyltransferase	10q26	Involving recognition and repair of damaged DNA and subsequent synthesis of new DNA	Piperi et al. (2010)
TMS1	Target of methylation-induced silencing	16p11.2-12	Apoptosis; inflammation	Gordian et al. (2009)
BRCA1	Breast cancer type 1	17q21	Tumor suppressor; DNA damage sensor; signal transducers proliferation; apoptosis; chromatin remodeling	Stefansson et al. (2011), Snell et al. (2008)
ESR1	Estrogen receptor 1	6q25.1	DNA-binding transcription factor; plays an important role in cell division and DNA replication	Martínez-Galán et al. (2008)
pRB	Retinoblastoma protein	13q14.2	Steroid receptor; tumor suppressors; plays an important role in cell growth by inhibiting cell cycle progression	Stefansson et al. (2011)
CCND2	Cyclin D2	12p13.3	Regulator of cyclin-dependent kinases whose activity is required for cell cycle G1/S transition	Suijkerbuijk et al. (2011)
CDKN2A	Cyclin-dependent kinase inhibitor 2A	9p21	Negative regulator of cyclin-dependent kinases	Dębniak et al. (2005)

(Continued)

TABLE 3.10 (*CONTINUED*)

Methylation Markers in Blood, Their Chromosomal Location, and Their Role

Methylation Markers	Full Forms	Chromosome Location	Role	References
p16	—	9p21	Acts as a tumor suppressor; regulating the cell cycle	Hu et al. (2003)
p14	—	9p21	Acts as a tumor suppressor; stabilizes nuclear p53	Radpour et al. (2012)
SLIT2	Slit homolog 2 protein	4p15.3	Antiproliferative; antimetastasis	Dallol et al. (2002)
14-3-3σ	Stratifin	1p36.11	G2 checkpoint	Martínez-Galán et al. (2008)
RUNX3	Runt-related transcription factor 3	1p36	Acts as a tumor suppressor; antiproliferative	Xiao Yuan Fan et al. (2011)
TWIST1	Twist homolog 1	7p21.2	Cancerous cell dissemination	Swift-Scanlan et al. (2011)
SCGB3A1	Scretoglobin3A1	5q35	Cell growth, cell migration, invasion	Suijkerbuijk et al. (2010)
ATM	Ataxia telangiectasia mutated	11q22-q23	Role in cell division and DNA repair	Brennan et al. (2012)
HSD17β4	Type 4 17-beta-hydroxysteroid dehydrogenase	17q21.2	Steroid hormone receptor	Christensen et al. (2010)

3.7.2 MicroRNAs as Biomarkers

MicroRNAs (miRNAs or miRs) are a major class of small endogenous noncoding RNA molecules, 22 nucleotides long, and were described in 1993 by Lee et al. (1993). Many miRNAs have been found to be involved in several human cancers, including breast cancer (Farazi et al., 2011). The loss of several tumor suppressor miRNAs (miR-206, miR-17-5p, miR-125a, miR-125b, miR-200, let-7, miR-34a miR-335, miR-27b, miR-126, miR-101, miR-145, miR-146a/b, miR-205, miR-31) as well as overexpression of certain oncogenic miRNAs (miR-21, miR-155, miR-10b, miR-373, miR-520c, miR-27a, miR-221/222) has been observed in many breast cancers (Heneghan et al., 2010; Day et al., 2010). The gene networks implicated by these miRNAs are still largely unknown although their key targets have been identified (Thomas et al., 2010). Measurement of the miRs in plasma or serum from the cancer patients is a promising approach for the prognosis, diagnosis, and theragnosis of breast and other cancers (Heneghan et al., 2011). Lawrie et al. (2008) first identified serum miRNAs in patients with diffuse large B-cell lymphoma (Lawrie et al., 2008). In a study done by Schrauder et al. in 2012, microarray-based miRNA profiling on whole blood of 48 early-stage breast cancer patients was performed and 57 healthy individuals were kept as control. They found that 59 miRNAs were differentially expressed in whole blood of the early-stage patients compared with the healthy controls, out of which 13 were upregulated and 46 were downregulated. These results suggest that breast cancer is associated with changes in the expression of multiple miRNAs (Schrauder et al., 2012) that may disturb the functioning of network of genes in normal cell signaling pathways. Table 3.9 enlists various early-stage miRNAs that may function as tumor suppressors or activators in breast cancer.

3.7.2.1 Tumor Suppressor miRNAs Involved in Breast Cancer

3.7.2.1.1 miR-206

miR-206 plays an important role in the regulation of the estrogen receptor gene *ERα* (*ESR1*) (Day et al., 2010). It has been shown to be upregulated in ERα-negative breast cancers indicating its possible role in the regulation of *ESR1* (Adams et al., 2007). ERα agonists have been shown to be involved in repressing the expression of miR-206, whereas ERβ agonists have not been found to possess any inhibitory effect on the expression of miR-206 (Adams et al., 2007).

3.7.2.1.2 miR-17-5p

miR-17-5p, also known as miR-91, has been reported to be involved in the regulation of cell proliferation in breast cancer (Eiriksdottir et al., 1998). It has been reported to repress the expression of *AIB1* (oncogene amplified in breast cancer), thereby inhibiting the function of E2F1 and ERα. This further results into inhibition of estrogen-stimulated as well as estrogen/ER-independent proliferation of breast cancer cells through downregulation of *AIB1* (Hossain et al., 2006; Quin et al., 2006). The gene cyclin D1 (*CCND1*), which is involved in the proliferation, has also been identified as a direct target of miR-17-5p (Day et al., 2010).

3.7.2.1.3 miR-125a and miR-125b

miR-125a and miR-125b are downregulated in HER2-overexpressing breast cancers (Mattie et al. 2006). In SKBR3 cells (an HER2-dependent human breast cancer cell line), they have been reported to reduce the anchorage dependence, growth, cell motility, and invasive potential (Scott et al., 2007).

3.7.2.1.4 miR-200 Family

miR-200 family of miRNAs include miR-200c and miR-141 (located on chromosome 12) as well as miR-200a/b and miR-429 (located on chromosome 1) (Park et al., 2008). miR-200 family plays an important role in regulating the tumor progression and metastasis in breast cancer (Korpal and Kang, 2008). It has been reported to suppress *epithelial–mesenchymal transition* (EMT) through downregulation of ZEB1 and ZEB2 (zinc finger E-box-binding homeobox 1 and 2), which are repressors of the cell–cell contact protein, E-cadherin (Spaderna et al., 2008). EMT is responsible for the malignant transformation of many human cancers by allowing detachment of cells, thereby increasing tumor cell mobility and metastasis (Day et al., 2010). Downregulation of miR-200 has been shown to increase the tumor metastasis in breast cancer (Day et al., 2010). The functional pathway for miR-200 is TGF-β signaling. Gregory et al. (2008) found that TGF-β induced EMT in human Madin Darby canine kidney (MDCK) epithelial cells resulted in the downregulation of miR-200.

3.7.2.1.5 let-7 Family

The microRNA let-7 (lethal-7) is a widely studied tumor suppressor whose expression is downregulated in many cancers, including breast cancer. let-7 family microRNAs are critical regulators of proliferation, cell differentiation, self-renewal, as well as tumorigenicity of breast cancer cells (Yu et al., 2007). Reports suggest that let-7 represses the expression of Harvey rat sarcoma viral oncogene (*H-RAS*), high-mobility group AT-hook 2 (*HMGA2*), *LIN28*/zinc finger CCHC domain-containing protein 1, and phosphatidylethanolamine-binding protein 1 (*PEBP*) oncogenes involved in tumorigenesis (Lee and Dutta, 2007;

Yu et al., 2007). Recently, let-7 and HMGA2 have also been reported to be associated with the Raf kinase inhibitory protein (RKIP)–mediated inhibition of invasion and metastasis in breast cancer (Dangi-Garimella et al., 2009, 2010). Zhao et al. performed microarray screening of RNA samples obtained from formalin-fixed paraffin-embedded (FFPE) breast tissues of 13 benign, 16 DCIS, and 15 IDC. They were found that the expression of let-7 family miRNAs was significantly downregulated in DCIS and IDC breast tissues compared to benign tissues. There was an inverse correlation between ER-α expression and several members of let-7 family in the FFPE tissues. These results suggest that Let-7 family miRNAs regulate estrogen receptor alpha signaling in estrogen receptor–positive breast cancer (Zhao et al., 2010).

3.7.2.1.6 *miR-34a*

miR-34a plays an important role in regulation of DNA damage and cellular proliferation in breast cancer (Kato et al., 2009). It has been reported as a direct transcriptional target of p53 and has been found to be downregulated in a number of cancers, including breast cancer (Calin and Croce, 2006; Chang et al., 2007). miR-34a downregulates the expression of CCND1 (cyclin D1), *cyclin-dependent kinase 6* (CDK6), E2F transcription factor 3 (E2F3), and V-myc myelocytomatosis viral oncogene (MYC), thereby inducing cell cycle arrest in cancer (Sun et al., 2008). Low expression of miR-34a has been found in the cell lines derived from ER/PR/HER2-negative tumors (Kato et al., 2009). Studies have shown the role of miR-34 in governing the expression of genes such as CDK4, CDK6, and BCL2 that are involved in the regulation of cell cycle, proliferation, and survival in breast cancer (Zuoren et al., 2010).

3.7.2.1.7 *miR-31*

miR-31 is expressed in normal breast cells and has been shown to inhibit the metastasis by repressing the expression of prometastatic breast cancer genes (Zhu et al., 2007; Day et al., 2010). It is moderately decreased in nonmetastatic breast cancer cell lines and is barely detectable in metastatic breast cancer cell lines (Valastyan et al., 2009). The reported target prometastatic genes that are downregulated by miR-31 are frizzled3 (*Fzd3*), integrin α-5 (*ITGA5*), myosin phosphatase-rho-interacting protein (*M-RIP*), matrix metallopeptidase 16 (*MMP16*), radixin (*RDX*), and the ras homolog gene family member A (*RhoA*) (Baranwal and Alahari, 2010). Expression of *ITGA5*, *RDX*, and RhoA in the breast cancer cells has been shown to abolish the functions mediated by miR-31 such as inhibition of motility and invasion as well as induction of apoptosis (Day et al., 2010). Thus, miR-31 may prove as an attractive therapeutic target for breast cancer.

3.7.2.2 Oncogenic miRNAs Involved in Breast Cancer

3.7.2.2.1 *miR-21*

miR-21 functions as an oncogene and is one of the most studied miRNAs in cancer (Iorio et al., 2005; Volinia et al., 2006). It regulates the tumor suppressor genes *BCL-2*, tumor suppressor protein tropomyosin 1 (TPM1), programmed cell death protein 4 (*PDCD4*), phosphatase and tensin homolog (*PTEN*), and mammary serine protease inhibitor (*MASPIN*). In breast cancer cell line MCF-7, inhibition of miR-21 has been reported to sensitize the tumor cells to anticancer agents. Overexpression of miR-21 in breast cancer has been correlated to advanced tumor stage, lymph node metastasis, and poor survival of the patient (Yan et al., 2008).

TABLE 3.11

List of miRNAs and Their Role in Breast Cancer

Role	Tumor Suppressor miRs	Tumor Activator miRs
Regulation of cell proliferation	miR-17-5p, Let-7, miR-34a	—
Regulation of cell signaling	miR-206, miR-200c	miR-155
Regulation of cell cycle progression	miR-126	miR-27a
Regulation of metastasis and cell invasion	miR-31, miR-335, miR-101, miR-145, miR-27b, miR-126, miR-146a/b, miR-205	miR-10b, miR-373/520c

3.7.2.2.2 *miR-155*

miR-155 expression is elevated in a number of human malignancies, including breast cancer (Iorio et al., 2005; Volinia et al., 2006). It has been reported to inhibit the expression of *RhoA*, a gene that plays an important role in many cellular processes such as cell adhesion, motility, polarity, cell junction formation, and stability (Boureux et al., 2007; Dagan et al., 2012). It has also been shown to mediate TGF-β-induced EMT and cell invasion in various cells by disrupting the tight junction formation and promoting cell migration and invasion (Kong et al., 2008). Oncogenic role of miR-155 in breast cancer progression has recently been described (Mattiske et al., 2012).

3.7.2.2.3 *miR-10b*

miR-10b is overexpressed in metastatic cancer cells (Ma et al., 2007). It promotes cell invasion through RhoC-AKT signaling pathway by downregulating the Homeobox D10 (HOXD10) gene. Downregulation of HOXD10 activates pro-metastatic gene RHOC (ras homologue gene family member C) that involved in cell migration and invasion in breast cancer (Liu et al., 2012).

3.7.2.2.4 *miR-373/520c*

miR-373/miR-520c promote tumor invasion and metastasis, and their reported target gene is *CD44* (Huang et al., 2008; Keklikoglou et al., 2012). Huang et al., in their study, have reported the role of miR-373 and miR-520c in metastasis and invasion of breast cancer cells. In the study, a nonmetastatic, human breast tumor cell line was transduced with an miRNA-expression library and subjected to a trans-well migration assay. The study demonstrated that the ectopic expression of human miR-373 and miR-520c in the cancer cells stimulated the migratory and invasive phenotype (Huang et al., 2008). Table 3.11 enlists different tumor suppressor and activator miRNAs along with their putative role in breast cancer.

3.8 Proteomic Biomarkers of Breast Cancer

Proteomics can be defined as the identification, characterization, and quantification of the proteins in a wide variety of biological samples such as tissues or body fluids (Abhilash, 2009; Bantscheff et al., 2007; Laronga and Drake 2007). The analysis of proteins in early-stage cancers has provided new insights into the changes that occur during tumorigenesis (Wulfkuhle et al., 2003). Proteomics is the choice for discovery of biomarkers as it can bridge the gap between the genetic alterations underlying cancer and cellular physiology (Gast et al., 2009; Roy and Shukla, 2008). The recent comprehensive technologies that include protein microarrays, MS, such as matrix-assisted laser desorption/ionization time-of-flight mass spectrometry (MALDI-TOFMS) and its variant SELDI-TOFMS, and capillary zone electrophoresis (CZE) for proteome analysis have led to the identification of biomarkers that can be specifically applied in clinical diagnosis (Aebersold and Mann, 2003; Kann 2007; Simpson and Smith, 2005; Neubauer et al., 2007; Pusztai and Hess, 2004). A hierarchical cluster analysis of protein profiles in normal and malignant breast tissues has shown the ability of the proteomic biomarkers to differentiate between normal, benign, and different stages of breast cancer (Bertucci et al., 2006).

Tumor tissues as well as their microenvironment are the richest source of potential biomarkers. ER, PR, HER-2, BRCA1, Ki-67, and p53 are well-established invasive protein biomarkers that are in routine use (Ross et al., 2004). Investigational biomarkers under development include SMAR1, CUX, SATB1, cyclin D1, BTG3, mitosin, heat shock proteins, adhesion molecules, insulin-like growth factors, and plasminogen activators and inhibitors. Recent studies have identified and validated some more proteomic biomarkers for breast cancer. Elevated levels of galectin-3-binding protein, ALDH1A1, CK19, transferrin, transketolase, thymosin β4 and β10, enolase, vimentin, peroxiredoxin 5, Hsp 70, periostin precursor, RhoA, cathepsin D, and annexin have been reported in breast cancer patients (He et al., 2007). These could serve as promising candidates in guiding tumor classification and predicting response. Ou et al. (2008) identified and validated four novel, differentially expressed breast cancer biomarkers ANX1, CRAB, 6-phosphogluconolactonase (6PGL), and CAZ2 by integrative proteomic and gene expression mapping. Despite valuable sample source, there are limitations in tissue sampling due to high invasive procedures involved. This invites attention toward the protein profiling of body fluids (noninvasive procedures involved) to identify more specific biomarkers.

Circulating protein markers are widely accepted because they are easy to sample, readily accessible, reproducible, and sensitive than other markers (Van De Voorde et al., 2012). These include autoantibodies, tumor antigens, cytokeratins, tumor-secreted proteins, normal tissue, and plasma proteins digested by tumor proteases that are found in the serum and plasma (Malati, 2007). The circulating biomarkers that have been validated by protein profiling include RS/DJ-1, heat shock proteins, MUC1, CA 15-3, CEA, CA 27.29, MCA, MSA and CA 549, cytokeratins, HER-2/neu, p53, α1-acid glycoprotein 2, monocyte differentiation antigen CD14, biotinidase (BTD), glutathione peroxidase 3, HSP27, 14-3-3 sigma, afamin, apolipoprotein E, isoform 1 of inter-alpha trypsin inhibitor heavy chain H4 (ITIH4), alpha-2-macroglobulin, ceruloplasmin, and others (Perkins et al., 2003). NAF and ductal lavage fluid (DLF) are traditionally used biological samples for diagnosis of the breast cancer (Misek et al., 2011b). However, proteomic profiling of breast NAF and DLF biomarkers could help in identifying specific proteins as potential diagnostic or prognostic markers of breast cancer (Li et al., 2005). Currently available NAF and DLF biomarkers include GCDFP-15, apolipoprotein D (apoD), alpha1-acid glycoprotein (AAG), α-2-HS-glycoprotein, lipophilin b, beta-globin, hemopexin, and vitamin D–binding protein (Alexander et al., 2004; Teng et al., 2010). A panel of protein markers can reflect breast cancer complexity, thereby yielding improved sensitivity and specificity in early detection of the disease.

3.9 Glycobiomarkers

Glycosylation is one of the most important modifications of proteins and lipids and plays an important role in the regulation of many cellular events such as cell–cell and cell–substrate interactions, bacterial adhesion, membrane organization, cell immunogenicity, and protein targeting (Li and d'Anjou, 2009; Zhang and Chen, 2011). For example, sialyl-Lewisx (sLex) antigens are the ligands for selectins and are involved in the recruitment of leukocytes to lymphoid tissues and inflammation sites (Varki, 1994; Cazet et al., 2010).

Alteration in glycosylation is a common phenotypic change observed in cancer cells that mainly affects the outer part of glycans, leading to the expression of tumor-associated carbohydrate antigens (TACAs) (Wang, 2005; Cazet et al., 2010). For example, increased β1, six-branching or increase in sLe^x or sialyl-$Lewis^a$ (sLe^a) antigens or increased sialylation have been observed in *N*-linked and *O*-linked glycans present on cancer cells. These are usually associated with grade, invasion, metastasis, and poor prognosis (Wang, 2005). Alteration of glycosylation has been observed in a variety of cancers (Varki et al., 2009; Cazet et al., 2010). These modified glycoforms including glycoproteins, proteoglycans, and glycolipids may serve as the potential glycobiomarkers for the early detection of the disease (Kim et al., 2009a). The altered expression of glycoforms on cell surface or in the circulation has highlighted their role in cancer research (Drake et al., 2010). Currently, CA 15-3, CEA, and CA 27.29 are the most common serum glycoproteins with altered glycan profiles that are used as biomarkers for breast cancer (Meany and Chan, 2011). Alterations in the expression of glycosyltransferase (GT) genes result in change in glycosylation pattern that leads to overexpression of tumor-associated antigens sLe^x, s-Le^a and sialyl-Thomsen-nouvelle (sTn) on the surface of breast cancer cells (Ura et al., 1992; Narita et al., 1993; Soares et al., 1996). These are usually associated with poor prognosis and reduced overall survival of the patients (Miles et al., 1994).

Nakagoe et al. (2002) analyzed the expression of ABH/Lewis-related antigens immunohistochemically from breast cancer tissue samples as an independent prognostic factor of survival without clincopathological features of the primary tumor. Raval et al. (2003) evaluated alterations in serum levels of sialic acid forms, sialyltransferase, and sialoproteins from 225 breast carcinoma patients to investigate the potential clinical utility of these markers in diagnosis, prognosis, and treatment of breast carcinoma.

Saldova et al. (2002) observed the high levels of specific serum *N*-glycans containing sialyl Lewis x (sLe^x) epitopes (A2F1G1, A3F1G1, A4F1G1, and A4F2G2) from sera of 51 breast cancer patients were associated with CTCs that could provide a new noninvasive approach for prognosis and prediction. Moreover, glycobiomarkers are more stable, thereby making them more suitable for wide population screening (Saldova et al., 2010). Glycan profiling of human sera, blood, and tissue samples by MALDI FT-ICR, MALDI-TOF, electrospray ionization (ESI), and LC-MS/MS techniques is an important approach in the emerging potential field of glycobiomarkers (Neubauer et al., 2007).

3.10 Lipid Biomarkers

Lipids are the important components of our body and regulate various biological functions including energy metabolism and various signal transduction mechanisms (Simons and Toomre, 2000). They have been reported to participate in many human diseases including cancer (Chajès et al., 2011). Various studies have shown a direct association between lipids and incidence of breast cancer. Since altered lipid metabolism and profiling have shown a significant correlation with breast cancer risk, disease status, recurrence, and treatment outcome, lipidomics provides an opportunity to identify reliable lipid markers associated with breast cancer (McGrowder et al., 2011). Lipid profiling of cell extracts, body fluids, and biopsy specimens by using isotope labeling, thin-layer chromatography (TLC), high-performance liquid chromatography (HPLC), MS technology, matrix-assisted laser desorption ionization (MALDI), and electro-spray ionization (ESI) techniques has helped in isolation of lipid biomarkers for breast cancer (Wenk, 2005; Hou et al., 2008).

Lipid rafts are cholesterol-enriched, highly dynamic, heterogeneous microdomains of the cell membrane that regulate cell adhesion and membrane signaling through proteins located within these rafts (Simons and Toomre, 2000; Simons and Sampaio, 2011). Recent studies have shown critical role of lipid rafts in cancer cell adhesion and migration. The lipid molecules include fatty acids, triglycerides, cholesterol, phosphoglycerides, sphingomyelins, glycosphingolipids, ceramide, sphingosine, phosphate phosphatidylcholine (PC), phosphatidylethanolamine (PE), as well as lipoproteins including high-density lipoprotein (HDL), low-density lipoprotein (LDL), and very-low-density lipoprotein (VLDL). These could be used as potential biomarkers for prognosis, diagnosis, as well as treatment of cancer.

Shah et al. analyzed plasma lipid profile including cholesterol, high-density lipoprotein, low-density lipoprotein, very-low-density lipoprotein, and triglycerides of 70 healthy controls, 30 patients with benign breast disease (BBD), 125 untreated breast cancer patients, and 93 posttreatment follow-up samples by highly sensitive and specific spectrophotometric methods. They found a positive correlation between altered lipid profile levels and breast cancer risk (Shah et al., 2008).

Owiredu et al. investigated lipid profile in 100 breast cancer patients and 100 healthy controls. There was a significant increase in total cholesterol, triglyceride, and low-density lipoprotein (LDL-cholesterol) in the breast cancer patients compared to the controls, thereby suggesting that the alterations in lipid profile are associated with risk of developing breast cancer (Owiredu et al., 2009).

Analysis of breast tissue samples by immunohistochemistry, ultra-performance LC/MS, and other techniques is routinely used for the analysis of invasive lipid biomarkers. Hilvo et al. analyzed the global lipid profiles in 267 human breast cancer tissues. They observed the increased expression of palmitate-containing phosphatidylcholines in breast estrogen receptor–negative and grade 3 tumors that was associated with cancer progression and patient survival (Hilvo et al., 2011). Immunohistochemical analyses of lipid metabolism regulating genes acetyl-CoA carboxylase α (ACACA), elongation of very long chain fatty acid-like 1 (ELOVL1), fatty acid synthase (FASN), insulin-induced gene 1 (INSIG1), sterol regulatory element-binding protein cleavage-activating protein (SCAP), stearoyl-CoA desaturase (SCD), and thyroid hormone–responsive protein (THRSP) showed that they are highly expressed in clinical breast cancer samples (Hilvo et al., 2011). These findings suggest the diagnostic potential of these lipid makers that could provide early therapeutic options.

Borrelli et al. compared the serum concentrations of cholesterol, HDL-cholesterol, triglycerides, and total lipids of women having breast cancer with the patients having benign breast disease. The higher serum concentration of HDL-cholesterol was observed in breast cancer patients as compared to benign patients, whereas there was no difference observed in the serum concentration of total cholesterol, triglycerides, and total lipids between the two groups. Their results suggest that high serum HDL-cholesterol could be a biochemical index of increased breast cancer risk. They have also shown that the changes in the lipid profile could be associated with increased estrogen activity that is involved in the development of breast cancer (Borrelli et al., 1993). Thus, lipid profile is a promising biomarker for the early detection of breast cancer.

3.11 Metabolomic Biomarkers

Metabolomics includes profiling of the endogenous metabolites present in biological cells and tissues or shed into the body fluids such as serum, plasma, urine, cerebrospinal fluid, tears, saliva, and nipple aspirate fluid (Jordan et al., 2009; Serkova and Glunde, 2009). It may play an important role in identification of new prognostic and predictive markers associated with breast cancer progression (Denkert et al., 2012). The altered metabolic activities of cancer cells may generate wide range of metabolites that may help in distinguishing them from their healthy counterparts (Locasale et al., 2010). The analytical platforms used for metabolomic studies are based on nuclear magnetic resonance spectroscopy (NMR), mass spectroscopy or LC/MS, Fourier-transform infrared (FT-IR) spectrometry and ultra-performance liquid chromatography combined with mass spectroscopy (UPLC-MS) (Griffin and Schockcor, 2004).

Nam et al. proposed a systematic computational method for the identification of metabolic biomarkers in urine samples by selecting candidate biomarkers from altered genome-wide gene expression signatures of cancer cells. They have analyzed gene expression profiles in cancer cells and urine samples of 50 breast cancer patients and 50 healthy controls by this method. From the gene expression profiles, they found that nine metabolic pathways (pyrimidine, purine metabolism, valine, leucine and isoleucine, tyrosine metabolism, arachidonic acid metabolism, metabolism of xenobiotics, butanoate metabolism, tryptophan metabolism, and fatty acid metabolism) were altered. Out of these, four metabolic biomarkers that include homovanillate, 4-hydroxyphenylacetate, 5-hydroxy indoleacetate, and urea were found to be altered in breast cancer patients compared to their normal counterparts (Nam et al., 2009). Thus, metabolic markers from urine samples of cancer patients could help not only in discriminating them from their healthy control subjects but also in detecting the early stage of the disease.

Silva et al. studied the urinary metabolomic profile of 26 breast cancer patients and 21 healthy individuals with the aim of investigating the volatile organic metabolites (VOMs) as biomarkers in early diagnosis. They detected the presence of 79 VOMs, belonging to distinct chemical classes, in control as well as breast cancer groups. They observed a significant increase in the levels of (−)-4-carene, 3-heptanone, 1,2,4-trimethylbenzene, 2-methoxythiophene, and phenol, in VOMs of cancer patients compared to that of controls. They also identified the presence of dimethyl disulfide in lower amounts in cancer patients. Their study, thus, provided an evidence for the use of VOMs as valuable biomarkers for breast cancer detection (Silva et al., 2012).

3.12 Imaging Biomarkers

Imaging biomarkers play a key role in evaluating the efficacy, activity, and response of new candidate drugs and/or innovative therapeutic regimens that would improve clinical outcome (Silberman et al., 2012). Imaging biomarkers have the ability to assess the molecular events at an early stage and hence in predicting the treatment outcome (Moffat et al., 2006). Anatomic imaging modalities include mammography, planar x-ray, ultra sounds, CT, and magnetic resonance imaging (MRI) (Herranz and Ruibal, 2012). Evidences have suggested that diffusion-weighted (DW) and dynamic contrast-enhanced (DCE) MRI are reliable and quantitative measures implemented in clinical research to noninvasively predict the response in patients with breast cancer following neoadjuvant chemotherapy (Whitcher and Schmid, 2011). Xing et al. (2008) have proposed, quantified, and tested two MRI imaging biomarkers such as parenchyma volume and parenchyma enhancement for their ability to assess the breast cancer risk. MRI has also been shown to improve the detection of early breast cancers in patients with hereditary BRCA mutations (Saslow et al., 2007). However, a few disadvantages of these biomarkers include low specificity, limited sensitivity in detecting DCIS, association with false positive results, and their inability to determine accurate response to drugs.

Valuable contribution has been made by noninvasive molecular imaging techniques in clinical evaluation and targeted therapeutic interventions (Shankar, 2012). They help to visualize and quantify cellular and physiologic processes in vivo for accurate tumor staging, design individually suited therapies, assess the drug response, and early detection of disease recurrence (Pouliot et al., 2009). Positron emission tomography (PET), scintimammography (SMM), electrical impedance tomography (EIT), T-scan electrical impedance imaging, and galactography are the recent noninvasive molecular imaging tools. Among these, PET molecular imaging gained widespread acceptance for the diagnosis, staging as well as management of a variety of malignancies, including breast cancer. Molecules related to tumor microenvironment, angiogenesis, hypoxia, metabolisms, apoptosis, proliferation, tumor receptors, and transport proteins are the PET imaging molecular biomarkers (Penuelas et al., 2012).

FDG-PET is a primary PET radioactive tracer that includes glucose analogs (FDG) as biomarkers for initial diagnosis and staging of primary breast cancer (Rosen et al., 2007). It accurately differentiates cancerous tissue from its benign counterpart based on the glycolysis rate and glucose avidity of malignant cells (Quon and Gambhir, 2005). FDG PET along with CT is another biomarker that contributes in defining the extent of the disease with improved sensitivity, early assessment of therapeutic response, as well as relapse in patients with advanced tumors (Rosen et al., 2007).

3′-Deoxy-3′-[18F] fluorothymidine (18FLT-PET) is a clinically used biomarker for in vivo imaging of cell proliferation that could predict lesion response with good sensitivity after initiating chemotherapy. Studies have shown that 18FLT-PET positively correlates with Ki67, a proliferation marker in cancer tissues (Vesselle et al., 2002; Shah et al., 2009; Richard et al., 2011).

Apoptosis imaging marker [F-18]–labeled annexin V is widely studied agent for in vivo study to assess apoptosis. Studies have shown the potential applications of [F-18]-labeled annexin V as imaging marker for early response to therapy in cancer, acute cerebral and myocardial ischemic injury and infarction, immune-mediated inflammatory disease, and transplant rejection (Toretsky et al., 2004; Li et al., 2008).

16α-[18F]-fluoro-17β-estradiol (18F-FES-PET) is a biomarker that noninvasively assesses the molecular information of ER expression in both primary and tumor metastasis cases and helps in the therapeutic management and prognostic evaluation (Tsuchida et al., 2007).

TABLE 3.12

Imaging Biomarkers for Breast Cancer

Imaging Biomarker	Uses	References
FDG-PET	Initial diagnosis of primary breast cancer and the staging of axillary lymph nodes	Rosen et al. (2007)
18FLT-PET	In vivo imaging of cell proliferation	Shah et al. (2009)
[F-18]-labeled annexin V	Apoptosis imaging marker	Li et al. (2008)
18F-FES-PET	Detection of ER expression in primary and metastasis breast cancer	Tsuchida et al. (2007)
18 FMISO-PET	Imaging biomarker for angiogenesis	Yoo et al. (2005)

Imaging biomarker [18F] fluoromisonidazole (18 FMISO-PET) is used to image hypoxia generated by the tumors, thereby improving the diagnostic understanding and providing information regarding antiangiogenic therapy in breast cancer patients (Penuelas et al., 2012).

N-[11C] methyl-choline (11C-choline) imaging biomarker has been used to assess the altered choline metabolism in breast cancer (Contractor et al., 2011). 11C/99m Tc-methionine amino acid–based radiotracer is used to detect breast cancer (Sharma et al., 2009). ^{99m}Tc-NC100692 and ^{18}F-galacto-RGD are radiolabeled RGD peptides (peptide sequence that consists of arginine–glycine–aspartic acid) that are used for the breast cancer imaging (Axelsson et al., 2010). Apart from these, some other radioactive tracers that are used for the breast cancer imaging include ^{99m}Tc-methylene diphosphonate, ^{99m}Tc-Pentavalent DMSA, ^{18}F-fluoride, ^{18}F-fluciclatide, and Tc-99m sestamibi, which offer great promise in breast cancer patients (Massardo et al., 2005; Doot et al., 2010; Tomasi et al., 2011). Table 3.12 enlists various imaging biomarkers used for breast cancer detection.

3.13 Integrative Omics–Based Molecular Markers for Early Diagnosis, Prognosis, and Therapy

Genomics, transcriptomics, proteomics, epigenomics, lipidomics, metabolomics, PG, and bioinformatics are the platforms for identification of novel cancer biomarkers (Sikaroodi et al., 2010; Palsson and Zengler, 2010) (Figure 3.6). All these approaches play an important role in oncology research with differing strengths and limitations. Integration of all these *omics-based approaches* would lead to a better understanding of the disease and would help in discovery and initial characterization of candidate biomarkers for cancer staging, prediction of recurrence, prognosis, as well as treatment selection.

Cancer is now recognized as systems dysfunction of cellular regulatory pathways caused due to combination of environmental/lifestyle-related factors and genetic defects such as somatic or germline mutations, SNPs, copy number alternations, and epigenetic modifications (Shimokawa et al., 2010). Recent developments in high-throughput omic-based technologies have shifted the focus from identification of genes and proteins to mapping the networks of interactions that take place among them (Zhang and Chen, 2011). Thus, detailed clinical/environmental information together with the molecular

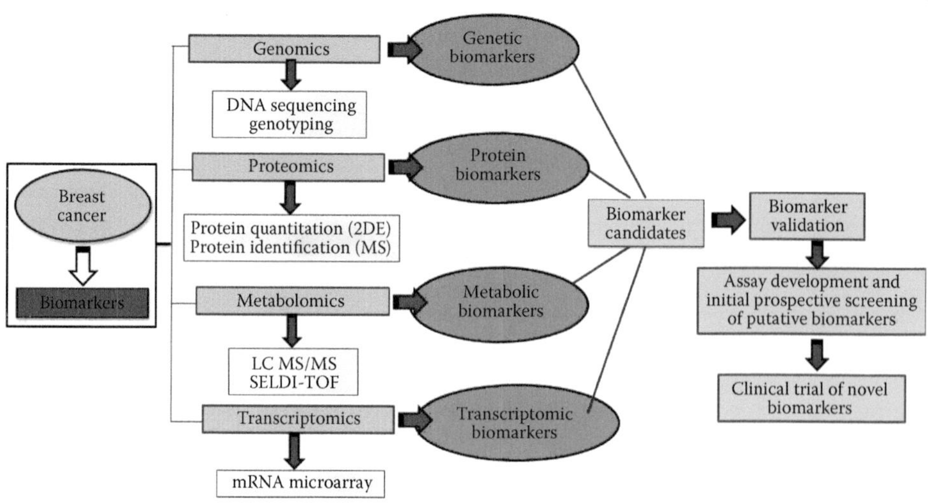

FIGURE 3.6
Integrative omics-based approaches for identifying biomarkers for early diagnosis of breast cancer. Omic-based approaches include genomics, proteomics, metabolomics, and transcriptomics that are platforms for identification of novel and breast cancer–specific biomarker.

networks is required to elucidate the process of carcinogenesis. Recently, the field of systems biology is gaining significance in elucidation of complex molecular interactions within a cell by combining computational, engineering, and physical analyses along with biological and medical inputs (Wang et al., 2010). The effectiveness of such network-based approaches in the identification of multiple disease markers has been demonstrated in human breast cancer (Pujana et al., 2007). Pujana et al. have identified genes through network modeling strategy that could be potentially associated with higher risk of developing breast cancer. They started with four known tumor suppressor genes of breast cancer (ATM, BRCA1, BRCA2, and CHEK2), and by combining gene expression profiles with functional genomic and proteomic data from various species, they could generate a network containing 118 genes linked by 866 potential functional associations (Pujana et al., 2007). Barh et al. have recently shown the presence of more than one cross-talking signaling pathways and targets in most of the breast cancer cases by combining various omics data for breast cancer with integrative bioinformatics approach. They have shown the association between various transcription factors, miRNAs, fetal oncogenes, and pluripotent stem cell factors in the regulation of tumorigenesis. The identified transcription factors and miRNAs are differentially expressed in breast cancer and thus have been proposed to be used as early diagnostic and prognostic markers (Barh et al., 2013).

Various open-access as well as commercial tools such as Georgetown Database of Cancer (G-DOC), Oncomine, ArrayExpress, the Stanford Microarray Database, the Gene Expression Omnibus, integrated clinical omics database (iCOD), International Cancer Genome Consortium (ICGC), and The Cancer Genome Atlas (TCGA) have been developed for storage, analysis, and interpretation of omics-based data. G-DOC is an open-access tool that allows physicians, scientists, and translational researchers to mine and analyze a variety of *omics* data (Madhavan et al., 2011). This would help basic and clinical research through integration of patient characteristics and clinical outcome data with various high-throughput research data. It mainly provides data related to mRNA and miRNA expression, CNV, and metabolite MS (Madhavan et al., 2011). At present, G-DOC contains data from 24 different studies that include more than 3600 breast cancer patients and around 4400 biospecimens (Georegetown, Lombardi Comprehensive Cancer Center 2013). Oncomine is another microarray database and web-based data mining platform that provides data related to differentially expressed genes across multiple microarray experiments from various cancers (Rhodes et al., 2007). Unlike G-DOC, Oncomine provides only transcriptome data, of which majority of datasets are not openly accessible. Array Express, Stanford Microarray Database, and the Gene Expression Omnibus repositories provide cancer microarray data but do not allow the user to efficiently mine and analyze the data (Sherlock et al., 2001; Edgar et al., 2002; Rocca-Serra et al., 2003). The other two agencies, ICGC and TCGA, contain omics (genomic) data that are openly accessible and allow us to understand the molecular mechanisms underlying cancer (Zang et al., 2011). The iCOD includes not only molecular omics data such as comparative genomic hybridization (CGH) and gene expression profiles but also consists clinical information that includes clinical manifestations, medical images (CT, x-ray, ultrasounds, etc.), laboratory tests, drug history, pathological findings, and even lifestyle/environmental information (Shimokawa et al., 2010).

3.13.1 Challenges in Translation of Cancer Omics Findings

The increased availability of omics data poses new challenges both for the data management and analysis (Zhang et al., 2012). The major challenge, at bioinformatics level, for example, arises during integration of a transcriptomics dataset with a proteomics dataset wherein it becomes difficult to map transcript identifiers to protein identifiers. For example, the integration of transcriptional and translational data in prokaryotic and some lower eukaryotic organisms becomes easier as per one gene one protein hypothesis. However, in higher eukaryotes, it becomes difficult to integrate the two datasets because the one gene one protein hypothesis does not stand true. In them, a single gene encodes multiple transcripts by means of alternative splicing; transcripts can be translated into multiple protein isoforms and posttranslational modifications are also involved. The problem becomes even more complex when one tries to integrate a transcriptomics or proteomics dataset with a metabolomic, glycomic, or lipidomic dataset (Choi and Pavelka, 2011). However, such challenges could be overcome by mapping the enzymes responsible for synthesis or chemical conversion of metabolites with the help of metabolic networks as provided by Kyoto encyclopedia of genes and genomes (KEGG) (Kanehisa and Goto, 2000) or Reactome (Joshi-Tope et al., 2005). Besides, the systems biology markup language (SBML) is one of the successful efforts to develop a unified language to represent complex models of interacting biological molecules (Hucka et al., 2003). However, only few genes encode metabolic enzymes, the rest being structural, regulatory, or signal transduction proteins (Choi and Pavelka, 2011). Thus, it becomes a challenge for the integrative omics data analysis methods to deal with molecules that cannot be directly mapped between the two types of datasets.

Lack of well-defined data standards and standardized nomenclature across different data repositories makes the retrieval and assembly of integrated datasets difficult.

Semantic Web technologies offer an immediate integration of data, which can be easily queried across different databases (Choi and Pavelka, 2011). They also allow a precise characterization of the *semantics* of the data, that is, the integration between represented entities and their relations. However, use of such technology depends upon implementation by developers of primary omics databases.

Due to complexity of the available models from multilayered omics data, statistical analysis becomes a big challenge (Ideker et al., 2011). Thus, the models should be established in a way that would ensure highly sensitive, specific, and reproducible results. Other practical challenges include lack of availability of well-defined, clinically characterized cohorts for biomarker evaluation along with information related to collection, handling, and storage of specimens. These challenges can be efficiently overcome by integrative computational methods that include development of new designs for databases, new software, and workflows for integration of heterogeneously distributed data, well-defined mathematical and statistical tools, and analytical methods to identify complex signals in different datasets and upgradation of standards for generating, maintaining, and sharing data. This would ultimately help in identification of authentic omics-based biomarkers that would help in early diagnosis and prognosis of breast cancer.

3.14 Ethnic-Specific Markers

Human kallikreins, hK2 and hK3, the members of human kallikrein family, are the serine proteases that are downregulated in breast cancer (Borgoño et al., 2004). hK3 is also known as PSA and is a marker of breast as well as prostate cancer (Becker et al., 2001). hK2 and hK3 share significant homology at both DNA and protein levels, and hK2 may also regulate the activity of hK3 (Yousef and Diamandis, 2001). Studies have shown that systemic progesterone levels, which appear to upregulate hK3, are significantly influenced by ethnicity (Sauter et al., 2002). Thus, Sauter et al. analyzed the expression of hK2/hK3 in NAF collected from 285 (244 white and 41 black) women who were categorized into risk groups, with no risk factors, having a history of first-degree relative with breast cancer, history of cancer in the breast contralateral to that being studied, biopsy-proven atypical hyperplasia (AH), biopsy-proven LCIS, biopsy-proven DCIS, or biopsy-proven invasive carcinoma. They found that the expression of hK2 and hK3 and the ratio of hK2/hK3 were lower in breast cancer patients than in normal subjects. Moreover, the expression of hK2 and hK3 was significantly lower in black than in white population and was higher in pre- than in postmenopausal whites. hK3 level was lower in postmenopausal women with breast cancer, regardless of ethnicity (Sauter et al., 2002).

Recent study by Liang et al. evaluated the ethnic-specific expression of 10 differentially expressed hydrophobic proteins from breast cancer patients of three different ethnicities, that is, Chinese, Malay, and Indian. They found significantly elevated expression levels of four hydrophobic proteins that include peroxiredoxin-2, heat shock protein 60, protein disulfide isomerase, and calreticulin in cancerous tissues as compared with the normal controls. They concluded that these four hydrophobic proteins may serve as ethnic-related potential markers for Chinese, Malay, and Indian cohorts (Liang et al., 2010).

3.15 Awards Won in Breast Cancer Research is Represented in Table 3.13

TABLE 3.13

List of Scientists Who Have Won Awards in Breast Cancer Research

Scientist Name	Won Research in This Field	Award Presented by	Year
Douglas Easton	• Establishment of the breast cancer lineage consortium. • Elucidated the genetic epidemiology of BRCA1 and BRCA2, which has provided definitive evidence for the localization of a breast cancer susceptibility locus on BRCA1 and provided the first estimates of the breast and ovarian cancer risks in BRCA1 mutation carriers.	Outstanding investigator award in breast cancer research funded by Komen for the cure	2008
Dr. Joan Massague	• Defined the mechanisms by which signals initiated by transforming growth factor-b (TGF-b) are conveyed from their receptors on the cell membrane to the nucleus to affect cell proliferation, differentiation, and cancer. • In his studies, he identified genes that define metastatic tissue tropism, providing a firm genetic basis for understanding the ability of breast cancer cells to colonize either the lung or bone.	AACR distinguished lectureship in breast cancer research	2009
Elizabeth H. Blackburn	• Discovered how chromosomes are protected by telomeres and the enzyme telomerase. • Blackburn co-discovered telomerase, the enzyme that replenishes the telomere.	Nobel Prize in physiology or medicine	2009
Charles M. Perou	• His seminal work has shown that breast cancer is not a single disease, but instead, represents a series of diseases that include the more favorable prognosis luminal A subtype and multiple worse prognosis subtypes including the luminal B, HER2 positive (HER2+), basal-like, and claudin-low groups.	AACR outstanding investigator award for breast cancer	2009
Klaus Pantel	• The pioneer work of Prof. Pantel in the field of cancer micometastasis and CTCs is reflected by more than 300 publications in excellent high-ranking biomedical and scientific journals (including NEJM, Lancet, Nature Journals, PNAS, JCO, JNCI, and Cancer Res.) and has been awarded recently.	AACR outstanding investigator award 2010, German cancer award 2010, ERC advanced investigator grant 2011	2010
Ramon E. Parsons	• Dr. Parsons has made the seminal discovery of the PTEN tumor suppressor and showed that PTEN was inactivated by mutation in a wide variety of human malignancies including breast cancer and in the rare breast cancer predisposition syndrome, and Cowden disease.	AACR outstanding investigator award for breast cancer research	2011

3.16 Various Test Panels Commercially Available with High Specificity and Sensitivity

Biomarkers can promise outstanding prediction efficiency for the early detection of breast cancer, thereby enabling better patient therapy (Bhatt et al., 2010). A wide number of breast cancer diagnostic kits are readily available in the market, most of which rely on the gene expression profiles of the prognostic biomarkers (Ross et al., 2008). Some of the multigenic tests developed for breast cancer detection include Oncotype Dx, Theros Breast Cancer Index, Breast Bioclassifier, Celera Metastatic Score, eXagen, Mammostrat, ProEXTMBr, MammaPrint, MapQuant Dx, Breast Lymph Node (BLN) Assay, Invasive Gene Signature, Wound Response Indicator, Breast Cancer Gene Expression Ratio, 2-gene ratio, H/I or HOXB13/IL17BR, and Rotterdam Signature 76-Gene Panel (Pusztai, 2008) (Table 3.14). Of the aforementioned tests, the Oncotype DX assay is the most widely used one (Cronin et al., 2007). More than 135,000 tests have been performed by using this kit (Genomic Health Annual report, 2009). Besides the aforementioned tests, the test called *DirectHit*™ is a pharmacodiagnostic test that helps to determine the tumor sensitivity or resistance to drug regimens recommended for the treatment of breast cancer. It provides information about the presence of certain proteins in the tumor that helps to prescribe the most effective drug treatment. The presence of these proteins may be related to the mechanism of action of particular drugs. DirectHit™ is the only test of its kind that may be used to recommend effective treatment for both hormonal and chemotherapeutic drugs (http://directhittest.com/providers.html).

3.17 Recommended Tests/Panels in Combination with/without Imaging for Early Diagnosis of Breast Cancer

The American Cancer Society recommends the use of mammograms, MRI, clinical breast exams, and breast self-examination for early detection that may help in reduction of mortality. Table 3.15 describes various tests alone or in combination along with rationale that are used in early breast cancer detection.

3.18 Advantages and Challenges in Developing Molecular Biomarkers for Early Detection, Prognosis, and Therapy

Biomarkers provide a dynamic and powerful approach for understanding the biology of cancer. They are widely used in the risk assessment, diagnosis, prognosis, and monitoring of cancer progression and may contribute in understanding of the pathophysiology of the disease (Bhatt et al., 2010). Biomarkers play an important role in predicting the response of the patients to treatment, to guess the efficacy and safety of novel therapeutic agents, in determining the drug doses and in the development of more effective and disease-specific chemotherapeutic drugs with minimal undesired systemic toxicity (Morey et al., 2012). A panel of biomarkers may provide higher predictive power and may improve the

TABLE 3.14

Various Test Panels Commercially Available with Specificity and Sensitivity

Name	Description	Specificity (%)	Sensitivity (%)	References
Oncotype Dx	It is used to diagnose the patients with early-stage (stage I or II), node-negative, estrogen receptor–positive (ER+) invasive breast cancer.	68–93	48–73	Cronin et al. (2007)
Theros H/I℠ & MGI℠	This molecular diagnostic test is combination of two gene indexes, Theros H/I℠ and Theros MGI℠, that measures the ratio of HOXB13:IL17BR gene expression as a predictor of clinical outcome for breast cancer patients treated with tamoxifen. Theros MGI℠ is an additional test that uses a five-gene expression index to stratify ER+ breast cancer patients into high or low risk of recurrence by reclassifying tumors and also provides information about the tumor grade, proliferative status, sensitivity, or resistance to chemotherapy.	67	63	Ma et al. (2008)
Breast Bioclassifier™	It is a 55-gene qRTPCR assay that provides information about the biological subtype (luminal A, luminal B, HER2, and basal) of tumor and provides a risk score that enables physicians to make treatment decisions for the patients.	79–64	44	Perreard et al. (2006)
Celera Metastatic Score™	It is a 14-gene multiplex RT-PCR test that provides information about the tumor grade and quantifies the risk for metastasis for variable time periods in breast cancer patients.	94	88	Garber (2004)
CellSearch™	It is a simple blood test that captures and assesses CTCs to determine the prognosis of patients with metastatic disease.	93–99	27–57	Riethdorf et al. (2007)
eXagen™	It is a prognostic assay proposed for estrogen receptor/progesterone receptor positive (ER/PR+) and ER/PR− patients.	92	87	Ross et al. (2008)
Mammostrat	The assay is used for calculating risk index score for breast cancer patients. The higher the risk index score, the more likely is the cancer recurrence.	93	48	Bartlett et al. (2010)
ProEXTMBr	Score ≥2 associated with disease relapse in LN− and LN+ breast cancer patients.	—	—	Whitehead et al. (2004)
MammaPrint	It is a molecular diagnostic tool of 70-gene signature that is used for risk assessment in patients with node-negative breast cancer. It is recommended for patients upto 60 years with stage 1 or 2, lymph node-negative invasive breast cancer.	73	91	Buyse et al. (2006)

(Continued)

TABLE 3.14 (*CONTINUED*)

Various Test Panels Commercially Available with Specificity and Sensitivity

Name	Description	Specificity (%)	Sensitivity (%)	References
MapQuant Dx™	It is a gene expression assay used to diagnose the patients with estrogen receptor positive, grade II breast cancer. The test provides information about tumor grade and tumor aggressiveness.	42–50	68–90	Sotiriou et al. (2006)
BLN assay	The assay detects the presence of breast tumor metastasis in lymph nodes by detection of gene expression markers present in breast tissue but not in the nodal tissue.	71.4–83.9	80–98.1	Mansel et al. (2009)
Invasive gene signature	Risk prediction for death and metastasis in breast cancer.	100	96	Liu et al. (2007)
Wound response indicator	Here the set of genes represents the wound-healing response, provides improved risk prediction for death and metastasis.	48	93	Chang et al. (2005)
DirectHit™	It provides information about the presence of certain proteins in the tumor that helps to prescribe the most effective drug treatment for both hormonal and chemotherapeutic drugs.	87–91a		http://directhittest.com/providers.html
Rotterdam Signature 76-Gene Panel	The kit is used to evaluate estrogen-receptor positive as well as estrogen-receptor-negative samples.	48	93	Oakman et al. (2009), Pusztai (2008)
HERmark™ assay	Measures total HER2 expression and HER2 homodimers.	—	—	Larson et al. (2010)
OncoVue® Test	Combines the SNP patterns of 117 genes and personal history to predict breast cancer risk.	99.9a		Ralph et al. (2007), http://www.intergenetics.com/
GeneSearch™ breast lymph node	Detection of gene expression markers mammaglobin and cytokeratin 19 via qRT-PCR. Detects breast tumor cell metastasis in lymph nodes.	97.4	88.9	Viale et al. (2005), Sun et al. (2011)
DiaGenic BCtect®	Analyzes gene expression signatures from peripheral blood.	73	72	Imbeaud et al. (2005), Tobin et al. (2007)

[a] Accuracy combined values of specificity and sensitivity.

statistical performance compared with individual biomarkers (Tesch et al., 2010). They help in accurate detection of the presence of cancer, thereby resulting in fewer false positive and negative tests (Mayeux, 2004). They are powerful tools for the identification of potential drug targets and adapting therapies for individual needs by allowing the selection of patients who are most likely to respond or react adversely to a particular treatment (Tesch et al., 2010). Biomarker discovery is a boon for the medical and pharmaceutical communities as well as for the oncology researchers (Mayeux, 2004).

Despite all the potential benefits of biomarkers in cancer diagnosis, prognosis, and therapy, several biological as well as economical challenges are faced by the research and medical communities in the development of new biomarkers. Biological challenges such

TABLE 3.15

Recommended Tests/Panels in Combination along with Their Rationale

Categories of Women at Risk	Age (Year)	Test[a]	Screening Intervals	Rationale
Women at average risk	20	BSE	Monthly	The chance of breast cancer occurrence is very low for women in their 20s and gradually increases with age.
	20–30	CBE and mammography	Every 3 years	The chance of breast cancer occurrence is very low for women in their 20s and gradually increases with age.
	40	Mammography	Annually	Significant reduction in mortality due to mammography screening.
Women at high risk >20% lifetime risk	45–55	MRI and mammography	Annually	MRI is more sensitive than mammograms, but may miss some cancers that a mammogram would detect.
Women at moderately increased risk 15%–20% lifetime risk	<40	Mammography and/or MRI	Annually	MRI may miss some cancers that a mammogram would detect.
Women at low risk <15% lifetime risk	>60	Mammography	Annually	Significant reduction in mortality due to mammography screening.

Source: American Cancer Society last revised: August 30, 2012.

[a] BSE, breast self-examination; CBE, clinical breast exam; MRI, magnetic resonance imaging.

as cancer progression, natural history, heterogeneity of the disease, and biomarker performance are the barriers in biomarker development (Bensalah et al., 2008). One of the major challenges of biomarker development in clinical domain is the translation of the knowledge gained through animal studies to humans (Deyati et al., 2013). Although a number of biomarkers are available for cancer diagnosis and detection, none of them have been found to achieve 100% sensitivity and specificity (Bensalah et al., 2008). Moreover, development and validation of biomarkers through clinical evidence are time consuming, labor intensive, and financially challenging (Tesch et al., 2010). Another major drawback for the development of biomarkers is the limited availability of sufficient number of good quality samples for evaluation. Besides, the normal clinical range of these biomarkers is difficult to establish and is possibly associated with laboratory errors (Tworoger and Hankinson, 2006; Kotsopoulos, 2011). Some other drawbacks include nonuniform preparation and storage of sample, sample heterogeneity, as well as cost of analysis (Camillo et al., 2012).

3.19 Market and Market Players of the Molecular Biomarkers for Early Diagnosis, Prognosis, and Therapy

The worldwide market of biomarkers is increasing with several new companies coming into the scenario. The popularity and wide use of biomarkers in drug discovery, for example, use in medical areas such as cancer research, are highly increasing its demand. Moreover, the understanding of the importance of biomarkers in the early detection as well as treatment of cancer has boosted the growth of this market to a large extent. Table 3.16 enlists various market players as well as the gene signature kits commercially available and under development for breast cancer.

TABLE 3.16

Market and Market Players of the Molecular Biomarkers

Company	Kit Name	Available	Sample[a]	Technique[b]	Diagnostic Aim
Genomic Health	Oncotype Dx	USA	FFP	Q-RT-PCR	Prognosis, recurrence after tamoxifen therapy
Biotheranostics	Theros Breast Cancer Index	USA	FFP	Q-RT-PCR	Prognosis, recurrence after endocrine therapy
ARUP	Breast Bioclassifier	USA	FFP	RT-PCR	Prognosis
Applera	Celera Metastatic score	USA	FFP	RT-PCR	Prognosis, recurrence after tamoxifen therapy
eXagen diagnostics	eXagenBC	USA	FFP	FISH	Prognosis
Applied genomics	Mammostrat	USA	—	IHC	Prognosis
TriPath	ProEXTMBr	USA	—	IHC	Prognosis
Agendia	MammaPrint	USA	F/F	Microarray	Prognosis in patients over 61 years
Ipsoggen	MapQuant Dx	EU	F/F	Microarray	Prognosis
GeneSearch Veridex	BLN Assay	UK	F/F	Microarray	Intraoperative metastasis Identification
bioTheranostics	HOXB13/IL17BR (H/I) ratio	USA	FFP	IHC	Prognosis and diagnosis
Veridex	CellSearch™	USA	Blood	IS/IF	Risk stratification
Onco Med Pharmaceuticals	Invasive Gene Signature	CA	F/F	Microarray	Prognosis
Not commercialized	Wound response Indicator	—	F/F	Microarray	Prognosis
Veridex	Rotterdam Signature 76-Gene Panel)	USA	F/F	Microarray	To predict prognosis of breast cancer recurrence
Nuvera Biosciences	NuvoSelect™	USA	F/F	Microarray	Prognosis and response to therapy
In development	ARUP bioclassifier	—	FFPE	RT-PCR	Multigene predictors for breast cancer
Not commercialized	Sorlie-Perou classifier	—	F/F	Microarray	Breast cancer prediction
Roche Diagnostics/ Merck Medco/Lab	Roche AmpliChip (cytochrome P450 CYP2D6)	USA	F/F	Microarray	To study the response of tamoxifen in breast cancer patients

[a] F/F, fresh/frozen; FFP, formalin-fixed paraffin-embedded.

[b] IHC, immunohistochemistry; FISH, fish fluorescent in situ hybridization; IS/IF, immunostaining/immunofluorescence; Q-RT-PCR, quantitative real-time polymerase chain reaction; RT-PCR, reverse transcriptase-polymerase chain reaction.

3.20 Patent Information of Molecular Markers/Tests for Invasive, Noninvasive, Early Diagnostic, Prognostic, and Therapeutic Aspects Are Represented in Table 3.17

TABLE 3.17

List of the Patents of Molecular Markers/Tests and Methods for Early Diagnostic, Prognostic, and Therapeutics for Breast Cancer

Year	Application No.	Title of the Patent	Inventors	Description
2002	US 0137064	Id-1 and Id-2 genes and products as diagnostic and prognostic markers and therapeutic targets for the treatment of breast cancer and other types of carcinoma	Pierreyves D et al.	Concerns with the use of Id-1 and/or Id-2 genes or Id-1 and/or Id-2 products as diagnostic markers for diagnosis, prognosis, and treatment of breast cancer and other types of cancers.
2003	EP 0785216	Chromosome 13–linked breast cancer susceptibility gene BRCA2	Sean VT et al.	This invention relates to germline mutations in the BRCA2 gene, which can be used in the diagnosis of predisposition to breast cancer.
2004	US 6762020	Methods of diagnosing breast cancer	David HM et al.	The invention relates to the identification of expression profiles and the nucleic acids and their use in diagnosis and prognosis of breast cancer. The invention further relates to methods for identifying and using candidate agents and/or targets that modulate breast cancer.
2004	US 6737040	Method and antibody for imaging breast cancer	Yongming S et al.	This invention relates, in part, to newly developed assays for detecting, diagnosing, monitoring, staging, prognosticating, imaging, and treating cancers, particularly breast cancer.
2004	US 6730477	Method of diagnosing, monitoring, and staging breast cancer	Yongming S et al.	This invention relates to newly developed assays for detecting, diagnosing, monitoring, staging, prognosticating, imaging, and treating breast cancer.
2004	US 6780586	Methods of diagnosing breast cancer	Kurt CG et al.	The invention relates to the identification of expression profiles and the nucleic acids involved in breast cancer, and their use in diagnosis and prognosis of breast cancer.
2005	WO 083429	Breast cancer prognostics	Yixin W	This invention relates to breast cancer patient prognosis based on the gene expression profiles of patient biological samples.
2006	WO 015312	Prognosis of breast cancer patients	Hongyue DAI et al.	Present invention relates to the identification of marker genes useful in the diagnosis and prognosis of breast cancer.
2007	US 7306910	Breast cancer prognostics	Yixin W	Invention is a method of assessing the recurrence or metastasis of breast cancer in a patient diagnosed with or treated for breast cancer.

(Continued)

TABLE 3.17 (*CONTINUED*)

List of the Patents of Molecular Markers/Tests and Methods for Early Diagnostic, Prognostic, and Therapeutics for Breast Cancer

Year	Application No.	Title of the Patent	Inventors	Description
2007	US 0054271	Gene expression in breast cancer	Kornelia P et al.	The invention features nucleic acids encoding proteins that are expressed at a higher or a lower level in breast cancer cells. This invention relates to methods of diagnosing and treating breast cancers of various grades and stages.
2007	US 7229770	YKL-40 as a marker and prognostic indicator for cancers	Paul AP et al.	This invention is directed to assays for the detection and quantitation of molecules and fragments of YKL-40 whereby serum levels of YKL-40 are indicative of the presence and/or prognosis of cancer including breast cancer.
2008	US 7419785	Methods and compositions in breast cancer diagnosis and therapeutics	Suzanne F et al.	The present invention is directed to the determination of susceptibility to breast cancer and the diagnosis of invasive breast cancer.
2008	WO 132167	Diagnostic, prognostic, and/or predictive indicators of breast cancer	O'driscoll L et al.	The invention relates to a novel panel of mRNAs that have potential as diagnostic, prognostic, and/or predictive indicators and novel therapeutic targets of breast cancer.
2009	WO 074364	Novel prognostic breast cancer marker	Edgar D et al.	This invention relates to the epigenetic silencing of the DKK3 gene in breast cancers, and the uses of this marker in the prognosis, diagnosis, and selection of appropriate treatments against breast cancer.
2009	US 0239763	Markers for breast cancer	Cox DG et al.	Methods of diagnosing, prognosing, and treating breast cancer are provided.
2009	WO 138130	Breast cancer prognostics	Stocksund UM et al.	The present invention generally relates to breast cancer prognostics, and in particular to molecular markers having prognostic value and uses thereof.
2009	US 7504214	Predicting outcome with tamoxifen in breast cancer	Mark EG et al.	The invention relates to the identification and use of gene expression profiles, or patterns, with clinical relevance to the treatment of breast cancer using tamoxifen.
2009	WO 108917	Markers for improved detection of breast cancer	Herman J et al.	The present invention relates to the identification of a cell proliferative disorder of breast by determining aberrant DNA methylation patterns of particular genes in breast cancer and precancer.
2009	US 0092973	Grading of breast cancer	Mark EG et al.	The invention relates to the identification and use of gene expression profiles, or patterns used to identify different grades of breast cancer within and between stages thereof.
2010	US 7642050	Method for predicting responsiveness of breast cancer to antiestrogen therapy	Nevalainen MT et al.	The application relates to the use of activated Stat5 for diagnosing and monitoring cancer and predicting the prognosis of breast cancer patients and the outcome of cancer therapies.

(*Continued*)

TABLE 3.17 (*CONTINUED*)

List of the Patents of Molecular Markers/Tests and Methods for Early Diagnostic, Prognostic, and Therapeutics for Breast Cancer

Year	Application No.	Title of the Patent	Inventors	Description
2010	US 7695915	Molecular prognostic signature for predicting breast cancer distant metastasis, and uses thereof	Lau K et al.	The present invention relates to a unique 14-gene molecular prognostic signature for prognosis of breast cancer metastasis.
2010	US 0105087	Low-molecular-weight (LMW) peptides as early biomarkers for breast cancer	Petricoin EF et al.	The LMW peptides have been discovered that are useful in detecting breast cancer during its early stages.
2011	US 0015092	Markers for breast cancer	Cox DG et al.	Present invention provided the methods and systems and kits for diagnosis, prognosis, and treatment of breast cancer.
2011	US 0307427	Molecular markers predicting response to adjuvant therapy, or disease progression, in breast cancer	Linke S et al.	The present invention concerns a method for the prediction of response to adjuvant therapy or disease progression, in breast cancer and a kit consisting of a panel of antibodies the binding of which with breast cancer tumor samples has been correlated with breast cancer treatment outcome or patient prognosis.
2011	US 0251082	Biomarkers for breast cancer	Hong-lin Chou C et al.	The present invention uses two-dimensional differential gel electrophoresis gel (2D-DIGE) and mass spectrum techniques to identify breast cancer biomarkers from various stages of breast cancer. The invention aids in developing proteins identified as useful diagnostic and therapeutic candidates on breast cancer research.
2011	US 0144198	Breast cancer prognostics	Uhlén M et al.	The present invention provides new methods, uses, and means for breast cancer prognostics.
2011	US 7879614	Methods for detection of breast cancer	Krepinsky JJ et al.	The invention relates to a simple screening test for neoplasia or breast cancer to detect breast cancer marker in breast fluid.
2011	US 0217297	Methods for classifying and treating breast cancers	Kao K et al.	The present invention relates to a method of treating a breast cancer in a subject, comprising determining the molecular subtype of the breast cancer in the subject and administering to the subject a therapy that is effective for treating the molecular subtype of the breast cancer.
2011	US 7955848	MicroRNA biomarkers for human breast and lung cancer	Dmitrovsky E et al.	The present invention relates to novel molecular markers for diagnosis and classification of human breast cancer and lung cancer.
2011	WO 133770	Salivary protein markers for detection of breast cancer	Streckfus CF et al.	This invention relates to a method of diagnosing a patient's risk of breast cancer comprises measuring the protein marker from saliva sample of the patient.

(*Continued*)

TABLE 3.17 (*CONTINUED*)

List of the Patents of Molecular Markers/Tests and Methods for Early Diagnostic, Prognostic, and Therapeutics for Breast Cancer

Year	Application No.	Title of the Patent	Inventors	Description
2012	US 8101352	Detection of ESR1 amplification in breast cancer	Sauter G et al.	This invention provides an in vitro method of identifying an individual with a noncancerous proliferative breast disease who is at risk of developing breast cancer.
2012	WO 021887	Biomarkers for the early detection of breast cancer	Labaer J et al.	The present invention provides reagents and methods for breast cancer detection.
2012	US 0184560	Molecular diagnostic methods for predicting brain metastasis of breast cancer	Wong ST et al.	This invention provides the methods for predicting brain metastasis of breast cancer, as well as methods for drug repositioning to identify existing and new therapeutics for use in developing individualized, patient-specific treatment regimens for improving diagnoses and patient outcomes in individuals at risk for brain metastasis of breast cancer.
2012	US 8097423	MN/CA IX and breast cancer therapy	Harris AL et al.	This invention concerns methods of detecting and quantitating, MN antigen and/or MN gene expression in tumors, tumor samples or body fluids, of ER-positive breast cancer patients, which would help in predicting patient resistance to endocrine therapy for breast cancer, and for making clinical decisions concerning cancer treatment.
2012	WO 060760	Molecular marker for cancer	Parris T et al.	The present invention relates to the assessment of a gene in the 8p11-p12 chromosomal region and gene products thereof, and their use as powerful molecular markers in decisions related to the diagnosis and/or prognosis of cancer, and in particular breast cancer.
2012	US 8187889	Protein markers for the diagnosis and prognosis of ovarian and breast cancer	Lomnytska M et al.	The present invention is directed to new protein markers and their use in diagnosing and monitoring ovarian and breast cancer.

3.21 Conclusions and Possible Future Directions

The global burden of the breast cancer continues to increase despite of advances in therapeutics and clinical research. Thus, early detection would not only reduce the suffering but also the associated cost. Despite efficient screening modalities available to diagnose breast cancer, there is an urgent need for most efficient, sensitive, as well as cost-effective methodologies for early screening. Biomarkers are the useful tools that can help not only in diagnosis and detection but also in deciding treatment option at an early stage that would reduce the associated mortality as well as morbidity. Promising developments in integrative omics approaches have led to the discovery of novel, specific, sensitive, easily measurable, reliable, cost-effective, and less complex biomarkers (both invasive and non-invasive) for the detection of breast cancer. Noninvasive biomarkers have more potential for the detection of disease at an early stage due to their easy access as well as potential for repeated sampling. Among these, circulating biomarkers present in the peripheral blood and bone marrow are the promising candidates for population-based screening that facilitate easy detection. No single biomarker is likely to have perfect predictive accuracy; however, biomarkers in panels may provide higher predictive power and thus provide a promising potential in clinical research.

Current proteomic-based approaches help in characterizing molecular alterations that could help in early cancer detection, subclassification, and accurate prognosis. Advanced platforms such as Orbitrap MS, Fourier transform ion cyclotron resonance MS, and protein microarrays combined with advanced bioinformatics are currently being used to identify molecular signatures of individual tumors that may be amplified by using emerging nanotechnology strategies. However, DNA methylation–based biomarkers are probably the most attractive analytes for development because epigenetic changes in genome are considered as an early event in the process of carcinogenesis. Moreover, current reports suggest that abnormal DNA methylation occurs in asymptomatic patients before the appearance of the early symptoms of cancer, so the detection of methylated genes would help in the accurate early detection. Thus, epigenetic biomarkers may provide one of the best promising platforms to develop reliable, specific, and sensitive screening tests for early breast cancer detection. Besides, metabolomic-based markers may also play an essential role in early identification of breast cancer as it may help to identify metabolites that may be released in the early stages of the disease. Thus, the management of breast cancer would lie in the potency and efficacy of the biomarkers to identify the symptomatic and asymptomatic disease conditions. The accumulated knowledge about the correlative biomarkers would not only overcome the challenge of early detection and clinical diagnosis but would also provide appropriate therapeutic alternatives that would benefit the patients.

Acknowledgments

We thank our director, Dr. P.K. Ranjekar, as well as IRSHA for supporting this work. We also thank Mr. Amit S. Choudhari, CSIR-SRF, for helping us in the editing the manuscript.

References

Abba MC, Drake JA, Hawkins KA et al. (2004) Transcriptomic changes in human breast cancer progression as determined by serial analysis of gene expression. *Breast Cancer Res* 6:R499–R513.

Abeloff MD, Wolff AC, Weber BL, et al. Cancer of the Breast. In: Abeloff MD, Armitage JO, Lichter AS, et al, eds. *Clinical Oncology*. Elsevier; 2008: pp. 1875–1943.

Abhilash M (2009) Applications of proteomics. *Int J Genomic Proteomic* 4(1).

Adami HO, Hunter D, Trichopoulos D (2002) *Textbook of Cancer Epidemiology*. New York: Oxford University Press, Inc.

Adams BD, Furneaux H, White BA (2007) The micro-ribonucleic acid (miRNA) miR-206 targets the human estrogen receptor-alpha (ERalpha) and represses ERalpha messenger RNA and protein expression in breast cancer cell lines. *Mol Endocrinol* 21:1132–1147.

Aebersold R, Mann M (2003) Mass spectrometry-based proteomics. *Nature* 422(6928):198–207.

Ahn SK, Moon HG, Ko E et al. (2013) Preoperative serum tissue polypeptide-specific antigen is a valuable prognostic marker in breast cancer. *Int J Cancer* 132(4):875–881.

Alao JP (2007) The regulation of cyclin D1 degradation: Roles in cancer development and the potential for therapeutic invention. *Mol Cancer* 6:24.

Al-azawi D, Kelly G, Myers E et al. (2006) CA15-3 is predictive of response and disease recurrence following treatment in locally advanced breast cancer. *BMC Cancer* 6:220.

Albergaria A, Paredes J, Sousa B et al. (2009) Expression of FOXA1 and GATA-3 in breast cancer: The prognostic significance in hormone receptor-negative tumours. *Breast Cancer Res* 11(3):R4.

Albertson DG, Collins C, McCormick F, Gray JW (2003) Chromosome aberrations in solid tumors. *Nat Gen* 34(4):369–376.

Alexander H, Stegner AL, Wagner-Mann C et al. (2004) Proteomic analysis to identify breast cancer biomarkers in nipple aspirate fluid. *Clin Cancer Res* 10(22):7500–7510.

Allegra JC, Lippman ME (1978) Growth of a human breast cancer cell line in serum-free hormone-supplemented medium. *Cancer Res* 38:3823–3829.

Al-Tarawneh SK, Border MB, Dibble CF et al. (2011) Defining salivary biomarkers using mass spectrometry-based proteomics: A systematic review. *OMICS* 15(6):353–361.

American Cancer Society. Breast Cancer Facts & Figures 2011–2012.

Ana KCV, Achatz MIW, Santos EMM et al. (2012) Germline DNA copy number variation in familial and early-onset breast cancer. *Breast Cancer Res* 14:R24.

Anderson KS, Sibani S, Wallstrom G et al. (2011) Protein microarray signature of autoantibody biomarkers for the early detection of breast cancer. *J Proteome Res* 10(1):85–96.

Anghel A, Raica M, Marian C et al. (2006) Combined profile of the tandem repeats CAG, TA and CA of the androgen and estrogen receptor genes in breast cancer. *J Cancer Res Clin Oncol* 132:727–733.

Anna M. Bofin, Borgny Y, Cara M (2004) Detection and quantitation of HER-2 Gene amplification and protein expression in breast carcinoma. *Am J Clin Pathol* 122:110–119.

Antoniou AC, Spurdle AB, Sinilnikova OM et al. (2008) Common breast cancer-predisposition alleles are associated with breast cancer risk in BRCA1 and BRCA2 mutation carriers. *Am J Hum Genet* 82(4):937–948.

Aoki K and Taketo MM (2007) Adenomatous polyposis coli (APC):a multi-functional tumor suppressor gene. *J Cell Sci.* 120(19):3327–35.

Aravidis C, Panani AD, Kosmaidou Z et al. (2012). Detection of numerical abnormalities of chromosome 9 and p16/CDKN2A gene alterations in ovarian cancer with fish analysis. *Anticancer Res* 32(12):5309–5313.

Artandi SE, DePinho RA (2000) A critical role for telomeres in suppressing and facilitating carcinogenesis. *Curr Opin Genet Dev* 10:39–46.

Atoum MF, Hourani HM, Shoter A et al. (2010) TNM staging and classification (familial and nonfamilial) of breast cancer in Jordanian females. *Indian J Cancer* 47(2):194–198.

Axelsson R, Bach-Gansmo T, Castell-Conesa J et al. (2010) An open-label, multicenter, phase 2a study to assess the feasibility of imaging metastases in late-stage cancer patients with the alpha v beta 3-selective angiogenesis imaging agent 99mTc-NC100692. *Acta Radio* l51(1):40–46.

Azim HA, Azambuja E, Colozza M et al.(2011) Long-term Toxic Effects of Adjuvant Chemotherapy in Breast Cancer. *Ann Oncol.* 22(9):1939–1947.

Badve S, Turbin D, Thorat MA (2007) FOXA1 expression in breast cancer—Correlation with luminal subtype A and survival. *Clin Cancer Res* 13:4415–4421.

Baglietto L, Severi G, English DR et al. (2010) Circulating steroid hormone levels and risk of breast cancer for postmenopausal women. *Cancer Epidemiol Biomarkers Prev* 19(2):492–502.

Banerji S, Cibulskis K, Rangel-Escareno C et al. (2012) Sequence analysis of mutations and translocations across breast cancer subtypes. *Nature* 486(7403):405–409.

Bansal V, Kumar V, Medhi B (2005) Future challenges of pharmacogenomics in clinical practice. *JK Science* 7(3):176–179.

Bantscheff M, Chirle M, Sweetman G et al. (2007) Quantitative mass spectrometry in proteomics: A critical review. *Anal Bioanal Chem* 389:1017–1031.

Barak V, Goike H, Panaretakis KW et al. (2004) Clinical utility of cytokeratins as tumor markers. *Clin Biochem* 37(7):529–540.

Baranwal S, Alahari (2010) miRNA control of tumor cell invasion and metastasis. *Int J Cancer* 126(6):1283–1290.

Barh D and Vedamurthy AB (2013). Therapeutic potential of let-7, mir-125, mir-205, and mir-296 in breast cancer: an update. *IIOABJ* 4(1):25–26.

Bartlett JM, Bloom KJ, Piper T et al. (2012) Mammostrat as an immunohistochemical multigene assay for prediction of early relapse risk in the tamoxifen versus exemestane adjuvant multicenter trial pathology study. *J Clin Oncol* 30(36):4477–4484.

Bartlett JM, Thomas J, Ross DT et al. (2010) Mammostrat as a tool to stratify breast cancer patients at risk of recurrence during endocrine therapy. *Breast Cancer Res* 12(4):R47.

Bassiouny M, El-Marakby HH, Saber N et al. (2005) Quadrantectomy and nipple saving mastectomy in treatment of early breast cancer: Feasibility and aesthetic results of adjunctive latissmus dorsi breast reconstruction. *J Egypt Natl Cancer Inst* 17(3):149–157.

Breast and Cervical Cancer Screening (BCCP). Website: www.healthoregon.org/bcc. Accessed January 15, 2011.

Becker C, Noldus J, Diamandis E, Lilja H (2001) The role of molecular forms of prostate-specific antigen (PSA or hK3) and of human glandular kallikrein 2 (hK2) in the diagnosis and monitoring of prostate cancer and in extra-prostatic disease. *Crit Rev Clin Lab Sci* 38(5):357–399.

Bensalah, K, Lotan, Y, Karam, JA, Shariat, SF, (2008) New Circulating Biomarkers for Prostate Cancer. Prost. *Cancer Prostat. Dis.* 11(2):112–120.

Berger MS, Locher GW, Saurer S et al. (1988) Correlation of c-erb B2 gene amplification and protein expression in human breast carcinoma with nodal status and nuclear grading. *Cancer Res* 48:1238–1243.

Bernard-Marty C, Lebrun F, Awada A et al. (2006) Monoclonal antibody-based targeted therapy in breast cancer: Current status and future directions. *Drugs* 66(12):1577–1579.

Bernstein JL, Godbold JH, Raptis G et al. (2005) Identification of mammaglobin as a novel serum marker for breast cancer. *Clin Cancer Res* 11(18):6528–6535.

Bernstein JL, Godbold JH, Raptis G et al. (2005) Identification of mammaglobin as a novel serum marker for breast cancer" Clinical cancer research : an official journal of the American Association for Cancer Research." *Clin Cancer Res.* 11(18):6528–35.

Bertucci F, Birnbaum D, Goncalves A (2006) Proteomics of breast cancer: Principles and potential clinical applications. *Mol Cell Proteomic* 5(10):1772–1786.

Beverly H (2009) The clinical utility of tumor markers. *Labmedicine* 40(2):99–103.

Bhargava R, Beriwal S, Dabbs DJ (2007) An immunohistologic validation survey for sensitivity and specificity. *Am J Clin Pathol* 127:103–113.

Bhatt AN, Mathur R, Farooque A et al. (2010) Cancer biomarkers—Current perspectives. *Indian J Med Res* 132:129–149.

Bidard FC, Hajage D, Bachelot T (2012) Assessment of circulating tumor cells and serum markers for progression-free survival prediction in metastatic breast cancer: A prospective observational study. *Breast Cancer Res* 14:R29.

Bohm D, Keller K, Pieter J et al. (2012) Comparison of tear protein levels in breast cancer patients and healthy controls using a de novoproteomic approach. *Oncol Rep* 28:429–438.

Boone JM, Kwan AL, Yang K et al. (2006) Computed tomography for imaging the breast. *J Mammary Gland Biol Neoplasia* 11(2):103–11.

Borgan E, Sitter B, Lingjaerde OC et al. (2010) Merging transcriptomics and metabolomics—Advances in breast cancer profiling. *BMC Cancer* 10:628.

Borgono CA, Diamandis EP (2004) The emerging roles of human tissue kallikreins in cancer. *Nat Rev Cancer* 4:876–890.

Borrelli R, del Sordo G, De Filippo E et al. (1993) High serum HDL-cholesterol in pre-and post-menopausal women with breast cancer in southern Italy. *Adv Exp Med Biol* 348:149–153.

Bourdon JC, Khoury MP, Diot A et al. (2011) p53 mutant breast cancer patients expressing p53γ have as good a prognosis as wild-type p53 breast cancer patients. *Breast Cancer Res* 13:R7.

Boureux A, Vignal E, Faure S et al. (2007) Evolution of the Rho family of ras-like GTPases in eukaryotes. *Mol Biol Evol* 24(1):203–216.

Bowman-colin C, Xia B, Bunting S et al. (2013) Palb2synergizes with Trp53 to suppress mammary tumor formation in a model of inhereted breast cancer. Proceedings of the National Academy of Sciences of the United States of America. In Press.

Boyd NF, Melnichouk O, Martin LJ et al. (2011) Mammographic density, response to hormones, and breast cancer risk. *J Clin Oncol* 2011:2985–2992.

Braaten T, Weiderpass E, Kumle M, Adami HO, Lund E (2004) Education and risk of breast cancer in the Norwegian-Swedish women's lifestyle and health cohort study. *Int J Cancer* 110(4):579–583.

Braun S, Vogl FD, Naume B et al. (2005) A pooled analysis of bone marrow micrometastasis in breast cancer. *N Engl J Med* 353(8):793–802.

Brennan K, Garcia-Closas M, Orr N et al. (2012) Intrageneic ATM methylation in peripheral blood DNA as a biomarker of breast cancer risk. *Cancer Res.* 72(9):2304–13.

Brooks J, Cairns P, Zeleniuch-Jacquotte (2009) A promoter methylation and the detection of breast cancer. *Cancer Causes Control* 20(9):1539–1550.

Brooks MN, Wang J, Li Y et al. (2008) Salivary protein factors are elevated in breast cancer patients. *Mol Med Rep* 1(3):375–378.

Bull SB et al. (2004) The combination of p53 mutation and neu/erbB-2 amplification is associated with poor survival in node-negative breast cancer. *J Clin Oncol* 22:86–96.

Butt S, Harlid S, Borgquist S et al. (2012) Genetic predisposition, parity, age at first childbirth and risk for breast cancer. *BMC Res Notes* 5:414.

Buyse M, Loi S, van 't Veer L et al. (2006) Validation and clinical utility of a 70-gene prognostic signature for women with node-negative breast cancer. *J Natl Cancer Inst* 98(17):1183–1192.

Cadieux C, Fournier S, Peterson AC et al. (2006) Transgenic mice expressing the p75 CCAAT-displacement protein/Cut homeobox isoform develop a myeloproliferative disease-like myeloid leukemia. *Cancer Res* 66(19):9492–9501.

Cakir A, Gonul II, Uluoglu O (2012) A comprehensive morphological study for basal-like breast carcinomas with comparison to non basal-like carcinomas. *Diagn Pathol* 7:145.

Calin GA, Croce CM (2006) MicroRNA signatures in human cancers. *Nat Rev Cancer* 6:857–866.

Calvo RM, Asuncion M, Sancho J et al. (2000) The role of the CAG repeat polymorphism in the androgen receptor gene and of skewed X-chromosome inactivation, in the pathogenesis of hirsutism. *J Clin Endocrinol Metab* 85:1735–1740.

Cancer care: Counseling. Support Groups. Education. Financial Assistance. Website: http://www.cancercare.org/.

Cancer.Net. Website: http://www.cancer.net/.

Carey LA, Metzger R, Dees EC et al. (2005) American Joint Committee on Cancer tumor-node-metastasis stage after neo adjuvant chemotherapy and breast cancer outcome. *J Natl Cancer Inst* 97(15):1137–1142.

Carla AB, Iacovos PM, Eleftherios PD (2004) Human tissue kallikreins: Physiologic roles and applications in cancer. *Mol Cancer Res* 5:257–280.

Carney WP (2007) Circulating oncoproteins HER2/neu, EGFR and CAIX (MN) as novel cancer biomarkers. *Expert Rev Mol Diagn* 7(3):309–319.

Cavazzana-Calvo M, Bagnis C, Mannoni P et al. (1999) Peripheral stem cells in bone marrow transplantation. Peripheral blood stem cell and gene therapy. *Baillieres Best Pract Res Clin Haematol* 12(1–2):129–138.

Cazet A, Julien S, Bobowski M et al. (2010) Tumour-associated carbohydrate antigens in breast cancer. *Breast Cancer Res* 12:204.

Celis Julio E, Gromov P, Cabezón T et al. (2004) Proteomic characterization of the interstitial fluid perfusing the breast tumor microenvironment: A novel resource for biomarker and therapeutic target discovery. *Mol Cell Proteomics* 3: 327–344.

Cen P, Duvic M, Cohen PR et al. (2008) Increased cancer antigen 27.29 (CA27.29) level in patients with mycosis fungoides. *J Am Acad Dermatol* 58(3):382–386.

Chajès V, Jenab M, Romieu I et al. (2011) Plasma phospholipid fatty acid concentrations and risk of gastric adenocarcinomas in the European Prospective Investigation into Cancer and Nutrition (EPIC-EURGAST). *Am J Clin Nutr*. 94(5):1304–13.

Chan DW, Beveridge RA, Bruzek DJ et al. (1988) Monitoring breast cancer with CA 549. *Clin Chem* 34(10):2000–2004.

Chang CC, Yang SH, Chien CC et al. (2009) Clinical meaning of age-related expression of fecal cytokeratin 19 in colorectal malignancy. *BMC Cancer* 22(9):376.

Chang HY, Nuyten DS, Sneddon JB et al. (2005) Robustness, scalability, and integration of a wound-response gene expression signature in predicting breast cancer survival. *Proc Natl Acad Sci USA* 102:3738–3743.

Chang TC, Wentzel EA, Kent OA (2007) Transactivation of miR-34a by p53 broadly influences gene expression and promotes apoptosis. *Mol Cell* 26(5):745–752.

Chapman C, Murray A, Chakrabarti J et al. (2007) Autoantibodies in breast cancer: Their use as an aid to early diagnosis. *Ann Oncol* 18(5):868–873.

Chattopadhyay S, Kaul R, Charest A et al. (2000) SMAR1, a novel, alternatively spliced gene product, binds the Scaffold/Matrix-associated region at the T cell receptor beta locus. *Genomics* 68(1):93–96.

Cheang MC, Chia SK, Voduc D et al. (2009) Ki67 index, Her2 status and prognosis of patients with luminal B breast cancer. *J Natl Cancer Inst*. 101(10):736–50.

Chen F, Chen GK, Millikan RC et al. (2011a) Fine-mapping of breast cancer susceptibility loci characterizes genetic risk in African Americans. *Hum Mol Genet* 20(22):4491–4503.

Chen H, Takahara M, Oba J, Xie L et al. (2011b) Clinicopathologic and prognostic significance of SATB1 in cutaneous malignant melanoma. *J Dermatol Sci* 64(1):39–44.

Chen HW, Huang CH, Lin YS et al. (2008) Breast cancer comparison and identification of estrogen-receptor related gene expression profiles in breast cancer of different ethnic origins. *Breast Cancer (Auckl.)* 1:35–49.

Chen WY, Rosner B, Hankinson SE et al. (2011c) Moderate alcohol consumption during adult life, drinking patterns, and breast cancer risk. *JAMA* 306(17):1884–1890.

Chen Y, Zou TN, Wu ZP et al. (2010) Detection of cytokeratin 19, human mammaglobin, and carcinoembryonic antigen-positive circulating tumor cells by three-marker reverse transcription-PCR assay and its relation to clinical outcome in early breast cancer. *Int J Biol Markers* 25(2):59–68.

Chin K, deSolorzano CO, Knowles D et al. (2004) In situ analyses of genome instability in breast cancer. *Nat Genet* 36(9):984–988.

Choi H, Pavelka N (2011) When one and one gives more than two: Challenges and opportunities of integrative omics. *Front Genet* 2:105.

Chourb S, Mackness BC, Farris LR et al. (2011) Improved detection of the MUC1 cancer antigen CA 15-3 by ALYGNSA fluorimmunoassay. *Heath* 3(8):524–528.

Christensen BC, Kelsey KT, Zheng S et al. (2010) Breast cancer DNA methylation profiles are associated with tumor size and alcohol and folate intake. *PLoS Genet* 6(7):e1001043.

Christopoulou A, Spiliotis J (2006) The role of BRCA1 AND BRCA2 in hereditary breast cancer. *Gene Ther Mol Biol* 10:95–100.

Cianfrocca M, Goldstein LJ (2004) Prognostic and predictive factors in early-stage breast cancer. *Oncologist* 9(6):606–616.

Cîmpean AM, Suciu C, Ceauşu R et al. (2008) Relevance of the immunohistochemical expression of cytokeratin 8/18 for the diagnosis and classification of breast cancer. *Rom J Morphol Embryol* 49(4):479–483.

Clarke MF, Fuller M (2006) Stem cells and cancer: Two faces of eve. *Cell* 124:1111–1115.

Clegg LX, Li FP, Hankey BF et al. (2002) Cancer survival among US whites and minorities: A SEER (Surveillance, Epidemiology, and End Results) Program population-based study. *Arch Intern Med* 162:1985–1993.

Cohen SJ et al. (2008) Relationship of circulating tumor cells to tumor response, progression-free survival, and overall survival in patients with metastatic colorectal cancer. *J Clin Oncol* 26(19):3213–3221.

Colozza M, Azambuja E, Cardoso F (2005) Proliferative markers as prognostic and predictive tools in early breast cancer: Where are we now? *Ann Oncol* 16:1723–1739.

Contractor KB, Kenny LM, Stebbing J et al. (2011) 18F-3deoxy-3-fluorothymidine positron emission tomography and breast cancer response to docetaxel. *Clin Cancer Res* 17(24):7664–7672.

Costa NR, Paulo P, Caffrey T et al. (2011) Impact of MUC1 mucin downregulation in the phenotypic characteristics of MKN45 gastric carcinoma cell line. *PLoS One* 6(11):e26970.

Costello JF, Fruhwald MC, Smiraglia DJ (2000) Aberrant CpG-island methylation has non-random and tumour-type-specific patterns. *Nat Genet* 24(2):132–138.

Cowper-SalLari R, Zhang X, Wright JB et al. (2012) Breast cancer risk-associated SNPs modulate the affinity of chromatin for FOXA1 and alter gene expression. *Nat Genet* 44(11):1191–1198.

Cox DG, Blanche H, Pearce C et al. (2006a) A comprehensive analysis of the androgen receptor gene and risk of breast cancer: Results from the National Cancer Institute Breast and Prostate Cancer Cohort Consortium (BPC3). *Breast Cancer Res* 8:R54.

Cox DG, Tamimi RM, Hunter DJ (2006b) Gene x Gene interaction between MnSOD and GPX-1 and breast cancer risk: A nested case-control study. *BMC Cancer* 6:217.

Cronin M, Sangli C, Liu M-L et al. (2007) Analytical validation of the oncotype DX genomic diagnostic test for recurrence prognosis and therapeutic response prediction in node-Nngative, estrogen receptor–positive breast cancer. *Clin Chem* 53(6):1084–1091.

Crooke PS, Justenhoven C, Brauch H et al. (2011) Estrogen metabolism and exposure in a genotypic–phenotypic model for breast cancer risk prediction. *Cancer Epidemiol Biomarkers Prev* 20:1502–1515.

Csősz É, Boross P, Csutak A et al. (2012) Quantitative analysis of proteins in the tear fluid of patients with diabetic retinopathy. *J Proteomics* 75(7):2196–2204.

CV Krepischi A, W Achatz MI, MM Santos E et al. (2012). Germline DNA copy number variation in familial and early-onset breast cancer. *Breast cancer Res.* 14:R24.

Dagan LN, Jiang X, Bhatt S et al. (2012) miR-155 regulates HGAL expression and increases lymphoma cell motility. *Blood* 119(2):513–520.

Dalberg K, Hellborg H, Wärnberg F (2007) Paget's disease of the nipple in a population based cohort. *Breast Cancer Res Treat* 111(2):313–319.

Dallol A, DaSilva NF, Viacava P et al. (2002) SLIT2, a human homologue of the *Drosophila* Slit2 gene, has tumor suppressor activity and is frequently inactivated in lung and breast cancers. *Cancer Res* 62(20):5874–5880.

Dangi-Garimella S, Strouch MJ, Grippo PJ, Bentrem DJ, Munshi HG (2010) Collagen regulation of let-7 in pancreatic cancer involves TGF-β1-mediated membrane type 1-matrix metalloproteinase expression. *Oncogene* 30(8):1002–1008.

Dangi-Garimella S, Yun J, Eves EM et al. (2009) Raf kinase inhibitory protein suppresses a metastasis signalling cascade involving LIN28 and let-7. *EMBO J* 28(4):347–358.

Danila DC et al. (2007) Circulating tumor cell number and prognosis in progressive 17. Castration-resistant prostate cancer. *Clin Cancer Res* 13(23):7053–7058.

Davis LM, Harris C, Tang L et al. (2007) Amplification patterns of three genomic regions predict distant recurrence in breast carcinoma. *J Mol Diagn* 9(3):327–336.

Dębniak T, Górski B, Huzarski T et al. (2005) A common variant of CDKN2A (p16) predisposes to breast cancer. *J Med Genet* 42:763–765.

Deng CX (2006) BRCA1: Cell cycle checkpoint, genetic instability, DNA damage response and cancer evolution. *Nucleic Acids Res* 34(5):1416–1426.

Denkert C, Bucher E, Hilvo M et al. (2012) Metabolomics of human breast cancer: New approaches for tumor typing and biomarker discovery. *Genome Med* 4(4):37.

Desbiens C, Hogue JC, Lévesque Y (2011) Primary breast angiosarcoma: Avoiding a common trap. *Case Rep Oncol Med* 2011:5pp.
Desmetz C, Bibeau F, Boissière F et al. (2008) Proteomics-based identification of HSP60 as a tumor-associated antigen in early stage breast cancer and ductal carcinoma in situ. *J Proteome Res* 7(9):3830–3837.
Deyati A, Younesi E, Hofmann-Apitius M et al. (2013) Challenges and opportunities for oncology bioarker discovery. *Drug Discovery Today* 18(13/14):1359–6446.
Di Camillo B, Sanavia T, Martina M et al. (2012) Effect of size and Heterogeneity of samples on biomarker discovery: Synthetic and real data assesment. *PLOS ONE* 7(3):e32200.
Dnistrian AM, Schwartz MK, Greenberg EJ (1991) CA 549 as a marker in breast cancer. *Int J Biol Mark* 6:139–143.
Donegan WL, Spratt JS (1995) Introduction to the history of breast cancer. In: Donegan S. *Cancer of the Breast*. New York: WB Saunders.
Dooley WC, Ljung BM, Veronesi U et al. (2001) Ductal lavage for detection of cellular atypia in women at high risk for breast cancer. *J Natl Cancer Inst* 93:1624–1632.
Doot RK, Muzi M, Peterson LM et al. (2010) Kinetic analysis of 18F-fluoride PET images of breast cancer bone metastases. *J Nucl Med* 51(4):521–527.
Drake PM, Cho W, Li B et al. (2010) Sweetening the pot: Adding glycosylation to the biomarker discovery equation. *Clin Chem* 56:223–236.
Dressing GE, Lange CA (2009) Integrated actions of progesterone receptor and cell cycle machinery regulate breast cancer cell proliferation. *Steroids* 74:573–576.
Duffy MJ (2006) Serum tumor markers in breast cancer: Are they of clinical value? *Clin Chem* 52(3):345–351.
Dunna WB, Broadhurst D, Brown M et al. (2008) Metabolic profiling of serum using Ultra Performance Liquid Chromatography and the LTQ-Orbitrap mass spectrometry system. *J Chromatogr* B 871:288–298.
Early Detection Research Network Biomarkers: The key to early detection. Website: http://edrn.nci.nih.gov/.
Edgar R, Domrachev M, Lash AE (2002) Gene Expression Omnibus: NCBI gene expression and hybridization array data repository. *Nucleic Acids Res* 30:207–210.
Eheman CR, Benard VB, Blackman D et al. (2006) Breast cancer screening among low-income or uninsured women: Results from the National Breast and Cervical Cancer Early Detection Pogram, July 1995 to March 2002 (United States). *Cancer Causes Control* 17:29–38.
Eiriksdottir G, Johannesdottir G, Ingvarsson S et al. (1998) Mapping loss of heterozygosity at chromosome 13q: Loss at 13q12-q13 is associated with breast tumour progression and poor prognosis. *Eur J Cancer* 34:2076–2081.
Eroles P, Bosch A, Pérez-Fidalgo JA et al. (2012) Molecular biology in breast cancer: Intrinsic subtypes and signaling pathways. *Cancer Treat Rev* 38(6):698–707.
Esteller M (2008) Epigenetics in canc. *N Engl J Med* 358(11):1148–1159.
Euhus DM, Bu D, Ashfaq R et al. (2007) Atypia and DNA methylation in nipple duct lavage in relation topredicted breast cancer risk. *Cancer Epidemiol Biomarkers Prev.* 16:1812–1821.
Evans WE (2003) Pharmacogenomics: Marshalling the human genome to individualise drug therapy. *Gut* 52:ii10–ii18.
Fabian CJ, Kimler BF (2001) Breast cancer risk prediction: Should nipple aspiration fluid cytology be incorporated into clinical practice? *J Natl Cancer Inst* 93(23):1762–1763.
Fabian CJ, Kimler BF, Mayo MS (2005) Breast-tissue sampling for risk assessment and prevention. *Endocr Relat Cancer* 12(2):185–213.
Fajac A, Gligorov J, Rezai K et al. (2010) Effect of ABCB1 C3435T polymorphism on docetaxel pharmacokinetics according to menopausal status in breast cancer patients. *Br J Cancer* 103(4):560–566.
Falasca M (2012) Cancer biomarkers: The future challenge of cancer. *J Mol Biomark Diagn* S2:e001.
Farazi TA, Horlings HM, TenHoeve JJ et al. (2011) MicroRNA sequence and expression analysis in breast tumors by deep sequencing. *Cancer Res* 71(13):4443–4453.
Feinberg AP, Tycko B (2004) The history of cancer epigenetics. *Nat Rev Cancer* 4:143–153.

Ferlay J, Héry C, Autier P et al. (2010) Global burden of breast cancer. *Breast Cancer Epidemiol*:1–19.

Fernando LA, Aleksandra VL, Sant Ana, Israel Bendit et al. (2005) Systemic chemotherapy induces microsatellite instability in the peripheral blood mononuclear cells of breast cancer patients. *Breast Cancer Res* 7(1):R28–R32.

Fessing MY, Mardaryev AN, Gdula MR et al. (2011) p63 regulates Satb1 to control tissue-specific chromatin remodeling during development of the epidermis. *J Cell Biol* 194(6):825–839.

Fisher B, Anderson S, Bryant J et al. (2002) Twenty-year follow-up of a randomized trial comparing total mastectomy, lumpectomy, and lumpectomy plus irradiation for the treatment of invasive breast cancer. *N Engl J Med* 347(16):1233–1241.

Fiszman GL, Jasnis MA (2011) Molecular mechanisms of trastuzumab resistance in HER2 overexpressing breast cancer. *Int J Breast Cancer* 60:295–299.

Fonseca FL, SantAna AV, Bendit I et al. (2005) Systemic chemotherapy induces microsatellite instability in the peripheral blood mononuclear cells of breast cancer patients. *Breast Cancer Res* 7(1):R28–R32.

Fornier M, Norton L (2005) Dose-dense adjuvant chemotherapy for primary breast cancer. *Breast Cancer Res* 7(2):64–69.

Foster MC, Helvie MA, Gregory NE et al. (2004) Lobular carcinoma in situ or atypical lobular hyperplasia at core-needle biopsy: Is excisional biopsy necessary. *Radiology* 231:813–819.

Foulkes WD, Smith IE, Reis-Filho JS (2010) Triple-negative breast cancer. *N Engl J Med* 363:1938–1948.

Fritz P, Cabrera CM, Dippon J et al. (2005) c-erbB2 and topoisomerase IIα protein expression independently predict poor survival in primary human breast cancer: A retrospective study. *Breast Cancer Res* 7:R374–R384.

Fu XD, Goglia L, Sanchez AM et al. (2010a) Progesterone receptor enhances breast cancer cell motility and invasion via extranuclear activation of focal adhesion kinase. *Endocr Relat Cancer* 17(2):431–443.

Fu YP, Edvardsen H, Kaushiva A et al. (2010b) NOTCH2 in breast cancer: Association of SNP rs11249433 with gene expression in ER-positive breast tumors without TP53 mutations. *Mol Cancer* 9:113.

Futreal PA, Coin L, Marshall M et al. (2004) A census of human cancer genes. *Nat Rev Cancer* 4:177–183.

Gaforio JJ, Serrano MJ, Sanchez-Rovira P et al. (2003) Detection of breast cancer cells in the peripheral blood is positively correlated with estrogen-receptor status and predicts for poor prognosis. *Int J Cancer* 107:984–990.

Galande S, Purbey PK, Notani D et al. (2007) The third dimension of gene regulation: Organization of dynamic chromatin loop scape by SATB1. *Curr Opin Genet Dev* 17(5):408–414.

Garber K (2004) Genomic medicine. Gene expression tests foretell breast cancer's future. *Science* 303:1754–1755.

Gast MC, Schellens JH, Beijnen JH (2009) Clinical proteomics in breast cancer: A review. *Breast Cancer Res Treat* 116(1):17–29.

Gemayel R, Vinces MD, Legendre M et al. (2010) Variable tandem repeats accelerate evolution of coding and regulatory sequences. *Annu Rev Genet* 44:445–477.

Genomic Health Report (2009). Inc. 301 Penobscot Drive, Redwood City, CA 94063.

Ghasabeh HR, Keyhanian S (2013) Relationship between tumor markers CEA and CA15-3 and recurrence breast cancer. *J Paramed Sci* (JPS) 4(1):16–20.

Giguere V, Yang N et al. (1988) Identification of a new class of steroid hormone receptors. *Nature* 331:91–94.

Gion M, Plebani M, Mione R et al. (1994) Serum CA549 in primary breast cancer: Comparison with CA15.3 and MCA. *Br J Cancer* 69(4):721–725.

Giovanella L, Ceriani L, Giardina G et al. (2002) Serum cytokeratin fragment 21.1 (CYFRA 21.1) as tumour marker for breast cancer: Comparison with carbohydrate antigen 15.3 (CA 15.3) and carcinoembryonic antigen (CEA). *Clin Chem Lab Med* 40(3):298–303.

Giuliano M, Giordano A, Jackson S et al. (2011) Circulating tumor cells as prognostic and predictive markers in metastatic breast cancer patients receiving first-line systemic treatment. *Breast Cancer Res* 13:R67.

Glazebrook KN, Magut MJ, Reynolds C (2008) Angiosarcoma of the breast. *AJR* 190(2):533–538.
Gobbi MD, Viprakasit V, Hughes JR (2006) A regulatory SNP causes a human genetic disease by creating a new transcriptional promoter. *Science* 312(5777):1215–1217.
Gonzalez-Angulo AM, Chen H, Karuturi MS et al. (2013) Frequency of mesenchymal-epithelial transition factor gene (MET) and the catalytic subunit of phosphoinositide-3-kinase (PIK3CA) copy number elevation and correlation with outcome in patients with early stage breast cancer. *Cancer* 119(1):7–15.
Gonzalez-Quintela A, Mallo N, Mella C et al. (2006) Serum levels of cytokeratin-18 (tissue polypeptide-specific antigen) in liver diseases. *Liver Int* 26(10):1217–1224.
Gordian E, Ramachandran K, Singal R (2009) Methylation mediated silencing of TMS1 in breast cancer and its potential contribution to docetaxel cytotoxicity. *Anticancer Res* 29:3207–3210.
Gosden JR, Middleton PG, Rout D (1986) Localization of the human oestrogen receptor gene to chromosome 6q24— q27 by in situ hybridization. *Cytogenet Cell Genet* 43(3–4):218–220.
Gøtzsche PC, Jørgensen KJ (2013) Screening for breast cancer with mammography. Cochrane Database Syst Rev. 4;6:CD001877.
Goulet B, Sansregret L, Leduy L et al. (2007) Increased expression and activity of nuclear cathepsin L in cancer cells suggests a novel mechanism of cell transformation. *Mol Cancer Res* 5(9):899–907.
Gregory PA, Bert AG, Paterson EL et al. (2008a) ThemiR-200 family and miR-205 regulate epithelial to mesenchymal transition by targeting ZEB1 and SIP1. *Nat Cell Biol* 10(5):593–601.
Gregory PA, Bracken CP, Bert AG et al. (2008b) Micro RNAs as regulators of epithelial-mesenchymal transition. *Cell Cycle* 7(20):3112–3118.
Griffin JL, Shockcor JP (2004) Metabolic profiles of cancer cells. *Nat Rev Cancer* 4(7):551–561.
Gunsoy NB, Garcia-Closas M, Moss SM (2012) Modelling the over diagnosis of breast cancer due to mammography screening in women aged 40–49 in the United Kingdom. *Breast Cancer Res* 14(6):R152.
Gupta S, Knowlton AA (2005) HSP60, bax, apoptosis and the heart. *J Cell Mol Med* 9(1):51–58.
Gymrek M, Golan D, Rosset S et al. (2012) lobSTR: A short tandem repeat profiler for personal genomes. *Genome Res* 22(6):1154–1162.
Habets JM, Tank B, Vuzevski VD et al. (1988) Absence of cytokeratin 8 and inconsistent expression of cytokeratins 7 and 19 in human basal cell carcinoma. *Anticancer Res* 8(4):611–616.
Halushka MK, Fan JB, Bentley K et al. (1999) Patterns of single-nucleotide polymorphisms in candidate genes for blood-pressure homeostasis. *Nat Genet* 22(3):239–247.
Hamrita B, Nasr HB, Chahed K et al. (2010) Proteomic analysis of human breast cancer: New technologies and clinical applications for biomarker profiling. *J Proteomics Bioinform* 3:091–098.
Han HJ, Russo J, Kohwi Y et al. (2008) SATB1 reprogrammes gene expression to promote breast tumour growth and metastasis. *Nature* 452(7184):187–193.
Hanahan D, Weinberg RA (2000) The hallmarks of cancer. *Cell* 100:57–70.
Hanby AM, Hughes TA (2008) In situ and invasive lobular neoplasia of the breast. *Histopathology* 52(1):58–66.
Handy B (2009). The clinical utility of tumor markers. *Labmedicine* 40(2):99–103.
Hanker LC, Karn T, Mavrova-Risteska L et al. (2011) SATB1 gene expression and breast cancer prognosis. *Breast* 20(4):309–313.
Hanstein B, Djahansouzi S, Dall P et al. (2004) Insights into the molecular biology of the estrogen receptor define novel therapeutic targets for breast cancer. *Eur J Endocrinoly* 150(3):243–255.
Harnett A, Smallwood J, Titshall V et al. (2009) Diagnosis and treatment of early breast cancer, including locally advanced disease—Summary of NICE guidance. *BMJ* 338:b438.
Harris L, Fritsche H, Mennel R et al. (2007) American society of clinical oncology 2007 update of recommendations for the use of tumor markers in breast cancer. *JCO* 25(33):5287–5312.
Hausauer AK, Keegan TH, Chang ET et al. (2009) Recent trends in breast cancer incidence in US white women by county-level urban/rural and poverty status. *BMC Med* 7:31.
He J, Gornbein J, Shen D et al. (2007) Detection of breast cancer biomarkers in nipple aspirate fluid by SELDI-TOF and their identification by combined liquid chromatography-tandem mass spectrometry. *Int J Oncol* 30:145–154.

Heck KE, Pamuk ER (1997) Explaining the relation between education and postmenopausal breast cancer. *Am J Epidemiol* 145:366–372.

Heianbo J, Whelan SA, Lu M et al. (2011) Proteomic-based biosignatures in breast cancer classification and prediction of therapeutic response. *Int J Proteomic* 2011:1–16.

Heikkinen T, Greco D, Pelttari LM et al. (2011) Variants on the promoter region of PTEN affect breast cancer progression and patient survival. *Breast Cancer Res* 13(6):R130.

Heiko S (2009) Molecular imaging of cancer: Receptors, angiogenesis, and gene expression. *Curr Clin Oncol* 2009:107–114.

Heneghan HM, Miller N, Kerin MJ (2010) Role of microRNAs in obesity and the metabolic syndrome. *Obesity Rev* 11(5):354–361.

Heneghan HM, Miller N, McAnena OJ et al. (2011) Differential miRNA expression in omental adipose tissue and in the circulation of obese patients identifies novel metabolic biomarkers. *J Clin Endocrinol Metab* 96(5):E846–E850.

Hermelink K, Untch M, Lux MP et al. (2007) Cognitive function during neoadjuvant chemotherapy for breast cancer. *Cancer* 109:1905–1913.

Herranz M, Ruibal A (2012) Optical imaging in breast cancer diagnosis: The next evolution. *J Oncol* 2012:1–10.

Hicks C, Asfour R, Pannuti A et al. (2011) An integrative genomics approach to biomarker discovery in breast cancer. *Cancer Inform* 11(10):185–204.

Higgins MJ, Baselga J (2011) Targeted therapies for breast cancer. *J Clin Invest* 121(10):3797–3803.

Hilvo M, Denkert C, Lehtinen L et al. (2011) Novel theranostic opportunities offered by characterization of altered membrane lipid metabolism in breast cancer progression. *Cancer Res* 71(9):3236–3245.

Holmes FA, Liticker JD (2005) Pharmacogenomics of tamoxifen in a nutshell—And who broke the nutcracker? *J Oncol Pract* 1(4):155–159.

Hossain A, Kuo MT, Saunders GF (2006) Mir-17-5p regulates breast cancer cell proliferation by inhibiting translation of AIB1 mRNA. *Mol Cell Biol* 26:8191–8201.

Hou W, Zhou H, Elisma F et al. (2008) Technological developments in lipidomics. *Brief Funct Genomic Proteomic* 7:395–409.

Houssami N, Turner R, Macaskill P et al. (2014) An individual person data meta-analysis of preoperative magnetic resonance imaging and breast cancer recurrence. *J Clin Oncol*. 32(5):392–401.

Howard DH, Ekwueme DU, Gardner JG et al. (2010) The impact of a national program to provide free mammograms to low-income, uninsured women on breast cancer mortality rates. *Cancer* 116:4456–4462.

http://edrn.nci.nih.gov/.

http://www.cancercare.org/.

http://www.cancer.net/.

Hu XC, Wong IH, Chow LW (2003) Tumor-derived aberrant methylation in plasma of invasive ductal breast cancer patients: Clinical implications. *Oncol Rep* 10(6):1811–1815.

Huang Q, Gumireddy K, Schrier M et al. (2008) The microRNAs miR-373 and miR-520c promote tumour invasion and metastasis. *Nat Cell Biol* 10(2):202–210.

Huang Y, Hinds DA, Qi L et al. (2010) Pooled versus individual genotyping in a breast cancer genome-wide association study. *Genet Epidemiol* 34(6):603–612.

Hudson MJ, Stamp GW, Chaudhary KS et al. (2001) Human MUC1 mucin: A potent glandular morphogen. *J Pathol* 194(3):373–383.

Huo D, Zheng Y, Ogundiran TO et al. (2012) Evaluation of susceptibility loci of breast cancer in women of African ancestry. *Carcinogenesis* 33:835–840.

Hussain R, Lodhi FB, Ali M (2006) Serum tumor markers. *Prof Med J* 13(1):1–10.

Ideker T, Dutkowski J, Hood L (2011) Boosting signal-to-noise in complex biology: Prior knowledge is power. *Cell* 144:860–863.

Ignatiadis M, Xenidis N, Perraki M et al. (2007) Different prognostic value of cytokeratin-19 mRNA positive circulating tumor cells according to estrogen receptor and HER2 status in early-stage breast cancer. *J Clin Oncol* 25(33):5194–202.

Ikeda Y, Kuwano H, Ikebe M et al. (1994) Immunohistochemical detection of CEA, CA19-9, and DF3 in esophageal carcinoma limited to the submucosal layer. *J Surg Oncol* 56(1):7–12.

Imbeaud S, Graudens E, Boulanger V et al. (2005) Towards standardization of RNA quality assessment using user-independent classifiers of microcapillary electrophoresis traces. *Nucleic Acids Res* 33(6):e56.

Ingle JN (2008) Pharmacogenomics of tamoxifen and aromatase inhibitors. *Cancer* 112(3):695–699.

Iorio MV, Ferracin M, Liu CG et al. (2005) MicroRNA gene expression deregulation in human breast cancer. *Cancer Res* 65(16):7065–7070.

Iorio MV, Ferracin M, Liu CG et al. (2006) A microRNA expression signature of human solid tumors defines cancer gene targets. *Proc Natl Acad Sci* 103:2257–2261.

Iorns E, Hnatyszyn HJ, Seo P et al. (2010) The role of SATB1 in breast cancer pathogenesis. *J Nat Cancer Inst* 102(16):1284–1296.

Jacques TS, Swales A, Brzozowski MJ et al. (2010) Combinations of genetic mutations in the adult neural stem cell compartment determine brain tumour phenotypes. *EMBO J*. 6;29(1):222–35.

Jalota A, Singh K, Pavithra L et al. (2005) Tumor suppressor SMAR1 activates and stabilizes p53 through its arginine-serine-rich motif. *J Biol Chem* 280:16019–16029.

James CR, Quinn JE, Mullan PB et al. (2007) BRCA1, a potential predictive biomarker in the treatment of breast cancer. *Oncologist* 12(2):142–150.

Jansen MP, Sieuwerts AM, Look MP et al. (2007) HOXB13-to-IL17BR expression ratio is related with tumor aggressiveness and response to tamoxifen of recurrent breast cancer: A retrospective study. *J Clin Oncol* 25(6):662–668.

Jemal A, Bray F, Center MM et al. (2011) Global cancer statistics. *Ca Cancer J Clin* 61:69–90.

Jemal A, Center MM, Santis CD et al. (2010) Global patterns of cancer incidence and mortality rates and trends. *Cancer Epidemiol Biomarkers Prev* 19:1893.

Jensen A, Sharif H, Olsen JH et al. (2008) Risk of breast cancer and gynecologic cancers in a large population of Nearly 50,000 Infertile Danish Women. *Am J Epidemiol* 168(1):49–57.

Jin Z, Cheng Y, Olaru A (2008) Promoter hypermethylation of CDH13 is a common, early event in human esophageal adenocarcinogenesis and correlates with clinical risk factors. *Int J Cancer* 123:2331–2336.

Jones PA, Baylin SB (2007) The epigenomics of cancer. *Cell* 128(4):683–692.

Jordan KW, Nordenstam J, Lauwers GY et al. (2009) Metabolomic characterization of human rectal adenocarcinoma with intact tissue magnetic resonance spectroscopy. *Dis Colon Rectum* 52(3):520–525.

Joshi-Tope G, Gillespie M, Vastrik I et al. (2005) Reactome: A knowledgebase of biological pathways. *Nucleic Acids Res* 33:D428–D432.

Jung SY, Han W, Lee JW et al. (2009) Ki-67 expression gives additional prognostic information on St. Gallen 2007 and Adjuvant! Online risk categories in early breast cancer. *Ann Surg Oncol* 16(5):1112–1121.

Kamat N, Khidhir MA, Jaloudi M et al. (2012) High incidence of microsatellite instability and loss of heterozygosity in three loci in breast cancer patients receiving chemotherapy: A prospective study. *BMC Cancer* 12:373.

Kams K and Herr AE. (2011) Human tear protein analysis enabled by an alkine microfluidic homogenous immunoassay. *Anal Chem*. 83(21):8115–8122.

Kancha RK, von Bubnoff N, Bartosch N et al. (2011) Differential sensitivity of ERBB2 kinase domain mutations towards lapatinib. *PLoS One* 6(10):e26760.

Kanehisa M, Goto S (2000) KEGG: Kyoto encyclopedia of genes and genomes. *Nucleic Acids Res* 28:27–30.

Kann MG (2007) Protein interactions and disease: Computational approaches to uncover the etiology of diseases. *Brief Bioinform* 8:333–346.

Kapali AS, Singh M, Deo SVS et al. (2010) Aggressive palliative surgery in metastatic phyllodes tumor: Impact on quality of life. *Indian J Palliat Care* 16:101–104.

Kapp A, Jeffrey S, Langerød A et al. (2006) Discovery and validation of breast cancer subtypes. *BMC Genomics* 7:231.

Kato M, Paranjape T, Müller RU et al. (2009) The mir-34 microRNA is required for the DNA damage response in vivo in *C. elegans* and in vitro in human breast cancer cells. *Oncogene* 28:2419–2424.

Kaul R, Mukherjee S, Ahmed F et al. (2003) Direct interaction with and activation of p53 by SMAR1 retards cell-cycle progression at G2/M phase and delays tumor growth in mice. *Int J Cancer* 103(5):606–615.

Kaul-Ghanekar R et al. (2004) SMAR1 and Cux/CDP modulate chromatin and act as negative regulators of the TCRbeta enhancer (Ebeta). *Nucleic Acids Res* 32(16):4862–4875.

Kaul-Ghanekar R, Singhet S, Hitesh M et al. (2009) Tumor suppressor protein SMAR1 modulates the roughness of cell surface: Combined AFM and SEM study. *BMC Cancer* 9:350.

Keam B, Im SA, Lee KH et al. (2011) Ki-67 can be used for further classification of triple negative breast cancer into two subtypes with different response and prognosis. *Breast Cancer Res* 13:R22.

Keklikoglou I, Koerner C, Schmidt C et al. (2012) MicroRNA-520/373 family functions as a tumor suppressor in estrogen receptor negative breast cancer by targeting NF-κ B and TGF-β signaling pathways. *Oncogene* 31(37):4150–4163.

Kelly K, Amy EH (2011) Ophthalmologist-on-a-chip: Fully integrated icrofluidic tear osmolarity and protein biomarker quantification for dry eye stratification. *15th International Conference on Miniaturized Systems for Chemistry and Life Sciences*, Seattle, WA.

Kevin M. Kelly, Judy Dean, W. Scott Comulada, Sung-Jae Lee (2010). Breast cancer detection using automated whole breast ultrasound and mammography in radiographically dense breasts. *European Radiology* 20(3):734–742.

Keyhani M, Nasizadeh S, Ardeshir D (2005) Serum CA15-3 measurement in breast cancer patients before and after mastectomy. *Arch Iranian Med* 8(4):263–266.

Kim JK, Jung KH, Noh JH et al. (2009a) Targeted disruption of S100P suppresses tumor cell growth by down-regulation of cyclin D1 and CDK2 in human hepatocellular carcinoma. *Int J Oncol* 35(6):1257–1264.

Kim YS, Yoo HS, Ko JH (2009b) Implication of aberrant glycosylation in cancer and use of lectin for cancer biomarker discovery. *Protein Pept Lett* 16(5):499–507.

King MC, Marks JH, Mandell JB et al. (2003) Breast and ovarian cancer risks due to inherited mutations in BRCA1 and BRCA2. *Science* 302(5645):643–646.

Klee GG, Schreiber WE (2004) MUC1 gene-derived glycoprotein assays for monitoring breast cancer (CA15-3, CA27.29,BR): are they measuring the same antigen? *Arch. Pathol. Lab. Med.* 128:1131–1135.

Kobeissi L, Hamra R, Samari G et al. (2012) The 2009 Lebanese national mammography campaign: Results and assessment using a survey design. *Epidemiology* 2:1.

Köhrmann A, Kammerer U, Kapp M et al. (2009) Expression of matrix metalloproteinases (MMPs) in primary human breast cancer and breast cancer cell lines: New findings and review of the literature. *BMC Cancer* 9:188.

Kolusayin Ozar MO, Orta T (2005) The use of chromosome aberrations in predicting breast cancer risk. *J Exp Clin Cancer Res* 24(2):217–222.

Kong EH, Pike AC, Hubbard RE (2003) Structure and mechanism of the oestrogen receptor. *Biochem Soc Trans* 31:56–59.

Kong W, Yang H, He L et al. (2008) MicroRNA-155 is regulated by the transforming growth factor beta/Smad pathway and contributes to epithelial cell plasticity by targeting RhoA. *Mol Cell Biol* 28:6773–6784.

Kornegoor R, Moelans CB, Verschuur-Maes AHJ (2012) Promoter hypermethylation in male breast cancer: Analysis by multiplex ligation-dependent probe amplification. *Breast Cancer Res* 14:R101.

Korpal M, Kang Y (2008) The emerging role of miR-200 family of microRNAs in epithelial-mesenchymal transition and cancer metastasis. *RNA Biol* 5(3):115–119.

Kosacka M, Jankowska R (2009) Comparison of cytokeratin 19 expression in tumor tissue and serum CYFRA 21-1 levels in non-small cell lung cancer. *Pol Arch Med Wewn* 119(1–2):33–37.

Kotsopoulos J, Tworoger SS, Campos H, Chung F et al. (2011) Reproducibility of plasma and urine biomarkers among premenopausal and post menopausal women from the nurses health studies. *Cancer Epidemiol Biomarkers. Prev.* 19:938–936.

Krassentein R, Sauter E, Dulaimi et al. (2004) Detection of breast cancer in nipple aspirate fluid by CpG island hypermethylation. *Clin Cancer Res.* 10(1 Pt 1):28–32.

Kruit A, Gerritsen WB, Pot N et al. (2010) CA 15-3 as an alternative marker for KL-6 in fibrotic lung diseases. *Sarcoidosis Vasc Diffuse Lung Dis* 27(2):138–146.

Kumar KS, Kumar MMJ (2008) Antiestrogen therapy for breast cancer: An overview. *Cancer Ther* 6:655–664.

Kumpulainen EJ, Keskikuru R, Johansson RT (2002) Serum tumor marker CA 15.3 and stage are the two most important predictors of survival in primary breast cancer. *Breast Cancer Res Treat* 76:95–102.

Kurian AW, McClure LA, John EM et al. (2009) Second primary breast cancer occurrence according to hormone receptor status. *J Natl Cancer Inst* 101:1058–1065.

Kurian S, Khan M, Grant M (2008) CA 27–29 in patients with breast cancer with pulmonary fibrosis. *Clin Breast Cancer* 8(6):538–540.

Kwei KA, Kung Y, Salari K et al. (2010) Genomic instability in breast cancer: Pathogenesis and clinical implications. *Mol Oncol* 4(3):255–266.

Lacroix-Triki M, Lambros MB, Geyer FC et al. (2010) Absence of microsatellite instability in mucinous carcinomas of the breast. *Int J Clin Exp Pathol* 4(1):22–31.

Laronga C, Drake RR (2007) Proteomic approach to breast cancer. *Cancer Control* 14(4):360–368.

Larson JS, Goodman LJ, Tan Y et al. (2010) Analytical validation of a highly sensitive, accurate, and reproducible assay (HERmark) for the measurement of HER2 total protein and HER2 homodimers in FFPE breast cancer tumor specimens. *Pathol Res* 2010:814176.

Lawrie CH, Gal S, Dunlop HM et al. (2008) Detection of elevated levels of tumour-associated microRNAs in serum of patients with diffuse large B-cell lymphoma. *Br J Haematol* 141(5):672–675.

Lea R, Bannister E, Case A et al. (2004) Use of hormonal replacement therapy after treatment of breast cancer. *J Obstet Gynaecol Can* 26(1):49–60.

Lebrecht A, Boehm D, Schmidt M et al. (2009) Diagnosis of breast cancer by tear proteomic pattern. *Cancer Genomic Proteomic* 6(3):177–182.

Lee MC, Patel-Parekh L, Bland KI et al. (2007) Increased frequency of Estrogen Receptor (ER) negative and aneuploid breast cancer in African American women at all stages of disease: First analysis from the National Cancer Database. *Society of Surgical Oncology Breast Cancer Symposium* Abstract 121.

Lee RC, Feinbaum RL and Ambros V (1993) The *C. elegans* heterochronic gene lin-4 encodes small RNAs with antisense complementarity to lin-14. *Cell* 75:843–854.

Lee SC, Berg KD, Sherman M et al. (2001) Microsatellite instability is infrequent in medullary breast cancer. *Am J Clin Pathol* 115:823–827.

Lee YS, Dutta A (2007) The tumor suppressor microRNA let-7 represses the HMGA2 oncogene. *Genes Dev* 21(9):1025–1030.

Lehman CD, DePeri ER, Peacock S et al. (2005) Clinical experience with MRI-guided vacuum-assisted breast biopsy. *AJR* 184:1782–1787.

Lehtimäki T, Lundin M, Linder N et al. (2011) Long-term prognosis of breast cancer detected by mammography screening or other methods. *Breast Cancer Res* 13(6):R134.

Lemieux J, Maunsell E, Provencher L (2008) Chemotherapy-induced alopecia and effects on quality of life among women with breast cancer: A literature review. *Psycho-Oncology* 17:317–328.

Le Naour F, Misek DE, Krause MC et al. (2001) Proteomics-based identification of RS/DJ-1 as a novel circulating tumor antigen in breast cancer. *Clin Cancer Res.* Nov;7(11):3328–35.

Levenson VV, Melniko AA (2012) DNA methylation as clinically useful biomarkers—Light at the end of the tunnel. *Pharmaceuticals* 5:94–113.

Lewis CM, Cler LR, Bu DW et al. (2005) Promoter hypermethylation in benign breast epithelium in relation to predicted breast cancer risk. *Clin Cancer Res* 11:166–172.

Li H, d'Anjou M (2009) Pharmacological significance of glycosylation in therapeutic proteins. *Curr Opin Biotechnol* 20:678–684.

Li J, Zhao J, Yu X et al. (2005) Identification of biomarkers for breast cancer in nipple aspiration and ductal lavage fluid. *Clin Cancer Res* 11:8312–8320.

Li X, Link JM, Stekhova S et al. (2008) Site-specific labeling of annexin V with F-18 for apoptosis imaging. *Bioconjug Chem* 19(8):1684–1688.
Liang S, Singh M, Gam LH (2011) Potential hydrophobic protein markers of breast cancer in Malaysian Chinese, Malay and Indian patients. *Cancer Biomark* 8(6):319–330.
Lianidou ES, Markou A (2011) Circulating tumor cells as emerging tumor biomarkers in breast cancer. *Clin Chem Lab Med* 49:1579–1590.
Lim LY, Vidnovic N, Ellisen LW et al. (2009) Mutant p53 mediates survival of breast cancer cells. *Br J Cancer* 101:1606–1612.
Lin PI, Vance JM, Pericak-Vance MA et al. (2007) No gene is an island: The flip-flop phenomenon. *Am J Hum Genet* 80:531–538.
Lindberg K, Helguero LA, Omoto Y et al. (2011) Estrogen receptor β represses Akt signaling in breast cancer cells via downregulation of HER2/HER3 and upregulation of PTEN: Implications for tamoxifen sensitivity. *Breast Cancer Res* 13:R43.
Lipton A, Ali SM, Leitzel K et al. (2002) Elevated Serum HER-2/neu level predicts decreased response to hormone therapy in metastatic breast cancer. *J Clin Oncol* 20(6):1467–1472.
Liska V, Holubec L, Treska V et al. (2007) Tumor markers as useful predictors of survival rate after exploratory laparotomy for liver malignancies. *Anticancer Res* 27:1887–1892.
Liu R, Wang X, Chen GY et al. (2007) The prognostic role of a gene signature from tumorigenic breast-cancer cells. *N Engl J Med* 356(3):217–226.
Liu Z, Zhu J, Cao H et al. (2012) miR-10b promotes cell invasion through RhoC-AKT signaling pathway by targeting HOXD10 in gastric cancer. *Int J Oncol* 40(5):1553–1560.
Lkeda Y, Kuwano H, Ikebe M et al. (1994) Immunohistochemical detection of CEA, CA19-9 and DF3 in esophageal carcinoma limited to the submucosal layer. *J Surg Oncol*. 56(1):7–12.
Locasale Jason W, Cantley Lewis C (2010) Altered metabolism in cancer. *BMC Biol* 8:88.
Locke I, Kote-Jarai Z, Fackler MJ et al. (2007) Gene promoter hypermethylation in ductal lavage fluid from healthy BRCA gene mutation carriers and mutation-negative controls. *Breast Cancer Res* 9:R20.
Lopez F, Belloc F, Lacombe F et al. (1991) Modalities of synthesis of Ki67 antigen during the stimulation of lymphocytes. *Cytometry* 12(1):42–49.
Luqmani YA, Mathew M (2004) Allelic variation of BAT-25 and BAT-26 mononucleotide repeat loci in tumours from a group of young women with breast cancer. *Int J Oncol* 25(3):771–775.
Lynn JF (2004) ('Faslodex')-a new hormonal treatment for advanced breast cancer. *Eur J Oncol Nurs* (Suppl 2):S83–S88.
Ma L, Teruya-Feldstein J, Weinberg RA (2007) Tumour invasion and metastasis initiated by microRNA-10b in breast cancer. *Nature* 449:682–688.
Ma XJ, Salunga R, Dahiya S et al. (2008) A five-gene molecular grade index and HOXB13:IL17BR are complementary prognostic factors in early stage breast cancer. *Clin Cancer Res* 14(9):2601–2608.
Macdonald IK, Allen J, Murray A et al. (2012) Development and validation of a high throughput system for discovery of antigens for autoantibody detection. *PLoS One* 7(7):e40759.
Mackay J, Szecsei CM (2010) Genetic counseling for hereditary predisposition to ovarian and breast cancer. *Ann Oncol* 21(7):334–338.
MacMahon B (2006) Epidemiology and the causes of breast cancer. *Int J Cancer* 118(10):2373–2378.
Madhavan S, Gusev Y, Harris M et al. (2011) G-DOC: A systems medicine platform for personalized oncology. *Neoplasia* 13(9):771–783.
Madu CO, Lu Y (2010) Novel diagnostic biomarkers for prostate cancer. *J Cancer* 1:150–177.
Malati T (2007) Tumour markers: An overview. *Indian J Clin Biochem* 22(2):17–31.
Mann AM, Tighe BJ (2007) Tear analysis and lens-tear interactions: Part I. Protein fingerprinting with microfluidic technology. *Cont Lens Anterior Eye* 30(3):163–173.
Mansel RE, Goyal A, Douglas-Jones A et al. (2009) Detection of breast cancer metastasis in sentinel lymph nodes using intra-operative real time Gene Search BLN Assay in the operating room: Results of the Cardiff study. *Breast Cancer Res Treat* 115(3):595–600.
Marotta LL, Almendro V, Marusyk A (2011) The JAK2/STAT3 signaling pathway is required for growth of $CD44^+CD24^-$ stem cell-like breast cancer cells in human tumors. *J Clin Invest* 121(7):2723–2735.

Marrakchi R, Ouerhani S, Benammar S et al. (2008) Detection of cytokeratin 19 mRNA and CYFRA 21-1 (cytokeratin 19 fragments) in blood of Tunisian women with breast cancer. *Int J Biol Markers* 23(4):238–243.

Martelli AM, Evangelisti C, Chiarini F et al. (2010) The phosphatidylinositol 3-kinase/Akt/mTOR signaling network as a therapeutic target in acute myelogenous leukemia patients. *Oncotarget* 1(2):89–103.

Martínez-Galán J, Torres B, Del MR et al. (2008) Quantitative detection of methylated ESR1 and 14-3-3-sigma gene promoters in serum as candidate biomarkers for diagnosis of breast cancer and evaluation of treatment efficacy. *Cancer Biol Ther* 7(6):958–965.

Mas-Morey P, Visser MH, Winkelmolen L et al. (2013) Clinical Toxicology and Management of Intoxications With Synthetic Cathinones ("Bath Salts"), *J Pharm Pract* 26(4):353–7.

Massardo T, Alonso O, Llamas-Ollier A et al. (2005) Planar Tc99m – sestamibi scintimammography should be considered cautiously in the axillary evaluation of breast cancer protocols: Results of an international multicenter trial. *BMC Nucl Med* 5:4.

Matsuda S, Rouault J, Magaud J et al. (2001) In search of a function for the TIS21/PC3/BTG1/TOB family. *FEBS Lett* 497(2–3):67–72.

Mattie MD, Benz CC, Bowers J et al. (2006) Optimized high-throughput microRNAs expression profiling provides novel biomarker assessment of clinical prostate and breast cancer biopsies. *Mol Cancer* 5:24.

Mattiske S, Suetani RJ, Neilsen PM (2012) The oncogenic role of miR-155 in breast cancer. *Cancer Epidemiol Biomarkers Prev* 21(8):1236–1243.

Matuschek C, Bölke E, Lammering G (2010) Methylated APC and GSTP1 genes in serum DNA correlate with the presence of circulating blood tumor cells and are associated with a more aggressive and advanced breast cancer disease. *Eur J Med Res* 15:277–286.

Mayeux R (2004) Biomarkers: Potential uses and limitations. *NeuroRx* 1(2):182–188.

McCann J, Stockton D and Godward S (2002) Impact of false-positive mammography on subsequent screening attendance and risk of cancer. *Breast Cancer Res* 4:R11.

McGrowder D, Riley C, Y St A Morrison E et al. (2011) The role of high-density lipoproteins in reducing the risk of vascular diseases, neurogenerative disorders, and cancer. *Cholesterol* 2011:1–9.

Meany DL, Chan DW (2011) Aberrant glycosylation associated with enzymes as cancer biomarkers. *Clin Proteomic* 8:7.

Menasce LP, White GR, Harrison CJ (1993) Localisation of the estrogen receptor locus (ESR) to chromosome 6q25.1 by FISH and a simple post-FISH banding technique. *Genomics* 17:263–265.

Metcalfe K, Lubinski J, Lynch HT et al. (2010) Hereditary breast cancer clinical study group. Family history of cancer and cancer risks in women with BRCA1 or BRCA2 mutations. *J Natl Cancer Inst* 102(24):1874–1878.

Michl P, Downward J (2006) CUTL1: A key mediator of TGF beta-induced tumor invasion. *Cell Cycle* 5(2):132–134.

Michl P, Ramjaun AR, Pardo OE (2005) CUTL1 is a target of TGF (beta) signaling that enhances cancer cell motility and invasiveness. *Cancer Cell* 7(6):521–532.

Miglietta L, Vanella P, Canobbio L, Naso C et al. (2010) Prognostic value of estrogen receptor and Ki-67 index after neoadjuvant chemotherapy in locally advanced breast cancer expressing high levels of proliferation at diagnosis. *Oncology* 79(3–4):255–261.

Miles DW, Happerfield LC, Smith P et al. (1994) Expression of sialyl-Tn predicts the effect of adjuvant chemotherapy in node-positive breast cancer. *Br J Cancer* 70:1272–1275.

Miller LD, Smeds J, George J et al. (2005) An expression signature for p53 status in human breast cancer predicts mutation status, transcriptional effects, and patient survival. *Proc Natl Acad Sci* 102:13550–13555.

Miranda BT, Jones PA (2007) DNA methylation: The nuts and bolts of repression. *J Cell Physiol* 213:384–390.

Misek DE, Kim EH (2011a) Protein biomarkers for the early detection of breast cancer. *Int J Proteomic* 9:343582.

Misek DE, Kondo T, Duncan MW (2011b) Proteomics-based disease biomarkers. *Int J Proteomic*:894618.

Mitelman F, Johansson B, Mertens F (2004) Fusion genes and rearranged genes as a linear function of chromosome aberrations in cancer. *Nat Genet* 36:331–334.

Moffat Bradford A, Chenevert Thomas L, Meyer Charles R et al. (2006) The functional diffusion map: An imaging biomarker for the early prediction of cancer treatment outcome. *Neoplasia* 8(4):259–267.

Molina R, Auge JM, Farrus B et al. (2010) Prospective evaluation of carcinoembryonic antigen (CEA) and carbohydrate antigen 15.3 (CA15.3) in patients with primary locoregional breast cancer. *Clin Chem* 56(7):1148–1157.

Momparler RL (2003) Cancer epigenetics. *Oncogene* 22(42): 6479–6483.

Mote PA, Leary JA, Avery KA et al. (2004) Germ-line mutations in BRCA1 or BRCA2 in the normal breast are associated with altered expression of estrogen-responsive proteins and the predominance of progesterone receptor A. *Genes Chromosomes Cancer* 39(3):236–248.

Muggerud AA, Rønneberg JA, Wärnberg F et al. (2010) Frequent aberrant DNA methylation of ABCB1, FOXC1, PPP2R2B and PTEN in ductal carcinoma in situ and early invasive breast cancer. *Breast Cancer Res* 12(1):R3.

Mukhopadhyay P, Chakraborty S, Ponnusamy MP et al. (2011) Mucins in the pathogenesis of breast cancer: Implications in diagnosis, prognosis and therapy. *Biochim Biophys Acta* 1815(2):224–240.

Munagala R, Aqil F, Gupta RC (2011) Promising molecular targeted therapies in breast cancer. *Indian J Pharmacol* 43(3):236–245.

Murata H, Khattar NH, Kang Y et al. (2002) Genetic and epigenetic modification of mismatch repair genes hMSH2 and hMLH1 in sporadic breast cancer with microsatellite instability. *Oncogene* 21(37):5696–5703.

Nadal R, Fernandez A, Sanchez-Rovira P et al. (2012) Biomarkers characterization of circulating tumour cells in breast cancer patients. *Breast Cancer Res* 14:R71.

Naeim A, Wong FL, Pal SK et al. (2010) Oncologists' recommendations for adjuvant therapy in hormone receptor-positive breast cancer patients of varying age and health status. *Clin Breast Cancer* 10(2):136–143.

Nakagoe T, Itoyanagi T, Ikuta Y et al. (2002) Preoperative serum levels of Sialyl Lewisa, Sialyl Lewisx, and carcinoembryonic antigens as prognostic factors after resection for primary breast cancer. *Acta Med Nagasaki* 47:37–41.

Nakata B, Ogawa TY, Ishikawa T et al. (2004) Serum CYFRA 21-1 (cytokeratin-19 fragments) is a useful tumour marker for detecting disease relapse and assessing treatment efficacy in breast cancer. *Br J Cancer* 91:873–878.

Nam H, Chung BC, Kim Y et al. (2009) Combining tissue transcriptomics and urine metabolomics for breast cancer biomarker identification. *Bioinformatics* 25(23):3151–3157.

Narita T, Funahashi H, Satoh Y et al. (1993) Association of expression of blood group-related carbohydrate antigens with prognosis in breast cancer. *Cancer* 71:3044–3053.

National Cancer Institute at the National Institute of Health. Website: www.cancer.gov.

Nelson HD, Huffman LH, Fu R et al. (2005) Genetic risk assessment and BRCA mutation testing for breast and ovarian cancer susceptibility: Systematic evidence review for the US Preventive Services Task Force. *Ann Intern Med* 143:355–361.

Nepveu A (2001) Role of the multifunctional CDP/Cut/Cux homeodomain transcription factor in regulating differentiation, cell growth and development. *Gene* 270(1–2):1–15.

Neubauer H, Fehm T, Schütz C et al. (2007) Proteomic expression profiling of breast cancer. *Recent Results Cancer Res* 176:89–120.

Nguyen PL, Taghian AG, Katz MS et al. (2008) Breast cancer subtype approximated by estrogen receptor, progesterone receptor, and HER-2 is associated with local and distant recurrence after breast-conserving therapy. *J Clin Oncol* 26(14):2373–2378.

Nicolini A, Carpi A, Tarro G (2006) Biomolecular markers of breast cancer. *Front Biosci* 11:1818–1843.

Nielsen DL, Kümler I, Palshof JA et al. (2012) Efficacy of HER2-targeted therapy in metastatic breast cancer. Monoclonal antibodies and tyrosine kinase inhibitors. *Breast* S0960-9776(12)00194-4.

Nolen BM, Marks JR, Tasan S et al. (2008) Serum biomarker profiles and response to neoadjuvant chemotherapy for locally advanced breast cancer. *Breast Cancer Res.* 10(3):R45.

Norman SA, Berlin JA, Weber AL et al. (2003) Combined effect of oral contraceptive use and hormone replacement therapy on breast cancer risk in postmenopausal women. *Cancer Causes Control* 14(10):933–943.

Novak P, Jensen TJ, Garbe JC et al. (2009) Stepwise DNA methylation changes are linked to escape from defined proliferation barriers and mammary epithelial cell immortalization. *Cancer Res* 69(12):5251–5258.

Oakman C, Bessi S, Zafarana E et al. (2009) Recent advances in systemic therapy. New diagnostics and biological predictors of outcome in early breast cancer. *Breast Cancer Res* 11:205.

O'Day E and Lal A (2010). MicroRNAs and their target gene networks in breast cancer. *Breast cancer res.* 12(2):201.

Ogawa S, Inoue S, Watanabe T et al. (1998) The complete primary structure of human estrogen receptor beta (hER beta) and its heterodimerization with ER alpha in vivo and in vitro. *Biochem Biophys Res Commun* 243(1):122–126.

Ogawa Y, Ishikawa T, Ikeda K et al. (2000) Evaluation of serum KL-6, a mucin-like glycoprotein, as a tumor marker for breast cancer. *Clin Cancer Res* 6:4069–4072.

Olivier M et al. (2006) The clinical value of somatic TP53 gene mutations in 1,794 patients with breast cancer. *Clin Cancer Res* 12:1157–1167.

Olofsson MH, Ueno T, Pan Y et al. (2007) Cytokeratin-18 is a useful serum biomarker for early determination of response of breast carcinomas to chemotherapy. *Clin Cancer Res* 13(11):3198–3206.

Onay VU, Briollais L, Julia A Knight et al. (2006) SNP-SNP interactions in breast cancer susceptibility. *BMC Cancer* 6:114.

Onitilo AA, Engel JM, Greenlee RT et al. (2009) Breast cancer subtypes based on ER/PR and Her2 expression: Comparison of clinicopathologic features and survival. *Clin Med Res* 7(1–2):4–13.

Oremek GM, Sauer-Eppel H, Bruzdziak TH (2007) Value of tumour and inflammatory markers in lung cancer. *Anticancer Res* 27:1911–1916.

Ormandy CJ, Musgrove EA, Hui R et al. (2003) CyclinD1, EMS1 and 11q13 amplification in breast cancer. *Breast Cancer Res Treat* 78(3):323–335.

Ou K, Seow TK, Liang RC et al. (2001) Proteome analysis of a human heptocellular carcinoma cell line, HCC-M: An update. *Electrophoresis* 22(13):2804–2811.

Ou YH, Chung PH, Hsu FF (2007) The candidate tumor suppressor BTG3 is a transcriptional target of p53 that inhibits E2F1. *EMBO J* 26(17):3968–3980.

Owiredu WK, Donkor S, Addai BW et al. (2009) Serum lipid profile of breast cancer patients. *Pak J Biol Sci* 12(4):332–338.

Paik S, Hazan R, Fisher ER et al. (1990) Pathologic findings from the nations' surgical adjuvant breast and bowel project: Prognostic significance of erb B2 protein overexpression in primary breast cancer. *J Clin Oncol* 8:103–112.

Palma M, Ristori E, Ricevuto E et al. (2006) BRCA1 and BRCA2: The genetic testing and the current management options for mutation carriers. *Crit Rev Oncol/Hematol* 57(1):1–23.

Palsson B, Zengler K (2010) The challenges of integrating multi-omic data sets. *Nat Chem Biol* 11:787–789.

Park BW, Oh JW, Kim JH et al. (2008a) Preoperative CA 15-3 and CEA serum levels as predictor for breast cancer outcomes. *Ann Oncol* 19(4):675–681.

Park SM, Gaur AB, Lengyel E et al. (2008b) ThemiR-200 family determines the epithelial phenotype of cancer cells by targeting the E-cadherin repressors ZEB1 and ZEB2. *Genes Dev* 22(7):894–907.

Parsa P, Kandiah M, Rahman HA (2006) Barriers for breast cancer screening among Asian women: A mini literature review. *Asian Pacific J Cancer Prev* 7:509–514.

Patani N, Jiang W, Mansel R et al. (2009) The mRNA expression of SATB1 and SATB2 in human breast cancer. *Cancer Cell Int* 9:18.

Pathiraja TN, Shetty PB, Jelinek J et al. (2011) Progesterone receptor isoform-specific promoter methylation: Association of PRA promoter methylation with worse outcome in breast cancer patients. *Clin Cancer Res* 17:4177–4186.

Patnaik JL, Byers T, DiGuiseppi C et al. (2011) Cardiovascular disease competes with breast cancer as the leading cause of death for older females diagnosed with breast cancer. *Breast Cancer Res* 13(3):64.

Pawlik TM, Hawke DH, Liu Y et al. (2006) Proteomic analysis of nipple aspirate fluid from women with early-stage breast cancer using isotope-coded affinity tags and tandem mass spectrometry reveals differential expression of vitamin D binding protein. *BMC Cancer* 6:68.

Pecina-Slaus N (2003). Tumor suppressor gene E-cadherin and its role in normal and malignant cells. *Cancer Cell Int.* 3(1):17.

Pei Y, Zhang T, Renault V et al. (2009) An overview of hepatocellular carcinoma study by omics-based methods. *Acta Biochim Biophys Sin* 41(1):1–15.

Pennant M, Takwoingi Y, Pennant L, et al. (2010) A systematic review of positron emission tomography (PET) and positron emission tomography/computed tomography (PET/CT) for the diagnosis of breast cancer recurrence. *Health Technol Assess.* 14(50):1–103.

Penuelas I, Domınguez-Prado I, Garcıa-Velloso MJ et al. (2012) PET tracers for clinical imaging of breast cancer. *J Oncol* 2012:9pp.

Perkins GL, Slater ED, Sanders GK et al. (2003) Serum tumor markers. *Am Fam Physician* 68(6):1075–1082.

Perou CM, Sørlie T, Eisen MB et al. (2000) Molecular portraits of human breast tumours. *Nature* 406(6797):747–752.

Perreard L, Fan C, Quackenbush JF et al. (2006) Classification and risk stratification of invasive breast carcinomas using a real-time quantitative RT-PCR assay. *Breast Cancer Res* 8:R23.

Pijpe A, Andrieu N, Easton DF et al. (2012) Exposure to diagnostic radiation and risk of breast cancer among carriers of BRCA1/2 mutations: Retrospective cohort study (GENE-RAD-RISK). *BMJ* 345:e5660.

Piperi C, Themistocleous MS, Papavassiliou GA (2010) High incidence of MGMT and RARβ promoter methylation in primary glioblastomas: Association with histopathological characteristics, inflammatory mediators and clinical outcome. *Mol Med* 16(1–2):1–9.

Pouliot F, Johnson M, Wu L (2009) Non-invasive molecular imaging of prostate cancer lymph node metastasis. *Trends Mol Med* 15(6):254–262.

Prabasheela B, Arivazhagan R (2011) CA-15–3 and breast cancer. *Int J Pharma Bio Sci* 2(2):B 34–38.

Prasad SN, Houserkova D (2007) A comparison of mammography and ultrasonography in the evaluation of breast masses. *Biomed Pap Med Fac Univ Palacky Olomouc Czech Repub.* 151(2):315–322.

Pujana MA, Han JD, Starita LM et al. (2007) Network modeling links breast cancer susceptibility and centrosome dysfunction. *Nat Genet* 39:1338–1349.

Pusztai L (2008) Current status of prognostic profiling in breast cancer. *Oncologist* 13:350–360.

Pusztai L, Hess K (2004) Clinical trial design for microarray predictive marker discovery and assessment. *Ann Oncol* 15:1731–1737.

Qin H, Yu T, Qing T et al. (2007) Regulation of apoptosis and differentiation by p53 in human embryonic stem cells. *J Biol Chem* 282(8):5842–5852.

Quon A, Gambhir SS (2005) FDG-PET and beyond: Molecular breast cancer imaging. *JCO* 23(8):1664–1673.

Radpour R, Barekati Z, Kohler C et al. (2011) Integrated epigenetics of human breast cancer: Synoptic investigation of targeted genes, microRNAs and proteins upon demethylation treatment. *PLoS One* 6(11):e27355.

Rakha EA, Boyce RW, Abd El-Rehim D et al. (2005) Expression of mucins (MUC1, MUC2, MUC3, MUC4, MUC5AC and MUC6) and their prognostic significance in human breast cancer. *Mod Pathol* 18(10):1295–1304.

Ralhan R, Kaur J, Kreienberg R et al. (2007) Links between DNA double strand break repair and breast cancer: accumulating evidence from both familial and nonfamilial cases. *Cancer Lett* 248:1–17.

Ralph DA, Zhao LP, Aston CE et al. (2007) Age-specific association of steroid hormone pathway gene polymorphisms with breast cancer risk. *Cancer* 109(10):1940–1948.

Ramona FS, Massimo C (2011) Circulating tumor cells in breast cancer: A tool whose time has come of age. *BMC Med* 9:43.

Rampalli S et al. (2005) Tumor suppressor SMAR1 mediates cyclin D1 repression by recruitment of the SIN3/histone deacetylase 1 complex. *Mol Cell Biol* 25(19):8415–8429.

Raval GN, Patel DD, Parekh LJ et al. (2003) Evaluation of serum sialic acid, sialyltransferase and sialoproteins in oral cavity cancer. *Oral Dis* 9(3):119–128.

Rehman F, Nagi AH, Hussain M (2010) Immunohistochemical expression and correlation of mammaglobin with the grading system of breast carcinoma. *Indian J Pathol Microbiol* 53:619–623.

Rennstam K, Baldetorp B, Kytölä S et al. (2001) Chromosomal rearrangements and oncogene amplification precede aneuploidization in the genetic evolution of breast cancer. *Cancer Res* 61(3):1214–1219.

Rhodes DR et al. (2007) Oncomine 3.0: Genes, pathways, and networks in a collection of 18,000 cancer gene expression profiles. *Neoplasia* 9:166–180.

Richard SD, Bencherif B, Edwards RP et al. (2011) Noninvasive assessment of cell proliferation in ovarian cancer using [18F] 3′deoxy-3 fluorothymidine positron emission tomography/computed tomography imaging. *Nucl Med Biol* 38(4):485–491.

Riethdorf S, Fritsche H, Müller V et al. (2007) Detection of circulating tumor cells in peripheral blood of patients with metastatic breast cancer: A validation study of the CellSearch system. *Clin Cancer Res* 13(3):920–928.

Robert SA et al. (2004) Socioeconomic risk factors for breast cancer: Distinguishing individual-and community-level effects. *Epidemiology* 15:442–450.

Roberti MP, Arriaga JM, Bianchini M et al. (2012) Protein expression changes during human triple negative breast cancer cell line progression to lymphnode metastasis in a xenografted model in nude mice. *Cancer Biol Ther* 13(11):1123–1140.

Robertson DG, Watkins PB, Reily MD (2011) Metabolomics in toxicology: Preclinical and clinical applications. *Toxicol Sci* 120(S1):S146–S170.

Rocca-Serra P, Brazma A, Parkinson H et al. (2003) ArrayExpress: A public database of gene expression data at EBI. *Current Res Biol* 326:1075–1078.

Roden DM, Altman RB, Benowitz NL et al. (2006) Pharmacogenomics: Challenges and opportunities. *Ann Intern Med* 145(10):749–757.

Rofaiel S, Muo EN, Mousa SA (2010) Pharmacogenetics in breast cancer: Steps toward personalized medicine in breast cancer management. *Pharmacogenomics Pers Med* 3:129–143.

Ronckers CM, Erdmann CA, Land CE (2005) Radiation and breast cancer: A review of current evidencehttp://www.ncbi.nlm.nih.gov/pubmed/14750532. *Breast Cancer Res* 7:21–32.

Rose MC, Voynow JA (2006) Respiratory tract mucin genes and mucin glycoproteins in health and disease. *Physiol Rev* 86(1):245–278.

Rosen Eric L, Eubank William B, Mankoff David A (2007) FDG PET, PET/CT, and breast cancer imaging. *Radiographics* 27(1):S215–S229.

Ross JS (2008) Multigene predictors in early-stage breast cancer: Moving in or moving out? *Expert Rev Mol Diagn* 8(2):129–135.

Ross JS, Fletcher JA, Bloom KJ (2004) Targeted therapy in breast cancer: The HER-2/neu gene and protein. *Mol Cell Proteomic* 3(4):379–398.

Ross JS, Hatzis Christos, Symmans WF et al. (2008) Commercialized multigene predictors of clinical outcome for breast cancer. *The Oncologist* 13:477–493.

Ross JS, Linette GP, Stec J et al. (2004) Breast cancer biomarkers and molecular medicine: Part II. *Expert Rev Mol Diagn* 4(2):169–188.

Roy P, Shukla Y (2008) Applications of proteomic techniques in cancer research. *Cancer Ther* 6:841–856.

Sachdev D (2010) Targeting the type I insulin-like growth factor system for breast cancer therapy. *Curr Drug Targets* 11(9):1121–1132.

Sadikovic B, Al-Romaih K, Squire JA et al. (2008) Cause and consequences of genetic and epigenetic alterations in human cancer. *Curr Genomic* 9(6):394–408.

Saha A, Halder S, Upadhyay SK et al. (2011) Epstein-Barr virus nuclear antigen 3C facilitates G1-S transition by stabilizing and enhancing the function of cyclin D1. *PLoS Pathog* 7(2):e1001275.

Sakorafas GH, Farley DR, Peros G (2008) Recent advances and current controversies in the management of DCIS of the breast. *Cancer Treat Rev* 34:483–497.

Saldova R, Rueben JM, Abd H et al. (2010) Levels of specific serum N-glycans identify breast cancer patients with higher circulating tumor cell counts. *Ann Oncol* 22(5):1113–1119.

Saloustros E, Perraki M, Apostolaki S et al. (2011) Cytokeratin-19 mRNA-positive circulating tumor cells during follow-up of patients with operable breast cancer: Prognostic relevance for late relapse. *Breast Cancer Res* 13:R60.

Sarkar DK, Lahiri S, Kar RG et al. (2008) Utility of prognostic markers in management of breast cancer. *Internet J Surg* 17(1).

Saslow D, Boetes C, Burke W et al. (2007) American Cancer Society guidelines for breast screening with MRI as an adjunct to mammography. *CA Cancer J Clin* 57:75–89.

Sauter E, Welch T, Magklara A et al. (2002) Ethnic variation in kallikrein expression in nipple Aspirate fluid. *Int J Cancer* 100:678–682.

Sauter ER, Ross E, Daly M et al. (1997) Nipple aspirate fluid: A promising non-invasive method to identify cellular markers of breast cancer risk. *Br J Cancer* 76(4):494–501.

Schiff R, Massarweh SA, Shou J et al. (2005) Advanced concepts in estrogen receptor biology and breast cancer endocrine resistance: Implicated role of growth factor signaling and estrogen receptor coregulators. *Cancer Chemother Pharmacol* 56(l):10–20.

Schmid F, Burock S, Klockmeier K et al. (2012) SNPs in the coding region of the metastasis-inducing gene MACC1 and clinical outcome in colorectal cancer. *Mol Cancer* 11:49.

Schott AF, Hayes DF (2012) Defining the benefits of neoadjuvant chemotherapy for breast cancer. *J Clin Oncol* 30(15):1747–1749.

Schrauder MG, Strick R, Schulz-Wendtland R et al. (2012) Circulating micro-RNAs as potential blood-based markers for early stage breast cancer detection. *PLoS One* 7(1):e29770.

Schumann D, Huang J, Clarke PE et al. (2004) Characterization of recombinant soluble carcinoembryonic antigen cell adhesion molecule. *Biochem Biophys Res Comm* 318:227–233.

Scott GK, Goga A, Bhaumik D et al. (2007) Coordinate suppression of ERBB2 and ERBB3 by enforced expression of micro-RNA miR-125a or miR-125b. *J Biol Chem* 282:1479–1486.

Sebova K, Zmetakova I, Bella V et al. (2011–2012) RASSF1A and CDH1 hypermethylation as potential epimarkers in breast cancer. *Cancer Biomark* 10(1):13–26.

Senapati S, Das S, Batra SK (2010) Mucin interacting proteins: From function to therapeutics. *Trends Biochem Sci* 35:236–245.

Seregni E, Coli A, Mazzuca N (2008) Circulating tumour markers in breast cancer. *Breast Cancer*:33–42.

Serkova NJ, Glunde K (2009) Metabolomics of cancer. *Methods Mol Biol* 520:273–295.

Shah C, Miller TW, Wyatt SK et al. (2009) Therapy in preclinical models of breast cancer imaging biomarkers predict response to anti-HER2 (ErbB2). *Clin Cancer Res* 15:4712–4721.

Shah FD, Shukla SN, Shah PM et al. (2008) Significance of alterations in plasma lipid profile levels in breast cancer. *Integr Cancer Ther* 7(1):33–41.

Shankar LK (2012) The clinical evaluation of novel imaging methods for cancer management. *Nature Rev Clin Oncol* 9:738–744.

Sharma R, Tripathi M, Panwar P et al. (2009) 99mTc-methionine scintimammography in the evaluation of breast cancer. *Nucl Med Commun* 30(5):338–342.

Sherlock G et al. (2001) The Stanford microarray database. *Nucleic Acids Res* 29:152–155.

Shimokawa K, Mogushi K, Shoji S et al. (2010) iCOD: An integrated clinical omics database based on the systems-pathology view of disease. *BMC Genomic* (4):S19.

Siah SP, Quinn DM, Graeme DB et al. (2000) Microsatellite instability markers in breast cancer: A review and study showing MSI was not detected at 'BAT 25' and 'BAT 26' microsatellite markers in early-onset breast cancer. *Breast Cancer Res Treat* 60(2):135–142.

Sikaroodi M, Galachiantz Y, Baranova A (2010) Tumor markers: The potential of "omics" approach. *Curr Mol Med* 10:249–257.

Silberman S, Breitfeld P, Butzbach A (2012) Imaging biomarkers in oncology drug development. *J Clin Stud* 4(3):22–24.

Silva CL, Passos M, Câmara JS (2012) Solid phase microextraction, mass spectrometry and metabolomic approaches for detection of potential urinary cancer biomarkers—A powerful strategy for breast cancer diagnosis. *Talanta* 89:360–368.

Simons K, Sampaio JL (2011) Membrane organization and lipid rafts. *Cold Spring Harb Perspect Biol* 3:a004697.

Simons K, Toomre D (2000) Lipid rafts and signal transduction. *Nature Rev Mol Cell Biol* 1(1):31–39.

Simpson DC, Smith RD (2005) Combining capillary electrophoresis with mass spectrometry for applications in proteomics. *Electrophoresis* 26(7–8):1291–1305.

Singh K et al. (2009) Tumor suppressor SMAR1 represses IkappaBalpha expression and inhibits p65 transactivation through matrix attachment regions. *J Biol Chem* 284(2):1267–1278.

Singh K, Mogare D, Giridharagopalan RO et al. (2007) p53 target gene SMAR1 is dysregulated in breast cancer: Its role in cancer cell migration and invasion. *PLoS One* 2(8):e660.

Singletary SE, Allred C, Ashley P et al. (2002) Revision of the American joint committee on cancer staging system for breast cancer. *J Clin Oncol* 20:3628–3636.

Sinicrope FA, Dannenberg AJ (2011) Obesity and breast cancer prognosis: Weight of the evidence. *J Clin Oncol* 29(1):4–7.

Slamon DJ, Clark GM (1988) Amplification of C-ERB-B2 and aggressive breast tumors? *Science* 240:1795–1798.

Śliwowska I, Kopczyński Z, Grodecka-Gazdecka S (2006) Diagnostic value of measuring serum CA 15–3, TPA, and TPS in women with breast cancer. *Postepy Hig Med Dosw* 60:295–299.

Smart YC, Stewart JF, Bartlett LD et al. (1990) Mammary serum antigen (MSA) in advanced breast cancer. *Breast Cancer Res Treat* 16(1):23–28.

Smith GL, Xu Y, Buchholz TA et al. (2012) Association between treatment with brachytherapy vs whole-breast irradiation and subsequent mastectomy, complications, and survival among older women with invasive breast cancer. *JAMA* 307(17):1827–1837.

Snell C, Krypuy M, Wong EM et al. (2008) BRCA1 promoter methylation in peripheral blood DNA of mutation negative familial breast cancer patients with a BRCA1 tumour phenotype. *Breast Cancer Res* 10:R12.

Soares R, Marinho A, Schmitt F (1996) Expression of sialyl-Tn in breast cancer. Correlation with prognostic parameters. *Pathol Res Pract* 192:1181–1186.

Song M, Pan K, Su H et al. (2012) Identification of serum micrornas as novel non-invasive biomarkers for early detection of gastric cancer. *PLoS One* 7(3):e33608.

Sorlie T, Perou CM et al. (2001) Gene expression patterns of breast carcinomas distinguish tumor subclasses with clinical implications. *Proc Natl Acad Sci USA* 98(19):10869–10874.

Sotiriou C, Neo SY, McShane LM et al. (2003) Breast cancer classification and prognosis based on gene expression profiles from a population-based study. *Proc Natl Acad Sci USA* 100(18):10393–10398.

Sotiriou C, Wirapati P, Loi S et al. (2006) Gene expression pro-filing in breast cancer: Understanding the molecular basis of histologic grade to improve prognosis. *J Natl Cancer Inst* 98(4):262–272.

Souzaki M, Kubo M, Kai M et al. (2011) Hedgehog signaling pathway mediates the progression of non-invasive breast cancer to invasive breast cancer. *Cancer Sci* 102(2):373–381.

Spaderna S, Schmalhofer O, Wahlbuhl M et al. (2008) The transcriptional repressor ZEB1 promotes metastasis and loss of cell polarity in cancer. *Cancer Res* 68:537–544.

Stacey SN, Sulem P, Zanon C et al. (2010) Ancestry-shift refinement mapping of the C6orf97-ESR1 breast cancer susceptibility locus. *PLoS Genet* 6: e1001029.

Stacker SA, Thompson CH, Sacks NPM et al. (1988) Cancer patients using monoclonal antibody 3e1.2 detection of mammary serum antigen in sera from breast. *Cancer Res* 48:7060–7066.

Stathopoulou A, Vlachonikolis I, Mavroudis D et al. (2002) Molecular detection of cytokeratin-19 – positive cells in the peripheral blood of patients with operable breast cancer: Evaluation of their prognostic significance. *J Clin Oncol* 20(16):3404–3412.

Stefansson OA, Jonasson JG, Olafsdottir K et al. (2011) CpG island hypermethylation of BRCA1 and loss of pRb as co-occurring events in basal/triple-negative breast cancer. *Epigenetics* 6(5):638–649.

Stokłosa T, Gołąb J (2005) Prospects for p53-based cancer therapy. *Acta Biochimica Polonica* 52(2):321–328.

Stoklosa T, Golab J (2005). Prospects for p53-based cancer therapy. *Acta Biochim Pol.* 52(2):321–8.

Stoppa-Lyonnet D, Buecher B, Houdayer C et al. (2009) Implications of genetic risk factors in breast cancer: Culprit genes and associated malignancies. *Bull Acad Natl Med* 193(9):2063–2083.

Streckfus CF, Arreola D, Edwards C et al. (2012) Salivary Protein profiles amongHER2/neu-receptor-positive and -negative breast cancer patients: Support for using salivary protein profiles for modeling breast cancer progression. *J Oncol* 2012:1–9.

Sugita M, Geraci M, Gao B et al. (2002) Combined use of oligonucleotide and tissue microarrays identifies cancer/testis antigens as biomarkers in lung carcinoma. *Cancer Res* 62(14):3971–3979.

Suijkerbuijk KP, Pan X, van der Wall E et al. (2010) Comparison of different promoter methylation assays in breast cancer. *Anal Cell Pathol* (Amst) 33(3):133–141.

Suijkerbuijk KPM, van Diest PJE et al. (2011) Improving early breast cancer detection: Focus on methylation. *Ann Oncol* 22(1):24–29.

Suijkerbuijk KPM, Wall E, Vooijs M et al. (2008) Molecular analysis of nipple fluid for breast cancer screening. *Pathobiology* 75:149–152.

Sun F, Fu H, Liu Q et al. (2008) Down regulation of CCND1 and CDK6 by miR-34a induces cell cycle arrest. *FEBS Lett* 582(10):1564–1568.

Sun X, Liu JJ, Wang YS et al. (2011) Using intra-operative gene search TM breast lymph node assay to detect breast cancer metastases in sentinel lymph nodes: Results from a single institute in China. *Chin Med J (Engl)* 124(7):973–977.

Suryadevara A, Paruchuri LP, Banisaeed N et al. (2010) The clinical behavior of mixed ductal/lobular carcinoma of the breast: A clinicopathologic analysis. *World J Surg Oncol* 8:51.

Suter R, Marcum JA (2007) The molecular genetics of breast cancer and targeted therapy. *Biologics* 1(3):241–258.

Swaby RF, Cristofanilli M (2011) Circulating tumor cells in breast cancer: A tool whose time has come of age. *BMC Med* 9:43.

Swen JJ, Huizinga TW, Gelderblom H et al. (2007) Translating pharmacogenomics: Challenges on the road to the clinic. *PLoS Med* 4(8):e209.

Swift-Scanlan T, Vang R, Blackford A, Fackler MJ, Sukumar S (2011) Methylated genes in breast cancer: Associations with clinical and histopathological features in a familial breast cancer cohort. *Cancer Biol Ther* 11(10):853–865.

Tahir M, Hendry P, Baird L et al. (2006) Radiation induced angiosarcoma a sequela of radiotherapy for breast cancer following conservative surgery. *Int Semin Surg Oncol* 3:26.

Tchen N, Juffs HG, Downie FP et al. (2003) Cognitive function, fatigue, and menopausal symptoms in women receiving adjuvant chemotherapy for breast cancer. *J Clin Oncol* 21:4175–4183.

Teng P, Bateman NW, Hood BL et al. (2010) Conrads advances in proximal fluid proteomics for disease biomarker discovery. *J Proteome Res* 9(12):6091–6100.

Tesch G, Amur S, Schousboe JT et al. (2010) Successes achieved and challenges ahead in translating biomarkers into clinical applications. *AAPS J* 12(3):243–53.

Thomas M, Lieberman J, Lal A (2010) Desperately seeking microRNA targets. *Nat Struct Mol Biol* 17:1169–1174.

Tobin D, Lindahl T, Hagen N et al. (2007) Employing a blood based gene expression signature to detect early stage breast cancer. *J Clin Oncol* 25(18S):21117.

Tobin NP, Sims AH, Lundgren KL et al. (2011) CyclinD1, Id1 and EMT in breast cancer. *BMC Cancer* 11:417.

Tomasi G, Kenny L, Mauri F et al. (2011) Quantification of receptor-ligand binding with [18F]fluciclatide in metastatic breast cancer patients. *Eur J Nucl Med Mol Imaging* 38:2186–2197.

Toretsky J, Levenson A, Weinberg IN et al. (2004) Preparation of F-18 labeled annexin V: A potential PET radiopharmaceutical for imaging cell death. *Nucl Med Biol* 31(6):747–752.

Treon SP, Maimonis P, Bua D et al. (2000) Elevated soluble MUC1 levels and decreased anti-MUC1 antibody levels in patients with multiple myeloma. *Blood* 96:3147–3153.

Truscott M, Raynal L, Premdas P et al. (2003) CDP/Cux stimulates transcription from the DNA polymerase alpha gene promoter. *Mol Cell Biol* 23(8):3013–3028.

Tsuchida T, Okazawa H, Mori T et al. (2007) In vivo imaging of estrogen receptor concentration in the endometrium and myometrium using 18F-FES PET—Influence of menstrual cycle and endogenous estrogen level. *Nucl Med Biol* 34(2):205–210.

Tung N, Miron A, Schnitt SJ et al. (2010) Prevalence and predictors of loss of wild type BRCA1 in estrogen receptor positive and negative BRCA1-associated breast cancers. *Breast Cancer Res* 12(6):R95.

Turnpenny P, Ellard S (2005) *Emery's Elements of Medical Genetics*, 12th ed. London, U.K.: Elsevier.

Tworoger SS and Hankinson SE (2006). Collecxtion, processing and storage of biological samples in epidemiologic studie:s sex harmones, caratenoids, inflammatory markers and proteomics as examples. *Cance Epid. Bio. Prev.* 15:1578–1581.

Ura Y, Dion AS, Williams CJ et al. (1992) Quantitative dot blot analyses of blood-group-related antigens in paired normal and malignant human breast tissues. *Int J Cancer* 50:57–63.

Usary J, Llaca V, Karaca G et al. (2004) Mutation of GATA3 in human breast tumors. *Oncogene* 23(46):7669–7678.

Ushijima T (2005) Detection and interpretation of altered methylation patterns in cancer cells. *Nat Rev Cancer* 5:223–231.

Ushijima T, Asada K (2010) Aberrant DNA methylation in contrast with mutations. *Cancer Sci* 101(2):300–305.

Vadnais C, Davoudi S, Afshin M et al. (2012) CUX1 transcription factor is required for optimal ATM/ATR-mediated responses to DNA damage. *Nucleic Acids Res* 40(10):4483–4495.

Valastyan S, Reinhardt F, Benaich N et al. (2009) A pleiotropically acting microRNA, miR-31, inhibits breast cancer metastasis. *Cell* 137:1032–1046.

van de Vijver MJ, Peterse JL, Mooi WJ, Wisman P, Lomans J, Dalesio O, Nusse R (1988) Neu-protein overexpression in breast cancer. Association with comedo-type ductal carcinoma *in situ* and limited prognostic value in stage II breast cancer. *N Engl J Med* 319:1239–1245.

van de Vivjer MJ, Peterse JL, Mooi WJ et al. (1988) Neu-protein overexpression in breast cancer. *N Engl J Med* 319:1239–1245.

Van De Voorde L, Speeckaert R, VanGestel D et al. (2012) DNA methylation-based biomarkers in serum of patients with breast cancer. *Mutat Res* 751(2):304–325.

van den Akker EB, Verbruggen B, Heijmans BT et al. (2011) Integrating protein-protein interaction networks with gene-gene co-expression networks improves gene signatures for classifying breast cancer metastasis. *J Integr Bioinform* 8(2):188.

van der Auwera I, Peeters D, Benoy I H et al. (2010) Circulating tumour cell detection: A direct comparison between the CellSearch System, the AdnaTest and CK-19/mammaglobin RT–PCR in patients with metastatic breast cancer. *Br J Cancer* 102(2):276–284.

van der Auwera I, Van Laere SJ, Van den Bosch SM et al. (2008) Aberrant methylation of the Adenomatous Polyposis Coli (APC) gene promoter is associated with the inflammatory breast cancer phenotype. *Br J Cancer* 99:1735–1742.

Varghese C (2007) The significance of oestrogen and progesterone receptors in breast cancer. *J Clin Diagn Res* 1:198–203.

Varki A (1994) Selectin ligands. *Proc Natl Acad Sci USA* 91:7390–7397.

Varki A, Cummings RD, Esko JD et al. (2009) *Essentials of Glycobiology*, 2nd ed. Cold Spring Harbor, NY: Cold Spring Harbor Laboratory Press.

Vaughan Christopher L (2012) New developments in medical imaging to detect breast cancer. *CME* 30(1).

Veeck J, Esteller M (2010) Breast cancer epigenetics: From DNA methylation to microRNAs. *J Mammary Gland Biol Neoplasia* 15(1):5–17.

Verma S, Lavasani S, Mackey J et al. (2010) Optimizing the management of her2-positive early breast cancer: The clinical reality. *Curr Oncol* 17(4):20–33.

Verma S, Miles D, Gianni L et al. (2012) Trastuzumab emtansine for HER2-positive advanced breast cancer. *N Engl J Med* 367(19):1783–1791.

Verring A, Clouth A, Ziolkowski P et al. (2011) Clinical usefulness of cancer markers in primary breast cancer. *Pathology*: 4pp.

Vesselle H, Grierson J, Muzi M et al. (2002) in vivo validation of 3′deoxy-3′-[18F]fluorothymidine ([18F]FLT) as a proliferation imaging tracer in humans: Correlation of [18F]FLT uptake by positron emission tomography with Ki-67 immunohistochemistry and flow cytometry in human lung tumors. *Clin Cancer Res* 8(11):3315–3323.

Viale G, Maiorano E, Pruneri G et al. (2005) Predicting the risk for additional axillary metastases in patients with breast carcinoma and positive sentinel lymph node biopsy. *Ann Surg* 241(2):319–325.

Viale G, Regan MM, Maiorano E et al. (2007) Prognostic and predictive value of centrally reviewed expression of estrogen and progesterone receptors in a randomized trial comparing letrozole and tamoxifen adjuvant therapy for postmenopausal early breast cancer: BIG1-98. *J Clin Oncol* 25(25):3846–3852.

Vogel CL, Cobleigh MA, Tripathy D (2002) Efficacy and safety of trastuzumab as a single agent in first-line treatment of HER2-overexpressing metastatic breast cancer. *J Clin Oncol* 20(3):719–726.

Volinia S, Calin GA, Liu CG et al. (2006) A microRNA expression signature of human solid tumors defines cancer gene targets. *Proc Natl Acad Sci* 103(7):2257–2261.

Voyatzi S, Desiris K, Paikos DA et al. (2010) Promoter methylation of p16^{INK4A}, RASSF1A, and RAR2b genes in tumor DNA from patients with breast cancer (BC) in correlation with clinical recurrence. *J Clin Oncol* 28:15.

Wajapeyee N, Somasundaram K (2004) Pharmacogenomics in breast cancer: Current trends and future directions. *Curr Opin Mol Ther* 6(3):296–301.

Wang K, Lee I, Carlson G et al. (2010) Systems biology and the discovery of diagnostic biomarkers. *Dis Markers* 28: 199–207.

Wang L (2010) Pharmacogenomics: A systems approach. *Wiley Interdiscip Rev Syst Biol Med* 2(1):3–22.

Wang P-H (2005) Altered glycosylation in cancer: Sialic acids and sialyltransferases. *J Cancer Molecules* 1(2):73–81.

Wang SP, Wang WL, Chang YL et al. (2009a) p53 controls cancer cell invasion by inducing the MDM2-mediated degradation of slug. *Nat Cell Biol* 11:694–704.

Wang Z, Gerstein M, Snyder M (2009b) RNA-Seq: A revolutionary tool for transcriptomics. *Nature Rev Genetics* 10:57–63.

Weaver DL (2010) Pathology evaluation of sentinel lymph nodes in breast cancer: Protocol recommendations and rationale. *Mod Pathol* (Suppl 2):S26–S32.

Weigel MT, Dowsett M (2010) Current and emerging biomarkers in breast cancer: Prognosis and prediction. *Endocr Relat Cancer* 17(4):R245–R262.

Wenk MR (2005) The emerging field of lipidomics. *Nat Rev Drug Discov* 4(7):594–610.

Whitcher B, Schmid VJ (2011) Quantitative analysis of dynamic contrast-enhanced and diffusion-weighted magnetic resonance imaging for oncology in R. *J Stat Softw* 44:5.

Whitehead CM, Nelson R, Hudson P et al. (2004) Selection and optimization of a panel of early stage breast cancer prognostic molecular markers. *Mod Pathol* 17:50A.

Wiechmann L, Kuerer HM (2008) The molecular journey from ductal carcinoma in situ to invasive breast cancer. *Cancer* 112(10):2130–2142.

Wiedswang Gro, Borgen Elin, Kåresen Rolf et al. (2004) Isolated tumor cells in bone marrow three years after diagnosis in disease-free breast cancer patients predict unfavorable clinical outcome. *Clin Cancer Res* 10(16):5342–5348.

Williams-Jones B, Carriyan OP (2003) Rheotoric and type: Where's the ethics in pharmacogenomics? *Am J Pharmacogenomic* 3(6):375–383.

Wood AJJ, Shapiro CL, Recht A (2001) Side effects of adjuvant treatment of breast cancer. *N Engl J Med* 344(26).

Wu K, Zhang Y (2007) Clinical application of tear proteomics: Present and future prospects. *Proteomics–Clin Appl* 1(9):972–982.

Wulfkuhle JD, Paweletz CP, Steeg PS et al. (2003) Proteomic approaches to the diagnosis, treatment, and monitoring of cancer. *Adv Exp Med Biol* 532:59–68.

www.cancer.gov.

Xenidis N, Ignatiadis M, Apostolaki S et al. (2009) Cytokeratin-19 mRNA-positive circulating tumor cells after adjuvant chemotherapy in patients with early breast cancer. *JCO* 27(13):2177–2184.

Xiao-yuan Fan, Xin-lei Hu, Tie-mei Han et al. (2011) Association between RUNX3 promoter methylation and gastric cancer: A meta-analysis. *BMC Gastroenterol* 11:92.

Xing Y, Xue Z, Englander S et al. (2008) Improving parenchyma segmentation by simultaneous estimation of tissue property T1 map and group-wise registration of inversion recovery MR breast images. *Med Image Comput Comput Assist Interv.* 11(1):342–350.

Xu J, Wang B, Zhang Y (2012) Clinical implications for BRCA gene mutation in breast cancer. *Mol Biol Rep* 39(3):3097–3102.

Yan LX, Huang XF, Shao Q et al. (2008) MicroRNA miR-21 overexpression in human breast cancer is associated with advanced clinical stage, lymph node metastasis and patient poor prognosis. *RNA* 14(11):2348–2360.

Yan PS, Venkataramu C, Ibrahim A et al. (2006) Mapping geographic zones of cancer risk with epigenetic biomarkers in normal breast tissue. *Clin Cancer Res* 12(22):6626–6636.

Yang R, Cheung MC, Hurley J et al. (2009) A comprehensive evaluation of outcomes for inflammatory breast cancer. *Breast Cancer Res Treat* 117(3):631–641.

Yiannakopoulou EC (2012) Pharmacogenomics of breast cancer targeted therapy: Focus on recent patents. *Recent Pat DNA Gene Seq* 6:33–46.

Yin P, Roqueiro D, Huang L, Owen JK, Xie A et al. (2012) Genome-wide progesterone receptor binding: Cell type-specific and shared mechanisms in T47D breast cancer cells and primary leiomyoma cells. *PLoS One* 7(1):e29021.

Yong Li (2010) The detection of tear biomarkers for future prostate cancer diagnosis. *Open Biomark J* 3:26–29.

Yoo J, Dence CS, Sharp TL et al. (2005) Synthesis of an estrogen receptor beta-selective radioligand: 5-[18F] fluro-(2R,3S)-2,3-bis(4-hydroxyphenyl) pentanenitrile and comparision of in vivo distribution with 16alpha-[18F]fluoro-17beta-estradiol. *J Med Chem* 48(20):6366–6378.

Yousef GM, Diamandis EP (2001) The new human tissue kallikrein gene family: Structure, function, and association to disease. *Endocr Rev* 22(2):184 –204.

Yu F, Yao H, Zhu P et al. (2007) let-7 regulates self renewal and tumorigenicity of breast cancer cells. *Cell* 131(6):1109–1123.

Yu J, Zhang Y, Qi Z (2008) Methylation-mediated downregulation of the B-cell translocation gene 3 (BTG3) in breast cancer cells. *Gene Expr* 14(3):173–182.

Zehentner BK, Persing DH, Deme A et al. (2004) Mammaglobin as a novel breast cancer biomarker: Multigene reverse transcription-PCR assay and sandwich ELISA. *Clin Chem* 50(11):2069–2076.

Zeinab B, Ramin R, Qing L et al. (2012) Methylation signature of lymph node metastases in breast cancer patients. *BMC Cancer* 12:244.

Zelivianski S, Cooley A, Kall R et al. (2010) Cyclin-dependent kinase 4-mediated phosphorylation inhibits Smad3 activity in cyclin D-overexpressing breast cancer cells. *Mol Cancer Res* 8(10):1375–1387.

Zhang F, Chen JY (2011) Data mining methods in omics-based biomarker discovery. *Methods Mol Biol* 719:511–526.

Zhang J, Liu YJ (2008) HER2 over-expression and response to different chemotherapy regimens in breast cancer. *Zhejiang Univ Sci B* 9(1):5–9.

Zhang J, Baran J, Cros A et al. (2011a) International cancer genome consortium data portal: A one stop-shop for cancer genomics data. Database.

Zhang J, Bowers J, Liu L et al. (2012a) Esophageal cancer metabolite biomarkers detected by LC-MS and NMR methods. *PLoS One* 7(1):e30181.

Zhang L, Kelly G, Hagen T (2011b) The cellular microenvironment and cell adhesion: A role for O-glycosylation. *Biochem Soc Trans* 39(1):378–382.

Zhang L, Xiao H, Karlan S et al. (2010) Discovery and preclinical validation of salivary transcriptomic and proteomic biomarkers for the non-invasive detection of breast cancer. *Plos One.* 31:5(12):e15573.

Zhang L, Xiao H, Karlan S et al. (2010) Discovery and preclinical validation of salivary transcriptomic and proteomic biomarkers for the non-invasive detection of breast cancer. *PLoS One* 5(12):e15573.

Zhang S, Liu C, Li W et al. (2012b) Discovery of multi-dimensional modules by integrative analysis of cancer genomic data. *Nucleic Acids Res* 1–13.

Zhao H, Shen J, Medico L et al. (2010) A pilot study of circulating miRNAs as potential biomarkers of early stage breast cancer. *PLoS One* 5(10):e13735.

Zhao Y, Deng C, Wang J, Xiao J, Gatalica Z, Recker RR, Xiao GG (2010) Let-7 family miRNAs regulate estrogen receptor alpha signaling in estrogen receptor positive breast cancer. *Breast Cancer Res Treat* 127(1):69–80.

Zhao Y, Verselis S J, Klar N et al. (2001) Nipple fluid carcinoembryonic antigen and prostate-specific antigen in cancer-bearing and tumor-free breasts. *J Clin Oncol* 19(5):1462–1467.

Zheng Y, Huo D, Zhang J et al. (2012a) Microsatellites in the Estrogen Receptor (ESR1, ESR2) and Androgen Receptor (AR) genes and breast cancer risk in African American and Nigerian women. *PLoS One* 7(7):e40494.

Zheng YY, Xie L, Liu L et al. (2012b) BAT-25 polymorphism in Chinese from Jiangsu province and its implication for locus microsatellite instability screening. *Int J Biol Markers* 27(3):e227–e231.

Zhong Li, Ge K, Zu J-C et al. (2008) Autoantibodies as potential biomarkers for breast cancer. *Breast Cancer Res* 10:R40.

Zhou L, Beuerman RW, Chan CM et al. (2009) Identification of tear fluid biomarkers in dry eye syndrome using iTRAQ quantitative proteomics. *J Proteome Res* 8(11):4889–4905.

Zhu CS, Pinsky PF, Cramer DW et al. (2011) A framework for evaluating biomarkers for early detection: Validation of biomarker panels for ovarian cancer. *Cancer Prev Res* 4(3):375–383.

Zhu S, Si M, Wu H et al. (2007) MicroRNA-21 targets the tumor suppressor gene tropomyosin 1 (TPM1). *J Biol Chem* 282:14328–14336.

Zhu W, Qin W, Sauter ER (2004) Large-scale mitochondrial DNA deletion mutations and nuclear genome instability in human breast cancer. *Cancer Detect Prev* 28(2):119–126.

Zuoren Yu, Renato B, Lide C et al. (2010) microRNA, cell cycle, and human breast cancer. *Am J Pathol* 176(3):1058–1064.

4

Diagnostic and Prognostic Markers of Breast Invasive Lesions

Maria C. Calomarde, MD, Carlos Iglesias, MD, Elisa Moreno-Palacios, MD, Javier De Santiago, MD, PhD, and Ignacio Zapardiel, MD, PhD

CONTENTS

ABSTRACT Breast cancer is the most common cancer in women, the second most common cause of cancer death in women, and the main cause of death in women aged 40–59. Important risk factors are age, gender, reproductive history, hormonal factors, and family history. Diagnostic evaluation includes screening and diagnostic breast imaging and breast biopsy. There are several histologic kinds of breast cancer; however, 70%–80% of breast cancers are infiltrating ductal carcinomas. An assay of hormone receptors is important for both prognostic and predictive purposes as patients could benefit from endocrine treatments. Also, HER 2/neu expression should be assayed as it represents an important predictive factor because patients might benefit from treatments such as trastuzumab. Other prognostic factors include the status of the draining axillary lymph nodes, tumor size, tumor grade, markers of an elevated proliferative rate, and circulating tumor cells. Treatment of locoregional disease includes surgery, radiation therapy, or both, and treatment of systemic disease with unique or a combination of chemotherapy, endocrine therapy, or biologic therapy. In patients with clinically node-negative breast cancer, sentinel lymph node biopsy identifies the status of the axillary nodes. Primary tumor size, lymph node status, and histologic grade of differentiation are all important prognostic factors to help in the determination of an individual adjuvant systemic therapy.

4.1 Introduction

4.1.1 Epidemiology

Global cancer statistics show that breast cancer is the most frequently diagnosed cancer and the leading cause of cancer death among females, accounting for 23% of total cancer cases and 14% of cancer deaths (Siegel et al. 2011, Jemal et al. 2011). Breast cancer is now also the leading cause of cancer death among females in economically developing countries. Despite increasing incidence rates, annual mortality rates from breast cancer have decreased over the last decade (1.8% per year from 1998 to 2007) (Kohler et al. 2011). The decline has been more pronounced in Caucasian than in African-American women. The lifetime probability of developing breast cancer is one in six overall (one in eight for invasive disease).

In the early 1980s, breast cancer rates rose steeply by 3.7% per year over the baseline incidence. This was most likely the result of the increasing use of screening mammography, since the incidence of ductal carcinoma in situ (DCIS) and stage I carcinomas increased, while that of higher stages either decreased or remained stable. After increasing from 1994 to 1999, breast cancer incidence rates decreased from 1999 to 2007 by 1.8% per year (Kohler et al. 2011).

Potential contributory factors to this decline include discontinuation of hormone therapy (HT) according to the data from the Women's Health Initiative (WHI) linking HT and breast cancer and saturation/leveling off of mammography rates. Discontinuation of HT has probably had a greater effect. The WHI reported their data on breast cancer risk in the postintervention phase of the randomized trial (HT vs. placebo) and in the observational (HT users vs. nonusers) cohort. In both groups, there was a rapid decline in breast cancer incidence after discontinuation of HT. Changes in mammography utilization were unlikely to have contributed to the decrease, since postintervention mammography rates were similar in both the HT and control arms of the randomized trial, and mammography rates did not fluctuate over time in the observational cohort (Breen et al. 2007).

Globally, breast cancer is the most frequently diagnosed cancer and the leading cause of cancer death in females. Breast cancer incidence rates are highest in North America, Australia/New Zealand, and in western and northern Europe and lowest in Asia and sub-Saharan Africa. Despite the decreases in incidence rates in North America, breast cancer incidence has been increasing in other parts of the world, such as Asia and Africa. These international differences are thought to be related to societal changes occurring during industrialization (e.g., changes in fat intake, body weight, age at menarche and/or lactation, and reproductive patterns such as fewer pregnancies and later age at first birth).

Breast cancer mortality rates have declined since 1975, attributed to the increased use of screening mammography and greater use and improvements of adjuvant therapies. However, this trend has not been equally seen in all subgroups:

- Despite having a lower incidence rate than white women, black women have a higher mortality rate, which is attributable to both more advanced stage at diagnosis and higher stage-specific mortality.
- The mortality decline has been greater in women younger than age 50 (3.8% per year) compared to older women (2.2% per year).
- Declines have also been greater for women with ER-/PR-positive as compared to ER-/PR-negative tumors.

A significant portion of the decline in mortality is attributable to the impact of screening mammography, which permits diagnosis at an earlier stage of disease (Berry et al. 2005). Preinvasive breast cancer (DCIS) now accounts for 25%–30% of all newly diagnosed, mammographically detected breast cancers.

4.1.2 Types of Breast Cancer

Most breast malignancies arise from epithelial elements and are categorized as carcinomas. Breast carcinomas are a diverse group of lesions that differ in microscopic appearance and biologic behavior although these disorders are often discussed as a single disease.

The in situ carcinomas of the breast are either ductal (also known as intraductal carcinoma) or lobular. This distinction is primarily based upon the growth pattern and cytologic features of the lesions, rather than their anatomic location within the mammary ductal–lobular system.

The invasive breast carcinomas consist of several histologic subtypes; the estimated percentages are from a contemporary population-based series of 135,157 women with breast cancer reported to the Surveillance Epidemiology and End Results (SEER) database of the National Cancer Institute between 1992 and 2001 (Li et al. 2005): infiltrating ductal (76%), invasive lobular (8%), ductal/lobular in situ (7%), mucinous (colloid) (2.4%), tubular (1.5%), medullary (1.2%), and papillary (1%).

Other subtypes, including metaplastic breast cancer and invasive micropapillary breast cancer, all account for fewer than 5% of cases.

4.1.3 Diagnosis

The majority of breast cancers are diagnosed as a result of an abnormal mammogram, but not all mammographic findings represent cancer. Women who have an abnormal screening mammogram often need further diagnostic evaluation with magnification views, spot compression views, and/or targeted ultrasonography to determine the need for tissue sampling or biopsy. Additionally, not all cancers are detectable on mammography. A clinically suspicious mass should also be biopsied, regardless of imaging findings, as about 15% of such lesions can be mammographically occult. The goal of the initial biopsy is to obtain sufficient diagnostic material using the least invasive approach and to avoid surgical excision of benign lesions.

4.1.4 Treatment

The treatment of early stage breast cancer includes the treatment of locoregional disease with surgery, radiation therapy, or both and the treatment of systemic disease with one or a combination of chemotherapy, endocrine therapy, or biologic therapy. The need for timing and selection of therapy is based upon tumor variables such as histology, stage, and tumor markers; patient variables such as age, menopausal status, and comorbid conditions; and patient preference, such as a desire for breast preservation.

4.2 Diagnostic Evaluation

A suspicion of breast cancer requires that care be coordinated among clinicians in several specialties, a multidisciplinary care. An integrated approach with breast imagers and breast surgeons can minimize unnecessary biopsies and expedite diagnosis for the woman who receives a diagnosis of breast cancer. Similarly, once the diagnosis of cancer is made, multidisciplinary coordination among breast and reconstructive surgeons, radiation and medical oncologists, radiologists, and pathologists facilitates treatment planning and streamlines patient care.

4.2.1 Mammography

The majority of breast cancers are associated with abnormal mammographic findings (Smart et al. 1993). As an example, in the Breast Cancer Detection Demonstration Project (BCDDP), fewer than 10% of cancers were detected only by physical examination and over 90% were identified mammographically (Smart et al. 1993).

If an abnormality is found at mammographic screening, supplemental mammographic views and possibly ultrasound should be used for further characterization. A variety of mammographic techniques, including spot compression and magnification views (Figure 4.1) and varied angled views, may characterize a lesion more precisely prior to making a final recommendation for management (Figure 4.2).

Some of the most aggressive cancers appear between normal screening mammograms and are therefore termed interval cancers (Lin et al. 2009). Younger women may present with large tumors prior to the age at which screening is usually recommended. Accordingly, when women present with a suspicious new mass, diagnostic mammograms should be part of the initial work-up, despite young age or having had a negative routine screening mammogram.

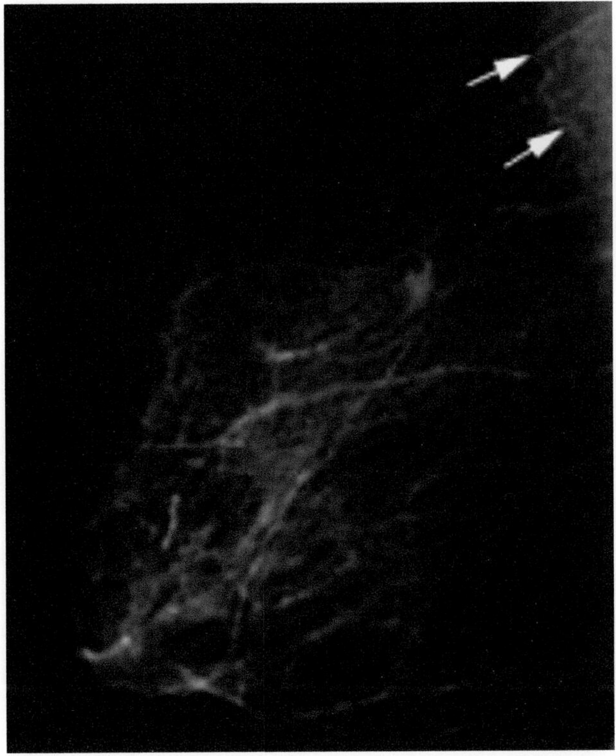

FIGURE 4.1
Medial lateral oblique mammographic view. There is a mass at the posterior edge of the film (arrows) that is incompletely characterized. The borders of the lesion can be better characterized with regional spot compression and magnification.

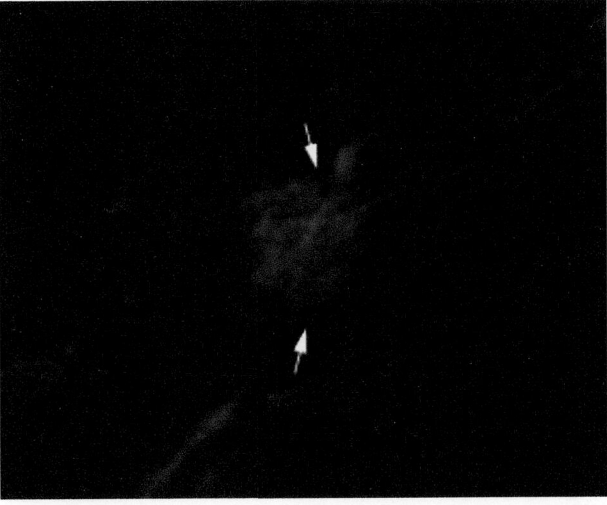

FIGURE 4.2
The spot magnification view shows that the lesion has irregular borders and spiculation. In addition, associated microcalcifications are seen. The lesion can now be characterized as suspicious, BI-RADS 4c, requiring biopsy. Pathology revealed infiltrating duct cell carcinoma with papillary features.

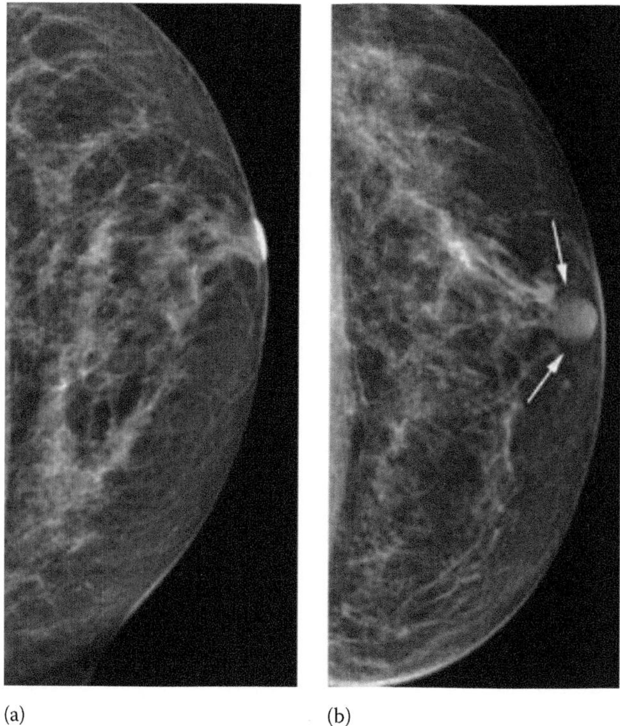

FIGURE 4.3
Technical factors. On a standard CC view performed during routine screening mammogram, the nipple (arrows) can appear as a nodule (a) if not properly positioned leading to additional work-up. When the CC view of the same breast is repeated with the nipple in profile (b), it becomes clear that there is no lesion.

Abnormalities on screening mammograms include nodules, calcifications, architectural distortion, and asymmetry. The abnormality could be related to technical factors such as motion, improper positioning, or artifacts (Figure 4.3). Alternatively, the finding might represent benign or malignant breast disease. Even when the abnormality seen on a screening mammogram is very suspicious for malignancy, additional evaluation is usually indicated to determine the extent of the lesion and to assess for the presence of any additional lesions (Kopans 1993). Availability of the abnormal screening mammogram at the time of diagnostic examination is crucial in obtaining correct views. This is particularly important when the screening mammogram is performed in a different institute.

The diagnostic examination is always supervised by a radiologist. The views obtained are tailored to work up of the specific abnormality, with the adjunctive use of ultrasound if needed in order to make an accurate diagnosis. The radiologist interprets the images and conveys the findings and recommendations directly to the patient at the time of the examination.

A focal spot compression view, one type of additional view, is performed by applying focal compression to the area of interest in the breast using small compression paddles. This view is helpful to further evaluate an area of asymmetry or a nodule seen on screening mammogram (Figure 4.4). Spot compression views of a palpable area have been shown to detect additional cancers (Faulk et al. 1992).

A magnification view is performed to further characterize calcifications. The size, distribution, and morphology of calcifications are seen best on magnification views. In addition, magnification views can provide details regarding margins of masses.

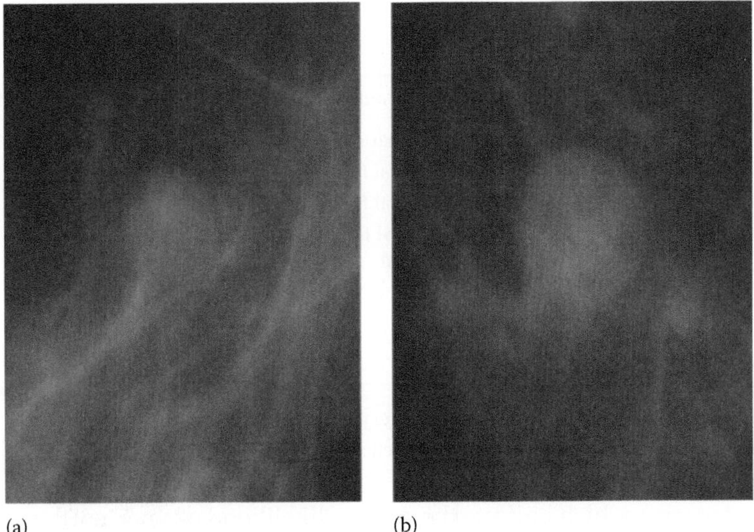

FIGURE 4.4
Diagnostic imaging allowed the probably benign assessment to be made with confidence. (a) Screening mammogram showing a partially obscured mass with somewhat indistinct margins. (b) Spot compression magnification mammogram displacing adjacent dense tissues so that the mass margins are less obscured and are depicted in finer detail. The mass now is seen to be circumscribed over at least 75% of its contour, supporting a probably benign assessment.

A 90° lateral view is a true lateral view of the breast. The x-ray beam can travel from either the medial (mediolateral) or from the lateral (lateromedial) side of the breast. This view is a direct orthogonal view to the craniocaudal (CC) projection and is useful in triangulating lesions. A delayed lateral view is often performed in evaluating calcifications. The breast is held in compression for up to 2 min, and the image is obtained after the 2 min *delay*. This view may help in confirming the presence of a benign pattern of calcifications, called milk of calcium deposition, associated with benign breast microcysts.

Other views that may be obtained in a diagnostic work-up are tangential views, to confirm dermal calcifications, and rolled views. Rolled views are helpful in establishing the presence of a lesion and to better evaluate the lesion by moving or *rolling* the lesion away from dense breast parenchyma. For the rolled view, the patient is positioned similar to the view that represented the original lesion. The technologist places his or her hands on either side of the breast and *rolls* the breast tissue (medial and lateral for the CC view and superior and inferior for the medio lateral oblique [MLO] view). Compression is applied to keep the breast tissues rolled, and the image is obtained. The direction of the roll (medial, lateral, superior, or inferior) should be written on the film.

Diagnostic mammography is associated with higher sensitivity but lower specificity as compared to screening mammography. In one prospective study of women with signs or symptoms of breast cancer, 15% of diagnostic mammograms were abnormal (Barlow et al. 2002). The sensitivity and specificity of diagnostic mammograms declined with breast density, younger age, and mammographic examination.

4.2.1.1 Diagnostic Categories: BI-RADS

The radiologist summarizes the mammographic findings using the American College of Radiology (ACR) Breast Imaging Reporting and Data System (BI-RADS) final diagnostic

TABLE 4.1
BI-RADS

Assessment Category	Recommendation	Probability of Malignancy
0: Incomplete	Need for further evaluation.	Not applicable
1: Normal	Normal interval follow-up.	0%
2: Benign	Normal interval follow-up.	0%
3: Probably benign	A short-interval follow-up is recommended.	≤2%
4: Suspicious abnormality	A biopsy should be considered.	>2%–95% (a) Low risk (b) Intermediate risk (c) Moderate to high risk
5: Highly suggestive of malignancy	Biopsy or surgery should be performed.	≥95%
6: Biopsy-proven carcinoma	Appropriate action should be taken.	

assessment categories, which indicate the relative likelihood of a normal, benign, or malignant diagnosis (Reston, American College of Radiology 2003). The BI-RADS final assessment categories standardize both the reporting of mammographic findings and the recommendations for further management (i.e., routine screening, short-interval follow-up, or biopsy). Assessments are either incomplete (category 0) or final assessment categories (categories 1–6) as described in Table 4.1 (Reston, American College of Radiology 2003).

4.2.1.2 Clinical Decision Making

- *A positive mammography report*—All reports with BI-RADS 0, 4, or 5 need further intervention. In most institutions, the clinician is contacted to convey the need for biopsy, and both the clinician and patient are contacted to convey the need for further imaging. A BI-RADS designation of 4c or 5 should alert the pathologist that a malignant diagnosis is strongly suspected and that further evaluation of the specimen (and possible rebiopsy) is needed if the biopsy is initially interpreted as benign.
- *A negative mammography report*—A negative mammogram should not deter further intervention if there is clinical suspicion for malignancy. The false-negative rate of screening mammography has been reported between 10% and 30% (Ciatto et al. 2005). Up to 15% of cancers detected on clinical breast examination are not visible even on diagnostic mammography (Shaw et al. 2009). The addition of ultrasound decreases the false-negative rate, but still does not exclude the presence of breast cancer.

The final disposition of a palpable abnormality rests with the clinician in the presence of a negative mammogram.

4.2.1.3 Mammographic Features of Breast Cancer

There are two general categories of mammographic findings suggestive of a breast cancer: soft tissue masses and clustered microcalcifications.

- *Soft tissue mass/architectural distortion*—The most specific mammographic feature of malignancy is a spiculated soft tissue mass; nearly 90% of these lesions represent invasive cancer. Approximately one-third of noncalcified cancers appear as spiculated masses; 25% as irregularly outlined masses; 25% as less specific round, oval, or lobulated masses; less than 10% as well-defined round, oval, or lobulated masses; and 5% as areas of architectural distortion of dense tissue without an obvious mass. The positive predictive value for malignancy of well-defined solid masses with benign imaging features is between 0% and 7%, and biopsy or short-term (3–6 months) follow-up is considered an appropriate management (Harvey et al. 2009).

- *Clustered microcalcifications*—Clustered microcalcifications are calcium particles of various size and shape measuring between 0.1 and 1 mm in diameter and numbering more than 4–5 per cm^3. Microcalcifications are seen in approximately 60% of cancers detected mammographically. Histologically, these represent intraductal calcifications in areas of necrotic tumor (Figure 4.5) or calcifications within mucin-secreting tumors such as the cribriform or micropapillary subtype of intraductal cancer. Linear branching microcalcifications, most commonly associated with the comedo histologic subtype, have a higher predictive value for malignancy than do granular (i.e., nonlinear irregular calcifications of varying size and shape) microcalcifications, particularly for high-grade DCIS. However, breast cancers, including DCIS, more often present with the granular type of calcifications (Stomper et al. 2000). Calcifications that are not suspicious for malignancy and considered benign include vascular and skin calcifications, large coarse calcifications, and smooth round or oval calcifications.

Despite the association of microcalcifications with DCIS, mammographic appearance alone cannot differentiate between purely intraductal and invasive ductal breast cancers; there is no mammographic correlate of basement membrane invasion (Stomper et al. 2003). One-third of invasive carcinomas are associated with microcalcifications, with or without a soft tissue mass, and 10% of intraductal cancers present as a soft tissue mass without microcalcifications.

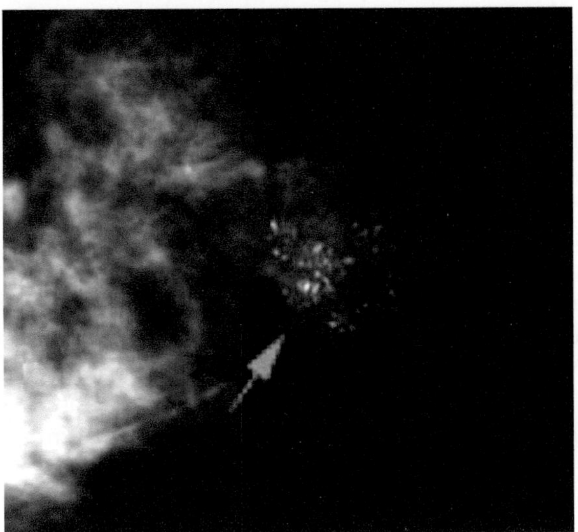

FIGURE 4.5
Mammogram clustered calcifications. Mammogram showing linear branching calcifications in a segmental distribution (arrow). These are highly suggestive of carcinoma; the linear branching is suggestive of a ductal lesion.

However, calcifications can also be stratified by risk for malignancy, and the BI-RADS 4a, 4b, and 4c categories are helpful in alerting the referring physicians, the pathologists, and surgeons to the underlying risk of malignancy. Low-risk calcifications are much more likely to be benign.

4.2.1.4 Assessing the Extent of Disease

Mammographic assessment of the extent of DCIS and early invasive carcinoma begins during diagnostic mammography and continues through the biopsy, specimen management, and the postexcision mammogram (Stomper et al. 2003). Mammography of both breasts is particularly important in the patient with DCIS or invasive cancer who is considering breast conservation. Preoperative diagnostic mammography can help to define the extent of disease and may identify multifocal or multicentric cancer that could exclude breast conservation or signal a potential difficulty in achieving clear surgical margins. Multifocal disease is usually defined as involvement of several areas within a breast quadrant, probably representing disease along an entire duct. In contrast, multicentric disease involves multiple areas within different quadrants, probably representing involvement of multiple ducts.

Although the extent of mammographic nonlinear branching microcalcifications frequently underestimates the pathologic extent of the malignancy, the discrepancy is less than 2 cm in 80%–85% of cases. Several clusters of microcalcifications separated by normal appearing tissue should not be interpreted as multifocal or multicentric disease. Often, these represent areas of contiguous tumor that is only partially calcified within a ductal lobule.

The combination of a mass and associated calcifications often indicates the presence of an extensive intraductal component (EIC). EIC is defined pathologically as DCIS found adjacent to an invasive carcinoma, accounting for more than 25% of the volume of disease. This finding can be a predictor for more widespread residual tumor (usually DCIS) following gross excision of the lesion.

Postoperative mammograms to look for residual calcifications after surgical resection should be considered when the microcalcifications are not clearly or completely documented on the specimen radiograph or when margins are close or positive. If a reexcision is to be recommended on the basis of residual calcifications, care should be taken to ensure that the calcifications are associated with malignancy on histopathology and not benign tissue. Multifocal disease is not necessarily a contraindication to breast conservation, but is one of the factors that should be taken into consideration along with breast size relative to the extent of disease on imaging.

A significant limitation of mammographic assessment of disease extent is the obscuring of the borders or extent of the primary tumor by dense overlying tissue. Dense breasts can limit the sensitivity of mammography both for detection of breast cancers and for delineating disease extent (Mandelson et al. 2000). In this setting, contrast-enhanced breast magnetic resonance imaging (MRI) may complement mammographic staging. If the clinical extent of disease is larger than what can be appreciated by mammography, MRI may be considered.

Mammographic assessment of tumor size for the staging of multifocal disease presents a unique dilemma. Most staging classifications require that the largest tumor mass be utilized for T staging, even in cases where multifocal disease is suspected. However, others suggest that the total surface area, volume, or aggregate measurements are a better indicator of prognosis. Accurate delineation of the extent of irregular or multifocal tumors is important for treatment planning.

For invasive cancers that are contiguous to the chest wall and not completely included on mammographic projections, ancillary imaging techniques such as MRI may be necessary to assess posterior tumor extension and pectoralis fascia or muscle involvement if that will determine a change in surgical approach or the use of neoadjuvant therapy.

4.2.1.5 Significance of Intramammary Lymph Nodes

Intramammary lymph nodes are detected in 1%–28% of patients with breast cancer (Shen et al. 2004). Benign nodes can often be distinguished from metastatic or infiltrated intramammary lymph nodes by their mammographic or sonographic appearance, but definitive assessment often requires histopathologic study. The presence of intramammary lymph node metastases appears to confer a worse prognosis, both in women who otherwise have stage I breast cancer based upon tumor size and axillary nodal status and in those with stage II disease. Isolated intramammary lymph node metastases are considered to represent stage II disease, even if the axillary nodes are uninvolved.

4.2.2 Ultrasonography

Ultrasound can be used to differentiate between solid and cystic breast masses that are palpable or detected mammographically. In addition, ultrasound evaluation of the axilla can be used to detect lymph nodes that are suspicious for axillary metastases. Ultrasound provides guidance for interventional procedures of suspicious areas in the breast or axilla.

4.2.2.1 Breast Ultrasound

Ultrasound (US) examination of the breast is an important diagnostic adjunct to mammography. In patients suspected of having a breast cancer, breast US is most useful in the following circumstances:

- To further characterize a mammographically detected mass or an area of architectural distortion—Breast US can help to characterize solid masses as either benign or malignant. In one report, the sensitivity of US for malignancy was 98.4% and the negative predictive value 99.5%. Similar results have been reported in other studies (Harvey et al. 2009). Similar findings have been noted in subsequent studies. However, US is highly operator dependent and significant variability in the ability of radiologists to characterize solid breast lesions by US has been reported (Berg et al. 2004). A benign solid appearance on US should not be used to avoid biopsy of a mammographically or clinically suspicious mass (Figure 4.6).
- To measure and clip a lesion prior to neoadjuvant chemotherapy—For patients who present with large or locally advanced tumors for which neoadjuvant (induction) chemotherapy is considered, careful anatomic localization is critical to ensure that the surgeon can localize the area of tumor after neoadjuvant therapy. Typically, the lesion is measured both clinically and ultrasonographically and reported in

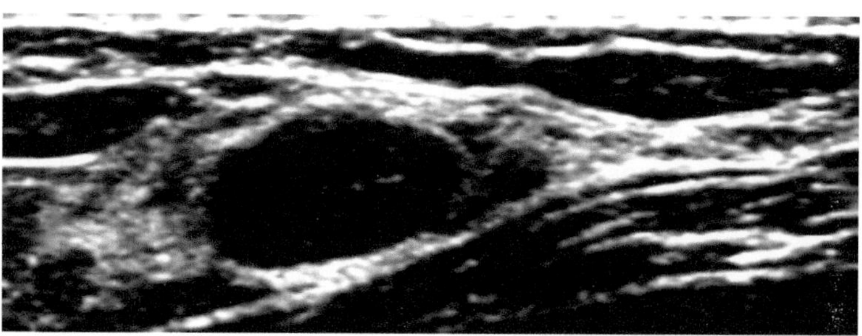

FIGURE 4.6
Benign solid nodule on US.

terms of size, the *o'clock* location on the breast surface, and the distance of the lesion from the nipple. The use of radio-opaque clips placed at the time of biopsy to localize the primary tumor in case there is a complete clinical and radiographic response to induction therapy is discussed below.

- To further characterize a lesion when a mass detected on clinical breast examination cannot be seen clearly on mammogram (often in women with dense breasts).
- To identify a cystic mass—Simple cysts need no further intervention because the risk of cancer is very low; one series found no malignancies in 223 cysts (Sickles et al. 1984). Indeterminate cysts can be aspirated under US guidance. The presence of an intracystic mass should prompt a fine needle aspiration (FNA) or core biopsy of the mass.
- To determine whether a mammographically suspicious lesion can be visualized and therefore sampled by US-guided biopsy.

Breast US is often added to the initial diagnostic evaluation for women with a suspected breast cancer if there is a palpable mass or a density is seen on mammogram. The benefit of this approach was suggested in a series of 2020 patients (470 with a palpable mass) who underwent clinical exam, mammography, and breast US (Flobbe et al. 2003). The systematic addition of breast US detected eight additional malignancies and correctly downgraded 332 cases of suspected malignancy to no suspected malignancy (predominantly cysts or fibroadenoma). Thus, the main benefit of breast US was improved specificity when used in a targeted manner. The sensitivity, specificity, and positive and negative predictive values for clinical examination plus mammography plus US were 96.9%, 94.8%, 39.2%, and 99.9%, while the corresponding values for clinical examination plus mammography were 91.5%, 87%, 19.7%, and 99.7%, respectively.

4.2.2.2 Axillary Ultrasound

For women with clinically suspicious lymph nodes, preoperative axillary US with FNA or core biopsy of suspicious areas provides a means to identify patients who have positive nodes. This information may be used to guide future additional surgery, radiation, or systemic therapy.

4.2.3 Breast MRI

Nearly all invasive breast carcinomas enhance on gadolinium contrast-enhanced MRI. The sensitivity of breast MRI for breast carcinomas is between 88% and 100%

(Bluemke et al. 2004). However, a major disadvantage is the limited specificity of MRI due to enhancement of benign breast lesions (Bluemke et al. 2004). In a meta-analysis of 44 studies evaluating diagnostic breast MRI in patients with breast lesions, pooled specificity was 72% (Peters et al. 2008). Specificity can be improved, to some extent, by alterations in technique. The technique of breast MRI is discussed elsewhere. However, even using optimal technique, specificity is still insufficient to obviate the need for biopsy confirmation of an MRI abnormality.

4.2.3.1 Assessment of Ipsilateral Disease with Breast MRI

MRI is more sensitive than mammography, ultrasound, or physical examination and identifies additional ipsilateral disease in about 16% of women with a known breast cancer (Liberman et al. 2003). Because MRI is so sensitive, it was assumed that preoperative MRI would estimate the extent of disease more accurately than conventional imaging, thereby improving surgical planning (e.g., prompting a change to mastectomy when breast conserving therapy had been previously considered) and enabling surgeons to better obtain clean margins in breast-conserving surgery. However, available data have shown that preoperative breast MRI has not improved outcomes, overestimates the extent of disease, and has overall limited value (Turnbull et al. 2010, Shin et al. 2012):

- It was already known from postmastectomy pathology studies that additional sites of tumor are frequently present in the ipsilateral breast. In fact, the entire purpose of RT in women undergoing breast conserving surgery is to eradicate sites of clinically occult disease in the ipsilateral breast. Multiple prospective randomized trials of breast conserving surgery with and without RT have demonstrated that the high risk of in-breast recurrence (40%) without RT is reduced to <10% with RT.
- There is no evidence that routine use of breast MRI results in fewer positive margins at the time of partial mastectomy or a lower rate of reoperation to achieve clear margins. A UK randomized trial (COMICE) evaluating the role of breast MRI in 1623 women with newly diagnosed breast cancer showed no difference in the reoperation rate with or without the use of preoperative MRI (18.7% and 19.3%, respectively). The lack of a difference in reoperation rates could reflect the UK's low reported reexcision rate of 10% in contrast to U.S. institutions where the rates are closer to 25%, presumably due to attempts at removing the smallest volume of tissue possible for breast conservation. In addition, many women had mastectomies (27.6% in the group randomized to MRI) without pathological verification of disease as not all centers in this trial performed MRI biopsy or localization (Turnbull et al. 2010).
- Because of its low specificity, MRI can delay treatment by necessitating additional biopsies. In one study, MRI was associated with a significant 22-day delay in definitive treatment.
- In a review of 1558 consecutive patients with invasive breast cancer and/or non-invasive breast cancer, MRI was not associated with an advantage to lower reexcision rate, improve the rate of breast conservation surgery achievement, or lower recurrence rate (Shin et al. 2012).

4.2.3.2 Assessment of Contralateral Disease with Breast MRI

MRI imaging of the contralateral breast identifies a suspicious, clinically occult finding in 9%–12% of women with a unilateral breast cancer, but cannot distinguish between benign and malignant lesions. In general, a synchronous clinically and mammographically inapparent malignancy will be found in 3%–5% of cases, approximately one-half of which are invasive cancer, and the remainder, intraductal cancer, results in about a 12% chance of biopsy.

As an example, in a meta-analysis of 22 studies (3253 women) of women with newly diagnosed breast cancer, the pooled estimate for detecting a suspicious abnormality that was occult on conventional imaging was 9.3% (Brennan et al. 2009). The incremental cancer detection rate with MRI was only 4% because more than half of the suspicious abnormalities detected by MRI alone proved to be benign. The summary estimate of positive predictive value was 48%. Interestingly, 10 women underwent contralateral mastectomy based upon MRI findings without a preoperative biopsy. Of these, only three had malignancy and the remaining seven were benign. Of the 42 women who underwent prophylactic mastectomy despite a negative MRI, 5 (12%) unexpected malignancies were identified on final pathology.

The clinical significance, especially the survival benefit, of detecting these cancers has not been addressed. As is the case with MRI of the affected breast, the finding of a contralateral malignancy on breast MRI may lead to overtreatment. Many of these subclinical cancers are effectively treated with the systemic therapy used for the treatment of the initial cancer.

Finally, the detection of these contralateral cancers must be weighed against the added time and additional costs associated with MRI and MRI-guided biopsy. For all of these reasons, the role of MRI to assess the contralateral breast is controversial and cannot be routinely recommended for the majority of women with a newly diagnosed breast cancer.

4.2.4 Breast Biopsy

In the patient with a suspicious mammographic abnormality or palpable breast mass, the obligatory diagnostic technique is biopsy. Surgical biopsy should not be utilized as a diagnostic tool unless percutaneous palpation-guided or image-guided biopsy is not feasible. A preoperative histologic diagnosis of invasive carcinoma may allow the surgeon to plan a single operation to treat the cancer, including SLN biopsy or full axillary dissection, depending upon the clinical circumstances.

4.2.4.1 Fine Needle Aspiratory Biopsy

Palpation-guided percutaneous fine needle aspiratory (FNA) biopsy has been used for years to evaluate a palpable breast mass. FNA biopsy is performed with a 10 or 20 mL syringe and a 23–27 gauge needle.

The main disadvantages of FNA cytology are the inability to distinguish between in situ and invasive cancers and the significant rate of nondiagnostic samples and false-negative results in inexperienced hands.

When performed by experienced operators, FNA has a sensitivity of 98% and a specificity of 97%; rates are much lower in the hands of clinicians who lack specific training. When a lesion is palpable, FNA can be rapidly performed as a non-image-guided procedure. When biopsy results are nonconcordant, image-guided biopsy should be pursued.

Ultrasound (US)-guided FNA of palpable lesions increases the level of confidence that needle placement has been accurate. In addition, it may be more prudent to perform an FNA rather than a core needle biopsy (CNB) of a lesion in a patient with coagulation abnormalities. In axillary lymph nodes, it is less painful and may be safer.

A major advantage of FNA is that it can be easily and quickly performed at the time of a diagnostic study, with potential for an immediate preliminary interpretation.

4.2.4.2 Core Needle Biopsy

Compared to FNA, CNB offers a more definitive histologic diagnosis, avoids inadequate samples, and may permit the distinction between invasive and in situ cancers. In most centers, stereotactic CNB has replaced wire localization and excision as the most common initial biopsy method for nonpalpable mammographic abnormalities. CNB is safe, even in patients receiving warfarin or aspirin anticoagulation therapy.

The use of US requires that the lesion can be well visualized by ultrasound and confidence that the ultrasound finding and mammographic finding represent the same thing. With US-guided CNB, the passage of the needle through the lesion can be directly visualized and confirmed; as a result, fewer samples (usually three to five) are needed to provide diagnostic material. If the lesion is better visualized mammographically and is difficult to reproduce reliably on US, then stereotactic guidance is the preferred method.

For patients with microcalcifications, stereotactically guided CNB is the standard approach, since these lesions cannot usually be visualized by US. Calcifications can be targeted sonographically if they can be visualized within a mass on US.

US-guided CNB may also be appropriate for palpable lesions. For example, a palpable abnormality does not always correspond to the true lesion, but instead may represent tissue anterior to the lesion. Image guidance can also be useful to successfully biopsy lesions that are small, deep, or mobile and those that are only vaguely palpable that may no longer be palpable after the administration of local anesthesia.

Some patients will have nonpalpable, mammographically occult lesions that are seen only on MRI. A proportion can be identified in on subsequent, targeted *second-look* US and may then be biopsied under US guidance. Ultrasound correlate findings have a high likelihood of malignancy. For the remaining lesions, targeting requires MRI guidance.

4.3 Prognostic Factors

Routine pathologic evaluation remains the most critical element in determining the prognosis of patients with breast cancer. Among the most potent prognostic factors available are lymph node status, tumor size and histologic grade, histologic tumor type, and lymphatic vascular invasion (Rakha et al. 2008).

It is important to distinguish between a *prognostic* factor and a *predictive* factor when evaluating either traditional or newer markers:

- A prognostic factor is capable of providing information on clinical outcome at the time of diagnosis, independent of therapy. Such markers are usually indicators of growth, invasion, and metastatic potential.
- A predictive factor is capable of providing information on the likelihood of response to a given therapeutic modality. Such markers either are within the target of the treatment or serve as modulators or epiphenomena related to expression and/or function of the target.

The following discussion will focus primarily upon prognostic factors.

A useful prognostic factor in breast cancer should have the following characteristics according to an NIH Consensus Conference:

- Provide significant and independent prognostic value, validated by clinical testing.
- Determination must be feasible, reproducible, and widely available, with quality control.
- Results should be readily interpretable by the clinician.
- Measurement of the marker must not consume tissue needed for other tests, particularly routine histopathologic evaluation.

4.3.1 Tests Done on Breast Tissue

4.3.1.1 HER2 Overexpression

Amplification or overexpression of the HER2 oncogene is present in approximately 18%–20% of primary invasive breast cancers. High levels of HER2 expression (3+ by immunohistochemistry [IHC] or an amplified HER2 gene copy number by fluorescence in situ hybridization [FISH]) represent an important predictive factor, identifying those patients who might benefit from treatments that target HER2, such as trastuzumab, both in the adjuvant and metastatic disease settings. The value of HER2 as a prognostic factor is more controversial. In most but not all studies, HER2 overexpression in primary tumor tissue (as determined by IHC) is associated with a worse prognosis in untreated patients (Gilcrease et al. 2009). In some, HER2 overexpression correlates with other factors associated with a poor prognosis (such as tumor grade, size, and nodal status).

The independent contribution of HER2 overexpression in tumor tissue as a marker of poor prognosis in patients with node-positive disease is fairly consistent. Although early studies were unclear about the prognostic role of HER2 in node-negative untreated patients, more recent studies have provided more clarity.

Thus, the bulk of the available data support the view that HER2 overexpression in tumor tissue is associated with a poorer prognosis in early node-positive as well as node-negative breast cancer. However, all of the relevant studies were performed prior to the publication of clinical trials demonstrating that adjuvant trastuzumab significantly improves outcomes when added to anthracycline- and taxane-based adjuvant chemotherapy in women with high-risk HER2-overexpressing tumors (the majority of which enrolled women with node-positive disease).

Assay for HER2 overexpression and/or amplification is recommended as a routine part of the diagnostic work-up on all primary breast cancers. The main benefit of HER2 testing is its predictive value. High levels of HER2 expression (3+ by IHC or an amplified HER2 gene copy number by FISH) identify those women who might benefit from trastuzumab both in the adjuvant and metastatic disease settings.

4.3.1.2 Hormone Receptors

The assay of hormone receptors has become a routine part of the evaluation of breast cancers, since the results predict the clinical response to HT, both in the adjuvant setting and for those with metastatic disease.

The prognostic importance of ER and PR expression has been a matter of debate for many years. However, taken together, the available evidence suggests that ER-/PR-negative tumors have a worse prognosis, at least in the first 5–10 years after treatment. On the other hand, other data suggest that as a result of sequential improvements in adjuvant chemotherapy (which disproportionately benefits those with hormone receptor–negative tumors) over time, the prognosis of individuals with ER-/PR-negative breast cancer now approaches that of patients with hormone receptor–positive disease.

In keeping with American Society of Clinical Oncology (ASCO) guidelines, ER/PR analysis should be performed routinely in all invasive breast cancers using either IHC or the now rarely used ligand-binding assay (Harris et al. 2007). The information should be used to select patients who are most likely to respond to HT.

4.3.1.3 Proliferation Markers

In general, markers of an elevated proliferative rate correlate with a worse prognosis in untreated patients. The proliferative rate of breast tumors may be assessed by a variety of methods, including mitotic counts, thymidine labeling index, bromodeoxyuridine (BrdU) labeling, S-phase fractions as determined by flow cytometry, IHC using monoclonal antibodies (MoAbs) to antigens found in proliferating cells (e.g., Ki-67 or proliferating cell nuclear antigen [PCNA/cyclin]), and the assessment of argyrophilic nucleolar organizer regions (AgNORs).

Most recent studies have assessed proliferative rate by determining S-phase fraction using flow cytometry or with IHC staining for Ki-67. However, because of the difficulty with methodology and inconsistency of the data, the ASCO tumor marker expert panel did not recommend the use of S-phase fraction or other flow-cytometry-based markers of proliferation to assign patients to prognostic groupings (Harris et al. 2007).

Several studies have investigated the value of IHC to detect antigens related to cell proliferation using MoAbs against Ki-67 or PCNA/cyclin. In general, IHC staining with these antibodies correlates with proliferative rate as determined by flow cytometric S-phase analysis. Cell kinetic analysis using tissue-based IHC may actually be more widely applicable than S-phase determination by flow cytometry, since accurate S-phase interpretation can be difficult in the presence of aneuploid cell populations and cellular debris.

Many studies have been undertaken to explore the relationship between Ki-67 status and prognosis in breast cancer (de Azambuja et al. 2007).

The authors concluded that evaluation of Ki-67 status should not be considered a routine part of breast cancer evaluation, reinforcing the position taken by the ASCO expert tumor marker committee in its 2007 updated guidelines.

4.3.1.4 Multigene Predictors

Gene expression profiling has identified molecular signatures, such as the 21-gene recurrence score (RS, Oncotype Dx®), the Amsterdam 70-gene prognostic profile (Mammaprint®), and the Rotterdam/Veridex 76-gene signature, which augment conventional prognostic indicators in their ability to predict breast cancer outcome and response to treatment.

The 21-gene recurrence score can be used to predict the risk of recurrence in patients with newly diagnosed, node-negative, estrogen receptor (ER)–positive disease and to identify patients who are likely to benefit from chemotherapy added to adjuvant endocrine therapy. Preliminary data also suggest utility of the 21-gene recurrence score in patients with node-positive, ER-positive breast cancer. Although use of the test has been cleared by the U.S. FDA for women with ER-positive early breast cancer and one to three positive nodes, further prospective validation in this group is awaited.

4.3.1.5 p53 Gene Analysis

Mutations in the p53 tumor suppressor gene or accumulation of p53 protein are reported in 20%–50% of human breast cancers. These abnormalities are more often seen in patients with hereditary breast cancer syndromes than in those with sporadic breast cancer. A number of studies suggest that high tissue p53 protein levels (as measured by IHC) or mutations or deletions in the p53 gene represent an independent predictor of decreased disease-free and overall survival in both node-positive and node-negative patients. However, other studies have failed to find an association between p53 abnormalities and clinical outcomes.

The ASCO panel on tumor markers concluded that IHC for p53 protein was unlikely to provide sufficiently accurate results to be clinically useful (Harris et al. 2007). At present, there is no role for p53 gene analysis in women with breast cancer.

4.3.2 Circulating Tumor Markers

4.3.2.1 CA 15.3

In the 2007 ASCO guidelines, monitoring selected patients with metastatic disease was the sole recommended use for circulating tumor markers (Harris et al. 2007).

4.3.2.2 HER2 ECD Levels

The presence of HER2 ECD is generally associated with a poorer prognosis. In early-stage disease, elevated levels of HER2 ECD also correlate with a worse prognosis. However, levels of circulating HER2 ECD are directly related to tumor burden, and there are no studies that suggest added value from knowledge of HER2 ECD in this setting. A review of 63 studies of patients with breast cancer concluded that concentrations of HER2 ECD are not consistently related to patient outcomes and that there is insufficient evidence to support the clinical use of serum HER2 ECD testing (Leyland-Jones et al. 2011). This position reinforces the recommendation of the 2007 ASCO expert panel on tumor markers against the use of serum ECD in any clinical setting (Harris et al. 2007).

4.3.2.3 Disseminated and Circulating Tumor Cells

Disseminated and/or circulating tumor cells are likely to play an important role in the development of distant metastases in breast cancer. In contrast to clinically overt metastases, which represent a relatively late event in the natural history of solid tumors such as breast cancer, circulation of tumor cells in the bloodstream, and/or their identification in bone marrow can be detected much earlier and is thought to be an early indicator of tumor spread. The 2007 ASCO expert panel concluded that measurement of CTCs should not be used to make a diagnosis of breast cancer or to influence treatment decisions in early-stage or metastatic disease (Harris et al. 2007). Despite the commercial availability of the CellSearch assay, the panel recommended against its use in patients with metastatic disease pending additional validation.

4.4 Patented Biomarkers

One of the most suitable types of cancer for early diagnosis biomarker discovery is breast cancer. The new biomarkers will improve early breast cancer detection mainly in patients where imagistic technologies cannot detect the onset of an early neoplastic event. In the best-case scenario, a biomarker panel, whether from the proteomic or genomic domain, can detect breast cancer even before imagistic investigations would point toward a diagnosis (Table 4.2) (Neagu et al. 2011).

4.4.1 Proteomic Biomarker Panels

Proteomics searches early diagnosis biomarkers by testing various body fluids, like serum/plasma, tears, and nipple aspirate. As an interesting novelty, the protein profile of tear fluid for breast cancer patients has recently been published. The new diagnostic pattern differentiated breast cancer patients from healthy controls with a specificity and sensitivity of approximately 70% (Lebrecht et al. 2009). A few years ago, the panel comprising carcinoembryonic (CEA) tissue polypeptide (TPA) cancer-associated (CA 15.3) antigens was reported to early detect breast cancer relapsing. Although the ASCO's recommendation is the use of biomarker combinations in order to enhance efficiency and sensitivity, only the combination of CA 15-3 and CA 27.29 is validated as markers for breast cancer in screening, diagnostic, or staging tests. The work of Goldknopf team spanned several patents in the field. Recently, the group has patented a group of 12 protein biomarkers detected in the serum of breast cancer patients. All their patents focus on immunoglobulin lambda chain, alpha-1-microglobulin, proapolipoprotein, four isoforms of inter-alpha-trypsin inhibitor family heavy chain–related proteins, apolipoprotein E3, serum albumin, lectin P35, transferrin, and complement component C4A.

4.4.2 Genomic Biomarker Panels

As in many types of cancer, the detection of circulating tumor cells is a recent and intriguing research domain. Using immunobead reverse transcription polymerase chain reaction (RT-PCR) method, a recent study reported a panel of five gene markers (E74-like factor 3 [ELF3], erythropoietin-producing hepatocellular receptor B4 [EPHB4], epithelial growth factor receptor [EGFR], mammaglobin-1 [MGB1], and tumor-associated calcium signal transducer protein 1 precursor [TACSTD1]) that detected circulating tumor cells in breast cancer patients. The markers were specific for epithelial cells, and the technique based on the mentioned panel could detect circulating tumor cells in early-stage breast cancer patients. Another approach detected circulating tumor cells in several types of mRNA. Thus, when mRNA for the pituitary tumor transforming gene 1, survivin, ubiquitin-conjugating enzyme (UbcH10), and thymidine kinase 1 was found in circulation, the test could detect breast cancer patients with a high sensitivity and specificity. In breast cancer early diagnosis, the most frequent approach in biomarker discovery is the improvement of the classical marker power of early discrimination by integrating them in complex panels and translating this improved standard combination toward clinical application.

TABLE 4.2

Recent Patent Applications in Cancer Biomarkers

Patent Number	Description	Assignee	Inventor	Priority Application Date	Publication Date
WO 2012061904	A method of diagnosing cancer in a subject, comprising measuring histone 2B protein monoubiquitination in a first cell of the subject, where decreased histone 2B protein monoubiquitination in the first cell compared to that of a second noncancerous cell is diagnostic of cancer	Northern Sydney Local Health District (St. Leonards, NSW, Australia)	Hahn MA, Marsh DJ	November 12, 2010	May 18, 2012
WO 2012021887	A method for detecting breast cancer, involving contacting a suitable bodily fluid sample obtained from a subject at risk of breast cancer with breast cancer biomarker, where the contacting occurs under conditions suitable for selective binding of antibodies in the bodily fluid sample to the biomarkers, and detecting the presence of antibodies to the biomarkers in the bodily fluid sample, where the presence of antibodies to the biomarkers indicates a likelihood of breast cancer in the subject	Dana-Farber Cancer Institute (Boston), Arizona State University (Scottsdale, AZ, USA)	Anderson KS, Labaer J, Ramachandran N, Sibani S, Wallstrom G	August 13, 2010	February 16, 2012; May 10, 2012
US 20120067742	A linker comprising a thiophene compound useful for joining an electrode and a capture probe on a biochip, where the capture probe is at least one protein, DNA, RNA, and enzyme, and the biochip is useful for point-of-care applications including cancer biomarkers	National Taiwan University (Taipei)	Chang K, Chen C, Chen Y, Lee AS, Lee BY, Lee C	September 17, 2010	March 22, 2012

(Continued)

TABLE 4.2 (*CONTINUED*)

Recent Patent Applications in Cancer Biomarkers

Patent Number	Description	Assignee	Inventor	Priority Application Date	Publication Date
WO 2012004565	A method of assessing an individual for cancer involving providing a sample obtained from the individual and determining the presence, amount, or expression of transcription factor Brf1 in at least one cell in the sample	Leung H, White R	Leung H, White R	July 6, 2010	January 12, 2012
US 20120003639	A method of characterizing a sample comprising scoring Ki-67 in a tissue sample from a DCIS lesion and scoring one of, for example, cyclooxygenase-2 and ER from the sample	Regents of the University of California (Oakland, CA, USA), Prelude (Laguna Hills, CA, USA)	Berman HK, Bremer T, Gauthier ML, Kerlikowske K, Molinaro AM, Tlsty TD	April 27, 2010	January 5, 2012
WO 2011162904	A single chain variable fragment or single domain variable fragment comprising a specific amino acid sequence, used in a biotag for targeting cancer biomarker and detecting and diagnosing cancer in a subject	Malecki M, Malecki R	Malecki M, Malecki R	May 24, 2010	December 29, 2011

4.5 Conclusions and Future Studies

Globally, breast cancer is the most frequently diagnosed cancer and the leading cause of death from cancer in females. For these reasons, it is fundamental to implement adequate screening, diagnosis, and treatment strategies. Breast cancer screening is accomplished with periodical mammography imaging, which identifies more than 90% of breast tumors.

Once a suspicious breast lesion has been detected by clinical exploration or mammography imaging, it is essential to diagnose and characterize it. Imaging techniques, such as mammography, US, or RMI, are essential for the diagnosis of suspicious breast lesions. Mammographic abnormal findings include nodules, calcifications, architectural distortion, and asymmetry. In some occasions, further mammographic views as focal compression, magnification, lateral view, and rolled view are needed to characterize breast lesions. It is important to acknowledge that the sensibility and specificity of diagnostic mammography decrease in high-density breasts and at younger age. US improves specificity when used to characterize suspicious breast lesions detected by mammography. US is useful to characterize breast masses, to measure and clip breast lesions prior to neoadjuvant chemotherapy, to visualize clinical masses not seen in mammography, to guide biopsies of not palpable breast lesions, and to establish axillary lymph node status in patients with clinical suspicion of axillary affection. Breast MRI has low specificity and high sensitivity and cannot distinguish between benign and malignant findings. MRI has not demonstrated clear benefit when it is used preoperatively.

Histological characterization is the most important diagnostic test. Mammographic or palpable suspicious breast masses must always have a biopsy due to the fact that histological characterization is the most important diagnostic and prognostic test. Two types of biopsy can be performed: FNA or CNB. FNA is easy and is quickly performed but cannot distinguish between in situ and invasive cancers. On the other hand, CNB gives more definitive histological diagnosis.

Pathologic evaluation is the most critical element in the determination of prognosis in breast cancer. Histological evaluation should always include lymph node status, tumor size, histological type and grade, linfovascular invasion status, hormone receptor status, and Her-2 expression.

Breast cancer diagnosis and treatment should be carried out by multidisciplinary teams, which include breast and reconstructive surgeons, radiotherapists, medical oncologists, and pathologists.

Further studies are needed to determinate concrete prognostic factors and treatments.

References

Barlow WE et al.; Performance of diagnostic mammography for women with signs or symptoms of breast cancer. *Cancer Inst.* 2002;94(15):1151.

Berg WA et al.; Diagnostic accuracy of mammography, clinical examination, US, and MR imaging in preoperative assessment of breast cancer. *Radiology.* 2004;233(3):830.

Berry DA et al.; Effect of screening and adjuvant therapy on mortality from breast cancer. Cancer Intervention and Surveillance Modeling Network (CISNET) Collaborators. *N Engl J Med.* 2005;353(17):1784.

Bluemke DA et al.; Magnetic resonance imaging of the breast prior to biopsy. *JAMA.* 2004;292(22):2735.

Breen N et al.; Reported drop in mammography: Is this cause for concern? *Cancer.* 2007;109(12):2405.

Brennan ME et al.; Magnetic resonance imaging screening of the contralateral breast in women with newly diagnosed breast cancer: Systematic review and meta-analysis of incremental cancer detection and impact on surgical management. *J Clin Oncol.* 2009;27(33):5640.

Ciatto S et al.; The role of arbitration of discordant reports at double reading of screening mammograms. *J Med Screen.* 2005;12(3):125.

de Azambuja E et al.; Ki-67 as prognostic marker in early breast cancer: A meta-analysis of published studies involving 12,155 patients. *Br J Cancer.* 2007;96(10):1504.

Faulk RM et al.; Efficacy of spot compression-magnification and tangential views in mammographic evaluation of palpable breast masses. *Radiology.* 1992;185(1):87.

Flobbe K et al.; The additional diagnostic value of ultrasonography in the diagnosis of breast cancer. *Arch Intern Med.* 2003;163(10):1194.

Gilcrease MZ et al.; Even low-level HER2 expression may be associated with worse outcome in node-positive breast cancer. *Am J Surg Pathol*. 2009;33(5):759.
Harvey JA et al.; Short-term follow-up of palpable breast lesions with benign imaging features: Evaluation of 375 lesions in 320 women. *Am J Roentgenol*. 2009;193(6):1723.
Harris L et al.; American Society of Clinical Oncology 2007 update of recommendations for the use of tumor markers in breast cancer. *J Clin Oncol*. 2007;25(33):5287.
Jemal A et al.; Global cancer statistics. *CA Cancer J Clin*. 2011;61(2):69.
Kohler BA et al.; Annual report to the nation on the status of cancer, 1975–2007, featuring tumors of the brain and other nervous system. *Cancer Inst*. 2011;103(9):714.
Kopans DB; Breast imaging and the standard of care for the symptomatic patient. *Radiology*. 1993;187(3):608.
Lebrecht A et al.; Diagnosis of breast cancer by tear proteomic pattern. *Cancer Genomics Proteomics*. 2009;6(3):177–182.
Leyland-Jones B et al.; Serum HER2 testing in patients with HER2-positive breast cancer: The death knell tolls. *Lancet Oncol*. 2011;12(3):286.
Li CI et al.; Clinical characteristics of different histologic types of breast cancer. *Br J Cancer*. 2005;93(9):1046.
Liberman L et al.; MR imaging of the ipsilateral breast in women with percutaneously proven breast cancer. *Am J Roentgenol*. 2003;180(4):901.
Lin C et al.; Detection of locally advanced breast cancer in the I-SPY TRIAL (CALGB 150007/150012, ACRIN 6657) in the interval between routine screening. *J Clin Oncol*. 2009;27:1503s.
Mandelson MT et al.; Breast density as a predictor of mammographic detection: Comparison of interval—and screen-detected cancers. *J Natl Cancer Inst*. 2000;92(13):1081.
Neagu M et al.; Patented biomarker panels in early detection of cancer. *Recent Patents on Biomarkers* 2011;1:10–24.
Peters NH et al.; Meta-analysis of MR imaging in the diagnosis of breast lesions. *Radiology*. 2008;246(1):116.
Rakha EA et al.; Prognostic significance of Nottingham histologic grade in invasive breast carcinoma. *J Clin Oncol*. 2008;26(19):3153.
Reston, American College of Radiology; *Breast Imaging Reporting and Data System (BI-RADS) Atlas*, 4th edn., Reston, VA, American College of Radiology, 2003.
Shaw CM et al.; Consensus review of discordant findings maximizes cancer detection rate in double-reader screening mammography: Irish National Breast Screening Program experience. *Radiology*. 2009;250(2):354.
Shen J et al.; Intramammary lymph node metastases are an independent predictor of poor outcome in patients with breast carcinoma. *Cancer*. 2004;101(6):1330.
Shin HC et al.; Limited value and utility of breast MRI in patients undergoing breast-conserving cancer surgery. *Ann Surg Oncol*. 2012;19(8):2572–2579. Epub Mar 24, 2012.
Sickles EA et al.; Benign breast lesions: Ultrasound detection and diagnosis. *Radiology*. 1984;151(2):467.
Siegel R et al.; Cancer statistics, 2011: The impact of eliminating socioeconomic and racial disparities on premature cancer deaths. *Cancer J Clin*. 2011;61(4):212.
Smart CR et al.; Insights into breast cancer screening of younger women. Evidence from the 14-year follow-up of the Breast Cancer Detection Demonstration Project. *Cancer*. 1993;72(4 Suppl):1449.
Stomper PC et al.; Mammographic detection and staging of ductal carcinoma in situ: Mammographic-pathologic correlation. *Semin Breast Dis*. 2000;3:1.
Stomper PC et al.; Mammographic predictors of the presence and size of invasive carcinomas associated with malignant microcalcification lesions without a mass. *Am J Roentgenol*. 2003;181(6):1679.
Turnbull L et al.; Comparative effectiveness of MRI in breast cancer (COMICE) trial: A randomised controlled trial. *Lancet*. 2010;375(9714):563.

5

Biomarkers for Early Detection of Familial Breast Cancer

Burak Yılmaz, MS, Catherine A. Moroski-Erkul, MS, Omer Faruk Hatipoglu, PhD, Esra Gunduz, DMD, PhD, Debmalya Barh, MSc, MTech, MPhil, PhD, and Mehmet Gunduz, MD, PhD

CONTENTS

ABSTRACT Breast cancer (BC) is classified as sporadic, familial, or hereditary. In familial BC, an unusual high number of members in a family are affected by breast, ovarian, or a related cancer. Family history is crucial in determining an individual's BC susceptibility. A person's risk of developing BC increases with an increasing number of affected family members. Only 5%–10% of all BC appears to have strong inheritance. Of these, 4%–5% is caused by genes with high penetrance and transmitted in an autosomal dominant manner. Testing for well-characterized mutations in blood based on a clinical suspicion of familial cancer is a well-known approach for genetic testing in cancer susceptibility. This review summarizes known genetic biomarkers, which may be used for early diagnosis of familial BC. Genes that serve as biomarkers for hereditary BC can be classified according to penetrance. *BRCA1* and *BRCA2*, two BC-associated genes with high penetrance, account for about 5% of all BCs, and mutation rates of these genes are variable across populations. Other BC susceptibility genes that have been described as having high to moderate penetrance are *CHEK2, PTEN, TP53, ATM, STK11/LKB1, CDH1, NBS1, RAD50, BRIP1*, and *PALB2*. A further 20 low-penetrance BC risk-modifying alleles have been identified to date. These genes all likely play a role in the development and progression in the wide spectrum of observed hereditary BCs.

5.1 Introduction

5.1.1 What is Familial Breast Cancer?

BC is classified as sporadic, familial, or hereditary. Sporadic BC accounts for 70%–75% of cases and is thought to be due to nonhereditary causes. Hereditary or familial terms are used to express BC caused by inheritable germline mutations in germ cells. According to National Institute for Health and Care Excellence (NICE) clinical guidelines, if there are an unusual high number of members in a family affected by breast, ovarian, or a related cancer, this is typically called familial or hereditary BC. Development of BC depends on the nature of the family history; the number of relatives who have developed breast, ovarian, or a related cancer; age at which relatives developed BC; and the age of the person (NICE clinical guideline 2013).

5.1.2 Why Is It Important?

BC remains the leading cause of cancer-related death in women despite a substantial decrease in BC mortality over the past two decades. This decrease in mortality is due, in part, to the development and use of adjuvant therapies as well as better and more widespread early screening programs (Peto et al. 2000; EBCTCG 2005). In addition to the pain suffered by cancer patients and their families, cancer places a significant economic burden on society as a whole. The estimated annual worldwide incidence is 1,383,000 (Lynch et al. 2012). Since cancer incidence is usually higher among older people, an aging population will increase the overall cost of cancer treatment in the future. Better diagnostic markers are needed to reduce the various personal and societal costs associated with this disease (Jemal et al. 2005; Lai et al. 2012).

There are many risk factors for BC development, including reproductive history, obesity, and hormonal factors (Turkoz et al. 2012). However, family history remains the most important associated factor, with risk increasing as the number of affected family members increases. Hereditary BC affects several family members across multiple generations. Most of these cancers are caused by mutations in the highly penetrant BC-associated genes. About 5%–10% of all BC has a strong inheritance while 25%–40% of BCs occurring before the age of 35 is hereditary in nature (Lux et al. 2006). Three to eight percent of all BC is caused by mutations in *BRCA1* and *BRCA2*, which are probably the best and most widely known BC-related genes. In familial BC cases, they account for up to 40% of all cases (Lux et al. 2006). Mutation rates of these highly penetrant genes vary from population to population (Kurian et al., 2010).

Other genes that have been described as high to moderately penetrant BC susceptibility genes are *CHEK2, PTEN, TP53, ATM, STK11/LKB1, CDH1, NBS1, RAD50, BRIP1,* and *PALB2* (Lalloo and Evans 2012). All of these genes play a role in the observed spectrum of hereditary BCs. Large number of genes with moderate to low penetrance may be responsible for BC cases, and a combination of these may contribute to a significant proportion of familial BC (Renwick et al. 2006; Rahman et al. 2007; Stratton and Rahman 2008; Mealiffe et al. 2010; Turnbull et al. 2010; Shuen and Foulkes 2011). Despite recent discoveries of new genetic susceptibility factors, there still remains a substantial portion of familial hereditary BC without any relationship to known BC susceptibility genes.

5.1.3 Early Detection of Familial BC

Easily detectable mutations in genes and proteins from patient blood samples are ideal diagnostic markers. Identifying biomarkers is immensely important to help medical doctors identify individuals who may be susceptible to certain cancer types. Biomarkers are also useful for distinguishing between different stages of cancer and providing more accurate prognoses. These biomarkers should be cancer-type specific and detectable in a wide range of specimens containing cancer-derived materials, including body fluids, tissues, and cell lines.

Mutations in several genes are associated with certain types of hereditary BC. As a gold standard, Sanger sequencing has been used to detect genetic-based mutations in blood. However, Sanger-based mutation detection faces difficulties of screening lots of samples at one time. Recent development of next-generation sequencing (NGS) provides the analysis of many genes at a time using commercial test panels. Testing for well-characterized mutations based on a clinical suspicion of familial cancer is through the approach of genetic testing for cancer susceptibility.

Early detection of cancer results in longer patient survival and reduces the amount of required treatment. There has been a considerable investment in the early detection of cancer over the past few decades. Screening programs for the early diagnosis of cancers that can detect asymptomatic malignancies or premalignant lesions are helpful for both patients and doctors. Early detection is one way to limit the human suffering associated with cancer as well as reduce the burden it places on society. Detection of cancer is related to how easily noticeable a tumor is. According to data from the Surveillance Epidemiology and End Results (SEER) Program of the National Cancer Institute, in the United States, a 5-year survival rate for patients diagnosed with skin cancer approaches 95%, and for BC patients, this figure ranges from 75% to 90%, while patients diagnosed with lung or pancreatic cancer have dramatically lower 5-year survival rates of 15% and 6%, respectively (http://seer.cancer.gov/statfacts/html/melan.html). This is due, in part, to the ease with which the former cancer types can be observed as compared with the latter types.

Detailed information regarding diagnosis of hereditary BC is available from several sources based in the United States, including American Society of Clinical Oncology (www.asco.org), the US Preventive Services Task Force (www.ahrq.gov/clinic/uspstfix.thm), and the National Comprehensive Cancer Network (www.nccn.org). Also available is a web-based tool offered by the US Department of Health and Human Services, which can be found at http://www.hhs.gov/familyhistory (Gage et al. 2012).

5.1.4 Genetics of BC

BRCA1 and *BRCA2* were the first genes to be linked to hereditary BC. They were discovered in the 1990s by linkage analysis and positional cloning using pedigrees with familial BC in successive generations (Miki et al. 1994; Wooster et al. 1995). *BRCA1* and *BRCA2* mutation carriers not only are susceptible to breast and ovarian cancers (Narod et al. 1991; Rigakos and Razis 2012) but also have an increased risk for developing melanoma (Cruz et al. 2011; Iscovich et al. 2002), as well as cancers of the fallopian tube (Kauff and Barakat 2007; Crum et al. 2012), colon and stomach (Brose et al. 2002), prostate (Kirchhoff et al. 2004; Moran et al. 2012), and pancreas (Hahn et al. 2003; Bartsch et al. 2012).

Although disease-related mutations in *BRCA1* and *BRCA2* have high penetrance and in individuals with mutations in these genes, the risk of BC increases by 10- to 20-fold; they are rare in the population with a frequency between 0.2% and 1% (Kurian 2010; Paradiso and Formenti 2011). The lifetime risk associated with mutations in various genes associated with BC varies from study to study depending on a variety of factors, including population studied, methods of sample selection, and methods of analysis. However, it is generally accepted that, in women, *BRCA1* mutations confer an overall lifetime risk of developing BC of about 65% and 40% for developing ovarian cancer. *BRCA2* mutations confer a risk of about 45% for BC in females and 6% in males and an approximately 11% risk of developing ovarian cancer.

Apart from the BRCA genes, there are a number of other genes that collectively account for some portion of non-*BRCA1*-/non-*BRCA2*-associated familial BC. Furthermore, it is possible that other low to moderate penetrance genes may account for the heterogeneity in tumor types associated with clearly *BRCA1*- or *BRCA2*-associated BCs, the so-called *polygenic model* (Shuen and Foulkes 2011). Furthermore, rare copy number variants (CNVs) that disrupt p53 and estrogen receptor pathways may contribute to hereditary BC risk in cases that are negative for mutations in genes known to confer increased BC risk (Pylkas et al. 2012). BC has been reported to be part of the Lynch syndrome in some families. Lynch syndrome is characterized by a predisposition to colon cancer, and the mismatch repair proteins MLH1, MSH2, and MSH6 are known to play a role in this condition. It is thought that the absence of MLH1 and MSH2 proteins may play a role in these BC cases. MSH6 may also be involved, but only one case has been reported thus far (Shanley et al. 2009; van der Groep et al. 2011).

5.2 High-Risk Genes

5.2.1 *BRCA1*

The early 1990s saw a number of papers published in which regions of chromosome 17q were identified as being associated with breast and/or ovarian cancer (Hall et al. 1990). In 1994, Miki et al. reported the positional cloning of a candidate *BRCA1* gene and identification of possible disease-associated mutations in patients with suspected 17q-associated breast or ovarian cancer (Miki et al. 1994). The *BRCA1* tumor suppressor is estimated to be responsible for approximately 8% of familial BC (Lalloo and Evans 2012). In the NCBI PubMed database, a search for *BRCA1* and BC retrieves over 7000 records, highlighting the significance of this gene in our understanding of this highly heterogeneous disease. Pathogenic mutation of *BRCA1* is observed in about 1 in every

1000 individuals (Lalloo et al. 2003), and such mutations increase the risk of developing BC in both women and men (Tai et al. 2007).

Based on a 2004 review of the literature by Liede et al., it appears that *BRCA1* mutations may account for approximately 4% of all male BC. Higher incidence has been reported in some studies, but these are typically based on cohorts that include patients who sought genetic counseling or were from families with known BRCA mutations (Liede et al. 2004). *BRCA1* mutations may also contribute somewhat to the risk of prostate cancer in men under 70 years of age; however, the relationship is not very strong. Evidence for the association of *BRCA2* mutations in both male breast and prostate cancers is much stronger (Liede et al. 2004).

A recently published multistage genome-wide association study (GWAS) of *BRCA1* carriers attempted to identify risk-modifying loci. Several loci that appear to significantly modify risk were found. The authors estimated that 5% of *BRCA1* carriers with the lowest risk have a lifetime risk of developing BC of 28%–50% and that the 5% of carriers with the highest risk have a lifetime risk of 81%–100% (Couch et al. 2013).

A retrospective study of radiation exposure from routine diagnostic tests carried out before the age of 30 was associated with higher incidence of BC in carriers of *BRCA1* and *BRCA2* mutations as compared to the general population (Pijpe et al. 2012). This result has very significant implications for the use of various diagnostic tests performed in families with known BRCA mutations.

BRCA1 is a large gene containing a total of 24 exons. It plays a key role in several cellular functions including DNA repair, chromatin remodeling, and transcriptional regulation (Poehlmann and Roessner 2010). Its role in DNA repair is primarily as part of homologous recombination (HR) repair that is required for the resolution of replication-associated double-strand breaks. In the absence of competent HR repair, the error-prone nonhomologous end joining (NHEJ) pathway is utilized thus compromising genome stability (Roy et al. 2012). Therapies that are aimed at multiple DNA repair pathways can sensitize otherwise therapy-resistant cancers (Stachelek et al. 2010; Yap et al. 2011). Targeted therapies capable of exploiting the HR repair deficiency in BRCA-deficient tumors have had some degree of success. An example is the use of poly ADP-ribose polymerase (PARP) inhibitors in combination with, for example, a drug-like temozolomide, to create a sort of *synthetic lethality*. PARP is involved in the repair of DNA via the base excision repair (BER) pathway. In the absence of PARP, lesions such as 3-methyladenine and 7-methylguanine that are normally repaired by BER are left unrepaired (Figure 5.1a). Subsequently, during replication, these normally nondeleterious lesions may be transformed into toxic lesions via replication fork stalling and collapse and the formation of single- and double-strand breaks (Figure 5.1b) (Trivedi et al. 2005, 2008; Fishel et al. 2007). Thus, PARP inhibition and BRCA deficiency combined with treatment using a DNA-damaging agent such as temozolomide lead to an overwhelming degree of damage that even cancer cells are incapable of tolerating (Yap et al. 2011).

5.2.1.1 Clinical Features of BRCA1

The breast tumors that develop in *BRCA1* carriers differ from those that develop in nonfamilial BCs. *BRCA1* BCs are generally characterized by an increased frequency of pushing margins, high degree of nuclear pleomorphism, and mitotic frequency (Lakhani et al. 2005; de la Cruz et al. 2012; Lalloo and Evans 2012). The diagnosis of BC in *BRCA1* carriers typically occurs at a younger age. Prognosis of these BCs is quite variable, with a range of disease-free survival similar to that seen in sporadic BCs. *BRCA1* tumors are typically hormone receptor negative and aggressive in nature (Paradiso and Formenti 2011).

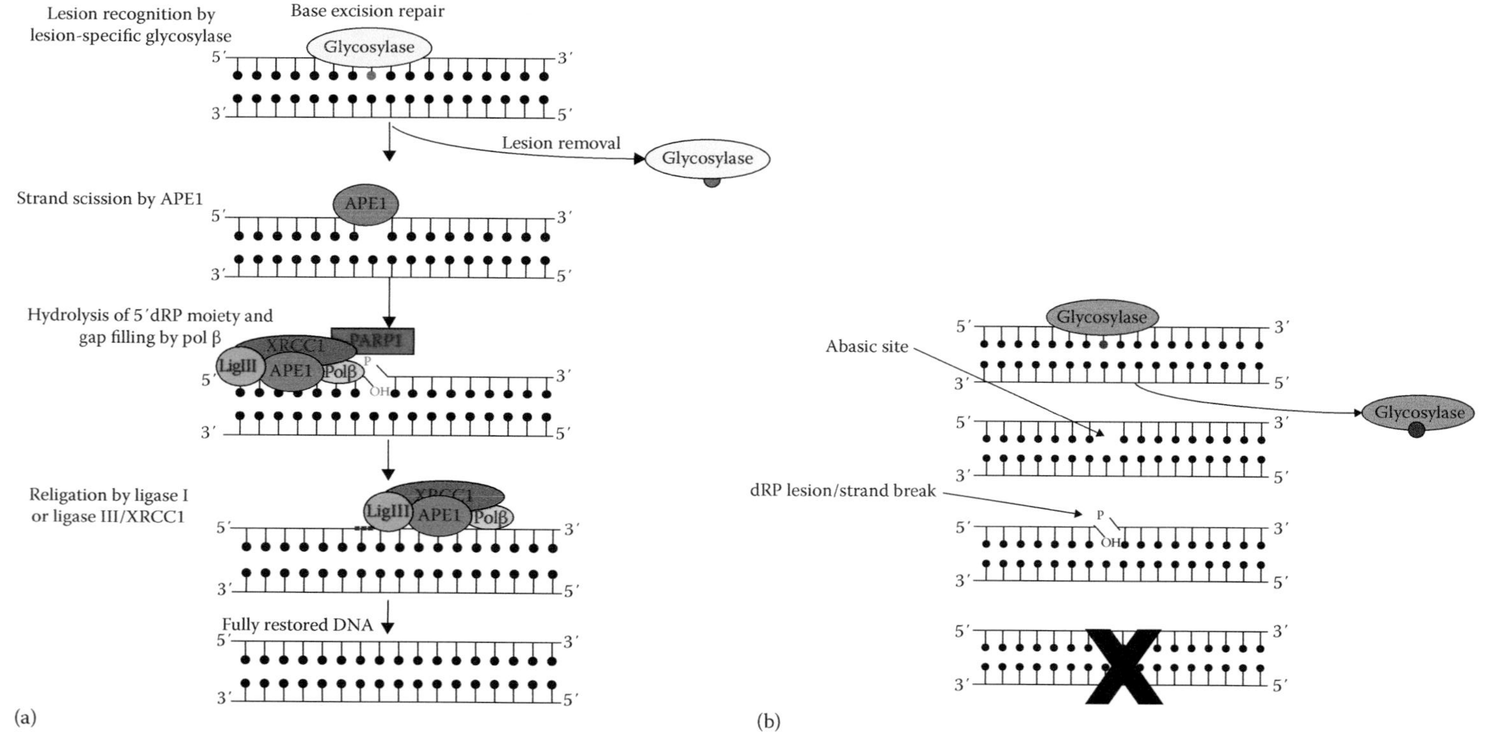

FIGURE 5.1
(a) Main steps involved in short-patch base excision repair. DNA lesions are recognized by lesion-specific DNA glycosylases. The base is excised, and an endonuclease cuts the sugar–phosphate backbone. DNA polymerase modifies DNA ends and fills gaps with appropriate base, and backbone is then religated, restoring DNA to its original state. In this model, PARP1 protects single-strand breaks during repair process. (b) Glycosylases recognize and remove damaged DNA base. In the absence of proteins required to carry out repair steps downstream of damage recognition (i.e., PARP inhibition), abasic sites and single-strand breaks accumulate. In tumor cells deficient in homologous recombination repair, exhibiting the so-called BRCAness, cells are overwhelmed with damage and cannot survive.

BRCA1 and triple-negative BCs frequently exhibit a similar genomic profile as assayed by array comparative genomic hybridization (aCGH) and share a similar presence of lymph node metastasis (Vollebergh et al. 2011). According to results from a comprehensive international epidemiological collaboration, the proportion of estrogen-receptor-negative and triple-negative tumors in *BRCA1* carriers appears to decrease with age at diagnosis (Mavaddat et al. 2012). The same study found that medullary tumors are more common in *BRCA1* carriers (Mavaddat et al. 2012).

BRCA1 cancers have a similar immunohistological profile to sporadic basal carcinoma and are positive for CK5/6/CK14 (Lakhani et al. 2005; Lalloo and Evans 2012). *BRCA1* tumors typically express basal markers like basal keratins, P-cadherin, and epidermal growth factor receptor (Palacios et al. 2008).

5.2.2 *BRCA2* (FANCD1)

Like *BRCA1*, *BRCA2* was identified in the early to mid-1990s amidst the search for BC susceptibility genes. After a second susceptibility locus was identified at 13q12, researchers began probing that region to find the associated gene. In 1995, Wooster et al. discovered *BRCA2* by positional cloning and identified germ line mutations in several BC families (Collins et al. 1995; Wooster et al. 1995). Also like *BRCA1*, *BRCA2* is associated with an increased risk of developing both breast and ovarian cancers. *BRCA2* mutations are found in 10% of families with a significant history of BC and confer an overall lifetime risk of about 40%–85% for women and 6% for men (Lalloo and Evans 2012). Note that the risk of developing BC in males with *BRCA2* mutations is much higher than in males with *BRCA1* mutations. *BRCA2* mutations have also been associated with an increased risk for developing other types of cancers such as pancreatic (Huang et al. 2013; Leung and Saif 2013; Mocci et al. 2013) and prostate (Sundararajan et al. 2011; Castro and Eeles 2012; Sandhu et al. 2013).

BRCA2 is a large gene with a total of 24 exons. Like *BRCA1*, it is involved in DNA repair by HR (Roy et al. 2012). Thus, cancers with *BRCA2* deficiency may also respond to therapies that target multiple DNA repair pathways (Clark et al. 2012). Interestingly, in a study that examined biopsies from patients whose cancers initially responded to PARP inhibition treatment and subsequently became resistant, secondary mutations in *BRCA2* were identified that actually resulted in restoration of full-length *BRCA2* protein (Barber et al. 2013).

BRCA2 has been shown to interact with a number of other proteins that have been implicated in the pathogenesis of BC, including RAD51, *TP53*, and *PALB2* (Clark et al. 2012; Roy et al. 2012). Biallelic mutations in *BRCA2* are responsible for a small percentage of children with Fanconi anemia (FA), a disease characterized by progressive marrow failure, congenital anomalies, and predisposition to malignancy (Myers et al. 2012). *BRCA2*-associated FA typically has an earlier age of onset, and patients are more likely to have leukemia and solid tumors (Myers et al. 2012).

5.2.2.1 Clinical Features of BRCA2

Unlike *BRCA1*, BCs with *BRCA2* mutations do not appear to have a specific characteristic pathology. However, they do tend to exhibit features more common to sporadic BCs than those associated with *BRCA1* (Roy et al. 2012). *BRCA2* tumors are more likely to be estrogen and progesterone receptor positive (Palacios et al. 2008). Both *BRCA1* and *BRCA2* mutation carriers are more likely than non-BRCA mutation carriers to have high expression of HIF1α (a key regulator of the response to hypoxia) in ductal carcinoma in situ (DCIS), a precancerous lesion known to progress to invasive BC (van der Groep et al. 2013).

Mitotic rates in *BRCA2* tumors range from being lower than those observed in sporadic tumors to higher (Lalloo and Evans 2012). There is an apparent negative correlation between age at diagnosis of *BRCA2* carriers and proportion of estrogen-receptor-negative/triple-negative status. The same study found that lobular tumors are more common in *BRCA2* carriers (Mavaddat et al. 2012). The same study found that lobular tumors are more common in *BRCA2* carriers (Mavaddat et al. 2012). A specific *BRCA2* mutation, 999del5, was found to be associated with high-grade, rapidly proliferating tumors in a study that compared 40 families harboring this mutation against an age-matched control group (Agnarsson et al. 1998). Thirty-four out of 40 *BRCA2* 999del5 mutation-harboring patients had ductal carcinoma. The *BRCA2* 999del5 tumors also had less tubule formation, more nuclear pleomorphism, and higher mitotic rates as compared with controls (Agnarsson et al. 1998).

5.2.3 *TP53*

In 1979, DeLeo et al. identified a protein with a molecular weight of 53 kDa in mouse cells transformed by various methods (DeLeo et al. 1979). In 1981, a protein of the same size was identified in both SV40-transformed human cell lines and cells derived from spontaneous tumors (Crawford et al. 1981). The gene that encodes the protein identified by these groups came to be known as *TP53* (or p53). *TP53* is a tumor suppressor and is the most frequently altered gene in human tumors. Somatic mutations in the *TP53* gene commonly occur in solid tumors, and at least 250 *TP53* germ line mutations have been identified to date (Ognjanovic et al. 2012). *TP53* mutations have been reported to be particularly common in triple-negative and *BRCA1*-associated BCs (Palacios et al. 2008; Walerych et al. 2012). Also, the spectrum of *TP53* mutations in BRCA-associated tumors is unique as compared to sporadic tumors, with differences in mutation distribution and base changes (Palacios et al. 2008).

Germ line mutations in *TP53* usually result in childhood cancers or early onset of tumors in adults. Autosomal dominant germ line *TP53* mutations are responsible for the majority (~80%) of families affected by Li–Fraumeni syndrome (LFS) (Ognjanovic et al. 2012) and is also associated with some cases (15%–25%) of Li–Fraumeni-like syndrome (LFL) (Ognjanovic et al. 2012). LFS is a cancer syndrome that was first described by Li and Fraumeni in 1969 (Varley 2003). It is characterized by early-onset cancer with a characteristic tumor spectrum including sarcomas, brain and breast tumors, and childhood adrenocortical carcinoma (Varley 2003). LFS families are highly radiosensitive, and about 50% of LFS individuals will develop some kind of cancer before the age of 30. This is in contrast to the 1% chance that individuals in the general population have of developing cancer by 30 years of age (Sorrell et al. 2013). Frebourg et al. began studying in earnest the link between germ line *TP53* mutations, LFS, and BC in 1991 (Frebourg et al. 1991). It is now known that about 30% of female mutation carriers will develop BC by 30 years of age. Furthermore, the development of secondary cancers later in life is also a high likelihood in LFS individuals (Sorrell et al. 2013). According to Masciari et al. (2012), most DCIS and invasive ductal carcinomas occurring in LFS patients who have *TP53* germ line mutations are hormone receptor positive and/or HER2 positive. Thus, hormone receptor status as well as the radiosensitivity associated with LFS should be taken into account when determining possible treatments. Although LFS is responsible for less than 0.1% of BC, there is an 18- to 60-fold increased risk of BC for individuals under 45 years of age as compared to the general population and therefore is an important BC syndrome to be aware of (Lalloo and Evans 2012).

TP53 has 11 exons with a core DNA-binding domain encoded by exons 4–8 (Lalloo and Evans 2012). *TP53* is often referred to as the *guardian of the genome* (Carson and Lois 1995; Sigal and Rotter 2000) and is involved in many cellular processes via transcription regulation and signaling networks including DNA damage response, regulation of cell cycle arrest, apoptosis, and senescence (Lalloo et al. 2003; Rubbi and Milner 2003). *TP53* has been reported to interact with as many as 100 different proteins. Because *TP53* is so essential to many cellular processes involved in maintaining genome integrity, it is hardly surprising that mutations in this gene are so common in human cancers. For this reason, it and the pathways that it is involved in are common targets for cancer therapy. As recently reviewed by Morandell and Yaffe (2012), therapeutic modalities that target tumor suppressors/oncogenes together with DNA damage pathways (much like the aforementioned PARP inhibitor plus DNA-damaging drug strategy) have been successfully applied both in vitro and in vivo, including treatment of human cancers.

5.2.4 *PTEN*

Phosphatase and tensin homolog (*PTEN*) is a tumor suppressor gene containing nine exons and is located at chromosome 10q23.3. *PTEN* encodes the protein phosphatidylinositol phosphate phosphatase protein. *PTEN* was identified in 1997 after deletions in the region of chromosome 10q23-24 were identified in greater than 90% of glioblastoma multiformes (Steck et al. 1997). Some 1900 different alterations, mutations, and deletions in *PTEN* have been identified thus far. Allelic or complete deletion of *PTEN* occurs in breast and prostate cancers. *PTEN*'s tumor suppressor activity is probably related to its function as a lipid phosphatase, which is involved in the regulation of the PI3K–AKT–mTOR pathway. It may also be related to its function as a protein phosphatase that is necessary for carrying out its activity in cell cycle arrest and inhibition of invasion in vitro (Hollander et al. 2011). *PTEN* localization to the nucleus may be necessary for repair of double-strand breaks mediated by RAD51, another gene that has been implicated in some types of BCs (Hollander et al. 2011). *PTEN* also regulates the tumor suppressor activity of APC and *CDH1* in the nucleus (Song et al. 2011).

Germ line mutations result in rare conditions that are collectively referred to as *PTEN* hamartoma tumor syndromes (PTHS). Two PTHS-inherited syndromes are Cowden syndrome (CS) and Bannayan–Riley–Ruvalcaba syndrome (BRRS). *PTEN* mutations have also been identified in brain and prostate cancers (Li et al. 1997). *PTEN* expression is downregulated in *BRCA1*-associated cancers exhibiting a basal-like phenotype (Campeau et al. 2008).

CS is an autosomal dominant disorder whose diagnosis is difficult (Eng 2010). While *PTEN* deletion in mice can cause Cowden-like phenotypes and spontaneous tumorigenesis in some tissues, it is likely that the combined disruption of several pathways is responsible for the development of most *PTEN*-associated cancers (Hollander et al. 2011). Eighty percent of CS patients harbor germ line mutations in *PTEN* and typically develop cancers of the breast, thyroid, and endometrium. Somatic *PTEN* mutations are also commonly seen in sporadic tumors of these same types (Hollander et al. 2011). In women with CS, the lifetime risk of developing BC is 25%–50%. In sporadic BCs, although only 5% has *PTEN* mutations, 40% exhibits loss of *PTEN* expression as determined by immunoreactivity (Hollander et al. 2011).

It is unclear whether BRRS is a distinct clinical condition or simply an early-onset type of CS (Gustafson et al. 2007; Lachlan et al. 2007). Lachlan et al. (2007) suggest that BRRS and CS are a single clinical entity, mostly differing in the age of onset, much like the tumor suppressor disorder neurofibromatosis type 1. On the other hand, Gustafson et al.

maintain that the two are clinically distinct syndromes as BRRS is not associated with an increased incidence of malignancy. However, they also recommend that any individuals identified as having *PTEN* mutations should follow cancer surveillance recommendations for CS (Gustafson et al. 2007).

5.2.5 *STK11*

Serine/threonine kinase 11 (*STK11*), also known as *LKB1*, is located on chromosome 19p13.3 and encodes a serine/threonine kinase that regulates cell polarity and functions as a tumor suppressor. As a kinase upstream of AMPK, it also is involved in the maintenance of metabolic homeostasis. Its loss may result in hyperactivation of the mTOR pathway in HER2-positive BC (Andrade-Vieira et al. 2013). In addition to BC, *STK11* has been studied in connection with non–small cell lung cancer (Shackelford et al. 2013) and colorectal cancer (Ngeow et al. 2013).

Germ line mutations in *STK11* occur in the autosomal dominant condition known as Peutz–Jeghers syndrome (PJS), which is characterized by perioral pigmentation and intestinal hamartomatous polyposis. PJS is also associated with a predisposition to various types of cancers including those of the breast, cervix, testicles, and ovarian sex cord (Hemminki 1999). Patients with this syndrome have an approximate risk of 30% of developing BC by the age of 60 (Lim et al. 2004; Hearle et al. 2006). In a study of cancer incidence in 240 PJS patients with *STK11* mutations, Lim et al. identified mutations in exon 3 of *STK11* that appear to be associated with the greatest risk of developing cancer. However, these mutations may only be related to gastrointestinal cancers and not those of the breast. Missense and truncating mutations in regions other than exon 3 all had similar degrees of cancer risk (Lim et al. 2004). Due to the function of *STK11* in the mTOR pathway, it is possible that rapamycin could be used to treat patients with PJS-associated cancers (Campeau et al. 2008).

5.2.6 E-Cadherin (*CDH1*)

Cadherin 1 (*CDH1*) or E-cadherin is located at chromosome 16q22.1 and encodes the protein E-cadherin, a calcium-dependent cell adhesion glycoprotein that is important for cell–cell adhesion (Becker et al. 1994). Approximately 30%–40% of familial diffuse gastric cancer (FDGC), an autosomal dominant syndrome, results from mutations in *CDH1*, and affected women are predisposed to lobular BC (Keller et al. 1999; Schrader et al. 2008). Patients with FDGC have an approximate risk of BC of between 39% and 52% (Schrader et al. 2011). Schrader et al. (2011) reported that in women with early-onset or familial lobular BC but *without* a family history of diffuse gastric cancer, mutations in *CDH1* are rare.

5.3 Moderate Penetrance Genes

5.3.1 *ATM*

Ataxia telangiectasia mutated (*ATM*) is located on chromosome 11q22.3 and encodes a checkpoint kinase involved in DNA damage signaling. Biallelic mutations cause a rare, autosomal recessive disorder called ataxia telangiectasia (AT) (Savitsky et al. 1995), which is characterized by a host of somatic disorders. Heterozygous mutations of *ATM* do not result in the AT phenotype; however, they increase an individual's sensitivity to radiation and raise the risk of BC by about 2.5-fold (Thompson et al. 2005; Renwick et al. 2006; Lalloo and Evans 2012).

The localization of p53 to the centrosome during mitosis is *ATM* dependent. Prodosmo et al. hypothesized that this feature could be used to distinguish between healthy A-T heterozygotes and A-T homozygotes. Indeed, by determining the percentage of mitotic lymphoblasts or PBMCs with p53 centrosomal localization, they were able to reliably, quickly, and inexpensively distinguish between these different genotypes. Healthy individuals had >75% p53 centrosomal localization, while A-T heterozygotes had 40%–56% and A-T homozygotes had <30%. In a preliminary study, their test confirmed that *ATM* is a BC susceptibility gene (Prodosmo et al. 2013).

A recently published study of the in vivo therapeutic potential of *ATM* siRNA was investigated. A gene-specific *ATM* siRNA was delivered using a well-characterized porous silicon-based multistage vector (MSV) delivery system (MSV/*ATM*). Treatment included biweekly administration of siRNA to BALB/c mice. Their immune response was monitored through serum measurement of cytokines, chemokines, and colony-stimulating factors. The drug delivery system/siRNA did not trigger any acute immune response in the mice, and other parameters such as body weight, blood chemistry, and major organ histology did not result in any significant changes even after 4 weeks of treatment. Furthermore, successful knockdown of *ATM* was achieved, and the growth of MDA-MB-231 orthotopic tumors in nude mice was inhibited. This report opens up future possibilities for modulation of DNA repair pathways for therapeutics in humans (Xu et al. 2013).

5.3.2 *CHEK2* (CHK2)

Checkpoint kinase 2 (*CHEK2*) is located on chromosome 22q12.1 and encodes a cell cycle checkpoint kinase involved in the DNA damage response (Matsuoka et al. 1998; Wu et al. 2001). It is located upstream of p53 and downstream of *ATM* in the DNA damage repair signaling network. *CHEK2* is a tumor suppressor gene, and somatic mutations as well as aberrant expression have been identified in a number of malignancies, including osteosarcoma and ovarian cancer (Miller et al. 2002), lymphomas (Hoglund et al. 2011; Ferrao et al. 2012), colon cancer (Meijers-Heijboer et al. 2003; Stawinska et al. 2008), and glioblastoma multiforme (Ferrao et al. 2012). In a study of uterine serous carcinoma (USC) employing targeted capture and massively parallel sequencing to assess the status of 30 different tumor suppressor genes, 5% of the 151 patients examined had germ line mutations in *BRCA1*, *CHEK2*, or *p53*. The authors thus concluded that a small number of USC cases appear to be associated with hereditary breast and ovarian cancer (Pennington et al. 2013).

It was previously thought that mutations in *CHEK2* might account for a small percentage of LFS cases in which *p53* mutations were not present (Bell et al. 1999; Lee et al. 2001; Varley 2003). However, after more thorough investigations, the case for this hypothesis was not able to be convincingly made (Tavor et al. 2001; Meijers-Heijboer et al. 2002; Stawinska et al. 2008; Hoglund et al. 2011).

Two germ line mutations, in particular, 1100delC and I157T, have been the focus of much research (Nevanlinna and Bartek 2006). The *CHEK2**1100delC mutation is a truncating mutation that results in reduced protein kinase activity. The mutation frequency was calculated to be 1.1% in healthy European and North American populations and 5.1% in a group of 718 BRCA-negative BC families (Meijers-Heijboer et al. 2002). *CHEK2* mutations are observed more often in patients with wild-type *BRCA1* and *BRCA2* than in patients who have mutations in these genes (Turnbull et al. 2012). When the *CHEK2**1100delC mutation *does* occur in BRCA mutation carriers, it does not result in any increased risk (Meijers-Heijboer et al. 2002). Based on a meta-analysis of 26,000 cases and 27,000 controls taken from unselected, early-onset, and familial BC studies, Weischer et al. (2008) concluded that the *CHEK2**1100delC mutation results in a 37% risk of BC by the age of 70 in heterozygous carriers. According to a recent publication (Adank et al. 2011), women from families with homozygous *CHEK2** 1100delC mutations have about a sixfold higher risk of developing BC. Based on these results, it may be recommended that patients in BC families be screened for *CHEK2* in addition to *BRCA1* and *BRCA2*. Kabacik et al. (2011) reported a potentially clinically useful test for assessing *ATM/CHEK2*/p53 pathway activity.

CHEK2 c.507delT is a loss-of-function mutation identified in a screen of *CHEK2* mutations in families with known BC predispositions (Manoukian et al. 2011).

5.3.3 *BRIP1/BACH1* (FANCJ)

The *BRIP1* gene encodes a protein that is a binding partner of *BRCA1* and has been investigated as a BC predisposing gene. As with *BRCA2* biallelic mutations, such mutations in *BRIP1/BACH1* also result in FA. In a study published by Tang et al., haplotype blocks constructed with 48 tag SNPs (tSNPs) were used to investigate the haplotypes of eight BC susceptibility genes (*TP53, PTEN, CHEK2, ATM, NBS1, RAD50, BRIP1,* and *PALB2*) in 734 female patients and 672 age-matched controls. Haplotypes within *NBS1, PTEN,* and *BRIP1* were associated with increased sporadic BC risk. However, in this study, only haplotypes within *NBS1* were found to be associated with increased familial BC risk (Tang et al. 2013).

In a study of high-risk individuals of Ashkenazi Jewish ethnic background, it was found that *BRIP1* mutations were only marginally associated with BC risk (Catucci et al. 2012). It is thought that mutations in *BRIP1* may also contribute to an increased risk for ovarian cancer (Rafnar et al. 2011).

5.3.4 *PALB2* (FANCN)

The *PALB2* gene encodes a protein that interacts with *BRCA2* during HR and double-strand break repair. Heterozygous mutations in *PALB2* result in increased risk for BC while homozygous mutations, as with *BRIP1* and *BRCA2*, result in FA. It is unclear why these FA genes confer an increased risk for BC while other FA genes do not. It may be that they are involved in or associate with proteins involved in DNA repair by HR (Campeau et al. 2008). *PALB2* mutations are found in about 1%–4% of families negative for *BRCA1* or *BRCA2* mutations (Poumpouridou and Kroupis 2012). Mutations in *PALB2* have also been associated with ovarian (Teo et al. 2013a; Tischkowitz et al. 2013) and pancreatic cancers (Axilbund and Wiley 2012; Solomon et al. 2012).

A rare mutation, *PALB2* c.3113G>A (p.Trp1038*), which results in a protein-truncating mutation and is associated with a risk of BC similar in magnitude to that of *BRCA2*, has been identified in Australian patients (Teo et al. 2013b). In another study originating from the same lab, a previously unreported *PALB2* mutation, PALB2c.1947_1948insA, was identified in a mutation screen of 748 Australasian multiple-case BC families. In this study, it was also determined that the c.3113G>A mutation occurs at a frequency of 1.5% in this population. Most of the cancers arising in carriers of any one of the 22 *PALB2* mutations identified in this study were high-grade invasive ductal carcinomas (Teo et al. 2013b). Fibroblast cell lines derived from patients with heterozygous *PALB2* c.229delT mutation displayed evidence of chromosomal rearrangements and altered centromere distribution. However, due to extremely low sample size, the relevance of this result is not clear (Wark et al. 2013). Pathogenic truncating *PALB2* mutations previously identified in family studies were identified in mutations screening of lymphocyte DNA in a population-based study and were estimated to confer a 5.3-fold increase in risk of developing BC. They also reported that, at least based on their obtained results, *rare* missense mutations in *PALB2* do not confer a strong BC risk (Tischkowitz et al. 2012).

PALB2 1592delT is a mutation that has been observed in BC families negative for mutations in *BRCA1* and *BRCA2*. Most of these tumors were triple negative and ductal and exhibited a high-grade phenotype. They were also mostly CK5/6, CK14, and CK17 negative and showed high expression of Ki67 and low expression of cyclin D1 as compared to other familial cases and sporadic BCs (Heikkinen et al. 2009; van der Groep et al. 2011).

5.4 Low-Penetrance BC Genes

There have been many studies in recent years in which BC predisposing SNPs have been identified. Many of these have been extremely large collaborative efforts which, along with advances in sequencing technology, have allowed scientists to move closer to understanding the complicated genetics of hereditary and sporadic BC. Table 5.1 contains a list of SNPs identified as having some degree of risk for BC in *BRCA1* and *BRCA2* mutation carriers. The table includes some SNPs that confer a *decrease* in disease risk. Also included is the gene *BARD1*, as a recent report suggests that this gene has no association with BC risk and thus resources should be funneled away from its study and directed toward more promising genes.

According to initial reports, *RAD51C* was identified as a high-risk gene for both breast and ovarian cancers. Later, research showed this gene to be predominantly associated with increased risk of ovarian cancer while the risk of BC is not clearly elevated (Lalloo and Evans 2012).

5.5 Conclusion and Future Directions

People with familial BC need a special approach because of differences in the BC risk. Family history is the most important factor for determining BC risk, and this risk grows with an increasing number of affected relatives with BC. The first high-risk BC genes were discovered in the 1990s, and since then, there has been intense research to find more BC susceptibility genes. BC is highly heterogeneous disease, complicating our understanding, diagnosis, and treatment of it. Recent advances in technology have greatly improved our ability to probe the genome for subtle changes. Although many of the genes that have been associated with hereditary BC are known to play in role in DNA repair, particularly the repair of double-strand breaks by HR repair, it is likely that most of hereditary and sporadic BC is caused by multiple genes from more than one pathway. The massive population-based GWASs are increasing our understanding of this deadly disease with each passing day. In time, our understanding of the roles played by many of the genes described in this chapter may provide better diagnostic and therapeutic tools for those

TABLE 5.1

Low-Penetrance SNPs and Gene Mutations that Modify Hereditary BC Risk in *BRCA1* and *BRCA2* Mutation Carriers

(Nearby) Gene	Locus	SNP/Variant	Hazard Ratio (HR)/ Assoc. with *BRCA1* or *BRCA2* Carriers	References
	6p24	rs9348512	0.85/*BRCA2* reduced risk	Gaudet et al. (2013)
	12q24	rs1292011	0.92/*BRCA2*	Antoniou et al. (2012)
	9q31.2	rs865686	*BRCA2*	Antoniou et al. (2012)
	9q31	rs865686	0.99/*BRCA2*	Antoniou et al. (2012)
	11q13	rs614367	1.08/*BRCA2*	Antoniou et al. (2012)
	5p12	rs10941679	1.07/*BRCA2*	Antoniou et al. (2010)
	20q13	rs311498	0.95/*BRCA2*	Couch et al. (2012)
		rs13039229	0.90/*BRCA2*	Gaudet et al. (2013)
	8q24	rs13281615 rs4733664	1.03/*BRCA2* 1.10/*BRCA2*	Antoniou et al. (2009) Gaudet et al. (2013)
	19p13.1		1.17/*BRCA1*[b]	Couch et al. (2012)
	2q35	rs13387042	1.14/*BRCA1* 1.18/*BRCA2*	Antoniou et al. (2009)
	1q32	rs2290854	1.14/*BRCA1*	Couch et al. (2013)
	6q22.33	rs2180341	Weak effect—may decrease risk *BRCA1*	Kirchhoff et al. (2012)
CDKN2A/B	9p21	rs1011970	1.03/*BRCA2*	Antoniou et al. (2012)
		rs10965163	0.84/*BRCA2*	Gaudet et al. (2013)
ZNF365	10q21.2	rs10995190?	0.84/*BRCA2*	Antoniou et al. (2012)
		rs16917302	0.88/*BRCA2*	Couch et al. (2012)
		rs17221319	1.09/*BRCA2*	Gaudet et al. (2013)
MERIT40	19p13	rs8170	0.98/*BRCA2*	Couch et al. (2012)
ZMIZ1	10q22	rs704010	1.01/*BRCA2*	Antoniou et al. (2012)
STXBP4, COX11	17q23	rs6504950	1.04/*BRCA2*	Antoniou et al. (2010)
PTHLH	12p11	rs27633	1.14/*BRCA2*	Gaudet et al. (2013)
MAP3K1	5q11	rs889312 rs16886113	1.10/*BRCA2* 1.24/*BRCA2*	Gaudet et al. (2013)
PTHLH	12p11	rs10771399	0.87/*BRCA1*[a]	Antoniou et al. (2012)
FGFR2	10q26	rs2981582	1.26/*BRCA2*	Gaudet et al. (2010)
		rs2420946	0.96/*BRCA2*	Gaudet et al. (2013)
TOX3	16q12	rs3803662	1.20/*BRCA2*	Gaudet et al. (2010)
NOTCH2	1p11	rs11249433	1.05/*BRCA2*	Antoniou et al. (2011)
BARD1		Cys557Ser and haplotypes	*Not* assoc. with increased risk[c]	Spurdle et al. (2011)
XRCC1		pArg280His-rs25489	*BRCA2*[d]	Osorio et al. (2011)
MORF4L1		rs7164529 rs10519219	*BRCA2*—weak assoc.	Martrat et al. (2011)
ESR1	6q25.1	rs2046210	1.17/*BRCA1*	Antoniou et al. (2011)
		rs9397435	1.14/*BRCA2*	Antoniou et al. (2011)
		rs2253407	0.92/*BRCA2*	Gaudet et al. (2013)
RAD51L1	1p11.2		1.14/*BRCA2*	Antoniou et al. (2011)
BRCA1		rs16942	Decreased risk[e]	Cox et al. (2011)

(Continued)

TABLE 5.1 (*CONTINUED*)

Low-Penetrance SNPs and Gene Mutations that Modify Hereditary BC Risk in *BRCA1* and *BRCA2* Mutation Carriers

(Nearby) Gene	Locus	SNP/Variant	Hazard Ratio (HR)/ Assoc. with *BRCA1* or *BRCA2* Carriers	References
SMAD3	15q22	rs71660081	1.25/*BRCA2*	Walker et al. (2010)
		rs3825977	1.20/*BRCA2*	
RHAMM	HMMR		1.09/*BRCA1*	Maxwell et al. (2011)
LSP1		rs3817198	1.16/*BRCA2*[f]	Antoniou et al. (2009)
			1.11/*BRCA2*	Antoniou et al. (2010)
IRS1		rs1801278 (Gly972Arg)	1.86/class II *BRCA1* mutations	Ding et al. (2012)
			0.86/class I *BRCA1* mutations	
PHB		rs6917 (1630 C > T)	Rare homozygote genotype that may modify risk/*BRCA1*	Jakubowska et al. (2012)

[a] Risk restricted to mutations proven or predicted to lead to the absence of protein expression; associated primarily with estrogen receptor (ER)-negative BC in *BRCA1* carriers (HR 0.82).

[b] Associated mostly with ER-negative BC, in both *BRCA1* and *BRCA2*.

[c] As it is a *BRCA1/2* interactor, BARD1 has been commonly studied as possible modifier of BC risk.

[d] In a small series of samples (701 *BRCA1* carriers and 576 *BRCA2* carriers), in *BRCA2* mutations carriers, rare homozygotes for this mutation had increased risk (HR = 22.3). However, when repeated with larger sample size (4480 *BRCA1* and 3016 *BRCA2*), no evidence of an association was found.

[e] In *BRCA1* mutation carriers who also carry this rare SNP on the WT *BRCA1* allele, the risk of BC is decreased; SNP may cause nuclear proteins to have higher affinity for *BRCA1*. Low-penetrance variants, identified through genome-wide association studies (GWASs), are common but associated with smaller increases in risk (Turnbull et al. 2012). Some of these act as modifiers of *BRCA1* and *BRCA2*. A total of 19 validated SNPs have been reported thus far (Turnbull et al., 2010).

[f] Appears to act multiplicatively in *BRCA2* mutation carriers.

suffering from BC. NGS is a featured method for screening hereditary BC. It allows for the analysis of multiple genes at a time using commercial panels. In future, more biomarkers would be revealed to enlighten hereditary BC, and NGS panels would be more accessible and comprehensive to detect mutations from blood.

References

Agnarsson BA, Jonasson JG, Bjornsdottir IB, Barkardottir RB, Egilsson V, Sigurdsson H (1998) Inherited BRCA2 mutation associated with high grade breast cancer. *Breast Cancer Research and Treatment* 47 (2):121–127.

Andrade-Vieira R, Xu Z, Colp P, Marignani PA (2013) Loss of lkb1 expression reduces the latency of ErbB2-mediated mammary gland tumorigenesis, promoting changes in metabolic pathways. *PLoS One* 8 (2):e56567. doi:10.1371/journal.pone.0056567.

Antoniou AC, Beesley J, McGuffog L, Sinilnikova OM, Healey S, Neuhausen SL, Ding YC et al. (2010) Common breast cancer susceptibility alleles and the risk of breast cancer for BRCA1 and BRCA2 mutation carriers: Implications for risk prediction. *Cancer Research* 70 (23):9742–9754. doi:10.1158/0008-5472.can-10-1907.

Antoniou AC, Kartsonaki C, Sinilnikova OM, Soucy P, McGuffog L, Healey S, Lee A et al. (2011) Common alleles at 6q25.1 and 1p11.2 are associated with breast cancer risk for BRCA1 and BRCA2 mutation carriers. *Human Molecular Genetics* 20 (16):3304–3321. doi:10.1093/hmg/ddr226.

Antoniou AC, Kuchenbaecker KB, Soucy P, Beesley J, Chen X, McGuffog L, Lee A et al. (2012) Common variants at 12p11, 12q24, 9p21, 9q31.2 and in ZNF365 are associated with breast cancer risk for BRCA1 and/or BRCA2 mutation carriers. *Breast Cancer Research* 14 (1):R33. doi:10.1186/bcr3121.

Antoniou AC, Sinilnikova OM, McGuffog L, Healey S, Nevanlinna H, Heikkinen T, Simard J et al. (2009) Common variants in LSP1, 2q35 and 8q24 and breast cancer risk for BRCA1 and BRCA2 mutation carriers. *Human Molecular Genetics* 18 (22):4442–4456. doi:10.1093/hmg/ddp372.

Axilbund JE, Wiley EA (2012) Genetic testing by cancer site: Pancreas. *Cancer Journal (Sudbury, MA)* 18 (4):350–354. doi:10.1097/PPO.0b013e3182624694.

Barber LJ, Sandhu S, Chen L, Campbell J, Kozarewa I, Fenwick K, Assiotis I et al. (2013) Secondary mutations in BRCA2 associated with clinical resistance to a PARP inhibitor. *The Journal of Pathology* 229 (3):422–429. doi:10.1002/path.4140.

Bartsch DK, Gress TM, Langer P (2012) Familial pancreatic cancer—Current knowledge. *Nature Reviews Gastroenterology & Hepatology* 9 (8):445–453. doi:10.1038/nrgastro.2012.111.

Becker KF, Atkinson MJ, Reich U, Becker I, Nekarda H, Siewert JR, Hofler H (1994) E-cadherin gene mutations provide clues to diffuse type gastric carcinomas. *Cancer Research* 54 (14):3845–3852.

Bell DW, Varley JM, Szydlo TE, Kang DH, Wahrer DC, Shannon KE, Lubratovich M et al. (1999) Heterozygous germ line hCHK2 mutations in Li-Fraumeni syndrome. *Science (New York, NY)* 286 (5449):2528–2531.

Brose MS, Rebbeck TR, Calzone KA, Stopfer JE, Nathanson KL, Weber BL (2002) Cancer risk estimates for BRCA1 mutation carriers identified in a risk evaluation program. *Journal of the National Cancer Institute* 94 (18):1365–1372.

Campeau PM, Foulkes WD, Tischkowitz MD (2008) Hereditary breast cancer: New genetic developments, new therapeutic avenues. *Human Genetics* 124 (1):31–42. doi:10.1007/s00439-008-0529-1.

Carson DA, Lois A (1995) Cancer progression and p53. *Lancet* 346 (8981):1009–1011.

Castro E, Eeles R (2012) The role of BRCA1 and BRCA2 in prostate cancer. *Asian Journal of Andrology* 14 (3):409–414. doi:10.1038/aja.2011.150.

Catucci I, Milgrom R, Kushnir A, Laitman Y, Paluch-Shimon S, Volorio S, Ficarazzi F et al. (2012) Germline mutations in BRIP1 and PALB2 in Jewish high cancer risk families. *Familial Cancer* 11 (3):483–491. doi:10.1007/s10689-012-9540-8.

Clark CC, Weitzel JN, O'Connor TR (2012) Enhancement of synthetic lethality via combinations of ABT-888, a PARP inhibitor, and carboplatin in vitro and in vivo using BRCA1 and BRCA2 isogenic models. *Molecular Cancer Therapeutics* 11 (9):1948–1958. doi:10.1158/1535-7163.mct-11-0597.

Collins N, McManus R, Wooster R, Mangion J, Seal S, Lakhani SR, Ormiston W et al. (1995) Consistent loss of the wild type allele in breast cancers from a family linked to the BRCA2 gene on chromosome 13q12–13. *Oncogene* 10 (8):1673–1675.

Couch FJ, Gaudet MM, Antoniou AC, Ramus SJ, Kuchenbaecker KB, Soucy P, Beesley J et al. (2012) Common variants at the 19p13.1 and ZNF365 loci are associated with ER subtypes of breast cancer and ovarian cancer risk in BRCA1 and BRCA2 mutation carriers. *Cancer Epidemiology, Biomarkers & Prevention* 21 (4):645–657. doi:10.1158/1055-9965.epi-11-0888.

Couch FJ, Wang X, McGuffog L, Lee A, Olswold C, Kuchenbaecker KB, Soucy P et al. (2013) Genome-wide association study in BRCA1 mutation carriers identifies novel loci associated with breast and ovarian cancer risk. *PLoS Genetics* 9 (3):e1003212. doi:10.1371/journal.pgen.1003212.

Cox DG, Simard J, Sinnett D, Hamdi Y, Soucy P, Ouimet M, Barjhoux L et al. (2011) Common variants of the BRCA1 wild-type allele modify the risk of breast cancer in BRCA1 mutation carriers. *Human Molecular Genetics* 20 (23):4732–4747. doi:10.1093/hmg/ddr388.

Crawford LV, Pim DC, Gurney EG, Goodfellow P, Taylor-Papadimitriou J (1981) Detection of a common feature in several human tumor cell lines—A 53,000-dalton protein. *Proceedings of the National Academy of Sciences of the United States of America* 78 (1):41–45.

Crum CP, McKeon FD, Xian W (2012) The oviduct and ovarian cancer: Causality, clinical implications, and "targeted prevention". *Clinical Obstetrics and Gynecology* 55 (1):24–35. doi:10.1097/GRF.0b013e31824b1725.

Cruz C, Teule A, Caminal JM, Blanco I, Piulats JM (2011) Uveal melanoma and BRCA1/BRCA2 genes: A relationship that needs further investigation. *Journal of Clinical Oncology* 29 (34):e827–e829. doi:10.1200/jco.2011.37.8828.

de la Cruz J, Andre F, Harrell RK, Bassett RL, Jr., Arun B, Mathieu MC, Delaloge S, Gilcrease MZ (2012) Tissue-based predictors of germ-line BRCA1 mutations: Implications for triaging of genetic testing. *Human Pathology* 43 (11):1932–1939. doi:10.1016/j.humpath.2012.02.002.

DeLeo AB, Jay G, Appella E, Dubois GC, Law LW, Old LJ (1979) Detection of a transformation-related antigen in chemically induced sarcomas and other transformed cells of the mouse. *Proceedings of the National Academy of Sciences of the United States of America* 76 (5):2420–2424.

Ding YC, McGuffog L, Healey S, Friedman E, Laitman Y, Paluch-Shimon S, Kaufman B et al. (2012) A nonsynonymous polymorphism in IRS1 modifies risk of developing breast and ovarian cancers in BRCA1 and ovarian cancer in BRCA2 mutation carriers. *Cancer Epidemiology, Biomarkers & Prevention* 21 (8):1362–1370. doi:10.1158/1055-9965.epi-12-0229.

EBCTCG (2005) Effects of chemotherapy and hormonal therapy for early breast cancer on recurrence and 15-year survival: An overview of the randomised trials. *Lancet* 365 (9472):1687–1717. doi:10.1016/s0140-6736(05)66544-0.

Eng C (2010) Mendelian genetics of rare—And not so rare—Cancers. *Annals of the New York Academy of Sciences* 1214:70–82. doi:10.1111/j.1749-6632.2010.05789.x.

Ferrao PT, Bukczynska EP, Johnstone RW, McArthur GA (2012) Efficacy of CHK inhibitors as single agents in MYC-driven lymphoma cells. *Oncogene* 31 (13):1661–1672. doi:10.1038/onc.2011.358.

Fishel ML, He Y, Smith ML, Kelley MR (2007) Manipulation of base excision repair to sensitize ovarian cancer cells to alkylating agent temozolomide. *Clinical Cancer Research* 13 (1):260–267. doi:10.1158/1078-0432.ccr-06-1920.

Frebourg T, Malkin D, Friend S (1991) Cancer risks from germ line tumor suppressor gene mutations. *Princess Takamatsu Symposia* 22:61–70.

Gage M, Wattendorf D, Henry LR (2012) Translational advances regarding hereditary breast cancer syndromes. *Journal of Surgical Oncology* 105 (5):444–451. doi:10.1002/jso.21856.

Gaudet MM, Kirchhoff T, Green T, Vijai J, Korn JM, Guiducci C, Segre AV et al. (2010) Common genetic variants and modification of penetrance of BRCA2-associated breast cancer. *PLoS Genetics* 6 (10):e1001183. doi:10.1371/journal.pgen.1001183.

Gaudet MM, Kuchenbaecker KB, Vijai J, Klein RJ, Kirchhoff T, McGuffog L, Barrowdale D et al. (2013) Identification of a BRCA2-specific modifier locus at 6p24 related to breast cancer risk. *PLoS Genetics* 9 (3):e1003173. doi:10.1371/journal.pgen.1003173.

Gustafson S, Zbuk KM, Scacheri C, Eng C (2007) Cowden syndrome. *Seminars in Oncology* 34 (5):428–434. doi:10.1053/j.seminoncol.2007.07.009.

Hahn SA, Greenhalf B, Ellis I, Sina-Frey M, Rieder H, Korte B, Gerdes B et al. (2003) BRCA2 germline mutations in familial pancreatic carcinoma. *Journal of the National Cancer Institute* 95 (3):214–221.

Hall JM, Lee MK, Newman B, Morrow JE, Anderson LA, Huey B, King MC (1990) Linkage of early-onset familial breast cancer to chromosome 17q21. *Science (New York, NY)* 250 (4988):1684–1689.

Hearle N, Schumacher V, Menko FH, Olschwang S, Boardman LA, Gille JJ, Keller JJ et al. (2006) Frequency and spectrum of cancers in the Peutz-Jeghers syndrome. *Clinical Cancer Research* 12 (10):3209–3215. doi:10.1158/1078-0432.ccr-06-0083.

Heikkinen T, Karkkainen H, Aaltonen K, Milne RL, Heikkila P, Aittomaki K, Blomqvist C, Nevanlinna H (2009) The breast cancer susceptibility mutation PALB2 1592delT is associated with an aggressive tumor phenotype. *Clinical Cancer Research* 15 (9):3214–3222. doi:10.1158/1078-0432.ccr-08-3128.

Hemminki A (1999) The molecular basis and clinical aspects of Peutz-Jeghers syndrome. *Cellular and Molecular Life Sciences* 55 (5):735–750.

Hoglund A, Stromvall K, Li Y, Forshell LP, Nilsson JA (2011) Chk2 deficiency in Myc overexpressing lymphoma cells elicits a synergistic lethal response in combination with PARP inhibition. *Cell Cycle (Georgetown, TX)* 10 (20):3598–3607. doi:10.4161/cc.10.20.17887.

Hollander MC, Blumenthal GM, Dennis PA (2011) PTEN loss in the continuum of common cancers, rare syndromes and mouse models. *Nature Reviews Cancer* 11 (4):289–301. doi:10.1038/nrc3037.

Huang L, Wu C, Yu D, Wang C, Che X, Miao X, Zhai K et al. (2013) Identification of common variants in BRCA2 and MAP2K4 for susceptibility to sporadic pancreatic cancer. *Carcinogenesis*. doi:10.1093/carcin/bgt004.

Iscovich J, Abdulrazik M, Cour C, Fischbein A, Pe'er J, Goldgar DE (2002) Prevalence of the BRCA2 6174 del T mutation in Israeli uveal melanoma patients. *International Journal of Cancer Journal International du Cancer* 98 (1):42–44.

Jakubowska A, Rozkrut D, Antoniou A, Hamann U, Scott RJ, McGuffog L, Healy S et al. (2012) Association of PHB 1630 C > T and MTHFR 677 C > T polymorphisms with breast and ovarian cancer risk in BRCA1/2 mutation carriers: Results from a multicenter study. *British Journal of Cancer* 106 (12):2016–2024. doi:10.1038/bjc.2012.160.

Jemal A, Murray T, Ward E, Samuels A, Tiwari RC, Ghafoor A, Feuer EJ, Thun MJ (2005) Cancer statistics, 2005. *CA: A Cancer Journal for Clinicians* 55 (1):10–30.

Kabacik S, Ortega-Molina A, Efeyan A, Finnon P, Bouffler S, Serrano M, Badie C (2011) A minimally invasive assay for individual assessment of the ATM/CHEK2/p53 pathway activity. *Cell Cycle (Georgetown, TX)* 10 (7):1152–1161.

Kauff ND, Barakat RR (2007) Risk-reducing salpingo-oophorectomy in patients with germline mutations in BRCA1 or BRCA2. *Journal of Clinical Oncology* 25 (20):2921–2927. doi:10.1200/jco.2007.11.3449.

Keller G, Vogelsang H, Becker I, Hutter J, Ott K, Candidus S, Grundei T et al. (1999) Diffuse type gastric and lobular breast carcinoma in a familial gastric cancer patient with an E-cadherin germline mutation. *The American Journal of Pathology* 155 (2):337–342. doi:10.1016/s0002-9440(10)65129-2.

Kirchhoff T, Gaudet MM, Antoniou AC, McGuffog L, Humphreys MK, Dunning AM, Bojesen SE et al. (2012) Breast cancer risk and 6q22.33: Combined results from Breast Cancer Association Consortium and Consortium of Investigators on Modifiers of BRCA1/2. *PLoS One* 7 (6):e35706. doi:10.1371/journal.pone.0035706.

Kirchhoff T, Kauff ND, Mitra N, Nafa K, Huang H, Palmer C, Gulati T et al. (2004) BRCA mutations and risk of prostate cancer in Ashkenazi Jews. *Clinical Cancer Research* 10 (9):2918–2921.

Kurian AW (2010) BRCA1 and BRCA2 mutations across race and ethnicity: Distribution and clinical implications. *Current Opinion in Obstetrics & Gynecology* 22 (1):72–78. doi:10.1097/GCO.0b013e328332dca3.

Kurian AW, Sigal BM, Plevritis SK (2010) Survival analysis of cancer risk reduction strategies for BRCA1/2 mutation carriers. *Journal of Clinical Oncology* 28 (2):222–231.

Lachlan KL, Lucassen AM, Bunyan D, Temple IK (2007) Cowden syndrome and Bannayan Riley Ruvalcaba syndrome represent one condition with variable expression and age-related penetrance: Results of a clinical study of PTEN mutation carriers. *Journal of Medical Genetics* 44 (9):579–585. doi:10.1136/jmg.2007.049981.

Lai D, Visser-Grieve S, Yang X (2012) Tumour suppressor genes in chemotherapeutic drug response. *Bioscience Reports* 32 (4):361–374. doi:10.1042/bsr20110125.

Lakhani SR, Reis-Filho JS, Fulford L, Penault-Llorca F, van der Vijver M, Parry S, Bishop T et al. (2005) Prediction of BRCA1 status in patients with breast cancer using estrogen receptor and basal phenotype. *Clinical Cancer Research* 11 (14):5175–5180. doi:10.1158/1078-0432.ccr-04-2424.

Lalloo F, Evans DG (2012) Familial breast cancer. *Clinical Genetics* 82 (2):105–114. doi:10.1111/j.1399-0004.2012.01859.x.

Lalloo F, Varley J, Ellis D, Moran A, O'Dair L, Pharoah P, Evans DG (2003) Prediction of pathogenic mutations in patients with early-onset breast cancer by family history. *Lancet* 361 (9363):1101–1102. doi:10.1016/s0140-6736(03)12856-5.

Lee SB, Kim SH, Bell DW, Wahrer DC, Schiripo TA, Jorczak MM, Sgroi DC et al. (2001) Destabilization of CHK2 by a missense mutation associated with Li-Fraumeni Syndrome. *Cancer Research* 61 (22):8062–8067.

Leung K, Saif MW (2013) BRCA-associated pancreatic cancer: The evolving management. *Journal of the Pancreas* 14 (2):149–151. doi:10.6092/1590-8577/1462.

Li J, Yen C, Liaw D, Podsypanina K, Bose S, Wang SI, Puc J et al. (1997) PTEN, a putative protein tyrosine phosphatase gene mutated in human brain, breast, and prostate cancer. *Science (New York, NY)* 275 (5308):1943–1947.

Liede A, Karlan BY, Narod SA (2004) Cancer risks for male carriers of germline mutations in BRCA1 or BRCA2: A review of the literature. *Journal of Clinical Oncology* 22 (4):735–742. doi:10.1200/jco.2004.05.055.

Lim W, Olschwang S, Keller JJ, Westerman AM, Menko FH, Boardman LA, Scott RJ et al. (2004) Relative frequency and morphology of cancers in STK11 mutation carriers. *Gastroenterology* 126 (7):1788–1794.

Lux MP, Fasching PA, Beckmann MW (2006) Hereditary breast and ovarian cancer: Review and future perspectives. *Journal of Molecular Medicine (Berlin, Germany)* 84 (1):16–28. doi:10.1007/s00109-005-0696-7.

Lynch HT, Snyder C, Lynch J (2012) Hereditary breast cancer: Practical pursuit for clinical translation. *Annals of Surgical Oncology* 19 (6):1723–1731. doi:10.1245/s10434-012-2256-z.

Manoukian S, Peissel B, Frigerio S, Lecis D, Bartkova J, Roversi G, Radice P, Bartek J, Delia D (2011) Two new CHEK2 germ-line variants detected in breast cancer/sarcoma families negative for BRCA1, BRCA2, and TP53 gene mutations. *Breast Cancer Research and Treatment* 130 (1):207–215. doi:10.1007/s10549-011-1548-5.

Martrat G, Maxwell CM, Tominaga E, Porta-de-la-Riva M, Bonifaci N, Gomez-Baldo L, Bogliolo M et al. (2011) Exploring the link between MORF4L1 and risk of breast cancer. *Breast Cancer Research* 13 (2):R40. doi:10.1186/bcr2862.

Masciari S, Dillon DA, Rath M, Robson M, Weitzel JN, Balmana J, Gruber SB et al. (2012) Breast cancer phenotype in women with TP53 germline mutations: A Li-Fraumeni syndrome consortium effort. *Breast Cancer Research and Treatment* 133 (3):1125–1130. doi:10.1007/s10549-012-1993-9.

Matsuoka S, Huang M, Elledge SJ (1998) Linkage of ATM to cell cycle regulation by the Chk2 protein kinase. *Science* 282 (5395):1893–1897.

Mavaddat N, Barrowdale D, Andrulis IL, Domchek SM, Eccles D, Nevanlinna H, Ramus SJ et al. (2012) Pathology of breast and ovarian cancers among BRCA1 and BRCA2 mutation carriers: Results from the Consortium of Investigators of Modifiers of BRCA1/2 (CIMBA). *Cancer Epidemiology, Biomarkers & Prevention* 21 (1):134–147. doi:10.1158/1055-9965.epi-11-0775.

Maxwell CA, Benitez J, Gomez-Baldo L, Osorio A, Bonifaci N, Fernandez-Ramires R, Costes SV et al. (2011) Interplay between BRCA1 and RHAMM regulates epithelial apicobasal polarization and may influence risk of breast cancer. *PLoS Biology* 9 (11):e1001199. doi:10.1371/journal.pbio.1001199.

Mealiffe ME, Stokowski RP, Rhees BK, Prentice RL, Pettinger M, Hinds DA (2010) Assessment of clinical validity of a breast cancer risk model combining genetic and clinical information. *Journal of the National Cancer Institute* 102 (21):1618–1627. doi:10.1093/jnci/djq388.

Meijers-Heijboer H, van den Ouweland A, Klijn J, Wasielewski M, de Snoo A, Oldenburg R, Hollestelle A et al. (2002) Low-penetrance susceptibility to breast cancer due to CHEK2(*)1100delC in noncarriers of BRCA1 or BRCA2 mutations. *Nature Genetics* 31 (1):55–59. doi:10.1038/ng879.

Meijers-Heijboer H, Wijnen J, Vasen H, Wasielewski M, Wagner A, Hollestelle A, Elstrodt F et al. (2003) The CHEK2 1100delC mutation identifies families with a hereditary breast and colorectal cancer phenotype. *American Journal of Human Genetics* 72 (5):1308–1314.

Miki Y, Swensen J, Shattuck-Eidens D, Futreal PA, Harshman K, Tavtigian S et al. (1994) A strong candidate for the breast and ovarian cancer susceptibility gene BRCA1. *Science (New York, NY)* 266 (5182):66–71.

Miller CW, Ikezoe T, Krug U, Hofmann WK, Tavor S, Vegesna V, Tsukasaki K, Takeuchi S, Koeffler HP (2002) Mutations of the CHK2 gene are found in some osteosarcomas, but are rare in breast, lung, and ovarian tumors. *Genes, Chromosomes & Cancer* 33 (1):17–21.

Mocci E, Milne RL, Yuste Mendez-Villamil E, Hopper JL, John EM, Andrulis IL, Chung WK et al. (2013) Risk of pancreatic cancer in breast cancer families from the breast cancer family registry. *Cancer Epidemiology, Biomarkers & Prevention* 22 (5):803–811. doi:10.1158/1055-9965.epi-12-0195.

Moran A, O'Hara C, Khan S, Shack L, Woodward E, Maher ER, Lalloo F, Evans DG (2012) Risk of cancer other than breast or ovarian in individuals with BRCA1 and BRCA2 mutations. *Familial Cancer* 11 (2):235–242. doi:10.1007/s10689-011-9506-2.

Morandell S, Yaffe MB (2012) Exploiting synthetic lethal interactions between DNA damage signaling, checkpoint control, and p53 for targeted cancer therapy. *Progress in Molecular Biology and Translational Science* 110:289–314. doi:10.1016/b978-0-12-387665-2.00011-0.

Myers K, Davies SM, Harris RE, Spunt SL, Smolarek T, Zimmerman S, McMasters R et al. (2012) The clinical phenotype of children with Fanconi anemia caused by biallelic FANCD1/BRCA2 mutations. *Pediatric Blood & Cancer* 58 (3):462–465. doi:10.1002/pbc.23168.

Narod SA, Feunteun J, Lynch HT, Watson P, Conway T, Lynch J, Lenoir GM (1991) Familial breast-ovarian cancer locus on chromosome 17q12-q23. *Lancet* 338 (8759):82–83.

Nevanlinna H, Bartek J (2006) The CHEK2 gene and inherited breast cancer susceptibility. *Oncogene* 25 (43):5912–5919. doi:10.1038/sj.onc.1209877.

Ngeow J, Heald B, Rybicki LA, Orloff MS, Chen JL, Liu X, Yerian L et al. (2013) Prevalence of germline PTEN, BMPR1A, SMAD4, STK11, and ENG mutations in patients with moderate-load colorectal polyps. *Gastroenterology* 144 (7):1402–1409. doi:10.1053/j.gastro.2013.02.001.

NICE clinical guideline 164 (2013) Familial breast cancer: Classification and care of people at risk of familial breast cancer and management of breast cancer and related risks in people with a family history of breast cancer. NICE, London, U.K. Issued: June 2013, guidance.nice.org.uk/cg164.

Ognjanovic S, Olivier M, Bergemann TL, Hainaut P (2012) Sarcomas in TP53 germline mutation carriers: A review of the IARC TP53 database. *Cancer* 118 (5):1387–1396. doi:10.1002/cncr.26390.

Osorio A, Milne RL, Alonso R, Pita G, Peterlongo P, Teule A, Nathanson KL et al. (2011) Evaluation of the XRCC1 gene as a phenotypic modifier in BRCA1/2 mutation carriers. Results from the consortium of investigators of modifiers of BRCA1/BRCA2. *British Journal of Cancer* 104 (8):1356–1361. doi:10.1038/bjc.2011.91.

Palacios J, Robles-Frias MJ, Castilla MA, Lopez-Garcia MA, Benitez J (2008) The molecular pathology of hereditary breast cancer. *Pathobiology: Journal of İmmunopathology, Molecular and Cellular Biology* 75 (2):85–94. doi:10.1159/000123846.

Paradiso A, Formenti S (2011) Hereditary breast cancer: Clinical features and risk reduction strategies. *Annals of Oncology* 22 (Suppl 1):i31–i36. doi:10.1093/annonc/mdq663.

Pennington KP, Walsh T, Lee M, Pennil C, Novetsky AP, Agnew KJ, Thornton A et al. (2013) BRCA1, TP53, and CHEK2 germline mutations in uterine serous carcinoma. *Cancer* 119 (2):332–338. doi:10.1002/cncr.27720.

Peto R, Boreham J, Clarke M, Davies C, Beral V (2000) UK and USA breast cancer deaths down 25% in year 2000 at ages 20–69 years. *Lancet* 355 (9217):1822. doi:10.1016/s0140-6736(00)02277-7.

Pijpe A, Andrieu N, Easton DF, Kesminiene A, Cardis E, Nogues C, Gauthier-Villars M et al. (2012) Exposure to diagnostic radiation and risk of breast cancer among carriers of BRCA1/2 mutations: Retrospective cohort study (GENE-RAD-RISK). *BMJ (Clinical Research Ed)* 345:e5660. doi:10.1136/bmj.e5660.

Poehlmann A, Roessner A (2010) Importance of DNA damage checkpoints in the pathogenesis of human cancers. *Pathology, Research and Practice* 206 (9):591–601. doi:10.1016/j.prp.2010.06.006.

Poumpouridou N, Kroupis C (2012) Hereditary breast cancer: Beyond BRCA genetic analysis; PALB2 emerges. *Clinical Chemistry and Laboratory Medicine: CCLM/FESCC* 50 (3):423–434. doi:10.1515/cclm-2011-0840.

Prodosmo A, De Amicis A, Nistico C, Gabriele M, Di Rocco G, Monteonofrio L, Piane M, Cundari E, Chessa L, Soddu S (2013) p53 centrosomal localization diagnoses ataxia-telangiectasia homozygotes and heterozygotes. *The Journal of Clinical Investigation* 123 (3):1335–1342. doi:10.1172/jci67289.

Pylkas K, Vuorela M, Otsukka M, Kallioniemi A, Jukkola-Vuorinen A, Winqvist R (2012) Rare copy number variants observed in hereditary breast cancer cases disrupt genes in estrogen signaling and TP53 tumor suppression network. *PLoS Genetics* 8 (6):e1002734. doi:10.1371/journal.pgen.1002734.

Rafnar T, Gudbjartsson DF, Sulem P, Jonasdottir A, Sigurdsson A, Jonasdottir A, Besenbacher S et al. (2011) Mutations in BRIP1 confer high risk of ovarian cancer. *Nature Genetics* 43 (11):1104–1107. doi:10.1038/ng.955.

Rahman N, Seal S, Thompson D, Kelly P, Renwick A, Elliott A, Reid S et al. (2007) PALB2, which encodes a BRCA2-interacting protein, is a breast cancer susceptibility gene. *Nature Genetics* 39 (2):165–167. doi:10.1038/ng1959.

Renwick A, Thompson D, Seal S, Kelly P, Chagtai T, Ahmed M, North B et al. (2006) ATM mutations that cause ataxia-telangiectasia are breast cancer susceptibility alleles. *Nature Genetics* 38 (8):873–875. doi:10.1038/ng1837.

Rigakos G, Razis E (2012) BRCAness: Finding the Achilles heel in ovarian cancer. *The Oncologist* 17 (7):956–962. doi:10.1634/theoncologist.2012-0028.

Roy R, Chun J, Powell SN (2012) BRCA1 and BRCA2: Different roles in a common pathway of genome protection. *Nature Reviews Cancer* 12 (1):68–78. doi:10.1038/nrc3181.

Rubbi CP, Milner J (2003) p53—Guardian of a genome's guardian? *Cell Cycle (Georgetown, TX)* 2 (1):20–21.

Sandhu SK, Omlin A, Hylands L, Miranda S, Barber LJ, Riisnaes R, Reid AH et al. (2013) Poly (ADP-ribose) polymerase (PARP) inhibitors for the treatment of advanced germline BRCA2 mutant prostate cancer. *Annals of Oncology* 24 (5):1416–1418. doi:10.1093/annonc/mdt074.

Savitsky K, Bar-Shira A, Gilad S, Rotman G, Ziv Y, Vanagaite L, Tagle DA, Smith S et al. (1995) A single ataxia telangiectasia gene with a product similar to PI-3 kinase. *Science (New York, NY)* 268 (5218):1749–1753.

Schrader KA, Masciari S, Boyd N, Salamanca C, Senz J, Saunders DN, Yorida E et al. (2011) Germline mutations in CDH1 are infrequent in women with early-onset or familial lobular breast cancers. *Journal of Medical Genetics* 48 (1):64–68. doi:10.1136/jmg.2010.079814.

Schrader KA, Masciari S, Boyd N, Wiyrick S, Kaurah P, Senz J, Burke W, Lynch HT, Garber JE, Huntsman DG (2008) Hereditary diffuse gastric cancer: Association with lobular breast cancer. *Familial Cancer* 7 (1):73–82. doi:10.1007/s10689-007-9172-6.

Shackelford DB, Abt E, Gerken L, Vasquez DS, Seki A, Leblanc M, Wei L et al. (2013) LKB1 inactivation dictates therapeutic response of non-small cell lung cancer to the metabolism drug phenformin. *Cancer Cell* 23 (2):143–158. doi:10.1016/j.ccr.2012.12.008.

Shanley S, Fung C, Milliken J, Leary J, Barnetson R, Schnitzler M, Kirk J (2009) Breast cancer immunohistochemistry can be useful in triage of some HNPCC families. *Familial Cancer* 8 (3):251–255. doi:10.1007/s10689-008-9226-4.

Shuen AY, Foulkes WD (2011) Inherited mutations in breast cancer genes—Risk and response. *Journal of Mammary Gland Biology and Neoplasia* 16 (1):3–15. doi:10.1007/s10911-011-9213-5.

Sigal A, Rotter V (2000) Oncogenic mutations of the p53 tumor suppressor: The demons of the guardian of the genome. *Cancer Research* 60 (24):6788–6793.

Solomon S, Das S, Brand R, Whitcomb DC (2012) Inherited pancreatic cancer syndromes. *Cancer Journal (Sudbury, MA)* 18 (6):485–491. doi:10.1097/PPO.0b013e318278c4a6.

Song MS, Carracedo A, Salmena L, Song SJ, Egia A, Malumbres M, Pandolfi PP (2011) Nuclear PTEN regulates the APC-CDH1 tumor-suppressive complex in a phosphatase-independent manner. *Cell* 144 (2):187–199. doi:10.1016/j.cell.2010.12.020.

Sorrell AD, Espenschied CR, Culver JO, Weitzel JN (2013) Tumor protein p53 (TP53) testing and Li-Fraumeni syndrome: Current status of clinical applications and future directions. *Molecular Diagnosis & Therapy* 17 (1):31–47. doi:10.1007/s40291-013-0020-0.

Spurdle AB, Marquart L, McGuffog L, Healey S, Sinilnikova O, Wan F, Chen X et al. (2011) Common genetic variation at BARD1 is not associated with breast cancer risk in BRCA1 or BRCA2 mutation carriers. *Cancer Epidemiology, Biomarkers & Prevention* 20 (5):1032–1038. doi:10.1158/1055-9965.epi-10-0909.

Stachelek GC, Dalal S, Donigan KA, Campisi Hegan D, Sweasy JB, Glazer PM (2010) Potentiation of temozolomide cytotoxicity by inhibition of DNA polymerase beta is accentuated by BRCA2 mutation. *Cancer Research* 70 (1):409–417. doi:10.1158/0008-5472.can-09-1353.

Stawinska M, Cygankiewicz A, Trzcinski R, Mik M, Dziki A, Krajewska WM (2008) Alterations of Chk1 and Chk2 expression in colon cancer. *International Journal of Colorectal Disease* 23 (12):1243–1249. doi:10.1007/s00384-008-0551-8.

Steck PA, Pershouse MA, Jasser SA, Yung WK, Lin H, Ligon AH, Langford LA et al. (1997) Identification of a candidate tumour suppressor gene, MMAC1, at chromosome 10q23.3 that is mutated in multiple advanced cancers. *Nature Genetics* 15 (4):356–362. doi:10.1038/ng0497-356.

Stratton MR, Rahman N (2008) The emerging landscape of breast cancer susceptibility. *Nature Genetics* 40 (1):17–22. doi:10.1038/ng.2007.53.

Sundararajan S, Ahmed A, Goodman OB, Jr. (2011) The relevance of BRCA genetics to prostate cancer pathogenesis and treatment. *Clinical Advances in Hematology & Oncology* 9 (10):748–755.

Tai YC, Domchek S, Parmigiani G, Chen S (2007) Breast cancer risk among male BRCA1 and BRCA2 mutation carriers. *Journal of the National Cancer Institute* 99 (23):1811–1814. doi:10.1093/jnci/djm203.

Tang LL, Chen FY, Wang H, Hu XL, Dai X, Mao J, Shen ZT et al. (2013) Haplotype analysis of eight genes of the monoubiquitinated FANCD2-DNA damage-repair pathway in breast cancer patients. *Cancer Epidemiology* 37 (3):311–317. doi:10.1016/j.canep.2012.12.010.

Tavor S, Takeuchi S, Tsukasaki K, Miller CW, Hofmann WK, Ikezoe T, Said JW, Koeffler HP (2001) Analysis of the CHK2 gene in lymphoid malignancies. *Leukemia & Lymphoma* 42 (3):517–520. doi:10.3109/10428190109064610.

Teo ZL, Park DJ, Provenzano E, Chatfield CA, Odefrey FA, Nguyen-Dumont T, kConFab et al. (2013b) Prevalence of PALB2 mutations in Australasian multiple-case breast cancer families. *Breast Cancer Research* 15 (1):R17.

Teo ZL, Sawyer SD, James PA, Mitchell G, Trainer AH, Lindeman GJ, Shackleton K, Cicciarelli L, Southey MC (2013a) The incidence of PALB2 c.3113G>A in women with a strong family history of breast and ovarian cancer attending familial cancer centres in Australia. *Familial Cancer* 12 (4):587–595. doi:10.1007/s10689-013-9620-4.

Thompson D, Duedal S, Kirner J, McGuffog L, Last J, Reiman A, Byrd P, Taylor M, Easton DF (2005) Cancer risks and mortality in heterozygous ATM mutation carriers. *Journal of the National Cancer Institute* 97 (11):813–822. doi:10.1093/jnci/dji141.

Tischkowitz M, Capanu M, Sabbaghian N, Li L, Liang X, Vallee MP, Tavtigian SV et al. (2012) Rare germline mutations in PALB2 and breast cancer risk: A population-based study. *Human Mutation* 33 (4):674–680. doi:10.1002/humu.22022.

Tischkowitz M, Sabbaghian N, Hamel N, Pouchet C, Foulkes WD, Mes-Masson AM, Provencher DM, Tonin PN (2013) Contribution of the PALB2 c.2323C>T [p.Q775X] founder mutation in well-defined breast and/or ovarian cancer families and unselected ovarian cancer cases of French Canadian descent. *BMC Medical Genetics* 14:5. doi:10.1186/1471-2350-14-5.

Trivedi RN, Almeida KH, Fornsaglio JL, Schamus S, Sobol RW (2005) The role of base excision repair in the sensitivity and resistance to temozolomide-mediated cell death. *Cancer Research* 65 (14):6394–6400. doi:10.1158/0008-5472.can-05-0715.

Trivedi RN, Wang XH, Jelezcova E, Goellner EM, Tang JB, Sobol RW (2008) Human methyl purine DNA glycosylase and DNA polymerase beta expression collectively predict sensitivity to temozolomide. *Molecular Pharmacology* 74 (2):505–516. doi:10.1124/mol.108.045112.

Turkoz FP, Solak M, Petekkaya I, Keskin O, Kertmen N, Sarici F, Arik Z, Babacan T, Ozisik Y, Altundag K (2012) Association between common risk factors and molecular subtypes in breast cancer patients. *Breast (Edinburgh, Scotland)*. doi:10.1016/j.breast.2012.08.005.

Turnbull C, Ahmed S, Morrison J, Pernet D, Renwick A, Maranian M, Seal S et al. (2010) Genome-wide association study identifies five new breast cancer susceptibility loci. *Nature Genetics* 42 (6):504–507. doi:10.1038/ng.586.

Turnbull C, Seal S, Renwick A, Warren-Perry M, Hughes D, Elliott A, Pernet D et al. (2012) Gene-gene interactions in breast cancer susceptibility. *Human Molecular Genetics* 21 (4):958–962. doi:10.1093/hmg/ddr525.

van der Groep P, van der Wall E, van Diest PJ (2011) Pathology of hereditary breast cancer. *Cellular Oncology (Dordrecht)* 34 (2):71–88. doi:10.1007/s13402-011-0010-3.

van der Groep P, van Diest PJ, Smolders YH, Ausems MG, van der Luijt RB, Menko FH, Bart J, de Vries EG, van der Wall E (2013) HIF-1alpha overexpression in ductal carcinoma in situ of the breast in BRCA1 and BRCA2 mutation carriers. *PLoS One* 8 (2):e56055. doi:10.1371/journal.pone.0056055.

Varley J (2003) TP53, hChk2, and the Li-Fraumeni syndrome. *Methods in Molecular Biology (Clifton, NJ)* 222:117–129. doi:10.1385/1-59259-328-3:117.

Vollebergh MA, Lips EH, Nederlof PM, Wessels LF, Schmidt MK, van Beers EH, Cornelissen S et al. (2011) An aCGH classifier derived from BRCA1-mutated breast cancer and benefit of high-dose platinum-based chemotherapy in HER2-negative breast cancer patients. *Annals of Oncology* 22 (7):1561–1570. doi:10.1093/annonc/mdq624.

Walerych D, Napoli M, Collavin L, Del Sal G (2012) The rebel angel: Mutant p53 as the driving oncogene in breast cancer. *Carcinogenesis* 33 (11):2007–2017. doi:10.1093/carcin/bgs232.

Walker LC, Fredericksen ZS, Wang X, Tarrell R, Pankratz VS, Lindor NM, Beesley J et al. (2010) Evidence for SMAD3 as a modifier of breast cancer risk in BRCA2 mutation carriers. *Breast Cancer Research* 12 (6):R102. doi:10.1186/bcr2785.

Wark L, Novak D, Sabbaghian N, Amrein L, Jangamreddy JR, Cheang M, Pouchet C et al. (2013) Heterozygous mutations in the PALB2 hereditary breast cancer predisposition gene impact on the three-dimensional nuclear organization of patient-derived cell lines. *Genes, Chromosomes & Cancer* 52 (5):480–494. doi:10.1002/gcc.22045.

Weischer M, Bojesen SE, Ellervik C, Tybjaerg-Hansen A, Nordestgaard BG (2008) CHEK2*1100delC genotyping for clinical assessment of breast cancer risk: Meta-analyses of 26,000 patient cases and 27,000 controls. *Journal of Clinical Oncology* 26 (4):542–548. doi:10.1200/jco.2007.12.5922.

Wooster R, Bignell G, Lancaster J, Swift S, Seal S, Mangion J, Collins N, Gregory S, Gumbs C, Micklem G (1995) Identification of the breast cancer susceptibility gene BRCA2. *Nature* 378 (6559):789–792. doi:10.1038/378789a0.

Wu X, Webster SR, Chen J (2001) Characterization of tumor-associated Chk2 mutations. *Journal of Biological Chemistry* 276 (4):2971–2974.

Xu R, Huang Y, Mai J, Zhang G, Guo X, Xia X, Koay EJ et al. (2013) Multistage vectored siRNA targeting ataxia-telangiectasia mutated for breast cancer therapy. *Small (Weinheim an der Bergstrasse, Germany)* 9 (9–10):1799–1808. doi:10.1002/smll.201201510.

Yap TA, Sandhu SK, Carden CP, de Bono JS (2011) Poly(ADP-ribose) polymerase (PARP) inhibitors: Exploiting a synthetic lethal strategy in the clinic. *A Cancer Journal for Clinicians* 61 (1):31–49. doi:10.3322/caac.20095.

6

DNA Methylation: An Epigenetic Marker of Breast Cancer Influenced by Nutrients Acting as an Environmental Factor

Tarique N. Hasan, MSc, Gowhar Shafi, PhD, B. Leena Grace, PhD, Jesper Tegner, PhD, and Anjana Munshi, PhD

CONTENTS

ABSTRACT DNA methylation is an important regulator of gene expression and plays an essential role in maintaining cellular function. Its role in carcinogenesis has been a topic of considerable interest in recent years. Changes in DNA methylation patterns may contribute to the development of cancer in general and breast cancer in particular. Aberrant global methylation of DNA is frequently found in tumor cells. Global hypomethylation can result in chromosome instability, and hypermethylation has been associated with the inactivation of tumor suppressor genes. Several studies suggest that part of the cancer-protective effects associated with several bioactive components may involve modifications of the DNA methylation profile. Dietary factors that are involved in one-carbon metabolism provide the most compelling evidence supporting an interaction of nutrients and DNA methylation because these factors influence the supply of methyl groups and therefore the biochemical pathways of methylation processes. These nutrients include folate, vitamin B_{12}, vitamin B_6, methionine, and choline. This chapter examines alterations in DNA methylation in breast cancer, the effects on gene expression, and the role of nutrients in DNA methylation in the treatment of breast cancer.

6.1 Introduction

6.1.1 Epigenetics: Events Beyond Genetics

The concept of epigenetics was first introduced in 1942 by C. H. Waddington (Waddington, 1942), describing the influence of environmental factors on the development of specific traits through gene–environment interaction. Waddington's words, "the interaction of genes with their environment, which bring the phenotype into being," are fundamental to developmental biology, that is, the "idea that phenotype, or the morphologic and functional properties of an organism, arises sequentially under a program defined by the genome under the influence of the organism's environment" (Van Speybroeck, 2002). Modern aspects of epigenetics refer to the modification of DNA and/or related proteins without altering the nucleotide sequence, which passes the contained information to next generation. Only 6 years following Waddington's narration on epigenetics, DNA methylation was identified as an epigenetic marker (Hotchkiss, 1948). DNA methylation is currently the most studied and the best understood epigenetic modification. On the basis of many studies on a battery of housekeeping genes and growth regulator genes, DNA methylation is established as an additional mechanism for gene inactivation in different cell types including cancer cells (Lehmann et al., 2002).

6.2 DNA Methylation Stabilizes Chromatin Structure and Regulates Gene Expression Epigenetically

In normal cells, actively transcribing chromatin is hypomethylated, whereas nontranscribing chromatin is methylated in such a manner that it produces compact structures that sterically hinder RNA Pol II activities (Lorincz et al., 2004). The methylation of DNA is found to be involved in the stabilization of chromatin structure in an inactive conformation and inhibits gene transcription (Keshet et al., 1986). Therefore, it is believed that the

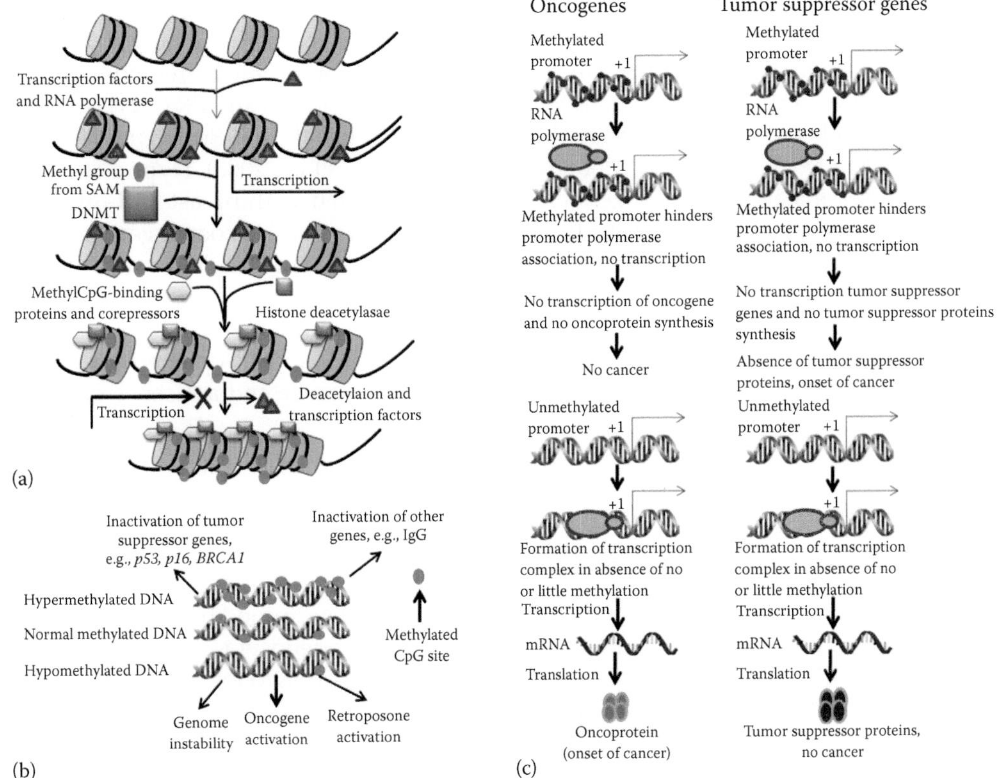

FIGURE 6.1
(a) Depiction of the epigenetic process in general methylation and, in particular, the subsequent stabilization of chromatin and inhibition of transcription. (b) Abnormal methylation of DNA leads either to inactivation of genes like tumor suppressor genes or activation of oncogenes, genome instability, and retroposon activation. (c) Methylation of oncogene promoters downregulates expression by blocking the formation of the transcriptional complex, while demethylation of oncogene promoters accelerates expression and leads toward cancer formation. Similarly, methylation of tumor suppressor genes downregulates expression by blocking the formation of the transcriptional complex, which in turn enhances the onset of cancer. Demethylation of tumor suppressor gene promoters facilitates transcriptional complex formation and increases tumor suppressor protein formation, thereby inhibiting tumor formation.

mechanism of gene regulation through DNA methylation is involved in essential genetic events including differentiation, genomic imprinting, and X-chromosome inactivation (Bernardino-Sgherri et al., 2002; Richardson and Yung, 2002) (Figure 6.1a).

The main target for DNA methylation is cytosine. The majority of 5′-methylcytosine in mammalian DNA is present in cytosine–guanine (CpG) dinucleotides, which are present in the promoter regions of several genes. Among all human promoters, 72% contain high CpG content, and 28% of promoters are those with CpG content characteristic of the overall genome, that is, low CpG content (Saxonov et al., 2006). As far as the whole human genome is concerned, CpGs are present approximately once per 80 dinucleotides in 98% of the genome; however, in the CpG islands, which comprise 1%–2% of the human genome, the frequency is five times higher (Bird, 1986).

Methylation and/or demethylation of DNA are essential features of a normal genome. But whenever DNA becomes abnormally methylated, several crucial functions become severely impeded. Abnormal DNA methylation accounts for (1) the excess of methylation (hypermethylation) of genes that must be transcriptionally active in normal conditions and (2) the excess of genome-wide demethylation (global hypomethylation) (Figure 6.1b). A major aberration associated with hypermethylation of the promoter regions of tumor suppressor genes and DNA repair genes (*p15, p16, p57, p53, SLC5A8,* and *BRCA1*) is the onset of different kinds of cancers including breast cancer (Dobrovic and Simpfendorfer, 1997; Chanda et al., 2006; Hayslip and Montero, 2006; Whitman et al., 2008). Hypomethylation of DNA causes instability of the genome and is also related with breast and other cancers. For example, a case–control study from Spain reports that leukocyte genomic DNA hypomethylation is associated with increased risk of developing bladder cancer (Moore et al., 2008) (Figure 6.1c). Hypermethylation takes place mostly at CpG islands of promoter region of a gene, but hypomethylation usually is associated with repeated DNA sequences, such as long interspersed nuclear elements (Ehrlich, 2002). Global hypomethylation also activates transposable elements (TEs) to transcribe in both sense and antisense directions (Roman-Gomez et al., 2005) (Figure 6.1b).

6.3 Essentials of DNA Methylation

The methylation status of DNA (hypo or hyper) is mainly determined by (1) availability of primary methyl group sources in diet, (2) availability of *S*-adenosyl-L-methionine (SAM), and (3) availability of functional DNA methyltransferases (DNMTs) to transfer methyl groups from SAM to DNA, specifically to 5-C of cytosine. This is explained in more detail in the following.

6.3.1 Methyl Group Source

The major methyl group sources in the human diet are methionine, choline, and de novo one-carbon metabolism via methylfolate, which provides the methyl groups for methionine synthesis (Institute of Medicine and National Academy of Sciences, USA, 1998). Homocysteine is also converted to methionine through two alternative pathways: (1) choline derivative betaine donates a methyl group to homocysteine in the presence of betaine homocysteine *S*-methyltransferase (Varela-Moreiras et al., 1992; Lu et al., 2001), and (2) homocysteine receives a methyl group from the de novo one-carbon pool by the action of 5-methyltetrahydrofolate (MTHF)–homocysteine *S*-methyltransferase (Barak and Kemmy 1982; Horne et al., 1989) to regenerate methionine (Figure 6.2).

6.3.2 S-Adenosyl-L-Methionine

Available methionine for the formation of SAM directly comes from food and via the conversion of homocysteine. Methionine adenosyltransferase converts methionine to SAM, which acts as a methyl group donor for DNA methylation (Lu et al., 2001).

6.3.3 Mammalian DNA Methyltransferase Families

The methylation of DNA is a product of the activities of a family of enzymes known as DNMTs, which take up the methyl group from cofactor SAM (Jeltsch et al., 2007) and mediate the transfer to a nucleotide (Bujnicki and Radlinska, 1999), particularly cytosine. Three families of mammalian DNMTs have been found, called DNMT1, DNMT2, and DNMT3 (Hermann et al., 2004). Among these, DNMT2 has little involvement in methyl group

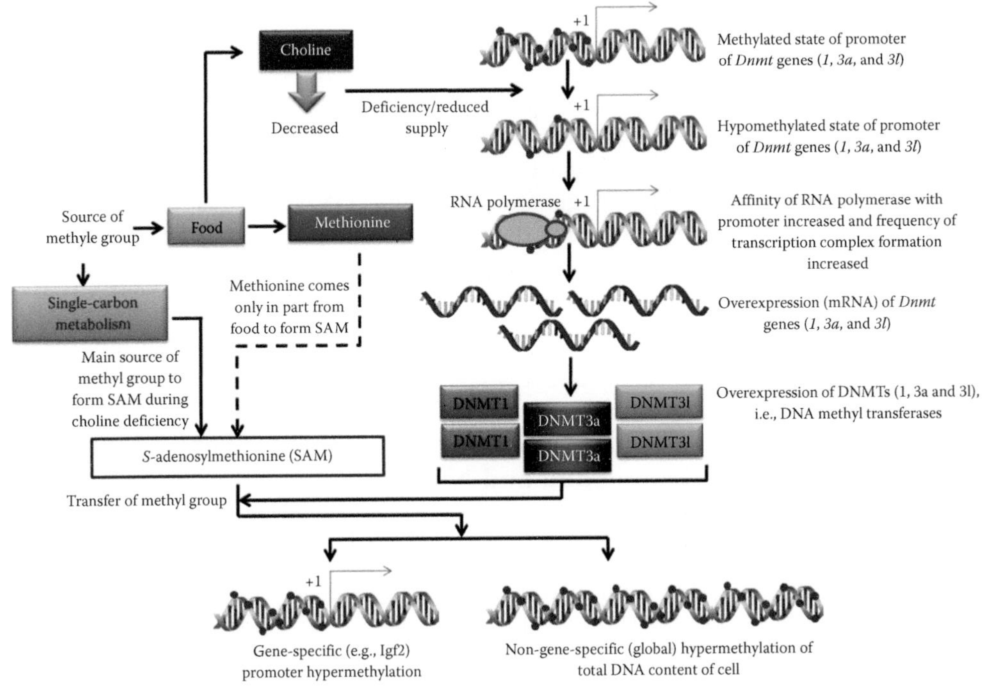

FIGURE 6.2
Methyl groups come from various sources in the human diet via methionine to be used in methylation process. This transfer of methyl groups is mediated by DNMT, while SAM is the final donor of the methyl group for the reaction.

transfer to DNA; recently, it has been found to be involved in the methylation of a cytosine residue in the anticodon loop of tRNAAsp (Goll et al., 2006).

DNMT1 is the first mammalian DNMT (Bestor et al., 1988). This is the sole mammalian DNMT identified biochemically and is responsible for copying the pattern of DNA methylation after each round of DNA replication. DNMT1 has a higher (5–30-fold) affinity to hemimethylated CpG sites (Yoder et al., 1997). This 1620-amino-acid-long protein has a C-terminal domain that more closely resembles many of the bacterial methyltransferases than those of either DNMT2 or DNMT3 (Bestor et al., 1988). The long N-terminal domain is involved in cellular targeting, protein–protein interaction, and catalytic domain regulation (Fatemi et al., 2001).

Three proteins have been recognized as member of DNMT3 family, namely, DNMT3A, DNMT3B, and DNMT3L. DNMT3L is not directly involved in methylation; rather, it is required for the activation of DNMT3A and DNMT3B. A long N-terminal is also found in DNMT3A and DNMT3B similar to that of DNMT1 and serves the same purpose. However, the isolated catalytic domain of DNMT3A and DNMT3B is enzymatically active, whereas that of DNMT1 is not (Gowher and Jeltsch, 2001; Reither et al., 2003). DNMT3A and DNMT3B are not capable of distinguishing between unmethylated or hemimethylated CpG sites. They do not show large sequence specificity except for CpG and a few flanking sequences (Gowher and Jeltsch, 2001; Handa and Jeltsch, 2005).

Although the roles of the availability of methyl group sources (choline, methionine, and 1-C metabolism mediated by MTHF), SAM, and functional DNMTs are primarily accounted for in DNA methylation, it is the availability of DNMTs specifically that governs the DNA methylation, given that SAM is a donor of methyl groups for more than 80 biological methylation reactions, including the methylation of DNA (Choi and Mason, 2002). *Hence, as far as the regulation of genes through methylation of DNA is concerned, the prime factor might be a process that regulates the presence of active DNMTs.*

In a nutshell, DNA methylation, along with histone tail modification and noncoding RNA expression, constitutes the cellular memory that stores the transcriptional profile of the cell, which is passed to the next generation. Hence, DNA methylation is involved in the regulation of gene expression during development and in response to environmental signals. In addition, DNA methylation is implicated in genetic imprinting, inactivation of one X-chromosome, and contributing to the stability of the genome.

6.4 Altered DNA Methylation May Cause Breast Cancer While Bioactive Components of Common Food and Nutrients Act as Epigenetic Factors

There is a battery of nutrients (Table 6.1) whose presence or absence to a large extent contributes to the determination of the methylation status of DNA globally and to certain genes in particular. For example, dietary zinc deficiency leads to the global hypomethylation of DNA in rat liver (Wallwork and Duerre, 1985), while hypomethylation of *c-Ha-ras* results from deficiency of methionine and choline (Zapisek et al., 1992). Here, we discuss the bioactive compounds present in common food and nutrients and their roles in DNA methylation and breast cancer (Table 6.1).

6.4.1 Alcohol

Alcohol is known for folate antagonist activities and is found to affect one-carbon metabolism adversely (Seitz and Stickel, 2007; Jung et al., 2008). Alcohol consumption was associated with DNA methylation in postmenopausal breast tumors, suggesting that the association of alcohol and breast cancer may be related, at least in part, to altered methylation and may differ by drinking pattern (Tao et al., 2011). It has been almost a half century since alcohol was recognized as risk factor for oral cancer (Wynder and Bross, 1957). Since then, several epidemiological studies have been carried out and have now established that alcohol is a major risk factor for head and neck cancers (Yokoyama et al., 2006; Freedman et al., 2007; Brooks et al., 2009) and laryngeal cancer (Bosetti et al., 2002; Altieri et al., 2005). Chronic alcohol consumption is found to induce genomic hypomethylation in rat colon (Choi et al., 1999). An interesting study by Bonsch et al. (2006) revealed that in patients with chronic alcoholism, DNMT (*Dnmt-3B*) mRNA expression is lowered and associated with genomic DNA hypermethylation. Furthermore, the chronic alcohol exposure was found to affect the genetic imprinting of sperm by altering the mRNA level of *Dnmt* (Bielawski et al., 2002). This may constitute one example of paternal sharing in abnormal fetal growth and development. Thus, chronic exposure of alcohol is associated with cancers, both somatically and autosomally.

6.4.2 Arsenic

Arsenic exposure is associated with increased risk of cancers of the breast, skin, liver, lung, and bladder (WHO, 2001). A study of the effects of long-term arsenic exposure on human HaCaT keratinocytes revealed that arsenic causes the depletion of

TABLE 6.1
Role of Dietary Factors in DNA Methylation

Dietary Factors	Effect	References
Alcohol	Float antagonist; adversely affects C1 metabolism.	Jung et al. (2008), Seitz and Stickel (2007)
Arsenic	DNMT inhibitor.	Benbrahim-Tallaa et al. (2005), Benbrahim-Tallaa and Waalkes, (2008), Reichard et al. (2007), Pilsner et al. (2007)
Cadmium	Noncompetitive DNMT inhibitor; increases the expression of *Dnmt1*, *Dnmt3a*, and *Dnmt3b* mRNAs.	Takiguchi et al. (2003), Zhang et al. (2009), Jiang et al. (2008)
Choline	Deficiency causes hypomethylation of CpGs of *Dnmt1*; *c-Ha-ras* increases the gene-specific and global DNA methylation.	Kovacheva et al. (2007), Xu et al, (2008), Zapisek et al. (1992)
Genistein	Modulates CpG methylation; inhibits cancer development in *BRCA1*-mutated cells.	Zheng et al. (2008), King-Batoon et al. (2008), Privat et al. (2009)
Lycopene	Modulates CpG methylation.	King-Batoon et al. (2008)
Folate	Aberrant genomic and site-specific DNA methylation, associated with adenomas; decreases SAM:SAH; affects one-carbon metabolism.	Kim (2004), Van den Donk et al. (2007), Balaghi and Wagner (1993), Kim et al. (2009)
Methionine	Inhibited proliferation of MCF-7 breast cancer cells; inhibits cellular growth dependent on the p53 status of cells; absence induces apoptosis of prostate cancer and hypomethylation of *c-Ha-ras*.	Larsson et al. (2007), Kim and Park (2003), Benavides et al. (2007), Lu et al. (2002), Zapisek et al. (1992)
Nickel	Induces carcinogenesis by manipulating DNA methylation, de novo DNA hypermethylation of tumor suppressor genes and senescence genes.	Lee et al. (1995, 1998), Costa (2002), Zhou et al. (2009)
Selenium	Deficiency led to liver and colon DNA hypomethylation.	Davis et al. (2000), Zeng and Combs (2008)
Vitamin A	Induces DNA hypomethylation in rat liver; hypomethylation of genes related to retinoid signaling; may play role in gastric carcinogenesis.	Vainio and Rautalahti (1999), Rowling et al. (2002), Shutoh et al. (2005)
Vitamin B_6	Restriction decreases the supply of single-unit carbon for thymidylate and methionine; higher intakes reduce the risk of colorectal cancer; may impair de novo methionine synthesis.	Perry et al. (2007), Zhang et al. (2006), Cravo et al. (1997)
Vitamin B_{12}	Elevated level associated with prostate cancer; plasma/blood level inversely associated with breast cancer among premenopausal women; one of the determinants of DNA hypomethylation.	Johansson et al. (2008), Zhang et al. (2003, 2008), Brunaud et al. (2003)
Zinc	Global hypomethylation of DNA in liver.	Wallwork and Duerre (1985)

S-adenosylmethionine, the main cellular methyl donor, and represses the expression of the DNMT genes *Dnmt1* and *Dnmt3A* (Reichard et al., 2007). Low-dose (5 μM) long exposure was found to transform the nonmalignant prostate cancer epithelial cell line (RWPE-1) to the tumorigenic (CAsE-PE) cell line with DNA hypomethylation and *K-Ras* expression as coevents (Benbrahim-Tallaa et al., 2005). Although the mechanism of the involvement of arsenic in DNA methylation has not been deciphered exactly, a population study indicates that the presence of adequate folate is essential for increased genomic DNA methylation (Pilsner et al., 2007).

6.4.3 Cadmium

Cadmium is a noncompetitive inhibitor of DNMTs. In vitro studies have shown that short-term cadmium exposure leads to genomic DNA hypomethylation, whereas long-term exposure results in hypermethylation of DNA (Takiguchi et al., 2003). Recent in vivo and in vitro studies demonstrate that chronic and subchronic exposures of cadmium cause the overexpression of *Dnmt1*, *Dnmt3A*, and *Dnmt3B* mRNAs (Jiang et al., 2008; Zhang et al., 2009). These findings suggest a possible underlying mechanism of cadmium carcinogenesis.

6.4.4 Choline

Choline is an essential micronutrient required for methyl group metabolism; it donates a methyl group to SAM via betaine (Varela-Moreiras et al., 1992; Lu et al., 2001). The nutritional role of choline is very well studied, and it also has been convincingly demonstrated in several studies that a deficiency of choline is associated with higher risk of breast cancer (Xu et al., 2008). However, the role in carcinogenesis and tumor progression is not well understood.

Choline deficiency results from the hypomethylation of *Dnmt1* CpG islands, consecutively increasing the expression of associated mRNAs including those mRNAs of *Dnmt3a* and *Dnmt3l*. Choline deficiency modulates fetal DNA methylation machinery in a complex fashion that includes hypomethylation of the regulatory CpGs within the *Dnmt1* gene, leading to overexpression, and the resultant increased global and gene-specific (e.g., *Igf2*) DNA methylation in fetal rat liver and brain (Kovacheva et al., 2007).

Findings from Kovacheva and coworkers (2007) suggest a tentative mechanism for DNA methylation that is modulated by choline, with the conclusion that (1) deficiency of choline does not cause global or gene-specific DNA hypomethylation, but rather hypomethylates *Dmnt1*; (2) choline deficiency is associated with overexpression of *Dnmt1*, *Dmnt3a*, and *Dmnt3l*; (3) choline is not the sole source of methyl groups for the formation of SAM, but rather the derivatives of one-carbon metabolism and homocysteine might be the sources; and (4) one-carbon metabolism is a housekeeping metabolism, and homocysteine comes only partially from diet. Thus, it seems that choline deficiency modulates global and gene-specific DNA methylation only by increasing the bioavailability of different DNMTs, while the major source of methyl groups is single-carbon metabolism derivatives (Figure 6.3).

This model of DNA methylation regulation by choline from Kovacheva and coworkers needs to be confirmed by using other animal models and in different organs. Additionally, a lot of work will be needed to ensure the fidelity of the hypothesized mechanism.

6.4.5 Genistein

Genistein is a phytoestrogen and is the main protein found in soy. It has been recognized for its antitumor properties. Genistein at very low, dietary-relevant concentrations can potentially mitigate tumorigenic processes via promoter methylation modulation of gene expression (King-Batoon et al., 2008). In a previous study, 0.5 mg of genistein was sufficient to hypermethylate the CpG islands of certain genes (e.g., glucose transporter 4, *GLUT4*)

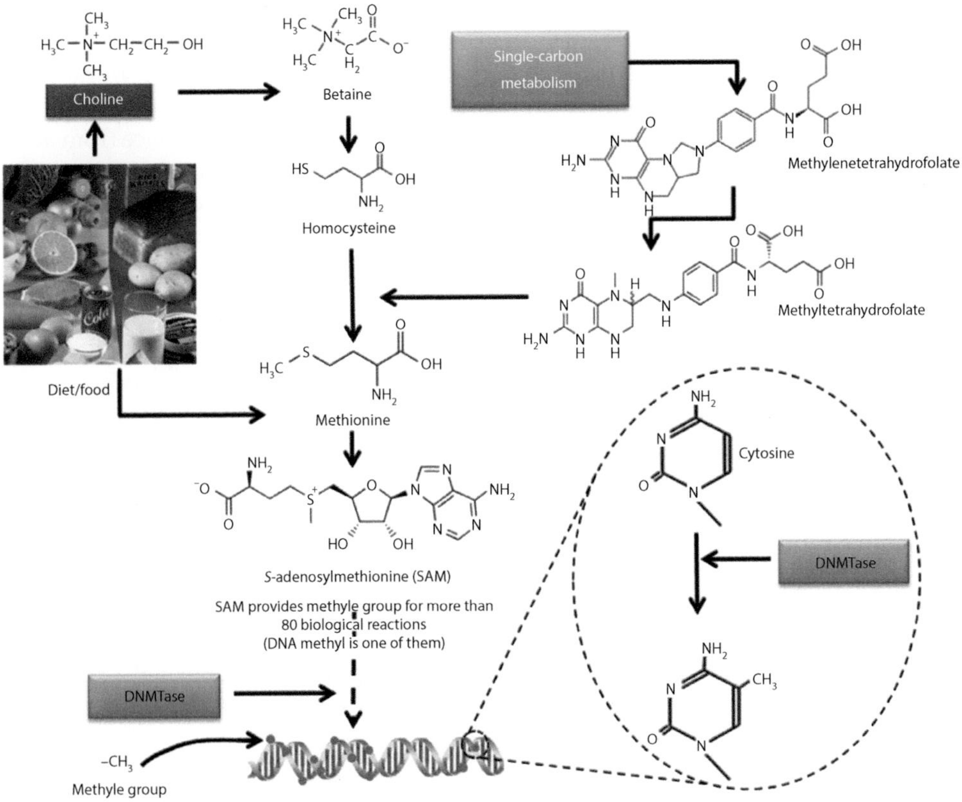

FIGURE 6.3
Deficiency of choline hypomethylates *Dnmts*, which in turn could increase the expression of DNMTs. This could lead to an increase in gene-specific and non-gene-specific global methylation. Because choline is deficient with only a little amount of methionine from food, the sole source of methyl groups could be *single-carbon metabolism*—a housekeeping metabolism.

and lower mRNA expression (Zheng et al., 2008). Genistein may, therefore, be an efficient inhibitor of cancer development in *BRCA1* mutant breast cancer cells (Privat et al., 2009). However, additional studies are required to support the role of genistein as an antitumorigenic and anticarcinogenic agent. Also, relevant dietary concentration must be established to determine the required physiologically available concentration sufficient to exert its anticancer actions.

6.4.6 Folate

Folate is one of the main components of single-carbon metabolism and the pathway for synthesis of SAM and SAM:SAH (*S*-adenosylhomocysteine) (Balaghi and Wagner, 1993), as folate in the form of MTHF provides methyl groups to homocysteine (Figure 6.1). Folate excess and deficiency both affect the formation of SAM and the status of more than 80 different biological methylation reactions, including DNA methylation. Folate intake in adenoma patients has been shown to be inversely associated with promoter methylation in case–case comparison, whereas it is positively associated with promoter methylation in case–control comparison (van den Donk et al., 2007). A recent study on maternal folate status in hyperhomocysteinemic rats concluded that folate status influences the homeostasis of folate-mediated one-carbon metabolism and the methyl pool, which would in turn affect placental DNA methylation by altering the methylation potential of the liver (Kim et al., 2009). Although large body of research has been performed addressing whether DNA hypomethylation is the mechanism through which folate deficiency leads to certain types of cancer (e.g., breast cancer, colorectal cancers), the details remain elusive. The evidence from animal, human, and in vitro studies suggests that the effects of folate deficiency on DNA methylation are highly complex and context dependent, since they appear to depend on cell type, target organ, and stage of transformation and are gene and site specific (Kim, 2004).

6.4.7 Methionine

Although little is known regarding the effect of dietary methionine supplementation on mammalian DNA methylation, the available data suggest that methionine supplementation can induce hypermethylation of DNA in specific genomic regions (Waterland, 2006). In vitro as well as in vivo studies have suggested that a higher dose of methionine interferes with expression of some crucial oncogenes like *p53* in MCF-7 breast cancer cells. Methionine suppresses the expression of *p53* up to 70%, hence interfering with *p53*-dependent cell growth (Kim and Park, 2003; Benavides et al., 2007). Methionine restriction induces apoptosis in prostate cancer cells via the c-Jun N-terminal kinase-mediated signaling pathway (Lu et al., 2002). Such data advocate the hypothesis that methionine restricts the growth of cancer cells through hypermethylation of oncogenes. This hypothesis has received support from a population study conducted by Larsson et al. (2007), which concludes with "higher methionine intake may reduce the risk of pancreatic cancer."

6.4.8 Nickel

Nickel is a heavy metal that has been reported for its carcinogenicity. Although nickel is not mutagenic, as confirmed by most bacterial and mammalian cell assays, it does produce a little genotoxicity because of the ability to induce small DNA damage. Lee et al. (1995) reported in the case of nickel carcinogenesis that it is DNA methylation that leads to the condensation of chromatin and does not allow the expression of certain genes. The finding from Lee et al. (1995) also explains that nickel carcinogenesis does not account for genetic alterations and DNA damage. It has been well studied and documented that nickel is involved in carcinogenesis through DNA hypermethylation of tumor suppressor genes and senescence genes (Lee et al., 1998), but the exact mechanism of involvement of nickel is still nebulous. Probably the nickel ion (Ni^{2+}) directly affects chromatin and leads to de novo DNA methylation (Costa, 2002; Zhou et al., 2009).

6.4.9 Selenium

Selenium is a micronutrient. A large amount of data suggest its possible role as an effective, naturally occurring, anticarcinogenic agent. It is found to be involved in hypomethylation of tumor suppressor genes like *p53* (Davis et al., 2000), which might be a possible mechanism through which selenium shows its anticancer property.

6.4.10 Vitamin A

Initially, it was Fujimaki (1926) who pulled the attention toward the possibility of the anticancer properties of vitamin A (Sporn and Roberts, 1983). In the past two decades, vitamin A has been extensively studied as a cancer chemopreventive agent. Retinol can activate nuclear retinoid receptors via some of its metabolites and may prevent or delay carcinogenesis at both the initiation and promotion steps (Vainio and Rautalahti, 1999). The mechanism involved in vitamin A acting as anticancer agent has not yet been detailed, but the work of Rowling et al. (2002) provides important clues. Glycine *N*-methyltransferase (GNMT) is the cytosolic enzyme that maintains the ratio of SAM and the SAM:SAH. Hence, inappropriate activation of GNMT may lead to the loss of methyl groups vital for many SAM-dependent transmethylation reactions, for example, DNA methylation. Vitamin A and its retinoic acid derivatives are able to induce GNMT. This observation suggests that hypomethylation or no further methylation of DNA because of inappropriate activation of GNMT in the presence of adequate vitamin A, and vice versa, may be the possible mechanism of methylation of DNA by vitamin A. This possibility got support by the finding that gastric carcinogenesis involves transcriptional inactivation by aberrant DNA methylation of genes related to retinoid signaling (Shutoh et al., 2005).

6.4.11 Vitamin B_6

Cravo and coworkers (1997) predicted that restriction of vitamin B_6 may interfere with DNA methylation status by impairing de novo methionine synthesis. Actually vitamin B_6 restriction decreases the activity and stability of serine hydroxymethyltransferase and may impair the supply of single-unit carbon for homocysteine remethylation for methionine formation (Perry et al., 1997) and probably affect the DNA methylation through restricting methionine availability for the formation of SAM, the ultimate donor of methyl groups to DNA via DNMT enzymes.

6.4.12 Vitamin B_{12}

Vitamin B_{12} is one of the determinants of one-carbon metabolism. Elevated circulating levels of vitamin B_{12} may be associated with risk for advanced stage prostate cancer (Johansson et al., 2008). Vitamin B_{12} and low methionine synthase activity also have been reported as the two determinants of DNA hypomethylation (Brunaud et al., 2003). Zhang et al. (2003) reported that plasma vitamin B_{12} levels were inversely associated with breast cancer risk among premenopausal women but not among postmenopausal women. Recently, it was found that treatment with vitamin B_{12} does not have any significant effect on the risk of breast cancer (Zhang et al., 2008).

6.5 Methylation of Genes Associated with Breast Cancer

Several recent studies have shown that DNA methylation is the most well-researched epigenetic mark that differs between normal cells and cancer cells in humans. In normal cells, CpG islands preceding gene promoters are generally unmethylated, while other individual CpG dinucleotides throughout the genome tend to be methylated. However, in cancer cells, CpG islands preceding tumor suppressor gene promoters are often hypermethylated, while CpG methylation of oncogene promoter regions and parasitic repeat sequences is often decreased. Hypermethylation of gene promoters can result in silencing of those genes. This type of epigenetic mutation is dangerous when genes that regulate the cell cycle are silenced, allowing cells to grow and reproduce uncontrollably, leading to tumorigenesis. Hundreds of hypermethylated genes have been described in breast cancer. Several genes involved in cell cycle regulation and apoptosis (*CCND2, CDKN2A/p16, RASSF1A*), DNA damage response (*BRCA1*), cell adhesion (*CDH1*), and cell signaling (*ER, RARβ 2*) have been reported to undergo promoter hypermethylation in breast carcinoma. DNA methylation has been reported to play diverse functions like genome imprinting, normal development, and repression of gene transcription.

6.5.1 *BRCA1* Gene Methylation and BRCA1

BRCA1 is located on chromosome 17q21 (Wakefield and Alsop, 2006). Its protein product is 1863 amino acid (NCBI amino acid sequence) and known for its association with tumor suppressor activity in breast and ovarian cancers. There is abundant evidence that BRCA1 plays a number of roles in maintenance of genome integrity. It is an important participant in the response to DNA damage, operating in both the repair of double-strand breaks (DSB) and in enaction of certain cell cycle checkpoint responses. There is considerable circumstantial evidence suggesting that at least part of its repair and/or checkpoint response function is linked to its tumor-suppressing activity (Boulton, 2006). Inherited mutations in *BRCA1* gene account for one-half of inherited breast carcinomas.

6.5.1.1 Breast Cancer and BRCA1 Hypermethylation

Southern analysis of the *BRCA1* promoter revealed methylation in 11% sporadic breast cancer cases (Catteau et al., 1999). Another study with 19% of breast cancer carcinoma demonstrated that *BRCA1* promoter is methylated in 13% of unselected primary breast tumors (Esteller et al., 2000). Loss of heterozygosity (LOH) for *BRCA1*, in familial breast cancer. Surprising fact is even in the presence of heterozygosity, and homozygosity of *BRCA1* occurrences of breast cancer had been reported, in the case of sporadic breast cancer cases. As expected, the normal tissues do not have the *BRCA1* gene with hypermethylated status. A study from Chinese population revealed that the frequency of *BRCA1* promoter hypermethylation is 32% (Jing et al., 2008). Hypermethylation of *BRCA1* is very rare to found outside breast cancer except ovarian cancers (Dobrovic and Simpfendorfer, 1997). Hence, it was strongly advocated that *BRCA1* promoter hypermethylation plays a significant role in breast cancer pathogenesis (Bianco et al., 2000).

6.5.1.2 Other Gene Hypermethylation in Breast Cancer

Lehmann et al. (2002) studied methylation status of some growth regulatory genes (e.g., *p16, RASSF1A, cyclinD2, 14-3-3σ*) in breast cancer patients in a German population. It was reported that promoter methylation is an early and frequent event in breast cancer development but displays great quantitative and gene-specific differences and changes in a gene-specific manner during tumor progression.

RAS association domain family protein 1A (*RASSF1A*), *adenomatous polyposis coli* (*APC*), and *death-associated protein* (*DAP*) *kinase* are three normally unmethylated and biologically significant genes. These three genes were studied by sensitive methylation-specific PCR in 34 breast tumors and paired preoperative serum DNAs. Collectively hypermethylation in one or more genes was found in 94% samples. *APC, RASSF1A*, and *DAP kinase* found individually as 47%, 65%, and 50% of samples, respectively (Dulaimi et al., 2004).

To evaluate whether hypermethylation identifies breast cancer with distinctive clinical and pathological features, Li et al. (2006) studied *RARβ2, CDH1, ER, BRCA1, CCND2, p16*, and *TWIST* genes in 193 breast carcinomas. It was found that methylation frequencies ranged from 11% for *CCND2* to 84% for *ER*. They concluded that gene methylation may be linked to various pathological features of breast cancer. Seniski et al. (2009) narrated that *ADAM33* gene promoter methylation may be a useful molecular marker for differentiating invasive lobular carcinoma and invasive ductal carcinoma.

E-cadherin gene located on chromosome 16 encodes a cell surface adhesion protein. It has an important role to play in maintaining hemophilic cell–cell adhesion in epithelial tissues (Ilyas and Tomlinson, 1997). Epigenetic silencing of E-cadherin gene by 5 CpG methylation has been reported to occur in some human breast cancer cell lines. Nass et al. (2000) demonstrated that hypermethylation of the E-cadherin CpG islands was evident in 30% ductal carcinomas in situ and increased significantly to nearly 60% of metastatic lesions suggestive of a role of methylation in tumor progression.

6.6 Sources of DNA for the Methylation Studies in Cancer Patients

Almost one decade earlier, the presence of abnormally high DNA concentration in the serum of patients of various malignant diseases was reported. Numerous studies showed tumor-specific alteration in cell-free DNA recovered from blood, plasma, or serum of patients. The nucleic acid markers described in plasma and serum include oncogene mutation, microsatellite alteration, gene rearrangements, and epigenetic alteration, such as aberrant promoter hypermethylation (Chen et al., 1999). Methylation status of certain genes (*RASSF1A* and *APC*) found in cell-free DNA from sera of breast cancer patients had been reported as more powerful prognostic marker than other prognostic parameters (Müller et al., 2003). Several other studies showed that the cell-free DNA isolated from sera of cancer patients can be used to study the methylation status of cancer-related genes (Widschwendter et al., 2004; Hu et al., 2006; Ikoma et al., 2006).

A good quality of cell-free DNA can be isolated from saliva. DNA from saliva had been used for the study of methylation of cancer-related genes for head and neck cancers as well as oral cancer (Viet and Schmidt, 2008). Saliva and urine were used as the source for studying methylation of cancer-related genes in breast cancer patients. But it was only the urine, not the saliva, that showed the significant alteration in the methylation of *BRCA1* gene (Hansmann et al., 2012). However, Bryan et al. (2013) had reported a differential methylation pattern in breast cancer genes assayed from saliva.

6.7 DNA Methylation–Based Biomarkers in Serum and Other Body Fluids of Breast Cancer Patients

Although DNA methylation analysis is a rapidly developing field, a reproducible epigenetic blood (serum) and other body fluids–based assay for diagnosis and follow-up of breast cancer has yet to be successfully developed into a routine clinical test. There is a tug nowadays to find and establish DNA methylation–based biomarkers in urine and saliva in addition to blood and serum (Viet and Schmidt, 2008; Hansmann et al., 2012; Bryan et al., 2013). With a little success with saliva and urine, blood and serum have been found more promising in terms of developing such markers. The use of such body fluids–based methylated DNA biomarkers is based on the fact that these fluids are readily available for molecular diagnosis. As far as the DNA methylation–based biomarkers in serum are concerned, the list of hypermethylated genes in breast cancer is heterogeneous, and no single gene is methylated in all breast cancer types. There is increasing evidence that a panel of epigenetic markers is essential to achieve a higher sensitivity and specificity in breast cancer detection.

6.7.1 Effect of Nutrients and Lifestyle on DNA Methylation–Based Biomarkers

The reported percentages of methylation in biomarkers are highly variable. This can be partly explained by the different sensitivities and the different intra-/interassay coefficients of variability of the analysis methods (De Voorde et al., 2012). Simultaneously, we know nutrients play a great role in maintaining and alteration of the DNA methylation pattern. Hence, they also can affect the DNA methylation–based biomarkers (Kim et al., 2010; Dominguez-Salas et al., 2013). These two are the main hurdles in developing efficient DNA methylation–based biomarkers in body fluids. So, while developing such biomarkers, one have to keep these issues in mind. Hence, developing such marker is still challenging while that is interesting as well as promising.

6.8 Conclusions and Future Perspective

Numerous scholarly investigations have demonstrated that DNA methylation is very dynamic and it is the most well-characterized epigenetic mark. DNA methylation, along with histone tail modifications, gives stability to the genome and is involved in cell differentiations and X-chromosome inactivation. DNA methylation (hypo- and hyper-) is a normal cellular event that determines the expression of genes according to the environment, at the transcriptional level. Hypo- and/or hypermethylation of DNA can initiate a cascade of abnormal events, which may be transcriptional activation and inactivation of oncogenes and tumor suppressor genes, respectively. As an outcome, cancer may occur. The source of the methyl groups (choline, homocysteine, and single-carbon metabolism), SAM, and families of DNMTs are the three main determinants of the DNA methylation status. The main target of DNMTs is the CpG island of promoters of different genes. Although SAM is the ultimate donor of methyl groups to cytosine residues in CpG islands, the reaction is mediated by DNMTs. However, SAM donates methyl groups to more than 80 biological reactions. Thus, the limiting factor for DNA methylation reactions is the presence of active DNMTs. Hence, the key factor for regulation of genes through methylation of DNA is something that regulates the presence of active DNMTs in appropriate concentrations. Further studies are needed to identify such factors.

There are large numbers of nutrients and food components that alter intracellular molecular environments, thus affecting DNA methylation machinery and mechanisms and, in turn, the methylation status of DNA. Several nutrients that have been studied with respect to the status of DNA methylation in cancers include alcohol, arsenic, cadmium, choline, folate, methionine, nickel, selenium, and vitamins like A, B_6, and B_{12}. Alcohol, arsenic, and cadmium interfere with DNA methylation processes and cause global hypomethylation. Choline is one of the methyl group sources that come from food. Choline deficiency causes gene-specific hypomethylation, for example, CpGs of *Dnmt1* and *c-Ha-ras*. A study in fetal rat liver and brain suggests that the modulation of DNA methylation machinery is performed by choline, and as a consequence of hypomethylation of *Dnmt1*, mRNA expression of *Dnmt1*, *Dnmt3a*, and *Dnmt3l* increases. There are global and gene-specific hypermethylation. Although this study does not give a complete picture of the complex mechanisms of modulation of DNA methylation, it supports some putative interpretations such as (1) choline deficiency does not cause hypomethylation; (2) choline is not the sole source of methyl groups; rather, it is a single-carbon metabolism because homocysteine is contributed in part from food; and (3) choline somehow modulates DNA methylation by stabilizing DNMTs in the intracellular environment. All of these assertions need to be carefully experimentally evaluated in order to decipher the exact mechanisms of DNA methylation. Both methionine and nickel have been demonstrated to induce gene-specific hypermethylation. It is assumed that methionine hypermethylates oncogenes, whereas nickel is involved in hypermethylation of tumor suppressor genes, both preventing and causing cancer, respectively. Selenium is anticarcinogenic via hypomethylation of tumor suppressor genes, thus altering expression of these genes. It is yet unclear how vitamins are involved in DNA methylation and, consequently, breast cancer. However, vitamins A, B_6, and B_{12} have been found to be involved in transcriptional inactivation by aberrant DNA methylation of genes related to retinoid signaling and impairing de novo methionine synthesis.

Although extensive research has been performed in the field of epigenetics and breast cancers where nutrients have been considered as environmental factors, there remain several challenges and questions to be answered. Among many crucial questions is determining the key factor(s) for regulation of genes through methylation of DNA through the regulation of the presence of active DNMT in appropriate concentrations.

References

Altieri A, Garavello W, Bosetti C et al. (2005) Alcohol consumption and risk of laryngeal cancer. *Oral Oncol* 41: 956–965.

Balaghi M, Wagner C (1993) DNA methylation in folate deficiency: Use of CpG methylase. *Biochem Biophys Res Commun* 193: 1184–1190.

Barak AJ, Kemmy RJ (1982) Methotrexate effects on hepatic betaine levels in choline-supplemented and choline-deficient rats. *Drug Nutr Interact* 1: 275–278.

Benavides MA, Oelschlager DK, Zhang HG et al. (2007) Methionine inhibits cellular growth dependent on the p53 status of cells. *Am J Surg* 193: 274–283.

Benbrahim-Tallaa L, Waalkes MP (2008) Inorganic arsenic and human prostate cancer. *Environ Health Perspect* 116: 158–164.

Benbrahim-Tallaa L, Waterland RA, Styblo M et al. (2005) Molecular events associated with arsenic-induced malignant transformation of human prostatic epithelial cells: Aberrant genomic DNA methylation and K-ras oncogene activation. *Toxicol Appl Pharmacol* 206: 288–298.

Bernardino-Sgherri J, Flagiello D, Dutrillaux B (2002) Overall DNA methylation and chromatin structure of normal and abnormal X chromosomes. *Cytogenet Genome Res* 99: 85–91.

Bestor TH, Laudano A, Mttialiano R et al. (1988) Cloning and sequencing of a cDNA encoding DNA methyl transferase of mouse cells: The carboxyl-terminal domain of the mammalian enzyme is related to the bacterial methyl transferase. *J Mol Biol* 203: 971–983.

Bianco T, Chenevix-Trench G, Walsh DC, Cooper JE, Dobrovic A (2000) Tumour-specific distribution of BRCA1 promoter region methylation supports a pathogenetic role in breast and ovarian cancer. *Carcinogenesis* 21(2): 147–151.

Bielawski DM, Zaher FM, Svinarich DM et al. (2002) Paternal alcohol exposure affects sperm cytosine methyltransferase messenger RNA levels. *Alcohol Clin Exp Res* 26: 347–351.

Bird AP (1986) CpG-rich islands and the function of DNA methylation. *Nature* 321: 209–213.

Bonsch D, Lenz B, Fiszer R et al. (2006) Lowered DNA methyltransferase (DNMT-3b) mRNA expression is associated with genomic DNA hypermethylation in patients with chronic alcoholism. *J Neural Transm* 113: 1299–1304.

Bosetti C, Gallus S, Franceschi S et al. (2002) Cancer of the larynx in non-smoking alcohol drinkers and in non-drinking tobacco smokers. *Br J Cancer* 87: 516–518.

Boulton SJ (2006) Cellular functions of the BRCA tumour-suppressor proteins. *Biochem Soc Trans* 34(Pt 5): 633–645.

Brooks PJ, Enoch MA, Goldman D et al. (2009) The alcohol flushing response: An unrecognized risk factor for esophageal cancer from alcohol consumption. *PLoS Med* 6: 258–263.

Brunaud L, Alberto JM, Ayav A et al. (2003) Effects of vitamin B12 and folate deficiencies on DNA methylation and carcinogenesis in rat. *Clin Chem Lab Med* 41: 1012–1019.

Bryan AD, Magnan RE, Hooper AE, Harlaar N, Hutchison KE. (2013) Physical activity and differential methylation of breast cancer genes assayed from saliva: A preliminary investigation. *Ann Behav Med* 45(1): 89–98.

Bujnicki MJ, Radlinska M (1999) Molecular evolution of DNA-(cytosine-N4) methyltransferases: Evidence for their polyphyletic. *Nucleic Acids Res* 27: 4501–4509.

Catteau A, Harris WH, Xu CF, Solomon E (1999) Methylation of the BRCA1 promoter region in sporadic breast and ovarian cancer: Correlation with disease characteristics. *Oncogene* 18: 1957–1965.

Chanda S, Dasgupta UB, Guhamazumder D et al. (2006) DNA Hypermethylation of promoter of gene *p53* and *p16* in arsenic-exposed people with and without malignancy. *Toxicol Sci* 89: 431–437.

Chen X, Bonnefoi H, Diebold-Berger S, Lyautey J, Lederrey C, Faltin-Traub E, Stroun M, Anker P (1999) Detecting tumor-related alterations in plasma or serum DNA of patients diagnosed with breast cancer. *Clin Cancer Res* 5(9): 2297–2303.

Choi SW, Mason JB (2002) Folate status: Effects on pathways of colorectal carcinogenesis. *J Nutr* 132: 2413S–2418S.

Choi SW, Stickel F, Baik HW et al. (1999) Chronic alcohol consumption induces genomic but not *p53*-specific DNA hypomethylation in rat colon. *J Nutr* 129: 1945–1950.

Costa M (2002) Molecular mechanisms of nickel carcinogenesis. *Biol Chem* 383: 961–967.

Cravo M, Gloria L, Camilo ME et al. (1997) DNA methylation and subclinical vitamin deficiency of folate, pyridoxal-Phosphate and vitamin B12 in chronic alcoholic. *Clin Nutr* 16: 29–35.

Davis CD, Uthus EO, Finley JW (2000) Dietary selenium and arsenic affect DNA methylation in vitro in Caco-2 cells and in vivo in rat liver and colon. *J Nutr* 130: 2903–2909.

Dobrovic A, Simpfendorfer D (1997) Methylation of the BRCA1 gene in sporadic breast cancer. *Cancer Res* 57: 3347–3350.

Dominguez-Salas P, Moore SE, Cole D, da Costa KA, Cox SE, Dyer RA, Fulford AJ et al. (2013) DNA methylation potential: Dietary intake and blood concentrations of one-carbon metabolites and cofactors in rural African women. *Am J Clin Nutr* 97(6): 1217–1227.

Dulaimi E, Hillinck J, Ibanez de Caceres I, Al-Saleem T, Cairns P (2004) Tumor suppressor gene promoter hypermethylation in serum of breast cancer patients. *Clin Cancer Res* 10(18 Pt 1): 6189–6193.

Ehrlich M (2002) DNA methylation in cancer: Too much, but also too little. *Oncogene* 21: 5400–5413.

Esteller M, Silva JM, Dominguez G, Bonilla F, Matias-Guiu X, Lerma E, Bussaglia E, Prat J, Harkes IC, Repasky EA, Gabrielson E, Schutte M, Baylin SB, Herman JG (2000) Promoter hypermethylation and BRCA1 inactivation in sporadic breast and ovarian tumors. *J Natl Cancer Inst* 92: 564–569.

Fatemi M, Hermann A, Pradhan S et al. (2001) The activity of the murine DNA methyltransferase Dnmt1 is controlled by interaction of the catalytic domain with the N-terminal part of the enzyme leading to an allosteric activation of the enzyme after binding to methylated DNA. *J Mol Biol* 309: 1189–1199.

Freedman ND, Schatzkin A, Leitzmann MF et al. (2007) Alcohol and head and neck cancer risk in a prospective study. *Br J Cancer* 96: 1469–1474.

Fujimaki Y (1926) Formation of gastric carcinoma in albino rats fed on deficient diets. *J Cancer Res* 10: 469.

Goll MG, Kirpekar F, Maggert KA et al. (2006) Methylation of t-RNA-Asp by the DNA methyltransferase homolog Dnmt2. *Science* 311: 395–398.

Gowher H, Jeltsch A (2001) Enzymatic properties of recombinant Dnmt3a DNA methyltransferase from mouse: The enzyme modifies DNA in a non-processive manner and also methylates non-CpG sites. *J Mol Biol* 309: 1201–1208.

Handa V, Jeltsch A (2005) Profound flanking sequence preference of Dnmt3a and Dnmt3b mammalian DNA methyltransferases shape the human epigenome. *J Mol Biol* 348: 1103–1112.

Hansmann T, Pliushch G, Leubner M, Kroll P, Endt D, Gehrig A, Preisler-Adams S, Wieacker P, Haaf T (2012) Constitutive promoter methylation of BRCA1 and RAD51C in patients with familial ovarian cancer and early-onset sporadic breast cancer. *Hum Mol Genet* 21(21): 4669–4679.

Hayslip J, Montero A (2006) Tumor suppressor gene methylation in follicular lymphoma: A comprehensive review. *Mol Cancer* 5: 44.

Hermann A, Gowher H, Jeltsch A (2004) Biochemistry and biology of mammalian DNA methyltransferases. *Cell Mol Life Sci* 61: 2571–2587.

Horne WD, Cook RJ, Wagner C (1989) Effect of dietary methyl group deficiency on folate metabolism in rats. *J Nutr* 119: 618–621.

Hotchkiss RD (1948) The quantitative separation of purines, pyrimidines, and nucleosides by paper chromatography. *J Biol Chem* 175: 315–332.

Hu S, Ewertz M, Tufano RP, Brait M, Carvalho AL, Liu D, Tufaro AP et al. (2006) Detection of serum deoxyribonucleic acid methylation markers: A novel diagnostic tool for thyroid cancer. *J Clin Endocrinol Metab* 91(1): 98–104.

Ikoma H, Ichikawa D, Koike H, Ikoma D, Tani N, Okamoto K, Ochiai T, Ueda Y, Otsuji E, Yamagishi H. (2006) Correlation between serum DNA methylation and prognosis in gastric cancer patients. *Anticancer Res* 26(3B): 2313–2316.

Ilyas M, Tomlinson IP (1997) The interactions of APC, E-cadherin and beta-catenin in tumour development and progression. *J Pathol* 182:128–137.

Institute of Medicine and National Academy of Sciences USA. *Dietary Reference Intakes for Folate, Thiamin, Riboflavin, Niacin, Vitamin B_{12}, Pantothenic Acid, Biotin, and Choline.* Washington, DC: National Academy Press, 1998.

Jeltsch A, Jurkowska RJ, Jurkowski TP (2007) Application of DNA methyltransferases in targeted DNA methylation. *Appl Microbiol Biotechnol* 75: 1233–1240.

Jiang G, Xu L, Song S et al. (2008) Effects of long-term low-dose cadmium exposure on genomic DNA methylation in human embryo lung fibroblast cells. *Toxicology* 244: 49–55.

Jing F, Jun L, Yong Z, Wang Y, Fei X, Zhang J, Hu L. (2008) Multigene methylation in serum of sporadic Chinese female breast cancer patients as a prognostic biomarker. *Oncology* 75(1–2): 60–66.

Johansson M, Appleby PN, Allen NE et al. (2008) Circulating concentrations of folate and vitamin B12 in relation to prostate cancer risk: Results from the European prospective investigation into cancer and nutrition study. *Cancer Epidemiol Biomarkers Prev* 17: 279–285.

Jung AY, Poole EM, Bigler J et al. (2008) DNA methyltransferase and alcohol dehydrogenase: Gene-nutrient interactions in relation to risk of colorectal polyps. *Cancer Epidemiol Biomarkers Prev* 17: 330–338.

Keshet I, Lieman-Hurwitz J, Cedar H (1986) DNA methylation affects the formation of active chromatin. *Cell* 44: 535–543.

Kim HH, Park CS (2003) Methionine cytotoxicity in the human breast cancer cell line MCF-7, in vitro cell. *Dev Biol Anim* 39: 117–119.

Kim JM, Hong K, Lee JH et al. (2009) Effect of folate deficiency on placental DNA methylation in hyperhomocysteinemic rats. *J Nutr Biochem* 20: 172–176.

Kim M, Long TI, Arakawa K, Wang R, Yu MC, Laird PW (2010) DNA methylation as a biomarker for cardiovascular disease risk. *PLoS One* 5(3): e9692.

Kim Y (2004) Folate and DNA methylation: A mechanistic link between folate deficiency and colorectal cancer? *Cancer Epidemiol Biomarkers Prev* 13: 511–519.

King-Batoon A, Leszczynska JM, Klein CB (2008) Modulation of gene methylation by genistein or lycopene in breast cancer cells. *Environ Mol Mutagen* 49: 36–45.

Kovacheva VP, Mellott TJ, Davison JM et al. (2007) Gestational choline deficiency causes global and Igf2 gene- DNA hypermethylation by upregulation. *J Biol Chem* 282: 31777–31788.

Larsson SC, Giovannucci E, Wolk A (2007) Methionine and vitamin B_6 intake and risk of pancreatic cancer: A prospective study of Swedish women and men. *Gastroenterology* 132: 113–118.

Lee YW, Broday L, Costa M (1998) Effects of nickel on DNA methyltransferase activity and genomic DNA methylation levels. *Mutat Res* 415: 213–218.

Lee YW, Klein CB, Kargacin B et al. (1995) Carcinogenic nickel silences gene expression by chromatin condensation and DNA methylation: A new model for epigenetic carcinogens. *Mol Cell Biol* 15: 2547–2557.

Lehmann U, Langer F, Feist H et al. (2002) Quantitative assessment of promoter hypermethylation during breast cancer development. *Am J Pathol* 160: 605–612.

Li S, Rong M, Iacopetta B (2006) DNA hypermethylation in breast cancer and its association with clinicopathological features. *Cancer Lett* 237(2): 272–280.

Lorincz MC, Dickerson DR, Schmitt M et al. (2004) Intragenic DNA methylation alters chromatin structure and elongation efficiency in mammalian cells. *Nat Struct Mol Biol* 11: 1068–1075.

Lu S, Hoestje SM, Choo EM et al. (2002) Methionine restriction induces apoptosis of prostate cancer cells via the c-Jun N-terminal kinase-mediated signaling pathway. *Cancer Lett* 179: 51–58.

Lu SC, Alvarez L, Huang ZZ et al. (2001) Methionine adenosyltransferase 1A knockout mice are predisposed to liver injury and exhibit increased expression of genes involved in proliferation. *Proc Natl Acad Sci USA* 98: 5560–5565.

Moore LE, Pfeiffer RM, Poscablo C et al. (2008) Genomic DNA hypomethylation as a biomarker for bladder cancer susceptibility in the Spanish bladder cancer study: A case—Control study. *Lancet Oncol* 9: 359–366.

Müller HM, Widschwendter A, Fiegl H, Ivarsson L, Goebel G, Perkmann E, Marth C, Widschwendter M (2003) DNA methylation in serum of breast cancer patients: An independent prognostic marker. *Cancer Res* 63(22): 7641–7645.

Nass SJ, Herman JG, Gabrielson E, Iversen PW, Parl FF, Davidson NE, Graff JR (2000) Aberrant methylation of the estrogen receptor and E-cadherin 5′ CpG islands increases with malignant progression in human breast cancer. *Cancer Res* 60: 4346–4348.

Perry C, Yu S, Chen J et al. (2007) Effect of vitamin B6 availability on serine hydroxymethyltransferase in MCF-7 cells. *Arch Biochem Biophys* 462: 21–27.

Pilsner JR, Liu X, Ahsan H et al. (2007) Genomic methylation of peripheral blood leukocyte DNA: Influences of arsenic and folate in Bangladeshi adults. *Am J Clin Nutr* 86: 1179–1186.

Privat M, Aubel C, Arnould S et al. (2009) Breast cancer cell response to genistein is conditioned by *BRCA1* mutations. *Biochem Biophys Res Commun* 379: 785–789.

Reichard JF, Schnekenburger M, Puga A (2007) Long term low-dose arsenic exposure induces loss of DNA methylation. *Biochem Biophys Res Commun* 352: 188–192.

Reither S, Li F, Gowher H et al. (2003) Catalytic mechanism of DNA-(cytosine-C5)-methyltransferases revisited: Covalent intermediate formation is not essential for methyl group transfer by the murine Dnmt3a enzyme. *J Mol Biol* 329: 675–684.

Richardson B, Yung R (2002) Role of DNA methylation in the regulation of cell function. *J Lab Clin Med* 134: 333–340.

Roman-Gomez J, Jimenez-Velasco A, Agirre X et al. (2005) Promoter hypomethylation of the LINE-1 retrotransposable elements activates sense/antisense transcription and marks the progression of chronic myeloid leukemia. *Oncogene* 24: 7213–7223.

Rowling MJ, McMullen MH, Schalinske KL (2002) Vitamin A and its derivatives induce hepatic glycine *N*-methyltransferase and hypomethylation of DNA in rats. *J Nutr* 132: 365–369.

Saxonov S, Berg P, Brutlag DL (2006) A genome-wide analysis of CpG dinucleotides in the human genome distinguishes two distinct classes of promoters. *Proc Natl Acad Sci* 103: 1412–1417.

Seitz HK, Stickel F (2007) Molecular mechanisms of alcohol-mediated carcinogenesis. *Nat Rev Cancer* 7: 599–612.

Seniski GG, Camargo AA, Ierardi DF, Ramos EA, Grochoski M, Ribeiro ES, Cavalli IJ et al. (2009) ADAM33 gene silencing by promoter hypermethylation as a molecular marker in breast invasive lobular carcinoma. *BMC Cancer* 9: 80. doi: 10.1186/1471-2407-9-80.

Shutoh M, Oue N, Aung PP et al. (2005) DNA methylation of genes linked with retinoid signaling in gastric carcinoma: Expression of the retinoid acid receptor beta, cellular retinol-binding protein 1, and tazarotene-induced gene 1 genes is associated with DNA methylation. *Cancer* 104: 1609–1619.

Sporn MB, Roberts AB (1983) Role of retinoids in differentiation and carcinogenesis. *Cancer Res* 43: 3034–3040.

Takiguchi M, Achanzar WE, Qu W et al. (2003) Effect of cadmium on DNA-(Cytosine-5) methyltransferase activity and DNA methylation status during cadmium-induced cellular transformation. *Exp Cell Res* 286: 355–365.

Tao MH, Marian, C, Shields PG et al. (2011) Alcohol consumption in relation to aberrant DNA methylation in breast tumors. *Alcohol* 45(7): 689–699.

Vainio H, Rautalahti M (1999) An international evaluation of the cancer preventive potential of vitamin A. *Cancer Epidemiol Biomarkers Prev* 8: 107–109.

Van De Voorde L, Speeckaert R, Van Gestel D, Bracke M, De Neve W, Delanghe J, Speeckaert M (2012) DNA methylation-based biomarkers in serum of patients with breast cancer. *Mutat Res* 751(2): 304–325.

van den Donk M, van Engeland M, Pellis L et al. (2007) Dietary folate intake in combination with *MTHFR* C677T genotype and promoter methylation of tumor suppressor and DNA repair genes in sporadic colorectal adenomas. *Cancer Epidemiol Biomarkers Prev* 16: 1562–1566.

Van Speybroeck L (2002) From epigenesis to epigenetics: The case of C. H. Waddington. *Ann N Y Acad Sci* 981: 61–81.

Varela-Moreiras G, Selhub J, da Costa K et al. (1992) Effect of chronic choline deficiency in rats on liver folate content and distribution. *J Nutr Biochem* 3: 519–522.

Viet CT, Schmidt BL (2008) Methylation array analysis of preoperative and postoperative saliva DNA in oral cancer patients. *Cancer Epidemiol Biomarkers Prev* 17(12): 3603–3611.

Waddington CH (1942) The epigenotype. *Endeavour* 1: 18–20.

Wakefield MJ, Alsop AE (2006) Assignment of BReast Cancer Associated 1 (BRCA1) to tammar wallaby (Macropus eugenii) chromosome 2q3 by in situ hybridization. *Cytogenet Genome Res* 112(1–2): 180C.

Wallwork JC, Duerre JA (1985) Effect of zinc deficiency on methionine metabolism, methylation reactions and protein synthesis in isolated perfused rat liver. *J Nutr* 115: 252–262.

Waterland RA (2006) Assessing the effects of high methionine intake on DNA methylation. *J Nutr* 136: 1706S–1710S.

Whitman SP, Hackanson B, Liyanarachchi S et al. (2008) DNA hypermethylation and epigenetic silencing of the tumor suppressor gene, *SLC5A8*, in acute myeloid leukemia with the *MLL* partial tandem duplication. *Blood* 112: 2013–2016.

WHO. *Arsenic and Arsenic Compounds*. 2nd edn. Geneva, Switzerland: Inter-Organization Programme for the Sound Management of Chemicals, World Health Organization 2001.

Widschwendter M, Jiang G, Woods C, Müller HM, Fiegl H, Goebel G, Marth C et al. (2004) DNA hypomethylation and ovarian cancer biology. *Cancer Res* 64(13): 4472–4480.

Wynder EL, Bross IJ (1957) Aetiological factors in mouth cancer; an approach to its prevention. *Br Med J* 18: 1137–1143.

Xu X, Gammon MD, Zeisel SH et al. (2008) Choline metabolism and risk of breast cancer in a population-based study. *FASEB J* 22: 2045–2052.

Yoder JA, Soman N, Verdin GV et al. (1997) DNA methyltransferase in mouse tissues and cells: Studied with a mechanism based probe. *J Mol Biol* 270: 385–395.

Yokoyama A, Omori T, Yokoyama T et al. (2006) Risk of squamous cell carcinoma of the upper aerodigestive tract in cancer-free alcoholic Japanese men: An endoscopic follow-up study. *Cancer Epidemiol Biomarkers Prev* 15: 2209–2215.

Zapisek WF, Cronin GM, Lyn-Cook BD et al. (1992) The onset of oncogene hypomethylation in the livers of rats fed methyl-deficient, amino acid-defined diets. *Carcinogenesis* 13: 1869–1872.

Zeng H, Combs Jr GF (2008) Selenium as an anticancer nutrient: Roles in cell proliferation and tumor cell invasion. *J Nutr Biochem* 19: 1–7.

Zhang J, Fu Y, Li J et al. (2009) Effects of subchronic cadmium poisoning on DNA methylation in hens. *Environ Toxicol Pharmacol* 27: 345–349.

Zhang SM, Cook NR, Albert CM et al. (2008) Effect of combined folic acid, vitamin B_6, and vitamin B_{12} on cancer risk in women. *JAMA* 300: 2012–2021.

Zhang SM, Moore SC, Lin J et al. (2006) Folate, Vitamin B6, multivitamin supplements, and colorectal cancer risk in women. *Am J Epidemiol* 163: 108–115.

Zhang SM, Willett WC, Selhub J et al. (2003) Plasma folate, vitamin B_6, vitamin B_{12}, homocysteine, and risk of breast cancer. *J Natl Cancer Inst* 95: 373–380.

Zheng S, Wang Z, Pan Y (2008) Oral intake of genistein changes DNA methylation at the promoters of rat colon genes. *FASEB J* 22: 885–886.

Zhou X, Li Q, Arita A et al. (2009) Effects of nickel, chromate, and arsenite on histone 3 lysine methylation. *Toxicol Appl Pharmacol* 236: 78–84.

Section III

Cervical Cancer

7

Biomarkers for Early Detection of Cervical Cancer

Ruchika Kaul-Ghanekar, MSc, PhD, Amit S. Choudhari, MSc, and Savita Pandita, MSc

CONTENTS

ABSTRACT Cervical cancer is the second most commonly diagnosed cancer among women worldwide with invasive cervical cancer being a leading cause of cancer death. Human papillomavirus (HPV) is the single most important etiological agent in cervical cancer that is responsible for neoplastic progression involving the main viral oncoproteins, E6 and E7. The most common cervical cancer screening program involves the Papanicolaou (Pap) smear test that has greatly reduced the cancer incidence as well as deaths, but still, cervical cancer remains a major global health problem. Biomarker profiling is one of the current challenges in clinical medicine that would not only help in early detection and diagnosis of cervical cancer but would reduce the cancer mortality rates immensely. The current chapter focuses on the recent developments in the noninvasive biomarkers involved in cervical cancer that could be targeted for early detection.

7.1 Introduction

Cervical cancer is the third most commonly diagnosed cancer and the fourth leading cause of cancer death in females worldwide (Jemal et al., 2011). Human papillomaviruses (HPVs) play a major role in the pathogenesis of cervical cancer wherein the viral oncogenes E6 and E7 have been shown to be critical for malignant transformation (Zur Hausen, 2000; Lomnytska et al., 2011). E6 has been shown to form complexes with the tumor suppressor protein p53 and promote its degradation through a ubiquitin-dependent protease system (Lee et al., 2010). On the other hand, the E7 protein has been shown to associate with the retinoblastoma protein (Rb), thereby interfering with its binding to the transcription factor E2F. This results into the release of E2F, leading to expression of the genes involved in cell proliferation (Huh et al., 2007). Besides HPVs, many other factors such as activation of proto-oncogenes and inactivation of tumor suppressor genes also contribute toward the induction of cervical cancer. The conventional cytological screening for early detection of cervical cancer using the Papanicolaou (Pap) test has greatly reduced the incidence as well as mortality rates (Bray et al., 2005). However, less specificity (SP) and sensitivity (SE) of Pap test (Schiffman et al., 2007; Nanda et al., 2000) have invited attention toward more specific markers for early detection and diagnosis of cervical cancer. Despite the introduction of preventive vaccines against HPV 16 and HPV 18, screening needs to be continued, since the vaccination can offer protection for only about 70% of cervical cancers (Franco and Cuzick, 2008). Thus, novel screening strategies need to be evaluated and followed. Due to advancement in technology and research, identification of new biomarkers for early detection has been gaining up recognition in the recent years.

Several candidate biomarkers including p16^{ink4a}, Ki-67, cyclin E, MCM2, TOP2A, carcino-embryonic antigen (CEA), and telomerase are gaining significance in the early detection of cervical cancer (Eun-Kyoung Yim and Jong-Sup Park, 2006). Moreover, different types of approaches based on genomics, proteomics, epigenetics, and recently metabolomics are being targeted to identify more biological markers for early detection as well as diagnosis. This chapter focuses on the different noninvasive biomarkers that are being utilized or are being proposed to be used for the early detection of cervical cancer so as to decrease the cancer risk as well as help in the management of the disease at an early stage.

7.1.1 Why Is It Important?

Cervical cancer has a major impact on the lives of women worldwide, particularly those in developing countries. It has been estimated to kill around 274,000 women every year (Zareen et al., 2009). Unlike other cancers, cervical cancer can be prevented through regular cytological screening programs that can detect and treat the precancerous lesions at an early stage. In developed countries, cervical cancer screening programs have dramatically reduced the incidence as well as death. However, in the majority of low-resource countries, cytological screening programs have proven difficult to sustain largely due to untrained cytotechnologists, inadequate laboratory facilities, and lack of colposcopic evaluation of abnormalities (Goldhaber-Fiebert and Goldie, 2006). The screening technologies that would help in detection of the cancer at early stages before it progresses to its invasive form should be cost effective. Even though, cytology screening has reduced cervical cancer morbidity and mortality, but it suffers from shortcomings in terms of SE and SP. An advance in molecular biology and high-throughput technologies has improved our understanding about the identification of molecular targets related to the process of carcinogenesis. These advancements would facilitate screening, early detection, and management as well as personalize the targeted therapy. Currently, the use of biomarkers has significantly increased the SP and the SE for early detection of cervical cancer. Thus, biomarker discovery represents one of the current challenges in clinical medicine and cytopathology.

7.1.2 Epidemiology

Cervical cancer mostly occurs in women that are less than 50 years of age (Chhabra et al., 2010). It is rarely observed in women younger than 20 years. Older women are also at the risk of developing cervical cancer wherein more than 20% of cases have been reported in women above 65 years (American Cancer Society, 2014). However, chances of cervical cancer have reduced with regular screening programs. According to the Human Papillomavirus and Related Cancers, Summary Report Update, 2010, global estimates for cervical cancer have been reported 529,409 new cases and 274,883 deaths in 2010. The age-standardized incidence rates (ASR) of cervical cancer differ significantly between high- and low-risk countries. The high-risk (HR) countries include Eastern and Western Africa (ASR greater than 30 per 100,000), Southern Africa (26.8 per 100,000), South–Central Asia (24.6 per 100,000), South America, and Middle Africa (ASRs 23.9 and 23.0 per 100,000, respectively), and the lowest-risk regions include Western Asia, Northern America, and Australia/New Zealand (ASRs less than 6 per 100,000) (GLOBOCAN 2008, International Agency for Research on Cancer) (Figure 7.1). More than 85% of the cervical cancer occurs in developing countries, thereby emphasizing the need for considerable preventive measures (WHO/ICO Information Center on Human Papillomavirus and Related Cancers, Summary Report Update, 2010). Table 7.1 describes the key cervical cancer statistics worldwide.

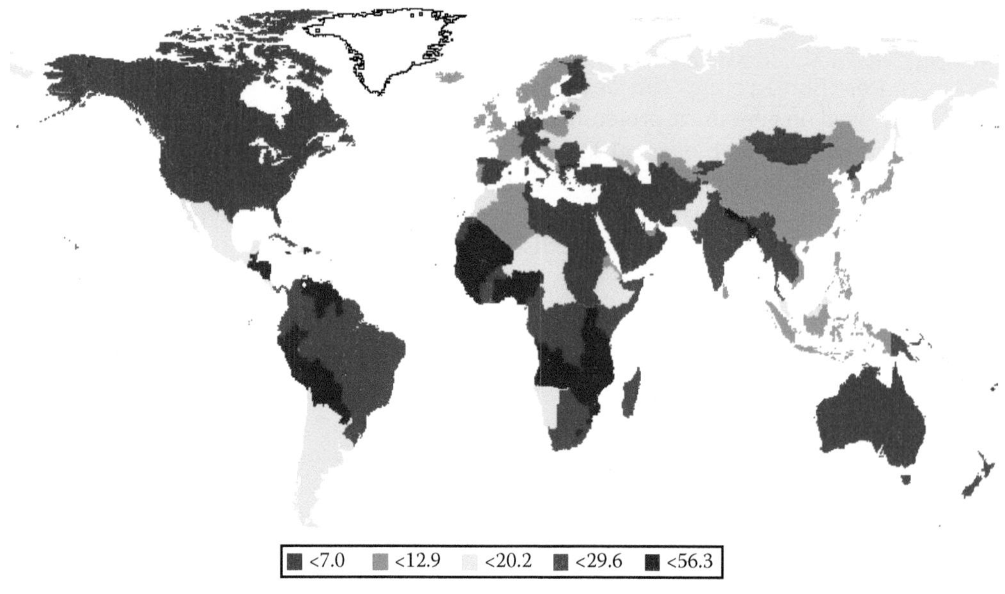

FIGURE 7.1
Reported cervical cancer age standard incident rates per 100,000 women. Figure shows the age-standardized incidence rates of cervical cancer in year 2008. The highest incidence rates (>30 per 100,000) in Eastern and Western Africa and the lowest (<6 per 100,000) in Australia/New Zealand. (From International Agency for Research on Cancer, GLOBOCAN, 2008.)

TABLE 7.1
Key Cervical Cancer Statistics Worldwide

Population	World	Developing Regions	Developed Regions
Number of women at risk for cervical cancer (female population aged ≥15 years) (in thousands)	2,336,986	1,811,867	525,120
Burden of Cervical Cancer (in Thousands)			
New cases recorded per year	529,828	453,321	76,507
Cervical cancer deaths per year	275,128	241,969	33,159
Number of new cervical cancer cases anticipated in 2025[a]	720,060	668,875	81,868
Number of cervical cancer deaths anticipated in 2025[a]	395,095	380,653	38,291
Burden of Cervical HPV Infection (in %)			
Incidence of HPV in the general population (women with normal cytology)	11.4	14.3	10.3
Incidence of HPV16/HPV18 among women with			
I. Normal cytology	3.8	4.6	3.6
II. Low-grade cervical lesions (LSIL/CIN I)	24.3	25.7	24.0
III. High-grade cervical lesions (HSIL/CIN II/CIN III/CIS)	51.1	46.8	52.4
IV. Cervical cancer	70.9	71.0	70.8

Source: WHO/ICO Information Center on Human Papillomavirus and Related Cancers, Summary Report Update, 2010.

LSIL, low-grade intraepithelial lesions; HSIL, high-grade squamous intraepithelial lesions; CIN II/III, CIN grade 2 or 3; CIS, carcinoma in situ.

[a] Projected burden in 2025 is estimated by applying current population forecasts for the country and assuming that current incidence/mortality rates of cervical cancer are constant over time.

7.1.3 Types of Cervical Cancer

Cervical cancer begins in the lining of the cervix at the lower narrow end of the uterus. Invasive cervical cancer develops slowly over the time as the cells change from normal to precancerous lesions called as cervical intraepithelial neoplasia (CIN) or dysplasia and eventually develop into the cancerous phenotype (Cervical Cancer Treatment [PDQ] National Cancer Institute, Patient Version, Last Modified: September 9, 2012 (Figure 7.2). In a large number of cases, these changes in cell structure are not harmful and go away over time (Cervical Cancer Fact Sheet—Centers for Disease Control and Prevention, 2012). During the normal virus life cycle, HPV genomes are found as episomes in the nucleus of infected cells of the normal cervix. However, in some low-grade and in most of the high-grade lesions, HPV genomes are integrated into the host cell genome (Lehn et al, 1988). The integration of HR-HPV DNA leads to the development of invasive cervical cancers (Peitsaro et al., 2002).

Based on the cytology, the Bethesda system (TBS) of classification has graded the changes in the cervical cells into several different categories: atypical squamous cells of undetermined significance (ASCUS), atypical glandular cells of undetermined significance (AGUS), low-grade squamous intraepithelial lesion (LSIL), and high-grade squamous intraepithelial lesion (HSIL). ASCUS is characterized by mild change in the cell cytology, the cause of which is unknown. AGUS refers to glandular cells that may originate in the cervical canal or uterus. LSIL is a mild dysplasia wherein HPV infection may get cleared up on its own within 2 years (Lisa Fayed, 2007). HSIL is an immediate precancerous lesion carrying a high risk of progression to invasive disease if left untreated. Based on the extent of spread of atypical cellular changes in the basal epithelium, CIN is histologically graded into mild dysplasia (CIN I), wherein one-third of the epithelium is affected; moderate dysplasia (CIN II), wherein two-thirds of the epithelium is affected; and severe dysplasia (CIN III), wherein more than two-thirds of the epithelium is affected and it includes full-thickness lesions (Holowaty et al., 1999) (Figure 7.2).

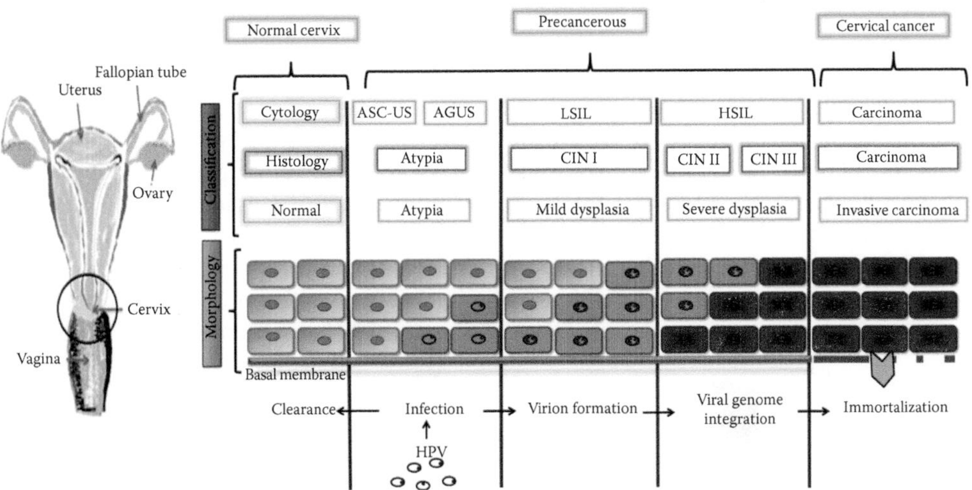

FIGURE 7.2
HPV progression from normal to cancerous with histological and cytological classification. Infection with high-risk HPV genotypes in the region of cervix is associated with viral DNA integration which if persist leads to development of precancerous and cancerous lesions; cytologically classified as ASC-US, AGUS, LSIL, HSIL, and histologically graded as CIN I, CIN II, and CIN III.

On the basis of origin, cervical cancer is characterized into two major types that include squamous cell carcinomas (SCCs) and adenocarcinomas (ACs), which accounts for about 70%–80% and 10%–15% of the carcinomas, respectively (Agnieszka et al., 2011). Even though SCC is more frequently observed, AC tends to grow much more rapidly than the SCC. The third form of the cancer is the mixed type of carcinoma that contains characteristic features of both SCC and AC.

7.1.4 Current Methods for Early Diagnosis, Prognosis, and Therapy with Specificity, Sensitivity, Advantages, and Disadvantages

7.1.4.1 Early Diagnosis

The main objective of cervical cancer screening is to prevent morbidity as well as mortality. Effective screening programs in developed countries have resulted in early diagnosis leading to effective treatment and high chances of recovery. There are various screening tests to identify precancerous lesions that include Pap test (cytology), visual inspection with acetic acid (VIA) and Lugol's iodine (VILI), and the HPV DNA test (Saxena et al., 2012). Cytological evaluation of the cervix by Pap smear test is an internationally accepted screening method in which cells are collected from the surface of the cervix and vagina and observed under microscope for any abnormal changes. Such screening program has substantially reduced the cervical cancer incidence and mortality rate in developed countries. However, in recent years, cervical cytological screening is less reliable because of a growing awareness of high rate of false negativity due to exfoliative variability in cell samples, irreproducibility, smear preparation and staining, microscopic reading, and variations in the reader's elucidation (Raab et al., 1998). VIA and VILI have overcome the limitations of Pap test with an increased SE values spanning from approximately 45.8% to 72.4% and 62.2% to 85.9%, respectively (Shastri et al., 2005). Visual screening methods have gained attention because of low cost, less infrastructure requirement, and fast results (Denny et al., 2000). HPV DNA testing is the most promising and reproducible technique compared to other cervical cancer screening tests. HPV DNA can be identified in invasive cervical cancer as well as in HSILs with high SE. Clinical studies have shown that HPV DNA testing is a better screening option in women aged above 30 years as it is more sensitive for detection of invasive cervical than the cytology tests (Petry and Petry, 2012). However, HPV DNA test cannot determine whether the infection is active, latent, or persistent. Moreover, it requires high technical skills for the sampling procedure and is thus expensive (Gutiérrez-Xicoténcatl et al., 2009). Combination of cytology and HPV testing has increased the SE and negative predictive values (NPVs) of cervical screening (Arbyn et al., 2005). The combination testing can detect more accurately cervical cell abnormalities than the individual tests. The SP and SE along with positive and negative prediction values of different diagnostic tests for the detection of HSIL are mentioned in Table 7.2.

TABLE 7.2

Accuracy of Screening Tests for the Detection of HSIL

Diagnostic Tests	SE (%)	SP (%)	PPV (%)	NPV (%)	Reference
VIA	59.7 (45.8–72.4)	88.4(87.4–89.4)	7.0	99.3	Shastri et al. (2005)
VILI	75.4 (62.2–85.9)	84.3(83.1–85.4)	6.5	99.6	Shastri et al. (2005)
Pap test (cytology)	57.4 (43.2–70.8)	98.6(98.2–99.0)	37.8	99.4	Shastri et al. (2005)
HPV DNA test	62.0 (47.2–75.4)	93.5(92.6–94.3)	12.1	99.4	Shastri et al. (2005)
Pap test with HPV DNA test	96	81	46	99	Arbyn et al. (2005)

7.1.4.2 Prognosis

Prognosis for cervical cancer is influenced by many factors such as the stage as well as the type of cervical cancer and the size of the tumor. Once the cancer has been formally diagnosed, it is staged depending upon the clinical examination of the patient. The current system of cervical cancer staging is based on the International Federation of Gynecology and Obstetrics (FIGO) classification. In stage I, carcinoma is strictly confined to the region of the cervix, and if detected, the 5-year survival rate would be at a higher end (80%–93%) (American Cancer Society, Cervical cancer, 2014). The next two stages, II and III, indicate the progression of the cancer to other areas around the pelvis. In stage II, the carcinoma extends beyond the cervix but not to the pelvic wall. The carcinoma spreads to the vagina but not as far as the lower one-third of the vagina, and the 5-year survival rate ranges between 58% and 63%. In stage III, the carcinoma extends to the pelvic wall as well as to the lower one-third of the vagina, and the 5-year survival rate ranges between 32% and 35% (American Cancer Society, Cervical cancer, 2014). In the final stage, that is, stage IV, the cancer extends beyond the true pelvis involving mucosa of bladder or rectum and the distant organs such as the lungs. Survival chances at this stage are slim, and mortality rates are high with an overall 5-year survival rate between 15% and 16% (American Cancer Society, Cervical cancer, 2014). Combination strategies that include surgery, chemotherapy, and radiation treatment can prolong the life, but often, it is too late to prevent death. The detailed description of the substages is mentioned in Table 7.3.

TABLE 7.3

Clinical Stages of Cervical Carcinoma according to FIGO with Treatment and 5-Year Survival Rate

Stage	Substages	Description	5-Year Survival Rate (%)	Treatment
Early stage	IA1	Carcinoma confined to the cervix, diagnosed only by microscopy. Measured invasion of stroma <3 mm in depth and lateral spread <7 mm.	93	LEEP, cryotherapy, laser therapy, radiotherapy
	IA2	Carcinoma confined to the cervix, diagnosed with microscopy. Measured invasion of stroma >3 mm and <5 mm with lateral spread <7mm.		
	IB1	Clinically visible lesion or greater than A2, <4 cm in the greatest dimension.	80	
	IB2	Clinically visible lesion, >4 cm in the greatest dimension.		
	IIA1	Involvement of the upper two-thirds of the vagina, without parametrial invasion, <4 cm in the greatest dimension.	63	
	IIA2	Involvement of the upper two-thirds of the vagina, without parametrial invasion, >4 cm in the greatest dimension.		
Late stage	IIB	Involvement of the upper two-thirds of the vagina, with parametrial invasion, >4 cm in the greatest dimension.	58	Radical hysterectomy, pelvic exenteration, chemotherapy, radiotherapy
	IIIA	Cancer spreads to lower third of vagina, but not to the pelvic wall.	35	
	IIIB	Cancer extends to pelvic wall and/or blocks urine flow to the bladder.	32	
	IVA	Cancer spreads to the bladder or rectum.	16	
	IVB	Cancer spreads to distant organs, for example, the lungs.	15	

Source: American Cancer Society, Cervical cancer; 2014.

7.1.4.3 Therapies

The treatment for cervical cancer depends upon the size and location of the tumor, stage of the disease, and age and general health of the patient. The various treatment options for cervical cancer include surgery, radiotherapy, and chemotherapy (Irish Cancer Society, 2014). Surgical treatments like cone biopsy or loop electrosurgical excision procedure (LEEP), radical trachelectomy, and hysterectomy are effective methods for treating early stages of the cervical cancer. Surgery is usually associated with several side effects such as cramping, pain, bleeding, and difficulty in emptying bladder. The advanced stage of cervical cancer is usually treated with radiation therapy that uses high-powered energy to destroy cancer cells (ref). Radiation therapy can be given externally using external beam radiation or internally (brachytherapy) by placing devices filled with radioactive material near the cervix. Chemotherapy that includes the use of cytotoxic drugs to kill or slow the growth of cancer cells is used in advanced cervical cancer. Chemotherapy is frequently associated with side effects such as myelosuppression, alopecia, and gastrointestinal symptoms. Mostly, the chemotherapy is combined with radiotherapy to make the radiotherapy more effective (*Treating Cervical Cancer—A Quick Guide*. Cancer Research UK, 2012).

7.1.5 Test Providers and Popular Tests with Cost

Cervical cancer screening tests (Pap and HVP DNA testing) can be performed by a variety of health-care providers including a local doctor or nurse, gynecologist/specialist, and family planning or sexual health clinician. In developing countries such as India, Kenya, Peru, South Africa, and Thailand, the direct medical costs of cervical cytology excluding laboratory transport and laboratory sample processing have been reported to be around \$2.34, \$2.67, \$3.65, \$16.27, and \$2.21, respectively. The costs for cytology test along with HPV DNA testing using Hybrid Capture 2 have been reported to be around \$4.22, \$5.60, \$6.21, \$21.21, and \$4.71 for India, Kenya, Peru, South Africa, and Thailand, respectively (Goldhaber-Fiebert et al., 2006). Recently, Ju-Fang Shi et al. estimated the costs of cervical cancer screening and diagnosis in China. Aggregated direct medical costs of screening were found to be around \$2.24, \$2.64, \$7.49, and \$7.95, respectively, for VIA, combined VIA/VILI, *care*HPV (self-sampling), and *care*HPV (clinician sampling). Moreover, the direct medical costs of diagnostic procedures were found to be around \$3.90, \$5.76, \$4.63, and \$10.6, respectively, for full colposcopy (with no biopsy), biopsy, endocervical curettage (ECC), and biopsy combined with ECC (Shi et al., 2012).

7.2 Treatment Strategy, Drug Targets, Targeted Therapy, and Pharmacogenomics

7.2.1 Treatment Strategy

Cervical cancer can be treated before it develops into a full-blown case when precancerous cells are detected through a cytological test. Precancerous cells of the cervix, often referred to as dysplasia, CIN, or carcinoma in situ (CIS), are treated by cryosurgery (freezing), laser treatment (high-energy light), and excision (surgical removal of the abnormal area) (Mann, 2012). Cryotherapy is a gynecological treatment used to freeze and destroy abnormal cervical cells and generally offers a safe treatment option for treating precancerous cervical

TABLE 7.4

Current Therapeutic Options and New Perspectives for Cervical Cancer Treatment

FIGO Stage	Current Therapeutic Options	New Perspectives
IA–IB1 IIA	S or RT	—
IB2 IIA	S + adjuvant RT CT (with cisplatin) + RT + adjuvant S	Neoadjuvant CT + S + RT Combination CT + RT Other CT agents[a] Biological agents[b]
IIB - IVA	CT (cisplatin) + RT	Neoadjuvant CT Combination CT + RT Other CT agents[a] Biological agents[b]
IVB	Palliative CT (cisplatin)	Combination CT Other CT agents[a] Biological agents[b]

Source: Daniela, B.C. et al., *Recent Pat. Anticancer. Drug. Discov.*, 4, 196, 2009.
S, surgery; RT, radiotherapy; CT, chemotherapy.
[a] Including carboplatin, nedaplatin, paclitaxel, gemcitabine, capecitabine, vinorelbine, ifosfamide, and topotecan.
[b] Including cetuximab, bevacizumab, erlotinib, gefitinib, lapatinib, sorafenib, and celecoxib.

lesions (Jacob et al., 2005). Lack of tissue specimen as well as ability to tailor the treatment to the size of the lesion remains a major disadvantage of cryotherapy. Neoadjuvant chemotherapy involving administration of anticancer drug to shrink the tumor before surgery is usually performed for early-stage or locally advanced cervical cancer (Rydzewska et al., 2010; Yin et al., 2011). Randomized trials have suggested use of chemotherapy prior to radical hysterectomy and radiation therapy (Bloss et al., 1993). However, in locally advanced disease, radiotherapy alone fails to control progression of cervical cancer. So, adjuvant cisplatin-based chemotherapy for patients undergoing radiotherapy is commonly practiced (Lee et al., 2012). Table 7.4 summarizes the current therapeutic options and the new perspectives for cervical cancer treatment according to FIGO stage.

In developing countries, diagnosis and treatment are done mostly by methods like cone biopsy and hysterectomy but are associated with a lot of complications and side effects that put women at risk. Moreover, these procedures require sophisticated infrastructure and are costly. Excision methods like LEEP and cryotherapy have advantages as these provide tissue specimen for histological observation that decreases the possibility of overlooking invasive cancer. Besides, these procedures are cost effective and lack side effects (Bishop et al., 1996).

7.2.2 Targeted Therapy

Conventional chemotherapy targets more differentiated and proliferating cancer cells. However, insufficient accumulation of the chemotherapeutic drug at the tumor region decreases its SP and increases the drug-associated side effects. Thus, there is a need to discover and design improved treatment strategies that would concentrate the drug at the specific tumor site, thereby, increasing the drug efficacy and reducing the associated adverse systemic effects.

Targeted therapy refers to a new generation of cancer drugs designed to interfere with a specific downstream protein or a metabolite that is believed to have a critical role in tumor

TABLE 7.5

Emerging Therapeutic Agents for Cervical Cancer

Molecular Targets	Antibody/Inhibitors	References
EGFR	Cetuximab (antibody)	Bellone et al. (2007)
	Gefitinib (inhibitor)	Goncalves et al. (2008)
	Erlotinib (inhibitor)	Nogueria-Rodrigues et al. (2008)
	Lapatinib (inhibitor)	Monk et al. (2010)
	Pazopanib (inhibitor)	Schutz et al. (2011)
VEGF	Bevacizumab (antibody)	Monk et al. (2009)
HSP90	Geldanamycin derivatives (17-DMAG), (17-AAG) (inhibitor)	Kummar et al. (2010)
CDKs	Roscovitine (inhibitor)	Vitali et al. (2002)

growth or progression (Coelho et al., 2007). In the last decade, increasing knowledge of the molecular pathways underlying the development of cervical carcinogenesis has led to the development of targeted agents for both diagnostic and therapeutic purposes (Zagouri et al., 2012). All the targeted anticancer drugs in the clinic and in development are either antibodies against the extracellular domains of growth factor receptors or enzyme inhibitors that target either the tyrosine kinase domains of receptors or intracellular protein tyrosine kinase (Arora et al., 2005). A number of reports have suggested the targeting of epidermal growth factor receptor (EGFR) and vascular endothelial growth factor (VEGF), heat shock protein (HSP90), and cyclin-dependent kinases (CDKs) (Table 7.5). The drugs that are commonly used or are under development for the targeted therapies include cetuximab (an anti-EGFR antibody) (Bellone et al., 2007); bevacizumab (an anti-VEGF antibody) (Monk et al., 2009); and gefitinib, erlotinib, lapatinib, and pazopanib (drugs targeting EGFR) (Goncalves et al., 2008; Nogueria-Rodrigues et al., 2008; Monk et al., 2010; Schutz et al., 2011). Furthermore, geldanamycin (HSP90 inhibitor) (Kummar et al., 2010) and roscovitine (CDK inhibitor) (Vitali et al., 2002) could also be promising drugs for targeting cervical cancer.

7.2.3 Pharmacogenomics

The evolving field of cancer pharmacogenomics uses genetic profiling to predict the response of the tumor as well as the normal tissue to therapy. The narrow therapeutic index and heterogeneity of patient responses to chemotherapy and radiotherapy imply that the efficacy of these treatments could be enhanced by understanding the genetic basis of interindividual differences. The cytotoxicity associated with chemotherapy and radiotherapy is largely related to their ability to induce DNA damage. The ability of cancer cells to recognize and repair this damage contributes to therapeutic resistance (Gossage and Madhusudan 2007). The goal of pharmacogenomics is to personalize the therapy based on an individual's genotype (Sauna et al., 2007). The promise of pharmacogenomics lies in maximizing the efficacy of a medical intervention while simultaneously minimizing the toxicity. Such approach is highly required in treatments due to the inherent toxicity of the drugs and the wide variability in individual responses (Desai et al., 2003). Genetic polymorphisms in drug-metabolizing enzymes, transporters, receptors, and other drug targets have been linked to interindividual differences in the efficacy and toxicity of many medications (William and Julie, 2001). Pharmacogenomic studies are rapidly elucidating the inherited nature of these differences in drug disposition and effects, thereby, enhancing drug discovery and providing a stronger scientific basis for optimizing drug therapy on the individual's genetic constitution (Evans and McLeod, 2003).

7.3 Invasive and Noninvasive Markers: Advantages and Disadvantages

Biomarkers/molecular markers are distinct biochemical indicators of normal biological or pathogenic processes or pharmacologic responses to a therapeutic intervention. A biomarker either might be a molecule secreted by a tumor or can be a specific response of the body to the presence of cancer. Biomarkers can be classified as invasive and noninvasive depending upon sampling technique. Invasive biomarkers are those that require sophisticated invasive interventions, whereas noninvasive biomarkers would be easily obtained from the body fluids such as serum, urine, or saliva. Even though invasive biomarkers have high SP and SE, an invasive intervention in the body may lead to several side effects such as anxiety and discomfort, prolonged recovery time, and high follow-up costs (Schönhofer, 2006; Schönhofer et al., 2008). On the other hand, noninvasive biomarkers reduce anxiety and discomfort and increase accessibility for clinical tests.

7.4 Noninvasive Molecular Biomarkers

Noninvasive tumor biomarkers are proteins or enzymes produced and released either by tumor cells or by host cells and whose presence may be detected in the serum or other biological fluids (Sharma, 2009). In the recent past, a number of markers have been assayed in noninvasively collected biofluids; however, only few biomarkers are highly sensitive and specific for cervical cancer detection at present. Identifying the reliable marker has still been a major concern. Scientific efforts have been ongoing to determine new prognostic indicators and tumor markers for cervical cancer. Integrated genomic, transcriptomic, proteomic, and epigenomic approaches provide platforms for the discovery of novel biomarkers. This would not only help in early detection and diagnosis of cervical cancer but would also help the oncologists to delineate the patients that need aggressive adjuvant, neoadjuvant, or combination therapy.

7.4.1 Serum Biomarkers

The ideal tumor marker should be secreted into the circulation in concentrations proportional to tumor burden and activity with a high SE and a high SP, in order to discriminate cancer patients from healthy subjects or patients with benign conditions (Lague et al., 2012). Several studies have suggested a positive correlationship between serum levels of squamous cell carcinoma antigen (SCC-Ag), cancer antigen (CA125), and cytokeratin fragments (CYFRA21-1), with tumor characteristics and outcome of the disease (Molina et al., 2005). These could be used as biomarkers in screening as well as evaluation of therapeutic response in cervical cancer. Here, we have addressed a few important serum markers that could be used for the effective diagnosis of cervical cancer.

7.4.1.1 Genetic Biomarkers

Carcinogenesis is a genetic disease initiated by alterations in genes, such as oncogenes and tumor suppressor genes that regulate cell proliferation, survival, and other homeostasis functions. Genetic gain and loss, that is, change in gene dosage, are predominantly responsible for oncogenic transformation. Identifying these defects could lead to early diagnosis and improved therapeutics. Recent advances in high-throughput genomics and the application of integrative approaches have accelerated gene discovery, thereby, facilitating the identification of molecular targets. Various studies have investigated genomic alterations in cervical cancer by means of metaphase comparative genomic hybridization (mCGH) and microsatellite marker analysis for the detection of loss of heterozygosity (LOH). Currently, high-throughput methods such as array comparative genomic hybridization (array CGH), single-nucleotide polymorphism array (SNP array), and gene expression arrays are available to study genome-wide alterations (Kloth et al., 2007).

7.4.1.1.1 Microsatellite Instability

Microsatellites are DNA sequences, wherein a short motif of around 1–5 nucleotides is tandemly repeated 10–100 times. Microsatellites are prone to mutations during replication due to transient split of the two helical strands and slippage of the DNA polymerase complex at reannealing, which generates either an insertion or a deletion loop depending on slippage direction (Jensen et al., 2009). Unless such a mismatch is corrected, the loss or gain of repeated units on the daughter strand results in length variation termed microsatellite instability (MSI). LOH as well as mutations within several proto-oncogenes can lead to MSI (Aaltonen et al., 1994). In one of the studies, MSI and cervical cancer association have been reported in Polish cervical cancer patients, wherein the MSI was observed in around 12.6% patients (Baay et al., 2009).

7.4.1.1.2 TNC, NCL, and ENO2

Sheng Jie et al. conducted a pilot study on 24 early-stage cervical cancer patients and 18 healthy controls to identify molecular biomarkers for cervical cancer in peripheral blood lymphocytes by using oligonucleotide microarrays. The expression of three genes, Tenascin-c (TNC), Nucleolin (NCL), and Enolase (ENO2), was found to be upregulated in patients with cervical cancer compared to that of healthy controls. The authors concluded that these genes may provide a promising and noninvasive method for the diagnosis of cervical cancer (Sheng and Zhang, 2010).

7.4.1.2 Epigenetic Markers

Epigenetics is described as a heritable change in gene expression without an alteration in the DNA sequence. DNA methylation and histone modification are the most important epigenetic changes that modulate gene expression (Vaissière et al., 2008). The advanced studies in the role of epigenetics in cancer have led to a strong focus on methylation markers. Methylation of CpG sites within the genome occurs at varying levels during cancer (Bell and Spector, 2011). While tumors are often hypomethylated in repetitive regions of DNA, promoter regions of tumor suppressor genes may become hypermethylated, frequently leading to decreased expression of important regulatory proteins (Jones and Baylin, 2002). DNA methylation could be a clinically useful biomarker to study changes in methylation patterns that occur early in the process of carcinogenesis. Over the last decade, a large variety of biomarkers have been investigated for the early detection of cervical cancer. Surprisingly, most of these markers have not yet come into the clinical application; the reason could be the presence of less and inconsistent data about the specific marker. Although methylation markers for cervical cancer screening have been analyzed in multiple studies (Feng et al., 2005; Niyazi et al., 2012), they have yet not come into use in the clinical domain. Thus, DNA methylation markers with high SE and SP are urgently needed to improve current population-based screening of premalignant cervical neoplasia. The availability of next-generation sequencing technology has recently allowed the survey of genome-wide epigenetic variations at a high resolution (Harris, 2010).

7.4.1.2.1 CDH1 and CDH13

Cadherins are transmembrane glycoproteins that interact with catenins for intercellular adhesion (Carien et al., 2011). Inactivation of cadherins due to methylation has been found to be associated with cervical cancer. Clinical utility of E-cadherin (CDH1) and H-cadherin (CDH13) was evaluated by Abida Abudukadeer et al. by investigating their DNA methylation status in serum samples of 49 cervical cancer patients and 40 patients with diseases other than cancer. Both these markers had low diagnostic SP and SE. The DNA methylation frequency of CDH1 and CDH13 in serum samples from cervical cancer patients was 55% and 10%, respectively. The multivariate analysis of the samples suggested that serum CDH1 methylation-positive patients were at a high risk (7.8-fold) of death, thereby suggesting importance of CDH1 methylation analysis in serum as a prognostic marker for cervical cancer patients (Abudukadeer et al., 2012).

7.4.1.2.2 DAPK, p16, and MGMT

Yang et al. investigated the frequency of promoter methylation of death-associated protein kinase (DAPK), p16, and O-6-methylguanine-DNAmethyltransferase (MGMT) genes in 40 pretreatment plasma samples of cervical cancers using methylation-specific polymerase chain reaction (MSP). Methylation frequency of DAPK, p16, and MGMT genes was found to be around 40%, 10%, and 7.5%, respectively. Moreover, in 55% (22/40) of cases, at least one of the three methylated genes was detected. Detection of the methylated genes in the circulation suggests that plasma DNA methylation could be used as a prognostic tool for studying the biomarkers (Yang et al., 2004).

7.4.1.2.3 CALCA, hTERT, MYOD1, PGR, and TIMP3

Widschwendter et al. investigated the methylation frequency of calcitonin-related polypeptide alpha (CALCA), human telomerase reverse transcriptase (hTERT), myoblast determination protein (MYOD1), progesterone receptor (PGR), and tissue inhibitor of metalloproteinases (TIMP3) in serum samples from 93 cervical cancer patients and 19 corresponding tissue samples using the MethyLight technique. They found that CALCA, hTERT, MYOD1, PGR, and TIMP3 were frequently methylated in both serum and tumor samples of cervical cancer patients. Methylation of PGR and MYOD1 was detected most frequently in all the investigated samples. Interestingly, in all the serum samples from the patients with grade 3 carcinoma, at least one gene was methylated (Widschwendter et al., 2004). Table 7.6 represents the methylation marker genes that have been studied in cervical cancer along with their function and chromosome location.

7.4.1.3 Proteomic Markers

Proteomics is the study of protein expression in tissue or biological fluids. It employs protein microarrays, electrophoresis, and mass spectrometry for the identification and characterization of proteins for biomarker development, target validation, diagnosis, prognosis, and optimization of treatment in medical care, especially in the field of clinical oncology. Proteomic technologies such as matrix-assisted laser desorption/ionization (MALDI) and surface-enhanced laser desorption/ionization–time-of-flight mass spectrometry (SELDI–TOFMS) have recently been developed that use the pattern of proteins within a clinical sample as a diagnostic fingerprint (Conrads et al., 2003).

TABLE 7.6

Methylation Markers Studied in Cervical Cancer

Gene Symbol	Gene Name	Function	Chromosome Location	Reference
APC	Adenomatous polyposis coli	Cell cycle arrest	5q21-q22	Reesink-Peters et al. (2004)
CADM1	Cell adhesion molecule 1	Cell recognition	11q22.3-23.2	Overmeer (2008)
CDH1	Cadherin 1, type 1, E-cadherin (epithelial)	Cell–cell signaling	16q22.1	Abida Abudukadeer et al. (2012)
CDH13	Cadherin 13, H-cadherin (heart)	Negative regulation of cell proliferation	16q24.2-q24.3	Abida Abudukadeer et al. (2012)
CDKN2A	Cyclin-dependent kinase inhibitor 2A (melanoma, p16, inhibits CDK4)	Cell cycle arrest	9p21	Yang et al. (2004)
DAPK1	Death-associated protein kinase 1	Induction of apoptosis by extracellular signals	9q34.1	Yang et al. (2004)
FHIT	Fragile histidine triad protein	Nucleotide metabolic process	3p14.2	Neyaz et al. (2008)
GSTP1	Glutathione S-transferase pi gene	Antiapoptosis	11q13	Pongtheerat et al. (2011)
HIC-1	Hypermethylated in cancer 1	Regulation of transcription, DNA dependent	17p13.3	Reesink-Peters et al. (2004)
MGMT	O-6-methylguanine-DNA methyltransferase	DNA ligation	10q26	Yang et al. (2004)
MLH1	Human mutL homolog 1	Mismatch repair	3p21.3	Wentzensen et al. (2009)
RARB	Retinoic acid receptor, beta	Signal transduction	3p24.2	Narayan et al. (2003)
RASSF1	Ras association domain-containing protein 1	Protein binding	3p21.31	Neyaz et al. (2008)
TERT	Telomerase reverse transcriptase	Telomere maintenance	5p15.33	Widschwendter et al. (2004)
TIMP3	TIMP metallopeptidase inhibitor 3	Transmembrane receptor protein tyrosine kinase signaling pathway	22q12.1-q13.2	Widschwendter et al. (2004)

7.4.1.3.1 *Squamous Cell Carcinoma Antigen*

SCC accounts for 80%–90% of cervical cancers, and thus its detection becomes important (Saonere, 2010). SCC-Ag, a subfraction of the glycoprotein TA-4, isolated from squamous cell cervical cancer tissues, is the most commonly used serum marker for clinical monitoring of SCC. Due to its higher SP and SE, serum SCC is useful in monitoring the early recurrence after treatment (Yoon et al., 2010). Esajas MD et al. analyzed the follow-up data of 225 patients with early-stage squamous cell cervical cancer treated with radical hysterectomy and pelvic lymphadenectomy with or without radiotherapy. Recurrent disease occurred in 35 (16%) out of 225 patients and was accompanied by an elevated serum SCC-Ag levels (SE, 74%). SCC-Ag analysis was able to detect early recurrence in a small proportion (14%) of patients (Esajas et al., 2001). Reesink-Peters et al. analyzed the utility of serum SCC-Ag as a preoperative marker to identify the early-stage cervical cancer patients with a low likelihood for adjuvant radiotherapy. The preoperative elevated level of SCC-Ag in 57% of IB1 and 74% of IB2/IIA squamous cell cervical cancers indicated for adjuvant radiotherapy compared to the normal SCC-Ag levels in 16% of IB1 and 29% of IB2/IIA patients (Reesink-Peters et al., 2005).

To increase the SE of SCC-Ag detection in patients with SCC, other markers have been evaluated, however, with contradictory results. Molina R et al. analyzed the serum levels of cytokeratin fragment (CYFRA 21.1), carcinoembryonic Ag (CEA), and SCC-Ag in 156 patients diagnosed with carcinoma of the uterine cervix. Histology revealed SSC in 119 patients, AC in 25 patients, and adenosquamous carcinoma in the remaining 12 patients. The SE of CYFRA 21.1, CEA, and SCC-Ag was 26%, 25%, and 43%, respectively, at diagnosis. The level of SSC-Ag was found to be higher in squamous tumors. The authors stated that the SCC-Ag alone was a sensitive marker for tumor with SSC histology, whereas addition of CYFRA 21.1 and CEA did not enhance its SE (Molina et al., 2005).

7.4.1.3.2 *Cytokeratin Fragment CYFRA 21.1*

CYFRA 21.1 is a tumor marker that measures the cytokeratin 19 fragment (Molina et al., 2005). Serum CYFRA 21.1 was reported to be significantly higher in stage IIb–IV as compared to stage Ib–IIa disease (Gaarenstroom et al., 1995). Serum CYFRA 21.1 assay was found to be positive in 20.0% of patients with CIN, 41.7% of patients with SSC, 62.5% of patients with AC, 45.8% of patients with endometrial cancer, and only 13% of patients with benign uterine diseases, thereby, suggesting a positive association of antigen levels with the tumor stage (Ferdeghini et al., 1993).

In another study, including 79 patients, positive SCC-Ag and negative CYFRA 21.1 (cutoff = 1.1 ng/mL) assays were found in 22.8% of the cases, and the inverse was observed in 11.4% cases. A positive or negative concordance between serum SCC-Ag and CYFRA 21.1 was found in 65.8%. The mean concentrations of SCC-Ag and CYFRA 21.1 were related to the stage of the cancer with CYFRA 21.1 being elevated in 100% of stage III–IV tumors (Callet et al., 1998).

7.4.1.3.3 *Insulin-Like Growth Factor*

Overexpression of growth factors and/or their receptors is a hallmark of malignancy (Yang et al., 2011). Insulin-like growth factor II (IGF-II) is an important regulator of tumor growth in many solid tumors (Fiore et al., 2010). Mathur et al. measured serum IGF-II levels in 20 controls, 26 CIN lesion positive, and 12 cervical cancer patients. The IGF-II level was elevated in cervical cancer and in advanced CIN stage and was similar to that of control group in CIN I stage (Mathur et al., 2000). Further work by the same group suggested the importance of serum vascular endothelial growth factor C (VEGF-C) as a unique marker for the early diagnosis of cervical cancer metastasis. VEGF-C positively correlated with IGF-II levels and negatively correlated with IGF-binding protein 3 (IGF-BP3) (Mathur et al., 2005), thus suggesting the use of serum IGF-BP3, VEGF-C, and IGF-II as early diagnosis markers and for predicting better prognosis (Mathur et al., 2000, 2003, 2005).

7.4.1.3.4 *MCM5 and MCM7*

Minichromosome maintenance proteins (MCM5 and MCM7), which belong to helicase family, function in the early stages of DNA replication and have been found to be evolutionarily conserved in all the eukaryotes. They are essential for initiating eukaryotic DNA replication and serve as useful markers for proliferating cells (Rodins et al., 2002).

Studies have shown that the MCM proteins, particularly MCM5, stain abnormal cells in cervical smears and sections with remarkably high SP and SE that could be useful for the detection of cervical cancer (Williams et al., 1998). It has been shown that MCM5 could detect HSIL with high SE (100%) and SP (67%) (Douglas et al., 2005).

7.4.1.4 Metabolomic Markers

The study of different patterns of metabolites within living organisms is known as metabolomics. Metabolites are stable, measurable entities in biological fluids, and their levels could reflect the response of biological systems to genetic or environmental stimuli (Carsten et al., 2006). An advantage of the metabolomic approach in the identification of novel biomarkers is that it encompasses cellular integration of the transcriptome, proteome, and interactome. For example, in many tumors, increased glucose utilization is a predominant and fundamental alteration in metabolism (Narayan et al., 2010). The mutations at the genetic level in the mitochondrial DNA result in functional impairment, upregulation of glycolysis, and enhanced expression of metabolic enzymes (Narayan et al., 2010). Metabolomics, when used as a translational research tool, can provide a link between the laboratory and clinic, particularly because metabolic and molecular imaging technologies enable the discrimination of metabolic markers noninvasively in vivo (Spratlin et al., 2009). The most common analytical technologies such as chromatographic separation (gas chromatography, liquid chromatography [LC], and capillary electrophoresis), followed by sensitive mass spectrometric detection, gas chromatography–time-of-flight mass spectrometry (GC–TOFMS), have probably eased the chromatographic resolution, for detection and identification of metabolites even at less concentrations.

7.4.1.4.1 Tu M2-PK

Pyruvate kinase is a key enzyme in glycolysis that is expressed in different cell types (Mazurek, 2012). Tetrameric isoenzyme pyruvate kinase type M2 (M2-PK) is generally present in proliferating cells, which during tumor development is decomposed to dimeric form, Tu M2-PK. Overexpression of Tu M2-PK has been reported in various tumor cells and has also been reported to be released into body fluids (Mazurek, 2012). Thus, monitoring its level in the body fluids could be a useful marker for prognosis of cervical cancer. Babita Kaura et al. quantified the plasma levels for the presence of Tu M2-PK in 50 cervical carcinoma patients, 10 chronic cervicitis patients, and 10 healthy controls. The level of Tu M2-PK could discriminate malignant from nonmalignant condition with high SE (82%) and SP (60%) (Kaura et al., 2004). In another study, plasma samples of 116 cervical cancer patients were investigated for Tu M2-PK levels that correlated with the disease stage (Kuemmel et al., 2006), thereby indicating Tu M2-PK to be a potential metabolomic marker in cervical carcinoma.

7.4.1.5 Glycobiomarkers

Glycobiomarkers are sugar molecules that are an integral feature of nearly all biomolecules. Glycans are carbohydrate chains that modify a protein's surface and play a major role in protein function. Glycosylation is the most common posttranslational modification of secreted proteins and occurs during or after protein synthesis (Raman et al., 2005). The identification of novel serum glycobiomarkers has become a topic of increasing interest as the glycan-processing pathways are frequently disturbed in cancer cells (Arnold et al., 2008). The most common glyco-analytical techniques used for characterization of glycan structures are high-/ultra-performance liquid chromatography (HPLC/UPLC), mass spectrometry, capillary electrophoresis, and lectin arrays (Marino et al., 2010).

7.4.1.5.1 Sialic Acids

Sialic acids (SAs) are a family of nine-carbon acidic monosaccharides that occur naturally at the outermost ends of the oligosaccharide chains of glycoconjugates (mucins, glycoproteins, and glycolipids) (Lehmann et al., 2006). Altered glycoprotein and glycolipid structure due to sialylation of sugar chains on the surface of the cells has been suggested to be a very important process during cancer (Ugorski and Laskowska, 2002). Researchers have tried to evaluate the changes of SA levels in the blood and/or urine of patients with cervical cancers (Wang, 2006). Earlier studies reported increased SA levels in serum and urine samples of patients with early stages of cervical carcinoma. Glycocomponents of glycoproteins were found to increase with cancer progression (Balasubramaniyan et al., 1994). In one of the studies, significant elevation in the serum total sialic acid (TSA), lipid-bound sialic acid (LBSA), corrected lipid sialic acid (CLSA), and free-form sialic acid (FSA) has been found in cancer patients compared to that of normal controls (Lagana et al., 1995).

7.4.1.5.2 YKL-40

YKL-40, also referred to as human cartilage glycoprotein-39 (HC gp-39), is a secreted glycoprotein belonging to the family of mammalian chitinases (Junker et al., 2005). The protein is expressed in many types of cancer cells, and the highest plasma YKL-40 level has been found to be positively associated with metastatic disease, short recurrence/progression-free intervals, and short overall survival (Hogdall et al., 2009). Mitsuhashi A et al. demonstrated serum YKL-40 level in SCC and AC cervical cancer. Compared to other markers (SCC-Ag, CA 125, and CA19-9), YKL-40 has been found to be significantly detected in SCC. Thus, YKL-40 seems to be a sensitive serum marker for early-stage cervical cancer of both AC and SCC types (Mitsuhashi et al., 2009).

7.4.1.5.3 Osteopontin

Osteopontin (OPN) is a secreted, cytokine-like matrix-associated phosphoglycoprotein present in extracellular fluids, at sites of inflammation and in the extracellular matrix of mineralized tissues. Increased expression of OPN has been correlated with the invasive and metastasis stage of cervical cancer (Song et al., 2009). Cho et al. compared plasma OPN levels of 81 cervical cancer patients and 34 patients having CIS of the uterine cervix with those of 283 healthy women using sandwich enzyme-linked immunosorbent assay (ELISA). In women with cervical cancer, plasma OPN levels (mean 355.8 ng/mL) were significantly higher ($P < 0.001$) than those of women with CIS (mean 185 ng/mL) and healthy controls (mean 100 ng/mL). OPN had a moderate SE (50.6%) and high SP (95.0%) in detecting cervical cancer (Cho et al., 2008).

7.4.2 Liquid-Based Cytology Biomarkers

Liquid-based cytology (LBC) is the method to prepare thin layer of cervical cells on a microscope slide for diagnosis of cytological abnormalities. Introduction of LBC has contributed to mitigate the problem of efficiency in processing samples. Liquid-based collection and processing provide more representative cervical sampling than conventional smearing of the specimen on a glass slide. It has been shown to increase the detection rate of preneoplastic squamous intraepithelial lesions that is equal to or greater than the conventional Pap smear method.

7.4.2.1 Genetic Biomarker

In order to understand the importance of DNA ploidy in malignant progression of disease, Singh et al. correlated aneuploid DNA patterns in cytologically diagnosed cases of mild (79), moderate (36), and severe dysplasia (12) as well as *ASCUS* (57) along with control subjects (69). The data suggested that a progressive increase in aneuploidy associated with severity of the lesions, wherein 49.36% was found in mild dysplasia, 77.77% in moderate dysplasia, and 91.66% in severe dysplasia (Singh et al., 2008). These results suggest the significance of DNA aneuploidy as a prognostic marker in cervical malignancies.

7.4.2.1.1 HPV DNA and E6/E7 mRNA

Prolonged cervical infection with HR-HPV genotypes is associated with viral DNA integration, which is a major factor responsible for the development of the precancerous (CIN) and cancerous lesions (Bosch et al., 2000). The HPV genome comprises early genes and late genes. Early genes (E1, E2, E4, E5, E6, and E7) encode for nonstructural proteins that participate in cell transformation, DNA replication, transcriptional regulation, and virus assembly as well as release, whereas late genes, L1 (major) and L2 (minor), encode for viral capsid proteins (Figure 7.3) (Zheng and Baker, 2006). The integration of viral DNA into host genome results in loss of viral E2 gene function that regulates E6/E7 gene function.

Nearly all the cervical cancer cases test positive for HPV (Walboomers et al., 1999) whose DNA is the most popular and extensively investigated biomarker in the management of cervical neoplasia. HPV DNA testing in combination with primary screening has been reported to increase diagnosis efficiency (Naucler et al., 2007). Lazcano et al., in a community-based study on 50,159 Mexican women, demonstrated HR-HPV test to be highly sensitive as compared to cytology study. The SE and SP of HR-HPV test for detecting histologically confirmed CIN II/III+ cases were 93.3% and 89.2%, respectively (Lazcano et al., 2010). Recent study reported HPV testing to be more cost effective than Pap cytology for cervical cancer screening (Flores et al., 2011).

The E6 and E7 genes of HPV are known to play an important role in cervical carcinogenesis (Zur Hausen et al., 1974). The E6 oncoprotein degrades and inactivates the tumor suppressor protein p53 (Scheffner et al., 1990). On the other hand, E7 oncoprotein binds to

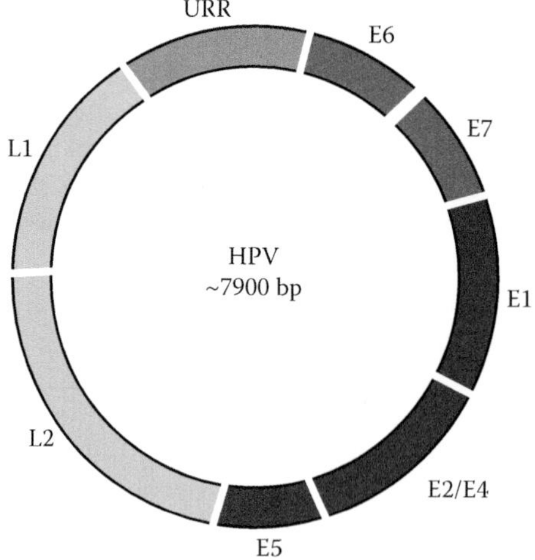

FIGURE 7.3
HPV genome showing early and late genes and upstream regulatory region (URR).

pRB and inhibits the formation of pRb–E2F complex, which regulates numerous cellular processes (Dyson et al., 1989). E6/E7 has been considered as a specific marker as it can be detected in both precancerous and milder lesions caused by HPV infection. Sorbye et al. demonstrated HPV E6/E7 mRNA testing to be more specific as compared to cytology test in postcolposcopy follow-up of women with negative cervical biopsy. The HPV mRNA test demonstrated 89.1% SE and 92.5% SP for detecting CIN of grade 2 (CIN II+) (Sorbye et al., 2011). Earlier, HPV fluorescence in situ hybridization (FISH) for E6/E7 mRNA demonstrated 83.3% SE and 91.3% SP for HSIL in 231 LBC samples (Narimatsu and Patterson, 2005). The detection of E6/E7 transcripts of HR-HPV types, thus, could serve as potential biomarkers for both detection of HSILs and progression of the cervical carcinoma.

7.4.2.1.2 Human Telomerase Gene

Invasive cervical carcinomas mostly carry extra copies of chromosome arm 3q, which results in gain of the human telomerase gene (TERC). Using a genomic probe for the TERC gene on chromosome band 3q26, it is possible to show the copy number increase of this locus and conversion of dysplastic lesions to invasive carcinomas, with gradual transition from ASCUS and CIN I to CIN II and CIN III. Kerstin et al. have reported that the detection of 3q gain and amplification of TERC in routinely collected Pap smears can help in identifying low-grade lesions with a high progression risk and in decreasing false-negative cytological screenings. They used FISH probe as a diagnostic tool for the direct detection of TERC gains in Pap smears. The results suggest that 3q gain is required for the transition from CIN I/CIN II to CIN III that predicted progression (Heselmeyer-Haddad et al., 2005).

7.4.2.2 Epigenetic Markers

7.4.2.2.1 APC, DAPK, MGMT, and GSTP1

Reesink-Peters et al. showed that cervical scrapings represent the hypermethylation status of underlying cervical epithelium for the tumor suppressor genes adenomatous polyposis coli (APC), DAPK, O-6-methylguanine-DNA methyltransferase (MGMT), and glutathione S-transferase pi (9GSTP1). All the scrapings obtained from cervical cancer patients as well as control groups were morphologically scored and analyzed with quantitative hypermethylation-specific polymerase chain reaction (QMSP) for all the four genes. It was found that methylated APC was detected in 26 (54%), DAPK in 35 (73%), MGMT in 5 (10%), and GSTP1 in 1 (2%) out of 48 cervical cancer scrapings. In 41 control scrapings, methylated APC was amplified in 16 (39%), DAPK in 2 (4.9%), MGMT in 6 (15%), and GSTP1 in none of the patients (Reesink-Peters et al., 2004). Thus, these genes could be used as epigenetic markers in cervical cancer scraping.

7.4.2.2.2 DAPK1 and IGSF4

Death-associated protein kinase 1 (DAPK1) is a calmodulin-regulated serine/threonine kinase and possesses apoptotic and tumor suppressor functions (Kuo et al., 2006). Immunoglobulin superfamily member 4 (IGSF4) has a key role in intercellular adhesion. It also serves as a cell surface recognition molecule involved in various cellular processes including morphogenesis, proliferation, differentiation, and migration (Watabe, 2003). Gustafson examined promoter methylation of 15 tumor suppressor genes in HSILs (n = 11), LSILs (n = 17), and negative tissues (n = 11) from LBC samples using multiplex, nested, MSP approach. Aberrant promoter methylation of DAPK1 and IGSF4 occurred at a high frequency in HSIL samples and was absent in LSIL and negative samples (Gustafson et al., 2004), thereby suggesting the two genes as biomarker for cervical cancer detection.

7.4.2.2.3 JAM3, TERT, EPB41L3, and C13ORF18

Eijsink et al. suggested a four-gene methylation marker panel as triage test in HR-HPV-positive patients. DNA methylation status of junctional adhesion molecule 3 (JAM3), telomerase reverse transcriptase (TERT), erythrocyte membrane protein band 4.1-like 3 (EPB41L3), and chromosome 13 open reading frame 18 (C13ORF18) in self-sampled cervicovaginal cells and cervical scrapings from 20 cervical cancer patients, followed by LBC, revealed that 95% (19/20) of the samples were positive for DNA methylation. Around 80% (12/15) of CIN II+ cervical scrapings were positive for DNA methylation and negative (0/8) for CIN0/1 cervical specimens (Eijsink et al., 2011).

7.4.2.2.4 DBC1, PDE8B, and ZNF582

Recently, Huang et al. analyzed the methylation profiles of deleted in bladder cancer protein 1 (DBC1), phosphodiesterase 8B (PDE8B), and zinc finger protein 582 (ZNF582) in human cervical carcinomas and normal cervix samples obtained from cervical scrapings of patients with different severities. DBC1, PDE8B, and ZNF582 were methylated in 93%, 29%, and 100% of cervical scrapings, respectively. Methylation frequency of DBC1 and ZNF582 in cervical scraping significantly correlated with the disease severity. The study further demonstrated ZNF582 as a potential biomarker for the detection of CIN III and worse lesion (Huang et al., 2012).

7.4.2.2.5 CCNA1 and C13ORF18

Methylation analysis of five markers that include C13ORF18, CCNA1 (cyclin A1), tissue factor pathway inhibitor 2 (TFPI-2), chromosome 10 open reading frame 166 (C13ORF166), and neuronal pentraxin-1 (NPTX1) showed that CCNA1 and C13ORF18 were frequently methylated in cervical scrapings from cancer patients (68/97). Methylation frequency for CCNA1 was found to be around 4.6%, 2.4%, 18.6%, and 51.1%, respectively, in CIN 0, CIN I, CIN II, and CIN III, whereas for C13ORF18, it was found to be around 18.6% and 51.1% in CIN II and CIN III, respectively, and nil in CIN 0 and CIN I. Both had low SE (37%) but high SP (96% for CCNA1 and 100% for C13ORF18) in CIN II+ with a positive predictive value (PPV) of 92% for CCNA1 and 100% for C13ORF18. Since these markers are strongly associated with high-grade cervical intraepithelial lesion and cervical cancer, they can be used for direct referral to gynecologists for evaluation in patients (Yang et al., 2009).

7.4.2.3 Proteomic Biomarkers

7.4.2.3.1 Ki-67

Ki-67 is a proliferation marker and is known as a predictive factor for tumor development. It is a nuclear antigen (associated with hetero- and euchromatin) that is expressed during all the active phases of the cell cycle (G1, S, G2, and M) except G0 (Ancuţa et al., 2009). The level of Ki-67 expression is used to determine the cell proliferation status. In a study on 147 patients, Sahebali et al. detected the expression of Ki-67 in cytological lesions by immunocytochemistry. A significantly higher number of Ki-67 immunopositive cells were found in the HSIL group compared with the other groups. Moreover, Ki-67 immunopositive cells were significantly associated with HPV 16-positive samples than in other HR-type samples. Thus, Ki-67 can be used as a cytology marker together with the routinely used LBC to identify HSIL and as a surrogate marker for HPV 16 infection (Sahebali et al., 2003). In another set of experiments, Dunton performed cytological screening in 101 patients with ASCUS and LSIL. Ki-67 was detected in high-grade CIN with an SE of 96%, SP of 67%, PPV of 49%, and NPV of 98% (Dunton et al., 2006) (Table 7.7).

TABLE 7.7

Specificity, Sensitivity, PPV, and NPV of Cytology Markers for Diagnosis of CIN II+

Markers	Detection	SP (%)	SE (%)	PPV (%)	NPV (%)	References
p16	Immunostaining	68.6	87.5	38.9	96	Ma et al. (2011)
Ki-67	Immunostaining	67	96	49	98	Dunton et al. (2006)
p16/Ki-67	Immunostaining	80.6	92.2	—	—	Schmidt et al. (2011)
ProExC	Immunostaining	82.4	98.8	—	—	Siddiqui et al. (2008)

7.4.2.3.2 p16

p16^{INK4a} is a tumor suppressor protein and a CDK inhibitor that is often inactivated in many cancers due to genetic deletion or hypermethylation (Liggett and Sidransky, 1998). Its overexpression is often associated with progression toward cervical carcinogenesis. p16^{INK4a} has been considered to be a possible diagnostic marker for cervical cancer. A number of studies have demonstrated overexpression of p16 in HSILs (Doeberitz, 2002; Bleotu et al., 2009). Hu et al. (2005) suggested p16 negative expression in cervicitis (inflammation) and squamous metaplastic epithelium (noncancerous). Horn et al. (2006) suggested predominant cytoplasm localization of p16 to be related with increasing histological grade of cervical lesion. Reports on immunohistochemical analysis of p16 have considered it as a powerful tool in the identification of HPV-mediated premalignant and malignant lesions of the uterine cervix. Yıldız et al. (2007) showed HR-HPV-positive cases to be p16 positive with no statistically significant relationship between HPV infection and the intensity and distribution of p16. A meta-analysis study performed by Tsoumpou I et al., which included 61 independent studies, demonstrated increase in p16^{INK4a} expression with severity of cytological abnormality. p16^{INK4a} expression was positive in 12% of normal smears as compared to 45% of ASCUS and LSIL and 89% of HSIL smears (Tsoumpou et al., 2009). Ma Yuan-Ying reported that p16 expression can help in predicting CIN II+ in ASCUS with high SE (87.5%), SP (68.6%), PPV (38.9%), NPV (96.0%), and accuracy (72.1%). Similarly, p16 expression could also help in predicting LSIL with high SE, SP, PPV, NPV, and accuracy (Ma et al., 2011) (Table 7.7).

7.4.2.3.3 TOPO2A and MCM2

DNA topoisomerase encoded by gene topoisomerase II-alpha (TOPO2A) is an enzyme that unwinds and decatenates DNA for replication, transcription, chromosome segregation, and cell cycle progression. Minichromosome maintenance protein-2 (MCM2) is a marker of cell proliferation in high-grade cervical dysplasia and carcinoma (Murphy et al., 2005). BD ProExC (ProExC) is a recently developed immunocytochemical assay that targets the expression of TOP2A and MCM2, two genes shown to be overexpressed in cervical cancers. Studies performed using ProExC on thin-layer cytology specimens have demonstrated that the ProExC test can efficiently differentiate between normal lesion and HSIL.

Kelly et al. used ProExC in 317 residual cytology samples to detect HSIL wherein it showed an SE of 85.3%, SP of 71.7%, PPV of 44.6%, and NPV of 94.8% (Kelly et al., 2006). In another study, ProExC staining was performed on 100 Atypical Squamous cells, cannot exclude high-grade squamous intraepithelial lesion (ASC-H) specimens, and results were compared with HR-HPV status. It was found that BD ProExC could detect CIN II+ in patients with ASC-H with a high SE (98.8%) and SP (82.4%) compared to Digene Hybrid Capture II HPV DNA Testing (SE 71.1% and SP 64.7%) (Siddiqui et al., 2008) (Table 7.7). The same group evaluated the utility of ProExC as a marker for HSIL CIN II+ and compared with HR-HPV status in Pap tests with ASCUS cytology. A study on 200 ASCUS patients showed that ProExC could detect CIN II+ with 98.04% SE and 74.50% SP (Siddiqui et al., 2008).

Another study on 624 cervical cytology samples showed that ProExC detected CIN II+/HSIL stage with high SP (84%) and SE (92%) (Tambouret et al., 2008). Depuydt et al. (2011) suggested that BD ProExC could be used as an adjunct molecular marker to improve the detection of CIN II+ in HPV screening.

7.4.2.3.4 Markers Tested in Combination (p16/Ki-67, p16/ProExC Dual Stain)

Several studies have reported the use of more than one biomarker in the same sample wherein p16, Ki-67, and ProExC have been used. In the recent years, several research groups have relied on p16/Ki-67 in immune-quantitative analysis of CIN II+ and CIN III+ grades. Petry et al. (2011), in 425 women with Pap-negative/HPV-positive test, performed p16/Ki-67 dual-stained cytology and correlated its expression with the presence of CIN II+ grade. They found that 108 (25.4%) Pap-negative/HPV-positive cases showed positive expression of p16/Ki-67 at baseline. The test could detect CIN II+ and CIN III+ in Pap-negative/HPV-positive cases with high SE (91.9% and 96.4%, respectively) and SP (82.1% and 76.9%, respectively) (Petry et al., 2011). In a study on 69 women, Yoshida et al. (2011) evaluated the utility of p16/Ki-67 for diagnosis of HPV-related cervical lesions for p16 and Ki-67 and found that the marker showed a significant correlation with HPV 16 compared to the lesser degree lesions.

In another LBC study on residual material from 776 retrospectively collected ASCUS/LSIL cases, p16/Ki-67 dual-stained cytology had a high SE of 92.2% (ASCUS) and 94.2% (LSIL) to confirm CIN II+ biopsy with SP rates of 80.6% (ASCUS) and 68.0% (LSIL) (Table 7.7). Figure 7.4 shows a representative study depicting the results of p16/Ki-67 dual-stained cytology, characterized by a brown cytoplasmic signal for p16 overexpression and a red nuclear signal for Ki-67 expression within the same cell. Positive cytology test results are shown for cells categorized as ASCUS, LSIL, and HSIL (Schmidt et al., 2011). Recently, Wentzensen et al. investigated utility of p16/Ki-67 immunostaining in the LBC samples of 625 women that had previously undergone colposcopy. The expression of p16/Ki-67 was positively associated with severity of histology with 26.8% in normal histology, 46.5% in CIN I, 82.8% in CIN II, and 92.8% in CIN III. p16/Ki-67 expression was highly associated with the HPV infection showing 100% positive expression in HPV 16-positive cases and 77.8% in HPV 16-negative infection. The p16/Ki-67 immunostaining had high SE (90.6%) and SP (48.6%) to detect CIN III in women with HR-HPV-positive ASCUS and LSIL (Wentzensen et al., 2012).

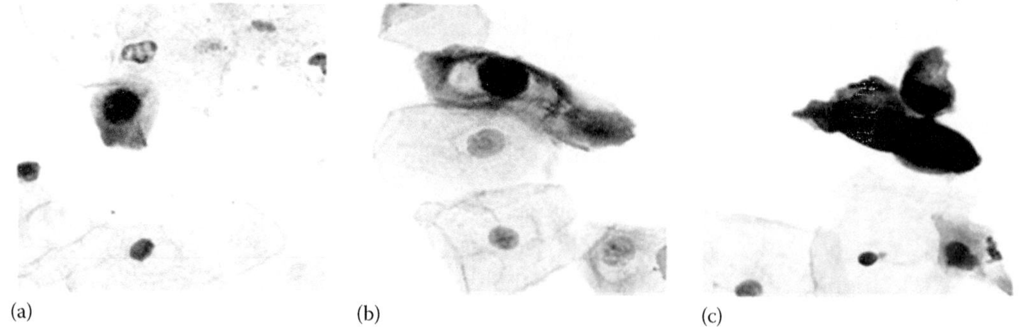

FIGURE 7.4
p16/Ki-67 dual-stained cytology. p16/Ki-67 dual-stained cytology, characterized by a brown cytoplasmic signal for p16 overexpression and a red nuclear signal for Ki-67 expression within the same cell. Positive cytology test results are shown for cells categorized as (a) ASCUS, (b) LSIL, and (c) HSIL. (From Schmidt, D. et al., *Cancer Cytopathol.*, 25, 119(3), 158(166), 2011.)

In a cohort of 469 women, 56% were positive for the dual stain with the SP of 51.3% in CIN II+ and 48.2% in CIN III+ patients (Waldstrøm et al., 2012). Donà et al. (2012) have also suggested the clinical utility of p16/Ki-67 in HR-HPV infection, particularly with HPV 16 and HPV 18. Sahebali et al. examined 500 LBC slides and found that Ki-67 occasionally stained normal proliferating cells, but that these cells were negative for p16. On the other hand, immunoreactivity for $p16^{INK4a}$ was seen in squamous metaplasia but not with Ki-67. The p16 and Ki-67 immunoreactive cells were high in HSIL compared to other cytological categories (Sahebali et al., 2006). Yimin et al. performed immunohistochemical stains for p16 and ProExC on 25 Pap specimens with menstrual contamination. HSIL cases expressed strong, diffused staining pattern for p16 and ProExC whereas LSIL cases expressed focal staining for p16 and were negative for ProExC. Further, the SE of p16 and ProExC was high for identifying significant lesions in Pap specimens with menstrual contamination (Yimin et al., 2012).

7.5 Imaging Biomarkers

Cervical cancer is a clinically staged disease where both invasive and noninvasive markers could be used for early detection of the cancer. Besides these, there are imaging technologies that could detect the cancer at an early stage and thus continue to reduce the incidence rates. Imaging markers such as lymphangiography (LA), ultrasonography (US), computed tomography (CT), magnetic resonance imaging (MRI), and positron-emission tomography (PET) are being routinely used for the diagnosis of cervical cancer at different stages (Table 7.8).

Recently, novel imaging techniques such as dynamic contrast-enhanced magnetic resonance imaging (DCE-MRI), diffusion-weighted MRI (DW-MRI), magnetic resonance spectroscopy (MRS), and F-18-fluorodeoxyglucose positron-emission tomography (FDG-PET) have come up that may help in characterizing biological specimens at the cellular level, thus providing molecular and metabolic information of the samples. These techniques could help in discovering early tumor biomarkers for deciding the therapeutic options (Harry, 2010). However, these techniques have not yet been explored in gynecological malignancies, but preliminary reports highlight their potential. In an effort to enhance the effectiveness of colposcopy and improve detection of cervical cancer at an early stage,

TABLE 7.8

Comparison of Diagnostic Ability of Different Imaging Tests

Detectable Diagnostic and Prognostic Features	LA	US	CT	MRI	PET
Depth and width of invasion				+	
Tumor size		+	+	+	+
Extension into parametria			+	+	
Extension into the vagina			+	+	+
Invasion of the bladder or rectum			+	+	
Metastases to distant organs			+	+	+
Lymph node metastasis	+		+	+	+
Intratumoral oxygenation				+	+
Tumor vascularity				+	+

Luma cervical imaging system (MediSpectra, Inc., Lexington, MA) was developed that is the first Food and Drug Administration (FDA)-approved optical detection system. It has been proposed to be used as an adjunct to colposcopy to identify areas of the cervix with the highest likelihood of high-grade CIN (Kendrick et al., 2007). The Luma system shines a light on the cervix and analyzes how different areas of the cervix respond to the light. The system produces a color map that distinguishes between healthy and potentially diseased tissues to indicate where from the biopsy samples should be taken (James et al., 2007). Another imaging system, LightTouch technology (Guided Therapeutics, Inc.), systematically and rapidly scans the cervix to identify cancer and precancer painlessly and noninvasively by analyzing the wavelengths of light reflected from cervical tissue. The technology distinguishes between normal and diseased tissues by detecting biochemical and morphological changes at the cellular level. Unlike Pap or HPV test, the LightTouch test does not require a tissue sample or laboratory analysis and is designed to provide results immediately that would save not only time but money as well (Vlaicu, 2009). The Resolve laboratory testing kit (Gynecor, Glen Allen, VA) is a new colposcopic method that uses cytobrush to obtain endocervical samples. However, there is not much evidence that is available on the effectiveness of the Resolve laboratory testing kit for cervical cancer screening or diagnosis.

7.6 Integrative Omics-Based Molecular Markers for Early Diagnosis, Prognosis, and Therapy

The early detection and accurate prediction of tumor evolution are one of the biggest challenges for clinical oncology of the disease. The recent concept of an *integrative omics model* that includes genomics, proteomics, transcriptomics, and metabolomics has accelerated the biomarker discovery for early diagnosis of human cancers (Zhang et al., 2007). The field of genomics includes the study of total analyses of DNA sequence changes, copy number aberrations, chromosomal rearrangements, and modifications in DNA methylation. It also helps in prospective identification of the candidate genes. A number of studies have investigated genomic alterations in cervical cancer mainly by means of mCGH and microsatellite marker analysis for the detection of LOH (Kersemaekers et al., 1999; Nishimura et al., 2000; Melsheimer et al., 2001; Narayan et al., 2003). Currently, high-throughput methods such as array CGH, SNP array, and gene expression arrays are available to reveal complex genetic alterations in cervical carcinogenesis (Kloth et al., 2007).

Transcriptomics includes the study of mRNA transcripts in a cell that frequently correlate with the expression of the corresponding proteins. There are several gene amplification–based techniques such as polymerase chain reaction (PCR), hybridization, and sequencing method that have facilitated the research in the field of transcriptomics. Nowadays, high-throughput techniques like serial analysis of gene expression (SAGE), massively parallel signature sequencing (MPSS), and DNA microarrays have a huge potential to fundamentally analyze the transcriptional regulatory networks. These are widely used due to their SP as well as high capacity for data management (Carlos et al., 2012).

Protein identification is central to most of the proteomics-based studies. Two-dimensional gel electrophoresis technique is used routinely for visualization of proteins. Mass spectrometry is used for identification of differentially expressed proteins in a given sample. Highly sensitive and specific techniques such as matrix-assisted laser desorption/ionization–time-of-flight mass spectrometry (MALDI–TOFMS), surface-enhanced laser desorption/ionization–mass spectrometry (SELDI–MS), liquid chromatography–mass spectrometry (LC–MS), isotope-coded affinity tags, and isobaric tags can detect very small amounts of protein in virtually all the clinical specimens (Giovanna Damia et al., 2011).

Genomic, transcriptomic, and proteomic approaches provide only a small snapshot of a tumor's presence in the body (Carlos et al., 2012). Gopeshwar Narayan et al. described the integrative genomic strategy utilizing information on recurrent copy number alterations (CNAs) at 5p, 20q11.2, and 20q13.13 loci to identify genes relevant to genomic copy number gains and amplifications. Such type of analysis has provided insights into the role of genes such as RNASEN (Ribonuclease 3), POLS (DNA polymerase), and S-phase kinase-associated protein 2 (SKP2) on 5p locus; KIF3B (kinase-like protein), RALY (RNA-binding protein), and E2F1 (transcription factor) at 20q11.2 locus; and CSE1L (chromosome segregation 1-like), ZNF313 (Zinc finger), and B4GALT5 (beta-1,4-galactosyltransferase 5) at 20q13.13 locus in cervical carcinogenesis (Narayan et al., 2010). Newer, sophisticated research tools have made it possible to study a broad range of substances such as sugars (glycomics), fats (lipidomics), and metabolites (metabolomics) in normal and diseased states. These could serve as biomarkers indicative of early disease phenotypes and subphenotypes or predictive of disease progression and outcome. Figure 7.5 shows the omics approaches and techniques used for the discovery of early detection biomarkers in cervical cancer.

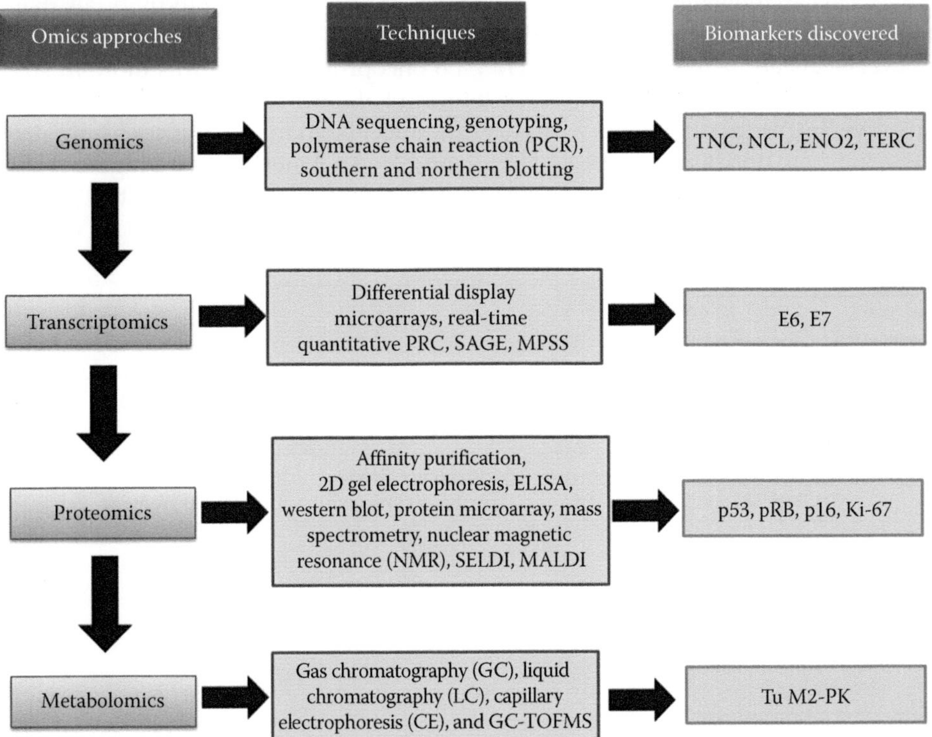

FIGURE 7.5
Omics approaches and techniques used for the discovery of early detection biomarkers for cervical cancer: genomics, transcriptomics, proteomics, and metabolomics are some of the approaches, together represented as integrative omics. Using these approaches and high-throughput techniques, a number of biomarkers have been discovered that have been explained in the respective sections.

7.7 Ethnic Group–Specific Markers with Specificity, Sensitivity, and Techniques

The burden of cervical cancer is not shared uniformly among women of all the races and ethnicities. While the age-adjusted incidence rate of cervical cancer for all US women is 8.1 per 100,000 women per year (Surveillance Epidemiology and End Results, SEER Stat Fact Sheet: Cervix Uteri, 2012), Latinas have a significantly higher incidence of cervical cancer (11.1 per 100,000 women) as do the African-American women (10.0 per 100,000) (National Cancer Institute, 2010). The incidence has been reported to be five times higher among Vietnamese American women than white women (Freeman and Wingrove, 2005). Table 7.9 represents the incidence and mortality rates of cervical cancer according to the different races.

7.7.1 p53 Polymorphism-Based Ethnic Group–Specific Markers

p53 is a well-known tumor suppressor protein that functions as a guardian of the genome (Lane, 1992). Storey et al. have demonstrated that polymorphism at codon 72 of p53 tumor suppressor protein, which codes for either arginine (Arg) or proline (Pro), was associated with cervical carcinogenesis in UK white women. It was found that individuals that were homozygous for the Arg variant of codon 72 of the p53 gene were at sevenfold increased risk of cervical cancer. The binding of HPV E6 oncoprotein to p53 was more in Arg/Arg genotype compared to Arg/Pro genotype (Storey et al., 1998). A number of studies on ethnically diverse groups of patients with cervical cancer from many countries have revealed that women from northern Europe and South and North America have a higher frequency of p53 Arg polymorphism than that observed in women from Asia, south Europe, and Central America. Table 7.10 represents frequency of p53 Arg polymorphism in different races/ethnic groups (Brenna et al., 2004).

TABLE 7.9

Incidence and Mortality Rate of Cervical Cancer by Race

Ethnic/Racial Group	Incidence Rates[a] (per 100,000 Women)	Mortality[b] (per 100,000 Women)
All races	8.1	2.4
White	8.0	2.2
Black	9.8	4.3
Asian/Pacific Islander	7.2	2.0
American Indian/Alaska Native	8.1	3.5
Hispanic	11.8	3.0

Source: SEER Stat Fact Sheet: Cervix Uteri, 2012.

[a] The rates are based on cases diagnosed in 2005–2009 from 18 SEER geographic areas.

[b] The rates are based on patients who died in 2005–2009 in the United States.

TABLE 7.10

Frequency of p53 Arg Polymorphism according to Ethnic/Racial Group

Ethnic/Racial Group	Frequency of p53 Arg (%)	References
Korean	40	Kim et al. (2001)
Japanese	44.8	Nishikawa et al. (2000)
Hong Kong	31	Wong et al. (2000)
Indian	27	Bhattacharya et al. (2002)
Jewish	34.8	Arbel-Alon et al. (2002)
North African	30.3	Arbel-Alon et al. (2002)
Italian	76.7	Zehbe et al. (2001)
White English	54	Rosenthal et al. (1998)
Dutch	69.4	Brady et al. (1999)
Swedish	62	Zehbe et al. (2001)
Peruvian	50.4	Klug et al. (2001)
Mexico	45	Suarez-Rincon et al. (2002)
Brazilian	67	Madeleine et al. (2000); Malcolm et al. (2000); Klug et al. (2001); Suarez-Rincon et al. (2002)

7.8 Author's Won Research in the Field

Dr. George Papanicolaou (1883–1962), father of the field of exfoliative cytology, discovered the atypical lesions in the cervix, which he identified as cancer cells in their early stage (Edmund, 2002). In late 1930s, he first reported vaginal smear as a means to diagnose uterine cancer. In 1940s, the introduction of vaginal smear (Pap test) saved millions of women worldwide from cervical cancer. The importance of his work was recognized in 1943 when Dr. Trout along with him published a classic book *Diagnosis of Uterine Cancer by the Vaginal Smear* (Papanicolaou et al., 1941).

Zur Hausen (1936 till date), a German virologist and professor emeritus, had hypothesized that the cervical cancer was caused by papillomaviruses. In 1974, he published his first report, demonstrating a cross-hybridization of the plantar wart virus DNA with some warts (Zur Hausen et al., 1974). He was awarded one-half of the Nobel Prize for medicine or physiology in the year 2008 *for his discovery of HPVs causing cervical cancer,* whereas the other half of the Nobel Prize was shared by Francoise Barre-Sinoussi and Luc Montagnier *for their discovery of human immunodeficiency virus.*

Frazer (1953 till date), an Australian immunologist, has contributed significantly to the health of mankind and is highly regarded for his work in developing the HPV cervical cancer vaccines. Dr. Frazer's work was focused on how the HPV worked in cells. During his research in late 1980s, Dr. Frazer met virologist Dr. Jian Zhou, and both engineered a synthetic noninfectious HPV to protect against HPV-associated cancer (Hodder, 2001). The vaccine has recently been licensed in many countries worldwide, which has the potential to eventually reduce the incidence of cervical cancer.

Thom Haubert, a medical device engineer in Battelle's Health and Life Science Global Business, manages a group of mechanical engineers, designers, and technicians who work to develop medical devices. Thom Haubert invented the ThinPrep® Pap Test, an automated diagnostic tool for screening of cervical cancer (Battelle, The Business of Innovation, 2012).

7.9 Various Test Panels Commercially Available for Early Diagnosis with Test Provider Detail and Cost

Test Name	SP (%)	SE (%)	Techniques	Test Provider	Reference
			DNA-Based Tests		
HC2	80.6	73.1	Hybrid capture/enzymatic luminescence	Qiagen, Valencia, CA, USA	Tsiodras et al. (2010)
Cervista Hr HPV	42.2	92.8	Invader method/fluorescence resonance energy transfer (FRET)	Hologic, Bedford, MA, USA	Dutra et al. (2012)
Cobas4800	70.5	90	Real-time PCR	Roche Molecular Diagnostics	Dutra et al. (2012)
careHPV	84.2	90	Signal-amplified hybridization	Qiagen	Dutra et al. (2012)
Linear Array HPV	32.8	98.2	Reverse line blot	Roche Molecular Diagnostics	Dutra et al. (2012)
AMPLICOR HPV Test	96.5	96.1	PCR/multiwell-plate hybridization, enzymatic color reaction	Roche Molecular Systems	Dutra et al. (2012)
HPV DNA chip	94	80	DNA microarray		Dutra et al. (2012)
			RNA-Based Tests		
APTIMA HPV mRNA Assay	98	92	Transcription-mediated amplification (TMA)	Gen-Probe, San Diego, CA, USA	Dutra et al. (2012)
HPV OncoTect® E6 E7 mRNA	94.5	89	In situ hybridization and flow cytometry	IncellDx, CA, USA	
PreTect Proofer	75.5	78.1	Nucleic acid sequence-based amplification (NASBA)/ molecular beacons real-time detection technology	NorChip AS, Klokkarstua, Norway	Dutra et al. (2012)
			Protein-Based Tests		
ProExC	74.50	98.04	Immunocytochemistry	Becton, Dickinson	Siddiqui et al. (2008)
CINtec® PLUS	68.0	94.2	Immunocytochemistry	Roche mtm laboratories AG	Schmidt et al. (2011)

7.10 Recommended Tests/Panels in Combination with/without Imaging for Early Diagnosis

Recently, US Preventive Services Task Force (USPSTF) and American Cancer Society (ACS) released new recommendations for cervical cancer screening. The guidelines address cervical cancer screening in the general population. These guidelines did not address special, HR populations such as women exposed to diethylstilbestrol (DES) in utero and with an immunocompromised status. Key recommendations in the guidelines are shown in Table 7.11.

TABLE 7.11
Current Recommendation with Rationale (USPSTF 2012)

Group	Recommendation	Rationale
Women aged <21	No screening.	Adequate evidence that screening women younger than age 21 years (regardless of sexual history) does not reduce cervical cancer incidence and mortality compared with beginning screening at age 21 years.
Women aged 21–29	Cytology every 3 years; HPV testing not recommended.	Adequate evidence that screening with HPV testing (alone or in combination with cytology) confers little to no benefit.
Women aged 30–65	Cytology every 3 years or cytology plus HPV testing every 5 years.	Adequate evidence that screening with a combination of cytology and HPV testing (co-testing) every 5 years provides benefits similar to those seen with cytology screening alone every 3 years.
Women aged >65	If adequately screened in the past, screening should be discontinued.	Adequate evidence that screening women older than age 65 years who have had adequate prior screening and are not otherwise at high risk provides little to no benefits.
Women with total hysterectomy and no prior history of high-grade CIN	Screening should be discontinued.	Convincing evidence that continued screening after hysterectomy with removal of the cervix for indications other than a high-grade precancerous lesion or cervical cancer provides no benefits.

Source: Screening for Cervical Cancer: Clinical Summary of U.S. Preventive Services Task Force Recommendation. AHRQ Publication No. 11-05156-EF-3, March 2012. http://www.uspreventiveservicestaskforce.org/uspstf11/cervcancer/cervcancersum.htm.

7.11 Advantages and Challenges in Developing Molecular Biomarkers for Early Detection, Prognosis, and Therapy

The use of morphology-based classification for cervical cancer poses a severe drawback for its accurate diagnosis. The factors that compromise the accuracy of Pap screening and cytology diagnosis include rare event detection; sample inadequacy; contamination of samples with blood, mucous, and debris; and subjective analysis of the technician. Thus, there is a need for diagnostic markers to improve the SE, SP, reproducibility, and utility of the current morphology-based diagnostics for the detection of high-grade cervical disease. The management of cervical cancer depends upon the prognostic and predictive biomarkers that would not only help to screen, detect, diagnose, prognosticate, treat, and predict recurrence but also play a major role in clinical decision making. Exploring the presence of such noninvasive markers secreted by cancer cells into the microenvironment not only will facilitate easy detection but will also be candidates for population-based screening. The recent advanced omics-based technologies including gene array technology, SAGE, improved 2-DE, and new mass spectrometric techniques together with advanced bioinformatic tools can help in the discovery of a variety of new biomarkers. This would help in the early detection of the disease, reduction of false-negative rates, selection of specific therapeutics, rational use of therapy, and understanding the process of carcinogenesis.

A major challenge in cervical cancer diagnosis is to establish the exact relationship between cancer biomarkers and the clinical pathology and to be able to noninvasively detect tumors at an early stage. Similarly, identification of subtle changes in the genomic and proteomic status specific to malignant transformation will allow molecular targets to be used for developing therapeutics. Moreover, development of statistical and mathematical tools for meaningful interpretation of different parameters to help the diagnosis is another future challenge in the biomarker development using integrative omics-based approach. Another major challenge in the biomarker development is setting up the validation as well as quality control procedures for using these markers with reliability and reproducibility.

7.12 Market and Market Players of the Molecular Biomarkers (Invasive, Imaging, and Noninvasive Molecular Markers) for Early Diagnosis, Prognosis, and Therapy

Early detection and intervention have substantially decreased the cervical cancer mortality rate. The overall global market for cervical cancer screening and diagnostics is about $2.1 billion (Roberta et al. 2012). Apart from the conventional Pap test, a number of different LBC techniques are in use worldwide. Recently, the use of thin-layer cytology has been widely implemented in many settings that increase the SE and SP of the testing. The lower rate of false-positive cervical cancer screening tests is one of the reasons for the rapid acceptance of the liquid-based tests. These include ThinPrep®, SurePath™, Cytoscreen™, Cyteasy®, Labonord Easy Prep, Cytoslide, SpinThin, and PapSpin. The first two of these are approved for use in the United States by the FDA and are the most widely used methods worldwide. The market players are Cytyc Corporation (ThinPrep®) and Becton, Dickinson and company (BD) acquired TriPath Imaging, Inc. (SurePath™).

The most current HPV molecular tests are DNA based, detecting the presence of the virus genome in the cervical cells of the patients. US FDA has approved three HPV tests: Aptima® Hpv Assay (Gen-Probe, San Diego, CA, USA), Cervista Hr HPV (Hologic, Bedford, Mass, USA), and Hybrid Capture 2 (Hc2) Test (Qiagen, Valencia, CA, USA), which are commercially available. However, none of the tests have been recommended for primary, stand-alone screening. In addition, *Roche and Abbott laboratories, Inc.* are some of the market players who have made considerable development in nucleic acid–based HPV test. Other well-validated tests such as AMPLICOR HPV, the Linear Array HPV Genotyping, the PapilloCheck, and the INNO-LiPA HPV are commercially available elsewhere in the world but have not been approved by the US FDA. The Cervista HPV 16/18 test (Hologic, Bedford, MA, USA) and Cobas 4800 HPV test (Roche Molecular Systems) are approved by the FDA for HPV genotyping. *OncoHealth Corp.*, a protein biomarker diagnostics company, is developing test for measurement of E6/E7 protein using multiple platforms. *IncellDx, CA, USA*, has a CE mark for E6/E7 mRNA and HPV OncoTect test that uses flow cytometry followed by FISH. *NorChip AS, Klokkarstua, Norway*, has developed an mRNA-based HPV test known as PreTect HPV-Proofer (Mark Ratner, 2011). *Quest Diagnostics* (NYSE:DGX), the world's leading provider of diagnostic testing, has come up with a new laboratory assay named TERC test that detects amplification of the human telomerase RNA component (TERC) gene and/or polysomy of chromosome 3. Apart from these molecular markers, the various diagnostic devices have come into the market. Recently, *Guided Therapeutics, Inc.* based upon biophotonic technologies has developed LightTouch™ noninvasive diagnostic device, for cervical cancer detection. Unlike Pap smear and HPV testing that require a tissue sample, LightTouch™ is designed as a fast, painless test that significantly improves the early detection of cervical precancerous and cancers, independent of the sample. LightTouch™ analyzes the light reflected from the cervix, thereby generating the image that highlights the location and severity of the disease (Michael, 2009).

7.13 Patent Information of Molecular Markers/Tests for Invasive, Noninvasive, Early Diagnostic, Prognostic, and Therapeutic Aspects (in Table 7.12, Information Can be Obtained from Patent Lens)

TABLE 7.12

List of Patents Disclosing Early Diagnostic Biomarkers Panel in Cervical Cancer

Patent Number	Patent Title	Patent for
US20100151466	Diagnosis and treatment of cervical cancer	hTERT, IGFBP-3, transferring receptor, beta-catenin, Myc-HPV E6 interaction, HPV E7, and telomere length, in cervical cells.
US20110224088	Biomarkers for subtyping of cervical cancer subjects	Biomarkers for subtyping of cervical cancer subjects.
US20120070837	CIP2A as a biomarker in detection of cervical cancer	Combined use of CIP2A with at least one additional biomarker selected from the group consisting of Ki67, TOP2A, MCM2, MCM5, p14ARF, and p16INK4a, to better serve as a detection means for cervical cancer.
WO/2011/112901A2	Hypermethylation biomarkers for detection of cervical cancer	GGTLA4, FKBP6, ZNF516, SAP 130, and INTS1.
US20100316990	Biomarkers for HPV-induced cancer	Cornulin, PA28 β, DJ-1, actin, transthyretin, HSPB1, Cl intracellular channel 1, cytokeratin 8, transferrin, Hspβ6 (HSP20), aflatoxin reductase, α2 type I collagen, creatine kinase B, cytokeratin 13, GST π, PA28 α, manganese SOD, lamin A/C, serpin B1 (elastase inhibitor), serpin B3 (SCAA1), cytokeratin 10, cytokeratin 6A, trp–tRNA synthetase.
US20090023137	ESR1 and cervical cancer	ESR1 DAP kinase, APC, TIMP-3, RAR-beta, CALCA, TSLC1, TIMP-2, DcR1, DcR2, BRCA1, p15, Rassf1A, MLH1, MGMT.
US20090170087	Gene methylation in cervical cancer diagnosis	DNA biomarker sequences that are differentially methylated in samples from normal individuals and individuals with cervical cancer.
US20100330558	Gene expression profiling for identification, monitoring, and treatment of cervical cancer	A method is provided for determining a profile dataset for a subject with cervical cancer or conditions related to cervical cancer based on a sample from the subject using amplification for measurement of amount of RNA in a panel of genes.
US20070128699	Methods of diagnosing cervical cancer	Invention provides reagents and methods for detecting pathogen infections in human samples.
US20050037342	Methods for determining risk of developing cervical cancer	Identifying a subject having an increased risk of developing cervical cancer based on levels of IGF-II in serum and levels of EGF-R and HPV-E6/E7 in cervical epithelial cells and in serum.
US20120264625	Compositions, kits, and methods for identification, assessment, prevention, and therapy of cervical cancer	The invention relates to nucleic acid molecules and proteins associated with cervical cancer including premalignant conditions such as dysplasia.

(Continued)

TABLE 7.12 (*CONTINUED*)

List of Patents Disclosing Early Diagnostic Biomarkers Panel in Cervical Cancer

Patent Number	Patent Title	Patent for
US20120129705	Diagnostic markers for determining the predisposition to the development of cervical cancer and oligonucleotides used for the determination	The invention relates to a method for predisposition prediction of a subject to the development of cervical cancer and/or cancer precursors in an infection with the HPV and/or for the detection of a persistent HPV infection, the method comprising the steps of obtaining a sample from the subject and detecting at least one of the diagnostic markers or fragments thereof in the sample obtained from the subject.
US 20100330558	Gene expression profiling for identification, monitoring, and treatment of cervical cancer	A method is provided in various embodiments for determining a profile dataset for a subject with cervical cancer or conditions related to cervical cancer based on a sample from the subject, wherein the sample provides a source of RNAs. The method includes using amplification for measuring the amount of RNA corresponding to at least 1 constituent from Tables 7.1 through 7.5. The profile dataset comprises the measure of each constituent, and amplification is performed under measurement conditions that are substantially repeatable.
US 20100316990	Biomarkers for HPV-induced cancer	Biomarkers include cornulin, PA28 β, DJ-1, actin, transthyretin, HSPB1, CV intracellular channel 1, cytokeratin 8, transferrin, Hspβ6 (HSP20), aflatoxin reductase, α2 type I collagen, creatine kinase B, cytokeratin 13 GST π, PA28 α, manganese SOD, lamin A/C, serpin B1 (elastase inhibitor), serpin B3 (SCAA1), cytokeratin 10, cytokeratin 6A, and trp–tRNA synthetase. Preferred biomarkers for HPV-induced cancer include cornulin, DJ-1, PA28 α and PA28 β, trp–tRNA synthetase, HSPβ6, creatine kinase B, aflatoxin reductase, GST π, transthyretin, transferrin, α2-type 1 collagen, and combinations thereof.
20100240049	Methods of detecting cervical cancer	Methods of detecting cervical dysplasia, such as cervical dysplasia likely to progress to carcinoma in a sample of human cervical cells, are provided. Methods of detecting changes in expression of one or more microRNAs (miRNAs) or mRNAs associated with cervical dysplasia or cervical cancer are also provided. Compositions and kits are also provided.
20100234445	Patterns of known and novel small RNAs in human cervical cancer	Small RNA sequences that are differentially expressed in squamous cell cervical cancer (SCCC) cells are provided. The sequences find use in diagnosis of cancer and classification of cancer cells according to expression profiles. The methods are useful for detecting cervical cancer cells, facilitating diagnosis of cervical cancer and the severity of the cancer (e.g., tumor grade, tumor burden, and the like) in a subject, facilitating a determination of the prognosis of a subject, and assessing the responsiveness of the subject to therapy.
20090186348	miRNAs differentially expressed in cervical cancer and uses thereof	The present invention concerns methods and compositions for identifying an miRNA profile for a particular condition, such as cervical disease, and using the profile in assessing the condition of a patient.

(*Continued*)

TABLE 7.12 (*CONTINUED*)

List of Patents Disclosing Early Diagnostic Biomarkers Panel in Cervical Cancer

Patent Number	Patent Title	Patent for
20090104597	Advanced cervical cell screening methods	Advanced cervical cancer screening methods that provide a molecular-based process of detecting HPV integration. The disclosed methods allow for a streamlined approach of conducting a Pap test and immunohistochemical test on the same slide.
20090087843	Molecular markers	A method for distinguishing between normal tissue and cervical cancer tissue comprising detecting differential expression of polynucleotide.
20070065810	Diagnosis and treatment of cervical cancer	In certain aspects, the invention relates to methods of diagnosing cervical cancer by using a combination of certain biomarkers such as hTERT, IGFBP-3, transferrin receptor, beta-catenin, Myc-HPV E6 interaction, HPV E7, and telomere length.
20060154275	Regulated genes in cervical cancer	Polynucleotides, as well as polypeptides encoded thereby, which are differentially expressed in SCCC cells are provided. The polynucleotides find use in diagnosis of cancer and classification of cancer cells according to expression profiles. The methods are useful for detecting cervical cancer cells, facilitating diagnosis of cervical cancer and the severity of the cancer (e.g., tumor grade, tumor burden, and the like) in a subject, facilitating a determination of the prognosis of a subject, and assessing the responsiveness of the subject to therapy.

7.14 Concluding Remarks and Future Perspectives

Biomolecular pathways of HPV-induced cervical carcinogenesis are well understood, thus being beneficial in the discovery of a number of potential biomarkers for early detection of cervical cancer. Recent developments in biomedicine have the potential to prevent as well as control cervical cancer. Despite this, advances in screening methods for cervical cancer are greatly needed, to provide an efficient, cost-effective screening tool that would quickly, accurately, and cheaply identify the women at risk for HPV-associated malignancies. A number of biomarkers available at present can efficiently detect the women at the greatest risk of cervical cancer. The recent introduction of FDA-approved prophylactic HPV vaccines will eventually reduce the incidence of cervical cancers, but it would take a few years to get the results.

Integrated genomic, transcriptomic, proteomic, and epigenomic approaches provide platforms for discovery of novel biomarkers. However, epigenomics (methylation) is the choice for discovery of biomarkers as changes in methylation patterns are considered as an early event in the process of carcinogenesis. A number of studies have suggested the use of gene panel instead of single gene for accurate and high-sensitive detection of cervical cancer. Despite their considerable promise for application in the investigation of cervical cancer, methylated markers still have limited utility in clinical practice. A main reason for this could be less sampling number as well as inconsistent information of the specific markers. Advancement in technology has led to the development of several new platforms (e.g., microarray format, bead array format, 454 sequencing format) that satisfies the demands of rapid and sensitive genome-wide DNA methylation profiling. This genome-wide scanning would help in identifying a novel panel of candidate genes methylated in cancer screening in the near future.

The use of noninvasive optical techniques for the early detection of precancerous conditions is a rapidly emerging area. Recent advances in fiber optics, sources, detectors, and computer-controlled instrumentation have motivated the research interest regarding the clinical applications of biophotonics in the early detection of precancer in several organs including the uterine cervix. These could serve as indicators of underlying biological processes, identifying asymptomatic individuals with a risk for cervical cancer in the following years. Only well-integrated, multidisciplinary studies in a concerted and systematic fashion would have the potential to discover relevant and new biomarkers in cervical cancer. Thus, the combination of traditional markers (Pap test, HPV detection) and recent invasive and noninvasive (genomics, transcriptomics, proteomics, epigenomics) markers, along with the optical techniques (imaging markers), could provide more robust biomarkers to be used in clinical practice. These biomarkers may identify the underlying biological processes of cervical carcinogenesis even prior to the onset of symptoms and offer the opportunity for early diagnosis.

References

Aaltonen LA, Peltomaki P, Mecklin JP, Jarvinen H, Jass JR, Green JS, Lynch HT, Watson P, Tallqvist G, and Juhola M. Replication errors in benign and malignant tumors from hereditary nonpolyposis colorectal cancer patients. *Cancer Res*, 54:1645–1648; 1994.

Abudukadeer A, Bakry R, Goebel G, Mutz-Dehbalaie I, Widschwendter A, Bonn G., and Fiegl H. Clinical relevance of CDH1 and CDH13 DNA-methylation in serum of cervical cancer patients. *J Mol Sci*, 13:8353–8363; 2012.

Acevedo-Rocha CG, Munguía-Moreno JA, Ocádiz-Delgado R, and Gariglio P. A transcriptome- and marker-based systemic analysis of cervical cancer, *Topics on Cervical Cancer With an Advocacy for Prevention*, Rajamanickam R (Ed.), ISBN: 978-953-51-0183-3, InTech, DOI: 10.5772/30866. 2012. Available from: http://www.intechopen.com/books/topics-on-cervical-cancer-with-an-advocacy-for-prevention/a-transcriptome-and-marker-based-systematic-analysis-of-cervical-cancer.

Agnieszka KW, Thomas CW, Alex Fy, Brigitte MR, and Robert JK. Carcinoma and other tumors of the cervix, *Blaustein's Pathology of the Female Genital Tract*, pp. 253–303; 2011. New York: Springer.

American Cancer Society, What are the key statistics about cervical cancer?, 2014, Available from http://www.cancer.org/cancer/cervicalcancer/detailedguide/cervical-cancer-key-statistics. Accessed September 11, 2014.

American Cancer Society, Cervical cancer. Available from: http://www.cancer.org/acs/groups/cid/documents/webcontent/003094-pdf.pdf. (2014). Accessed September 11, 2014.

Ancuţa E, Codrina A, Laurette GC, Cristina I, Ivona A-L, Anton E, Carasevici E, and Rodica C. Tumor biomarkers in cervical cancer: Focus on Ki-67 proliferation factor and E-cadherin expression. *Rom J Morphol Embryol*, 50(3):413–418; 2009.

Arbel-Alon S, Menczer J, Feldman N, Glezerman M, Yeremin L, and Friedman E. Codon 72 polymorphism of p53 in Israeli Jewish cervical cancer patients and healthy women. *Int J Gynecol Cancer*, 12:741–744; 2002.

Arbyn M, Paraskevaidis E, Martin-Hirsch P, Prendiville W, and Dillner J. Clinical utility of HPV-DNA detection: Triage of minor cervical lesions, follow-up of women treated for high-grade CIN: An update of pooled evidence. *Gynecol Oncol*, 99:7–11; 2005.

Arnold JN, Saldova R, Hamid UMA, and Rudd PM. Evaluation of the serum N-linked glycome for the diagnosis of cancer and chronic inflammation. *Proteomics*, 8:3284–3293; 2008.

Arora A, Eric M, and Scholar EM. Role of tyrosine kinase inhibitors in cancer therapy. *JPET*, 315(3):971–979; 2005.

Baay MF, Nakonieczny M, Wozniak I, Deschoolmeester V, Liss J, Lukaszuk K, Sotlar K, Emerich J, and Vermorken JB. Microsatellite instability and HPV genotype in Polish women with cervical cancer. *Eur J Gynaecol Oncol*, 30(2):162–166; 2009.

Balasubramaniyan N, Subramanian S, Sekar N, Bhuvarahamurthy V, and Govindasamy S. Diagnostic and prognostic role of plasma and urinary sialic acid in human carcinoma of uterine cervix. *Biochem Mol Biol Int*, 33:617–623; 1994.

Bell JT and Spector TD. A twin approach to unraveling epigenetics. *Trends Genet*, 27(3):116–125; 2011.

Bellone S, Frera G, Landolfi G et al. Overexpression of epidermal growth factor type-1 receptor (EGF-R1) in cervical cancer:Implications for Cetuximab-mediated therapy in recurrent/metastatic disease. *Gynecol Oncol*, 106(3):513–520; 2007.

Bhattacharya P, Duttagupta C, and Sengupta S. Proline homozygosity in codon 72 of p53: A risk genotype for human papillomavirus-related cervical cancer in Indian women. *Cancer Lett*, 188:207–211; 2002.

Bishop A, Sherris J, Tsu VD, and Kilbourne Book M. Cervical dysplasia treatment: Key issues for developing countries. *Bull PAHO*, 30(4); 1996.

Bleotu C, Botezatu A, Goia C, Socolov D, Cornişescu F, Teleman S, Huica I, Iancu I, and Anton G. p16INK4a—a possible marker in HPV persistence screening. *Roum Arch Microbiol Immunol*, 68(3):183–189; 2009.

Bloss JD, Liao SY, Buller RE, Manetta A, Berman ML, McMeekin S, Bloss LP, and DiSaia PJ. Extraovarian peritoneal serous papillary carcinoma: A case-control retrospective comparison to papillary adenocarcinoma of the ovary. *Gynecol Oncol*, 50(3):347–351; 1993.

Bosch FX, Rohan T, Schneider A et al. Papillomavirus research update: Highlights of the Barcelona HPV 2000 International Papillomavirus Conference. *J Clin Pathol*, 54:163–175; 2000.

Brady CS, Duggan-Keen MF, Davidson JA, Varley JM, and Stern PL. Human papillomavirus type 16 E6 variants in cervical carcinoma: Relationship to host genetic factors and clinical parameters. *J Gen Virol*, 80:3233–3240; 1999.

Bray F, Loos AH, McCarron P, Weiderpass E et al. Trends in cervical squamous cell carcinoma incidence in 13 European countries: Changing risk and the effects of screening. *Cancer Epidemiol Biomarkers Prev*, 14:677–686; 2005.

Brenna SMF, da Silva IDCG, Zeferino LC, Pereira J, Martinez EZ, and Syrjänen KJ. Prevalence of codon 72 P53 polymorphism in Brazilian women with cervix cancer. *Genetics Mol Biol*, 27(4):496–499; 2004.

Callet N, Cohen-Solal Le Nir CC, Berthelot E, and Pichon MF. Cancer of the uterine cervix: Sensitivity and specificity of serum Cyfra 21.1 determinations. *Eur J Gynaecol Oncol*, 19:50–56; 1998.

Carien MN, Deborah L, and Alpha SY. Tissue organization by cadherin adhesion molecules: Dynamic molecular and cellular mechanisms of morphogenetic regulation. *Physiol Rev*, 91(2):691–731; 2011.

Carsten DC, Jan BJ, Tobias KT, Wilko WW, Peter TP, Jalid SJ, Silvia NS, Dominique KD, Manfred DM, and Oliver FO. Mass spectrometry–based metabolic profiling reveals different metabolite patterns in invasive ovarian carcinomas and ovarian borderline tumors. *Cancer Res*, 66:10795; 2006.

Cervical Cancer Fact Sheet-Centers for Disease Control and Prevention, 2012. Available from http://www.cdc.gov/cancer/cervical/pdf/cervical_facts.pdf.

Chhabra S, Bhavani M, Mahajan N, and Bawaskar R. Cervical cancer in Indian rural women: Trends over two decades. *J Obstet Gynaecol*, 30:725–728; 2010.

Cho H, Hong SW, Oh YJ, Kim MA, Kang ES, Lee JM, Kim SW et al. Clinical significance of osteopontin expression in cervical cancer. *J Cancer Res Clin Oncol*, 134(8):909–917; 2008.

Coelho SM, Carvalho DP, and Vaisman M. New therapies for thyroid carcinoma. *Arq Bras Endocrinol Metab*, 51(4):612–624; 2007.

Conrads TP, Ming ZM, Petricoin EF III, Liotta L, and Veenstra TD. Cancer diagnosis using proteomic patterns. *Expert Rev Mol Diagn*, 3(4); 2003.

Daniela BC, Rafael R, and Gilberto S. Emerging therapeutic agents for cervical cancer. *Recent Pat Anticancer Drug Discov*, 4:196–206; 2009.

Denny L, Kuhn L, Pollack A, Wainwright H, and Wright TC Jr. Evaluation of alternative methods of cervical cancer screening for resource-poor settings. *Cancer*, 89:826–833; 2000.

Depuydt CE, Makar AP, Ruymbeke MJ, Benoy IH, Vereecken AJ, and Bogers JJ. BD-ProExC as adjunct molecular marker for improved detection of CIN2+ after HPV primary screening. *Cancer Epidemiol Biomarkers Prev*, 20(4):628–637; 2011.

Desai AA, Innocenti F, and Ratain MJ. Pharmacogenomics: Road to anticancer therapeutics nirvana? *Oncogene*, 22:6621–6628; 2003.

Doeberitz VKM. New markers for cervical dysplasia to visualise the genomic chaos created by aberrant oncogenic papillomavirus infections. *Eur J Cancer*, 38(17):2229–2242; 2002.

Donà MG, Vocaturo A, Giuliani M, Ronchetti L, Rollo F, Pescarmona E, Carosi M, Vocaturo G, and Benevolo M. p16/Ki-67 dual staining in cervico-vaginal cytology: Correlation with histology, human papillomavirus detection and genotyping in women undergoing colposcopy. *Gynecol Oncol* 126(2):198–202; 2012.

Douglas PM. Molecular diagnostic assays for cervical neoplasia: Emerging markers for the detection of high-grade cervical disease. *BioTechniques* 38:S17–S23; 2005.

Dunton CJ, Dooley M, Margaret CRNP, and Holtz DO. Early detection of cervical cancer by human papillomavirus DNA testing: Case reports. *J Low Genit Tract Dis*, 10(3):194; 2006.

Dutra I, Foroni I, Couto AR, Lima M, and Bruges-Armas J. Molecular diagnosis of human papillomavirus. *Human Papillomavirus and Related Diseases – From Bench to Bedside – Research Aspects*; 2012. Available from: http://www.intechopen.com/books/human-papillomavirus-and-related-diseases-from-bench-to-bedside-research-aspects/molecular-diagnosis-of-human-papillomavirus.

Dyson N, Howley PM, Münger K, and Harlow E. The human papilloma virus-16 E7 oncoprotein is able to bind to the retinoblastoma gene product. *Science*, 243(4893):934–937; 1989.

Edmund SC. *Cervical and Vaginal Cytology*. Philadelphia, PA: Elsevier/Saunders; 2002.

Eijsink JJH, Yang N, Lendvai A, Klip HG, Volders HH, Buikema HJ, van Hemel BM et al. Detection of cervical neoplasia by DNA methylation analysis in cervico-vaginal lavages, a feasibility study. *Gynecol Oncol*, 120:280–283; 2011.

Esajas MD, Duk JM, de Bruijn HW, Aalders JG, Willemse PH, Sluiter W, Pras B, ten Hoor K, Hollema H, and van der Zee AG. Clinical value of routine serum squamous cell carcinoma antigen in follow-up of patients with early-stage cervical cancer. *J Clin Oncol*, 19(19):3960–3966; 2001.

Eun-Kyoung Y and Jong-Sup P. Biomarkers in cervical cancer. *Biomarker Insights* 1:215–225; 2006.

Evans WE and McLeod HL. Pharmacogenomics—Drug disposition, drug targets, and side effects. *N Engl J Med*, 348:538–549; 2003.

Feng Q, Balasubramanian A, Hawes SE, Toure P, Sow PS et al. Detection of hypermethylated genes in women with and without cervical neoplasia. *J Natl Cancer Inst*, 97:273–282; 2005.

Ferdeghini M, Gadducci A, Annicchiarico C, Prontera C, Melagnino G, Castellani C et al. Serum CYFRA 21-1 assay in squamous cell carcinoma of the cervix. *Anticancer Res*, 13:1841–1844; 1993.

Fiore E, Campani D, Muller I, Belardi V, Giustarini E, Rossi G, Pinchera A, and Giani C. IGF-II mRNA expression in breast cancer: Predictive value and relationship to other prognostic factors. *Int J Biol Markers* 25(3):150–156; 2010.

Flores YN, Bishai DM, Lorincz A et al. HPV testing for cervical cancer screening appears more cost-effective than Papanicolaou cytology in Mexico. *Cancer Causes Control*, 22:261–272; 2011.

Franco EL and Cuzick J. Cervical cancer screening following prophylactic human papillomavirus vaccination. *Vaccine*, 26(S1):A16–A23; 2008.

Freeman HP and Wingrove BK. *Excess Cervical Cancer Mortality: A Marker for Low Access to Health Care in Poor Communities*. Rockville, MD: National Cancer Institute, Center to Reduce Cancer Health Disparities, May 2005. NIH Pub. No. 05-5282; 2005.

Gaarenstroom KN, Bonfrer JMG, Kenter GG, Korse CM, Hart AAM et al. Clinical value of pretreatment serum CYFRA 21-1, tissue polypeptide antigen and squamous cell carcinoma antigen levels in patients with cervical cancer. *Cancer*, 76:807–813; 1995.

Garcia M, Lemal A, Ward EM, and Center MM. *Global Cancer Facts and Figures*. Atlanta, GA: American Cancer Society; 2007.

Ge Y, Mody DR, Smith D, and Anton R. p16(INK4a) and ProEx C immunostains facilitate differential diagnosis of hyperchromatic crowded groups in liquid-based Papanicolaou tests with menstrual contamination. *Acta Cytol*, 56(1):55–61; 2012.

Giovanna DG, Massimo BM, Silvia MS, Sergio VS, and Daniele GD. New omics information for clinical trial utility in the primary setting. *J Natl Cancer Inst Monogr*, 43:128–133; 2011.

Goldhaber-Fiebert JD and Goldie SJ. Estimating the cost of cervical cancer screening in five developing countries. *Cost Eff Resour Alloc*, 4:13; 2006.

Gonçalves A, Fabbro M, Lhomme C et al. A phase II trial to evaluate gefitinib as second- or third-line treatment in patients with recurring locoregionally advanced or metastatic cervical cancer. *Gynecol Oncol*, 108(1): 42–46; 2008.

Gossage L and Madhusudan S. Cancer pharmacogenomics: Role of DNA repair genetic polymorphisms in individualizing cancer therapy. *Mol Diagn Ther*, 11(6):361–380; 2007.

Gustafson KS, Furth EE, Heitjan DF, Fansler ZB, and Clark DP. DNA methylation profiling of cervical squamous intraepithelial lesions using liquid-based cytology specimens: An approach that utilizes receiver-operating characteristic analysis. *Cancer*, 25;102(4):259–268; 2004.

Gutiérrez-Xicoténcatl L, Plett-Torres T, Madrid-González CL, and Madrid-Marina V. Molecular diagnosis of human papillomavirus in the development of cervical cancer. *Salud Publica Mex*, 51(suppl 3):S479–S488; 2009.

Harris JR. Sources of epigenetic variation at the MHC. *Twin Res Hum Genet*, 13:262; 2010.

Harry VN. Novel imaging techniques as response biomarkers in cervical cancer. *Gynecol Oncol*, 116(2):253–261; 2010.

Heselmeyer-Haddad K, Sommerfeld K, White NM, Chaudhri N, Morrison LE, Palanisamy N, et al. Genomic amplification of the human telomerase gene (TERC) in pap smears predicts the development of cervical cancer. *Am J Pathol*, 166(4):1229–1238; 2005.

Hilal A, Mark AM, Robert HP, Hubert S, Carlos S, Manuel Á, Julio M, Daron F, Jeffrey RL, and William SD. Characterization of molecular markers indicative of cervical cancer progression. *Proteomics Clin*, 3(5):516–527; 2009.

Hodder A. *Human Papillomaviruses: Clinical and Scientific Advances*; London, U.K.: Hodder Arnold Publication; 2001.

Hogdall EV, Ringsholt M, Hogdall CK, Christensen IJ, Johansen JS, Kjaer SK, Blaakaer J et al. YKL-40 tissue expression and plasma levels in patients with ovarian cancer. *BMC Cancer*, 9:8; 2009.

Holowaty P, Miller AB, Rohan T et al. Natural history of dysplasia of the uterine cervix. *J Natl Cancer Inst*, 91:252–258; 1999.

Horn LC, Lindner K, Szepankiewicz G, Edelmann J, Hentschel B, Tannapfel A, et al. p16, p14, p53, and cyclin D1 expression and HPV analysis in small cell carcinomas of the uterine cervix. *International Journal of Gynecologic Pathology*, 25(2):182–186; 2006.

Horn LC, Reichert A, Oster A, Arndal SF, Trunk MJ, Ridder R, Rassmussen OF et al. Immunostaining for p16INK4a used as a conjunctive tool improves interobserver agreement of the histologic diagnosis of cervical intraepithelial neoplasia. *Am J Surg Pathol*, 32:502–512; 2008.

Huang RL, Chang CC, Su PH, Chen YC, Liao YP, Wang HC, YO YT, Chao TK, Huang HC, Lin CY, Chu TY, and Lai HC. Methylomic analysis identifies frequent DNA methylation of zinc finger protein 582 (ZNF582) in cervical neoplasms. *PloS one*, 7(7):e41060; 2012.

Hu L, Guo M, He Z, Thornton J, McDaniel LS, Hughson MD. Human papillomavirus genotyping and p16INK4a expression in cervical intraepithelial neoplasia of adolescents. *Mod Pathol*, 18:267–273; 2005.

Huh K, Zhou X, Hayakawa H, Cho JY, Libermann TA, Jin J, Harper JW, and Munger K. Human papillomavirus type 16 E7 oncoprotein associates with the cullin 2 ubiquitin ligase complex, which contributes to degradation of the retinoblastoma tumor suppressor. *J Virol*, 81:9737–9747; 2007.

International Agency for Research on Cancer, Globocan (2008) Cancer Incidence and Mortality Worldwide. Available from http://www.iarc.fr/en/media-centre/iarcnews/2010/globocan2008.php. Accessed March 19, 2012.

Irish Cancer Society, Treatments for cervical cancer 2014. Available from http://www.cancer.ie/cancer-information/cervical-cancer/treatments#sthash.wJOR6LD4.dpbs. Accessed September 11, 2014.

Jacob M, Broekhuizen FF, Castro W, and Sellors J. Experience using cryotherapy for treatment of cervical precancerous lesions in low-resource settings. *Int J Gynecol Obstet*, 89(Suppl 2):S13–S20; 2005.

James EK, Warner KH, and Ronald DA. LUMA™ cervical imaging system—Spectra science. *Expert Rev Med Devices* 4(2):121–129; 2007.

Jemal A, Bray F, Center MM, Ferlay J, Ward E and Forman D. Global cancer statistics. *CA: A Cancer Journal for Clinicians*, 61(2):69–90; 2011.

Jensen SA, Vainer B, Kruhoffer M, and Sorensen JB. Microsatellite instability in colorectal cancer and association with thymidylate synthase and dihydropyrimidine dehydrogenase expression. *BMC Cancer*, 9:25; 2009.

Jones PA and Baylin SB. The fundamental role of epigenetic events in cancer. *Nat Rev Genet* 3:415–428; 2002.

Junker N, Johansen JS, Hansen LT, Lund EL, and Kristjansen PE. Regulation of YKL-40 expression during genotoxic or microenvironmental stress in human glioblastoma cells. *Cancer Sci*, 96(3):183–190; 2005.

Kaura B, Bagga R, and Patel FD. Evaluation of the Pyruvate Kinase isoenzyme tumor (Tu M2-PK) as a tumor marker for cervical carcinoma. *J Obstet Gynaecol Res*, 30(3):193–196; 2004.

Kelly D, Kincaid E, Fansler Z, Rosenthal DL, and Clark DP. Detection of cervical high-grade squamous intraepithelial lesions from cytologic samples using a novel immunocytochemical assay (ProEx C). *Cancer*, 108(6):494–500; 2006.

Kendrick JE, Huh WK, and Alvarez RD. LUMA cervical imaging system. *Expert Rev Med Devices*, 4:121–129; 2007.

Kersemaekers AM, van de Vijver MJ, Kenter GG, and Fleuren GJ. Genetic alterations during the progression of squamous cell carcinomas of the uterine cervix. *Genes Chromosomes Cancer*, 26:346–354; 1999.

Kim JW, Roh JW, Park NH, Song YS, Kang SB, and Lee HP. Polymorphism of TP53 codon 72 and the risk of cervical cancer among Korean women. *Am J Obstet Gynecol*, 184:55–58; 2001.

Kitchener HC, Castle PE, and Cox TJ. Chapter 7: Achievements and limitations of cervical cytology screening. *Vaccine*, 24S3:S3/63–S3/70; 2006.

Kloth JN, Oosting J, van Wezel T, Szuhai K, Knijnenburg J, Gorter A, Kenter GG, Fleuren GJ, and Jordanova ES. Combined array-comparative genomic hybridization and single-nucleotide polymorphism-loss of heterozygosity analysis reveals complex genetic alterations in cervical cancer. *BMC Genomics*, 8:53; 2007.

Klug SJ, Wilmotte R, Santos C, Almonte M, Herrero R, Guerrero I, Caceres E et al. TP53 polymorphism, HPV infection, and risk of cervical cancer. *Cancer Epidemiol Biomarkers Prev* 10:1009–1012; 2001.

Kuemmel S, Jeschke S, Landt S, Korlach S, Schmid P, Sehouli J, Blohmer J, Ulm K, Lichtenegger W, and Thomas A. *J Clin Oncol, ASCO Annu Meet Proc* Part I. Vol 24, No. 18S (June 20 Supplement), 5044; 2006.

Kummar S, Gutierrez ME, Gardner ER, Chen X, Figg WD, Zajac-Kaye M et al. Phase I trial of 17-dimethylaminoethylamino-17-demethoxygeldanamycin (17-DMAG), a heat shock protein inhibitor, administered twice weekly in patients with advanced malignancies. *Eur J Cancer*, 46(2):340–347; 2010.

Kuo JC, Wang WJ, Yao CC, Wu PR, and Chen RH. The tumor suppressor DAPK inhibits cell motility by blocking the integrin-mediated polarity pathway. The Rockefeller University Press. *J Cell Biol*, 172(4):619–631; 2006.

Lagana A, Martinez BP, Marino A, Fago G, and Bizzarri M. Correlation of serum sialic acid fractions as markers for carcinoma of the uterine cervix. *Anticancer Res*, (5B):2341–2346; 1995.

Lague M-N, Romieu-Mourez R, Bonneil É, Boyer A, Pouletty N et al. Proteomic profiling of a mouse model for ovarian granulosa cell tumor identifies VCP as a highly sensitive serum tumor marker in several human cancers. *PLoS One*, 7(8): e42470; 2012.

Lane DP. Cancer. p53, guardian of the genome. *Nature*, 358:15–16; 1992.

Lazcano-Ponce E, Lörincz AT, Salmerón J, Fernández I, Cruz A, Hernández P, Mejia I, and Hernández-Avila M. A pilot study of HPV DNA and cytology testing in 50,159 women in the routine Mexican Social Security Program. *Cancer Causes Control*, 21(10):1693–700. Epub; 2010.

Lee D, Kwon JH, Kim EH, Kim ES, and Choi KY. HMGB2 stabilizes p53 by interfering with E6/E6AP-mediated p53 degradation in human papillomavirus-positive HeLa cells. *Cancer Lett*, 292:125–132; 2010.

Lee SH, Lee SH, Lee KC, Lee KB, Shin, JW, Park CY, et al. Radiation therapy with chemotherapy for patients with cervical cancer and supraclavicular lymph node involvement. *Journal of Gynecologic Oncology*, 23(3):159-167; 2012.

Lehmann F, Tiralongo E, and Tiralongo J. Sialic acid-specific lectins: Occurrence, specificity and function. *Cell Mol Life Sci*, 63(12):1331–1354; 2006.

Lehn H, Villa LL, Marziona F, Hilgarth M, Hillemans HG, and Sauer G. Physical state and biological activity of human papillomavirus genomes in precancerous lesions of the female genital tract. *J Gen Virol*, 69:187–196; 1988.

Liggett WH and Sidransky D. Role of the p16 tumor suppressor gene in cancer. *Journal of Clinical Oncology*, 16(3):1197–1206; 1998.

Lisa FL. Cervical dysplasia. *About.com Guide*, Updated April 30, 2007.

Lomnytska MI, Becker S, Bodin I, Olsson A, Hellman K, Hellström A-C, Mints M, Hellman U, Auer G, and Andersson S. Differential expression of ANXA6, HSP27, PRDX2, NCF2, and TPM4 during uterine cervix carcinogenesis: Diagnostic and prognostic value. *Br J Cancer*, 104:110–119; 2011.

Madeleine MM, Shera K, Schwartz SM, Daling JR, Galloway DA, Wipf GC, Carter JJ, McKnight B, and McDougall JK. The p53 arg72pro polymorphism, human papillomavirus, and invasive squamous cell cervical cancer. *Cancer Epidemiol Biomarkers Prev*, 9:225–227; 2000.

Malcolm EK, Baber GB, Boyd JC, and Stoler MH. Polymorphism at codon 72 of p53 is not associated with cervical cancer risk. *Modern Pathol*, 13:373–378; 2000.

Marino K, Bones J, Kattla JJ, and Rudd PM. A systematic approach to protein glycosylation analysis: A path through the maze. *Nat Chem Biol*, 6(10):713–723; 2010.

Mark LR. Can E6E7 alter the competitive balance in the crowded HPV test market? *Invivo: Business Med Rep*; 2011. Available from: http://oncohealthcorp.com/IV_E6E7_Alter_The_Competitive_Balance_1111_WebReprint.pdf.

Mathur SP, Mathur RS, Gray EA, Lane D, Underwood PG, Kohler M, and Creasman WT. Serum vascular endothelial growth factor C (VEGF-C) as a specific biomarker for advanced cervical cancer: Relationship to insulin-like growth factor II (IGF-II), IGF binding protein 3 (IGF-BP3) and VEGF-A. *Gynecol Oncol*, 98(3):467–483; 2005.

Mathur SP, Mathur RS, Underwood PB, Kohler MF, and Creasman WT. Circulating levels of insulin-like growth factor-II and IGF-binding protein 3 in cervical cancer. *Gynecol Oncol*, 91:486–493; 2003.

Mathur SP, Mathur RS, and Young RC. Cervical epidermal growth factor-receptor (EGF-R) and serum insulin-like growth factor II (IGF-II) levels are potential markers for cervical cancer. *Am J Reprod Immunol*, 44(4):222–230; 2000.

Ma YY, Cheng XD, Zhou CY et al. Value of P16 expression in the triage of liquid-based cervical cytology with atypical squamous cells of undetermined significance and low-grade Squamous intraepithelial lesions. *Chin Med J*, 124:2443–2447; 2011.

Mazurek S. Pyruvate kinase M2: A key enzyme of the tumor metabolome and its medical relevance. *Biomed Res*, 23:SI 133–141; 2012.

Melsheimer P, Klaes R, Doeberitz MV, and Bastert G. Prospective clinical study comparing DNA flow cytometry and HPV typing as predictive tests for persistence and progression of CIN I/II. *Cytometry*, 46:166–171; 2001.

Meng-Ru S, Yueh-Mei H, Keng-Fu H, Yih-Fung C, Ming-Jer T, and Cheng-Yang C. Insulin-like growth factor 1 is a potent stimulator of cervical cancer cell invasiveness and proliferation that is modulated by αvβ3 integrin signalling. *Carcinogenesis* 27(5):962–971; 2006.

Mitsuhashi A, Matsui H, Usui H, Nagai Y, Tate S, Unno Y, Hirashiki K, Seki K, and Shozu M. Serum YKL-40 as a marker for cervical adenocarcinoma. *Ann Oncol*. 20(1):71–77; 2009.

Molina R, Filella X, Augé JM, Bosch E, Torne A, Pahisa J, Lejarcegui JA, Rovirosa A, Mellado B, Ordi J, and Biete. CYFRA 21.1 in patients with cervical cancer: Comparison with SCC and CEA. *Anticancer Res*, 25:1765–1772; 2005.

Monk BJ, Lopez LM, Zarba JJ et al. Phase II, open-label study of pazopanib or lapatinib monotherapy compared with pazopanib plus lapatinib combination therapy in patients with advanced and recurrent cervical cancer. *J Clin Oncol*, 28(22):3562–3569; 2010.

Monk BJ, Sill MW, Burger RA et al. Phase II trial of bevacizumab in the treatment of persistent or recurrent squamous cell carcinoma of the cervix: A gynecologic oncology group study. *J Clin Oncol*, 27(7):1069–1074; 2009.

Murphy N, Ring M, Heffron CCBB et al. p16INK4a, CDC6, and MCM5: Predictive biomarkers in cervical preinvasive neoplasia and cervical cancer. *J Clin Pathol*, 58:525–534; 2005.

Nanda K, McCrory DC, Myers ER, Bastian LA et al. Accuracy of the Papanicolaou test in screening for and follow-up of cervical cytologic abnormalities: A systematic review. *Ann Intern Med*, 132:810–819; 2000.

Narayan A, Mathur R, Farooque A, Verma A, and Dwarakanath BS. Cancer biomarkers—Current perspectives. *Indian J Med Res*, 132:129–149; 2010.

Narayan G and Murty VV. Integrative genomic approaches in cervical cancer: Implications for molecular pathogenesis. *Future Oncol*, 6(10):1643–1652; 2010.

Narayan G, Pulido HA, Koul S, Lu XY, Harris CP, Yeh YA, Vargas H et al. Genetic analysis identifies putative tumor suppressor sites at 2q35-q36.1 and 2q36.3-q37.1 involved in cervical cancer progression. *Oncogene*, 22:3489–3499; 2003.

Narimatsu R and Patterson BK. High throughput cervical cancer screening using intracellular human papillomavirus E6 and E7 mRNA quantification by flow cytometry. *Am J Clin Pathol*, 123(5):716–723; 2005.

Naucler P, Ryd W, Törnberg S. et al. Human papillomavirus and Papanicolaou tests to screen for cervical cancer. *N Engl J Med*, 357(16):1589–1597; 2007.

Neyaz MK, Suresh Kumar RS, Hussain S, Naqvi S, Kohaar I, Thakur N, et al. Effect of aberrant promoter methylation of FHIT and RASSF1A genes on susceptibility to cervical cancer in a North Indian population. *Biomarkers*, 13(6):597–606; 2008.

Nishikawa A, Fugimoto T, Akutagawa N, Iwasaki M, Takeuchi M, Fujinaga K, and Kudo R. P53 polymorphism (codon-72) has no correlation with the development and the clinical features of cervical cancer. *Int J Gynecol Cancer*, 10:402–407; 2000.

Nishimura M, Furumoto H, Kato T, Kamada M, and Aono T. Microsatellite instability is a late event in the carcinogenesis of uterine cervical cancer. *Gynecol Oncol*, 79:201–206; 2000.

Niyazi M, Liu XW, and Zhu KC. Death-associated protein kinase promoter (DAPK) hypermethylation in uterine cervical cancer and intraepithelial neoplasia in Uyghur nationality women. *Zhonghua Zhong Liu Za Zhi*, 34(1):31–34; 2012.

Nogueira-Rodrigues A, do Carmo CC, Viegas C et al. Phase I trial of erlotinib combined with cisplatin and radiotherapy for patients with locally advanced cervical squamous cell cancer. *Clin Cancer Res*, 14(19):6324–6329; 2008.

Overmeer RM, Henken FE, Snijders PJ, Claassen-Kramer D, Berkhof J, Helmerhorst TJ et al. Association between dense CADM1 promoter methylation and reduced protein expression in high-grade CIN and cervical SCC. *J Pathol*, 215:388–397; 2008.

Papanicolaou GN and Traut HF. The diagnostic value of vaginal smears in carcinoma of the uterus. *Am J Obstet Gynecol*, 42:193; 1941.

Peitsaro P, Johansson B, and Syrjanen S. Integrated human papillomavirus type 16 is frequently found in cervical cancer precursors as demonstrated by a novel quantitative real-time PCR technique. *J Clin Microbiol*, 40: 886–891; 2002.

Petry K and Petry U. Human papillomavirus testing in primary screening for cervical cancer. *Monographs in Virology*. Basel, Switzerland: Karger, vol. 28, pp. 120–126; 2012.

Petry KU, Schmidt D, Scherbring S, Luyten A, Reinecke-Luthge A, Bergeron C, Kommoss F, Loning T, Ordi J, Regauer S, and Ridder R. Triaging Pap cytology negative, HPV positive cervical cancer screening results with p16/Ki-67 Dual-stained cytology. *Gynecol Oncol*, 121(3):505–509; 2011.

Pongtheerat T, Pakdeethai S, Purisa W, Chariyalertsak S, and Petmitr S. Promoter methylation and genetic polymorphism of glutathione S-transferase P1 gene (GSTP1) in Thai breast-cancer patients. *Asian Pac J Cancer Prev*, 12; 2011.

Raab SS, Geisinger KR, Silverman JF, Thomas PA, and Stanley MW. Interobserver variability of a Papanicolaou smear diagnosis of atypical glandular cells of undetermined significance. *Am J Clin Pathol*, 110:653–659; 1998.

Raman R, Raguram S, Venkataraman G, Paulson JC, and Sasisekharan R. Glycomics: An integrated systems approach to structure-function relationships of glycans. *Nat Method*, 2(11); 2005.

Reesink-Peters N, van der Velden J, Ten Hoor KA, Boezen HM, de Vries EG, Schilthuis MS et al. Preoperative serum squamous cell carcinoma antigen levels in clinical decision making for patients with early-stage cervical cancer. *J Clin Oncol*, 23:1455–1462; 2005.

Reesink-Peters N, Wisman GB, Jéronimo C et al. Feasibility study hypermethylation assay on cervical scrapings: A detecting cervical cancer by quantitative promoter. *Mol Cancer Res*, 2:289–295; 2004.

Roberta Z, Maria IM, Andrea T et al. Detection of residual/recurrent cervical disease after successful LEEP conization: The possible role of mRNA-HPV test. *Curr Pharm Des*, 19(8):1450–1457; 2012.

Rodins K, Cheale M, Coleman N, and Fox SB. Minichromosome maintenance protein 2 expression in normal kidney and renal cell carcinomas: Relationship to tumor dormancy and potential clinical utility. *Clin Cancer Res*, 8(4):1075–1081; 2002.

Rosenthal AN, Ryan A, Al-Jehani RM, Storey A, Harwood CA, and Jacobs IJ. P53 codon 72 polymorphism and risk of cervical cancer in UK. *Lancet*, 352:871–872; 1998.

Rydzewska L, Tierney J, Vale CL, and Symonds PR. Neoadjuvant chemotherapy plus surgery versus surgery for cervical cancer. *Cochrane Database Syst Rev*, 1; 2010.

Sahebali S, Christophe E, Depuydt CE, Gaëlle A V Boulet GAV, Marc Arbyn M, Liliane M et al. Immunocytochemistry in liquid-based cervical cytology: Analysis of clinical use following a cross-sectional study. *Int J Cancer*, 118(5):1254–1260; 2006.

Sahebali S, Depuydt CE, Segers K, Vereecken AJ, Van Marck E, and Bogers JJ. Ki-67 immunocytochemistry in liquid based cervical cytology: Useful as an adjunctive tool? *J Clin Pathol*, 56:681–686; 2003.

Saonere JA. Awareness screening programme reduces the risk of cervical cancer in women. *Afr J Pharm Pharmacol*, 4(6):314–323; 2010.

Sauna ZE, Kimchi-Sarfaty C, Ambudkar SV, and Gottesman MM. Silent polymorphisms speak: How they affect pharmacogenomics and the treatment of cancer, *Cancer Res*, 67:9609; 2007.

Saxena U, Sauvaget C, and Sankaranarayanan R. Evidence-based screening, early diagnosis and treatment strategy of cervical cancer for national policy in low-resource countries: Example of India Asian Pacific. *J Cancer Prev*, 13:1699–1703; 2012.

Scheffner M, Werness BA, Huibregtse JM, Levine AJ, and Howley PM. The E6 oncoprotein encoded by human papillomavirus types 16 and 18 promotes the degradation of p53. *Cell*, 63:1129–1136; 1990.

Schiffman M, Castle PE, Jeronimo J, Rodriguez AC, and Wacholder S. Human papillomavirus and cervical cancer. *Lancet*, 370(9590):890–907; 2007.

Schmidt D, Bergeron C, Denton KJ, and Ridder R. p16/Ki-67 dual stain cytology in the triage of ASCUS and LSIL Papanicolaou cytology. *Cancer Cytopathol*, 119(3):158–166; 2011.

Schönhofer B, Kuhlen R, Neumann P, Westhoff M, Berndt C, Sitter H, and für die Projektgruppe. Nicht-invasive Beatmung bei akuter respiratorischer Insuffizienz. *Deutsches Ärzteblatt*, 105(24): 424–433; 2008.

Schönhofer B. *Nicht-invasive Beatmung—Grundlagen und Moderne Praxis*. Bremen, Germany: UNI-MED; 2006.

Schutz FA, Choueiri TK, and Sternberg CN. Pazopanib: Clinical development of a potent anti-angiogenic drug. *Crit Rev Oncol Hematol*, 77(3):163–171; 2011.

Screening for Cervical Cancer: Clinical Summary of U.S. Preventive Services Task Force Recommendation. AHRQ Publication No. 11-05156-EF-3, March 2012. http://www.uspreventiveservicestaskforce.org/uspstf11/cervcancer/cervcancersum.htm.

Sharma S. Tumor markers in clinical practice: General principles and guidelines. *Indian J Med Paediatr Oncol*, 30(1):1–8; 2009.

Shastri SS, Dinshaw K, Amin G, Goswami S, Patil S, Chinoy R, Kane S et al. Concurrent evaluation of visual, cytological and HPV testing as screening methods for the early detection of cervical neoplasia in Mumbai. *India, Bull World Health Org*, 83:186–194; 2005.

Sheng J and Zhang W. Identification of biomarkers for cervical cancer in peripheral blood lymphocytes using oligonucleotide microarrays. *Chin Med J*, 123(8):1000–1005; 2010.

Shi JF, Chen JF, Canfell K, Feng X X, Ma JF, Zhang YZ et al. Estimation of the costs of cervical cancer screening, diagnosis and treatment in rural Shanxi Province, China: A micro-costing study. *BMC Health Servs Res*, 12:123; 2012.

Siddiqui MT, Cohen C, Nassar A. Detecting high-grade cervical disease on ASC-H cytology: Role of BD ProEx C and Digene Hybrid Capture II HPV DNA testing. *Am J Clin Pathol*, 130(5):765–770; 2008.

Singh M, Mehrotra S, Kalra N, Singh U, and Shukla Y. Correlation of DNA ploidy with progression of cervical cancer. *J Cancer Epidemiol, Article ID* 298495; 2008.

Song JY, Lee JK, Lee NW, Yeom BW, Kim SH, and Lee KW. Osteopontin expression correlates with invasiveness in cervical cancer. *Aust N Z J Obstet Gynaecol*, 49:434–438; 2009.

Sorbye SW, Arbyn M, Fismen S, Gutteberg TJ, and Mortensen ES. HPV E6/E7 mRNA testing is more specific than cytology in post-colposcopy follow-up of women with negative cervical biopsy. *PLoS One*, 6(10):e26022; 2011.

Spratlin JL, Serkova NJ, and Eckhardt SG. Clinical applications of metabolomics in oncology: A review. *Clinical Cancer Research*, 15(2):431–440; 2009.

Storey A, Thomas M, Kalita A, Harwood C, Gardiol D, Mantovani F, Breuer J, Leigh Im, Matlashewski G, and Banks L. Role of a p53 polymorphism in the development of human papillomavirus-associated cancer. *Nature* 393:229–234; 1998.

Suarez-Rincon AE, Moran-Moguel MC, Montoya-Fuentes H, Allegos-Arreola MP, and Sanchez-Corona J. Polymorphism in codon 72 of the p53 gene and cervico-uterine cancer risk in Mexico. *Ginecol Obstet Mex*, 70:344–348; 2002.

Surveillance Epidemiology and End Results. SEER Stat Fact Sheet: Cervix Uteri. Available at: http://seer.cancer.gov/statfacts/html/cervix.html, 2012. Accessed March 19, 2012.

Tambouret RH, Misdraji J, and Wilbur DC. Longitudinal clinical evaluation of a novel antibody cocktail for detection of high-grade squamous intraepithelial lesions on cervical cytology specimens. *Arch Pathol Lab Med*, 132(6):918–925; 2008.

Treating Cervical Cancer-A Quick Guide. Cancer Research UK, 2012. Available from: http://www.cancerresearchuk.org/prod_consump/groups/cr_common/@cah/@gen/documents/generalcontent/treating-cervical-cancer.pdf.

Tsiodras S, Georgoulakis J, Chranioti A, Voulgaris Z, Psyrri A, Tsivilika A, Panayiotides J, and Karakitsos P. Hybrid capture vs. PCR screening of cervical human papilloma virus infections. Cytological and histological associations in 1270 women. *BMC Cancer*, 10:53; 2010.

Tsoumpou I, Kyrgiou M, Gelbaya TA, and Nardo LG. The effect of surgical treatment for endometrioma on in vitro fertilization outcomes: A systematic review and meta-analysis. *Fertil Steril*, 92(1):75–87; 2009.

Ugorski M and Laskowska W. Sialyl lewis(a): A tumor associated carbohydrate antigen involved in adhesion and metastatic potential of cancer cells. *Acta Biochem Pol*, 49:303–311; 2002.

U.S. Cancer Statistics Working Group. United States Cancer Statistics: 1999–2007 Incidence and Mortality Web-based Report. Atlanta (GA): Department of Health and Human Services, Centers for Disease Control and Prevention, and National Cancer Institute; 2010.

Vaissière T, Sawan C, and Herceg Z. Epigenetic interplay between histone modifications and DNA methylation in gene silencing. *Mutat Res Rev Mutat Res*, 659(1–2):40–48; 2008.

Vitali L, Yakisich JS, Vita MF, Fernandez A, Settembrini L, Siden A, Cruz M, Carminatti H, Casas O, and Idoyaga Vargas V. Roscovitine inhibits ongoing DNA synthesis in human cervical cancer. *Cancer Lett*, 180(1):7–12; 2002.

Vlaicu M. FDA Medical Device: Non-Invasive Cervical Cancer Detection (OTC:GTHP). Guided Therapeutics Inc. Available from: http://www.themarketfinancial.com/fda-medical-device-non-invasive-cervical-cancer-detection-otcgthp/666. Accessed September 11, 2014.

Walboomers JM, Jacobs MV, Manos MM et al. Human papillomavirus is a necessary cause of invasive cervical cancer worldwide. *J Pathol*, 189:12–19; 1999.

Waldstrøm M, Christensen RK, and Ørnskov D. Evaluation of p16INK4a/Ki-67 dual stain in comparison with an mRNA human papillomavirus test on liquid-based cytology samples with low-grade squamous intraepithelial lesion. *Cancer Cytopathol*; 2012.

Wang PH. Altered sialylation and its roles in gynecologic cancers. *J Cancer Mol*, 2(3):107–116; 2006.

Watabe K, Ito A, Koma Y, and Kitamura Y. IGSF4: A new intercellular adhesion molecule that is called by three names, TSLC1, SgIGSF and SynCAM, by virtue of its diverse function. *Histol Histopathol*, 18:1321–1329; 2003.

Wentzensen N, Schwartz L, Zuna RE, Smith K, Mathews C, Gold MA, Allen RA, Zhang R, Dunn ST, Walker JL, and Schiffman M. Performance of p16/Ki-67 immunostaining to detect cervical cancer precursors in a colposcopy referral population. *Clin Cancer Res*, 18:4154–4162; 2012.

Wentzensen N, Sherman ME, Schiffman M, and Wang SS. Utility of methylation markers in cervical cancer early detection: Appraisal of the state-of-the-science. *Gynecol Oncol*, 112:293–299; 2009.

WHO/ICO Information Center on Human Papillomavirus and Related Cancers, Summary Report Update (2010). Available from http://screening.iarc.fr/doc/Human%20Papillomavirus%20and%20Related%20Cancers.pdf. Accessed March 19, 2012.

Widschwendter A, Müller H, Fiegl H, Ivarsson L, Wiedemair A, Müller-Holzner E, Goebel G, Marth C, and Widschwendter M. DNA methylation in serum and tumors of cervical cancer patients. *Clin Cancer Res*, 10:565; 2004.

William E and Julie JA. Pharmacogenomics: The inherited basis for interindividual differences in drug response. *Annu Rev Genomics Hum Genet*, 2:9–39; 2001.

Williams GH, Romanowski P, Morris L, Madine M, Mills AD, Stoeber K, Marr J, Laskey RA, and Coleman N. Improved cervical smear assessment using antibodies against proteins that regulate DNA replication. *Proc Natl Acad Sci USA*, 95:14932–14937; 1998.

Wong YF, Chung TK, Cheung TH, Nobori T, Hamptom GM, Wang VW, Li YF, and Chang AM. P53 polymorphism and human papillomavirus infection in Hong Kong women with cervical cancer. *Gynecol Obstet Invest*, 50:60–63; 2000.

Wright TC. Cervical cancer screening in the 21st century: Is it time to retire the PAP smear? *Clin Obst Gynecol*, 50:313–323; 2007.

Xiaoxia Hu, Schwarz JK, Lewis JS Jr, Huettner PC, Rader JS, Deasy JO, Grigsby PW, and Wang X. A microRNA expression signature for cervical cancer prognosis. *Cancer Res*, 70:1441–1448; 2010.

Yang HJ, Liu VW, Wang Y, Chan KY, Tsang PC, Khoo US, Cheung AN, and Ngan HY. Detection of hypermethylated genes in tumor and plasma of cervical cancer patients. *Gynecol Oncol*, 93(2):435–440; 2004.

Yang N, Eijsink JJ, Lendvai A, Volders HH, Klip H, Buikema HJ, van Hemel BM, Schuuring E, van der Zee AG, and Wisman GB. Methylation markers for CCNA1 and C13ORF18 are strongly associated with high-grade cervical intraepithelial neoplasia and cervical cancer in cervical scrapings. *Cancer Epidemiol Biomarkers Prev*, 18(11):3000–3007; 2009.

Yang SY, Miah A, Pabari A, and Winslet M. Growth factors and their receptors in cancer metastases. *Front Biosci*, 16:531–538; 2011.

Yildiz IZ, Usubütün A, Firat P, Ayhan A, and Küçükali T. Efficiency of immunohistochemical p16 expression and HPV typing in cervical squamous intraepithelial lesion grading and review of the p16 literature. *Pathol Res Pract*, 203(6):445–449; 2007.

Yin M, Zhao F, Lou G, Zhang H, Sun M, Li C, et al. The long-term efficacy of neoadjuvant chemotherapy followed by radical hysterectomy compared with radical surgery alone or concurrent chemoradiotherapy on locally advanced-stage cervical cancer. *International Journal of Gynecological Cancer*, 21(1):92–99; 2011.

Yoon SM, Shin KH, Kim JY, Seo SS, Park SY, Moon SH, and Cho KH. Use of serum squamous cell carcinoma antigen for follow-up monitoring of cervical cancer patients who were treated by concurrent chemoradiotherapy. *Radiat Oncol*, 5:78; 2010.

Yoshida T, Sano T, Kanuma T, Inoue H, Itoh T, Yazaki C, Obara M, and Fukuda T. Usefulness of CINtec® PLUS p16INK4a/Ki-67 double-staining in cytological screening of cervical cancer. *Acta Cytologica*, 55:413–420; 2011.

Zagouri F, Sergentanis TN, Chrysikos D, Filipits M, and Bartsch R. Molecularly targeted therapies in cervical cancer. A systematic review. *Gynecol Oncol*, 126(2):291–303; 2012.

Zareen A, Kouser S, Begum A, and Tabassum Z. Cervical screening awareness and practice among medical personnel. *South Asian Feder Obstet Gynecol*, 1(2):34–37; 2009.

Zehbe I, Voglino G, Wilander E, Delius H, Marongiu A, Edler L, Klimek F, Anderson S, and Tommasino M. P53 codon 72 polymorphism and various human papillomavirus 16 E6 genotypes are risk factors for cervical cancer development. *Cancer Res*, 61:608–611; 2001.

Zhang X, Wei D, Yap Y, Li L, Guo S, and Chen F. Mass spectrometry-based "omics" technologies in cancer diagnostics. *Mass Spectrom Rev*, 26(3):403–431; 2007.

Zur Hausen H, Meinhof W, Scheiber W, and Bornkamm GW. Attempts to detect virus-specific DNA in human tumors. I. Nucleic acid hybridizations with complementary RNA of human wart virus. *Int J Cancer*, 13(5):650–656; 1974.

Zur Hausen H. Papillomaviruses causing cancer: Evasion from host-cell control in early events in carcinogenesis. *J Natl Cancer Inst*, 92:690–698; 2000.

8

Biomarkers in Cervical Cancer: DNA HR-HPV, p16INK4a, Ki-67, and RNA-m E6/E7

María Serrano,* MD, María-Dolores Diestro,* MD, PhD, Marcos Cuerva, MD, PhD, Ignacio Zapardiel, MD, PhD, Adolfo Loayza, MD, PhD, Alicia Hernández, MD, PhD, and Javier De Santiago, MD, PhD

CONTENTS

* María Serrano and María-Dolores Diestro have contributed equally to this chapter and shared first authorship credit.

ABSTRACT The relationship between infection with human papilloma virus (HPV) and cervical cancer is well defined. The detection of DNA in the cytology or biopsy in the infected patient is the first and most direct biomarker of exposure to the virus. Once the virus infects the basal layer cells, it uncoats and delivers its DNA to the cells' nucleus. The oncoproteins E6 and E7 are expressed and suppress the regulation of the cell cycle, inhibiting apoptosis. E6 and E7 bind to and inhibit p53 and Rb, which are tumor suppressor proteins. Pe6 and Pe7 should be considered as viral oncogenes and early biomarkers of cervical cancer, as well as p16 protein and cell proliferation marker Ki-67. The detection of intracellular mRNA HPV E6/E7 expression is of high relevance in medical practice; its quantification increases the specificity and positive predictive value of cervical cancer screening compared to DNA HR-HPV. Recent investigation in molecular biology has shown that the quantification of mRNA HPV E6/E7 in the affected cells is an indicator of progression to cancer development. There are already some screening tests using the detection of intracellular mRNA HPV E6/E7 expression. These tests can be used for the follow-up of patients after surgical conization and as a risk factor for treatment failure and recurrence. We proceed to the analysis by dual staining p16 protein and cell proliferation marker Ki-67, as biomarkers of tumor aggressiveness. Quantification of intracellular mRNA HPV E6/E7 expression is directly related as a biomarker to the tumor dissemination in early stages of cervical cancer. The test for mRNA HPV E6/E7 serves as the most sensitive diagnostic tool available for ultrastaging to detect micrometastases in the sentinel node biopsy. In addition, research on other biomarkers such as CK19 and SCC has promising results for a not-far-away future.

8.1 Introduction

8.1.1 Why Is It Important?

The relationship between HPV and cervical cancer is one of the most consistent in the field of oncology. HPV is a necessary condition but not enough for developing an oncogenic transformation alone (Bosch et al., 2002). Through translational research, several achievements have been reached, which will allow us to evaluate and manage patients with cervical cancer, selecting the most appropriate therapy for each case.

Cervical cancer is one of the few cancers that can be diagnosed in very early stages. Due to the natural history of cervical cancer, we are able to detect it in preinvasive stage. In the mid-twentieth century, cervical cytology or Pap test was introduced. Pap test has led to an important reduction in morbidity and mortality among the populations that have established a proper screening system. Pap test screening is a reliable, reproducible, convenient, and inexpensive method, but a minimum coverage of 70% of the population must be achieved and sustained. It also has a low sensitivity, with a wide range (30%–87%), which requires frequent repetitions of the test, in order to reduce the mortality in the general population (Puig-Tintoré et al., 2006).

The discovery of the HPV, as a necessary step in cervical oncogenesis, can be considered as the first biomarker discovered for the detection of cervical cancer and specially the DNA of the subtypes of HPV of high oncogenic risk (HR-HPV). The HR-HPV detection techniques, which will be discussed throughout this chapter, have a high sensitivity for detecting a moderate–severe cervical intraepithelial neoplasia (CIN2+), and their results are independent of age (Cuzick et al., 2006), which is an advantage when compared to cytology. Unfortunately, the HR-HPV detection techniques have a low specificity for CIN2+ (especially in young women, because of the high prevalence of HPV). So, HR-HPV detection techniques have a very low positive predictive value (PPV) and a high negative predictive value (NPV).

Other new specific biomarkers have been discovered due to the better understanding of the mechanism of action by which the virus persists in the epithelium of the cervix and starts the carcinogenesis. Some of these new specific biomarkers are as follows: the p16INK4a, the cell proliferation marker Ki-67, or the mRNA of E6 and E7. The new biomarkers indicate which preinvasive lesions are more likely to progress to cervical carcinomas and which carcinomas have an increased risk of recurrence. Most of these biomarkers are still under study, and their clinical use in order to integrate them into our care protocols has not been validated yet.

So far, the HR-HPV DNA and the biomarkers mentioned earlier can be used for the noninvasive diagnosis in the Pap tests or as invasive biomarkers when tissue samples are obtained by biopsy.

There has also been a huge progress in minimally invasive surgery related to the detection of cervical cancer. Although the detection techniques through minimally invasive surgery are considered as invasive biomarkers, they offer the possibility of reducing the aggressiveness of surgery and simultaneously the morbidity of the diagnosis. The sentinel lymph node biopsy in early-stage cervical carcinoma (FIGO stages Ia1 with lymphovascular invasion, IA2, IB1, and IIa1) allows immunohistochemical and molecular detection of nodal micrometastases (Sakuragi et al., 1999; Barranger et al., 2004; Opazo, 2009). Recent studies are focused on the detection of CK19, serum SCC antigen (SCC-ag), HR-HPV DNA, and HPV E6/E7 mRNA in the sentinel node, with very promising results.

8.1.2 Epidemiology of Cervical Cancer and HPV Infection

8.1.2.1 Cervical Cancer Epidemiology

Cervical cancer is the second most common cancer in women after breast cancer (Bosch et al., 2002) and is the fifth most common cancer worldwide. The average age at diagnosis is 48 years, although approximately 47% of all invasive cervical carcinomas are diagnosed before age 35. Only 10% of diagnoses are made in women over 65 years of age. The most common histological type is SCC, which is responsible for 80% of all invasive cervical carcinomas (Lowndes, 2006).

Eighty-three percent of all cervical cancers diagnosed every year occur in developing countries, being cervical cancer the most common cause of death caused by cancer in these countries. In developing countries, cervical cancer has a median survival of 5 years after diagnosis, while in developed countries the median survival is of 10 years after the diagnosis.

Different statistical models indicate that for women over 15 years of age, there are 27 million women with low-grade dysplasia, 1.5 million with high-grade dysplasia, and 400,000 with invasive cervical carcinoma worldwide (Bosch et al., 2006).

8.1.2.2 HPV Epidemiology

HPV infection is the most common sexually transmitted disease. Worldwide, it is responsible for 5.2% of all human tumors, corresponding to 2.2% of all human tumors in developed countries and 7.7% in developing countries (Parkin, 2006).

Seventy to eighty percent of sexually active women and men have been exposed to the HPV at some point in their lives (Syrjänen and Syrjánen, 2000).

Estimates suggest that there are 310 million carriers of HPV, and out of these 310 million carriers, 27 million suffer from genital warts and 68,400 people suffer from vulvar, vaginal, anal, pineal, or oropharyngeal cancer (Parkin, 2006).

The prevalence of HPV in women in developed countries is less than 10% and slightly more than 15% in developing countries (de Sanjosé et al., 2007). According to data from the International Agency for Research on Cancer (IARC), the HPV prevalence differs between geographical areas, following a similar distribution to the cervical cancer prevalence (Forslund et al., 2002; Molano et al., 2002; Ferreccio et al., 2004; Thomas et al., 2004).

A study conducted in the United Kingdom on 1075 women of the same age revealed that the cumulative risk of any HPV infection in 3 years is 44%, rising to 60% in 5 years, HPV 16 being the most common type of HPV (Woodman et al., 2001).

In Spain (Font et al., 2004), a study among 1383 women attending a family planning visit in Barcelona showed an incidence of new infections of 2% per year over a 3-year follow-up. Fifty percent of women with HR-HPV DNA at the beginning of the study had a negative result after 367 days (Diestro et al., 2007).

8.1.3 HPV and Cervical Cancer

There are approximately 100 types of HPV, out of them 30 or 40 infect regularly or sporadically the genital tract (Williers et al., 2004). The types of HPV are divided into groups of high and low oncogenic risk. Among the high-risk types, HPV 16 and 18 are the most important ones, and together are the cause of approximately 70% of cases of invasive cervical cancer (Bosch et al., 1995). HPV 16 and 18 are also present in more than 50% of all basaloid and verrucous vulvar and pineal and vaginal carcinomas and in over 50% of all anal carcinomas (Stanley, 2006a). The next types of HPV in frequency are types 31, 33, and 45, followed by types 35, 39, 51, 52, 56, 58, 59, 68, 73, and 82. Types 26, 53, and 66 have also high oncogenic risk. These viruses are also detected in high- and low-grade intraepithelial lesions.

8.1.3.1 Physiology of HPV Infection and Cervical Cancer

When an erosion or microtrauma in the surface layer of the target epithelia takes place, it facilitates the virus entry to the basal layer cells, where the virus amplifies its genome expressing the proteins E1, E2, E6, and E7 (Stanley, 2006a). In the intermediate layers, both cells and virus replicate themselves in tandem, without amplification of the viral copies with little expression of the E1, E2, E6, and E7 genes. In the upper layers, where the epithelium is more differentiated, the virus is amplified without cellular replication, reaching numbers of 1000 viral genome copies per cell. At this point, the expression of the structural protein genes (L1 and L2) as well as the E4 protein begins, producing the assembly of the virus capsid (Stanley, 1994).

The virus infects the cell, producing lesions in a time period that may last from weeks to months, inducing viral replication. During this viral replication, there is no detectable viremia, because the final target cells are the differentiated keratinocytes (Oriel, 1971). The keratinocytes are intended to peel in the surface layer of epithelium, and there are no obvious danger signals that alert the immune system, so that the injuries are not accompanied by inflammation.

Circulating antibodies against the viral protein capsid L1 are detectable after the infection, with decreasing trend in the next 2–3 weeks, remaining stable with low levels of antibodies, which are detectable over time (Stanley, 2006b).

Seroconversion confers type-specific immunity against future infections. Some degree of cross-immunity between viral types has been described (Frazer et al., 2006).

The cellular immunity against the viral infection is of main importance in controlling and clearing the HPV and, due to this, in the development, persistence and/or progression of dysplastic lesions (Chow and Broker, 2005). Langerhans cells are responsible for presenting viral antigens to keratinocytes, producing an immune response against infection (Padilla-Paz, 2005).

The estimated average duration of infection for high-risk virus is of 8–12 months; although types 16 and 18 tend to persist for longer periods, between 16 and 24 months (Bosch et al., 2006). Ninety percent of HPV infections are benign, subclinical, and self-limiting, and a high proportion of infections are associated with low-grade dysplasias, which regress spontaneously (Baseman and Koutsky, 2005). The low-grade squamous intraepithelial lesion (LSIL) can be caused by viruses of both high and low risk. Persistent cervical infection (defined by the viral detection more than once in a range of time equal or greater than 6 months) is produced by high-risk HPV types and is the most important risk factor for progression to high-grade dysplasia (Khan, 2005).

According to a study in Costa Rica, with results similar to those of other developed countries, the infections by HPV 16 and 18 that progressed to CIN3 were 17.7% and 13.6%, respectively (Castle et al., 2005). This can be seen in the curve of incidence of HPV, wherein after the initial peak in 20 years, there is a big drop and 10 years after, there is a new peak of incidence of premalignant lesions. It means that an LSIL that progresses to high-grade squamous intraepithelial lesion (HSIL) progresses after 10–20 years (age 40–50 years) to the peak incidence of cervical cancer, caused by viruses that created a persistent infection (Kjaer et al., 2002) (Figure 8.1).

8.1.3.2 HPV Viral Cycle: Oncogenesis E6/E7

The HPV is composed of a double-stranded circular DNA, inside an icosahedral protein capsid of two molecules (L1 and L2). E1 and E2 genes encode proteins responsible for modulating viral DNA replication. The proteins encoded by the E6 and E7 genes are those that have oncogenic transforming capacity (Figure 8.2).

In the HR-HPV infections, after the virus penetration in the basal cells of the cervical epithelium, it results in the breakage of the circular structure of the viral genome at the E1–E2 level so that it can be inserted into the host cell chromosome. This disruption alters the function of these genes. E1 and E2 proteins encode proteins that regulate in a repressor way the transcriptional activity of E6 and E7. E6 and E7 genes encode E6 and E7 proteins, which are involved in carcinogenesis (Diestro et al., 2007).

It is known that after the genome of HPV virus integration in host cells of the cervix, a continuous expression of viral E6 and E7 oncoproteins takes place. This persistent expression starts the process of cervical cancer, affecting the cell cycle control and producing a cell proliferation, which make these proteins reliable markers of early cervical cancer (Molden et al., 2007).

Transcription of the E6 and E7 genes of HR-HPV genotypes and production of functional oncogenes E6 and E7 are recognized as a necessary step in the conversion of malignant cells. The E6/E7 oncogenes are present in almost all cervical carcinomas and

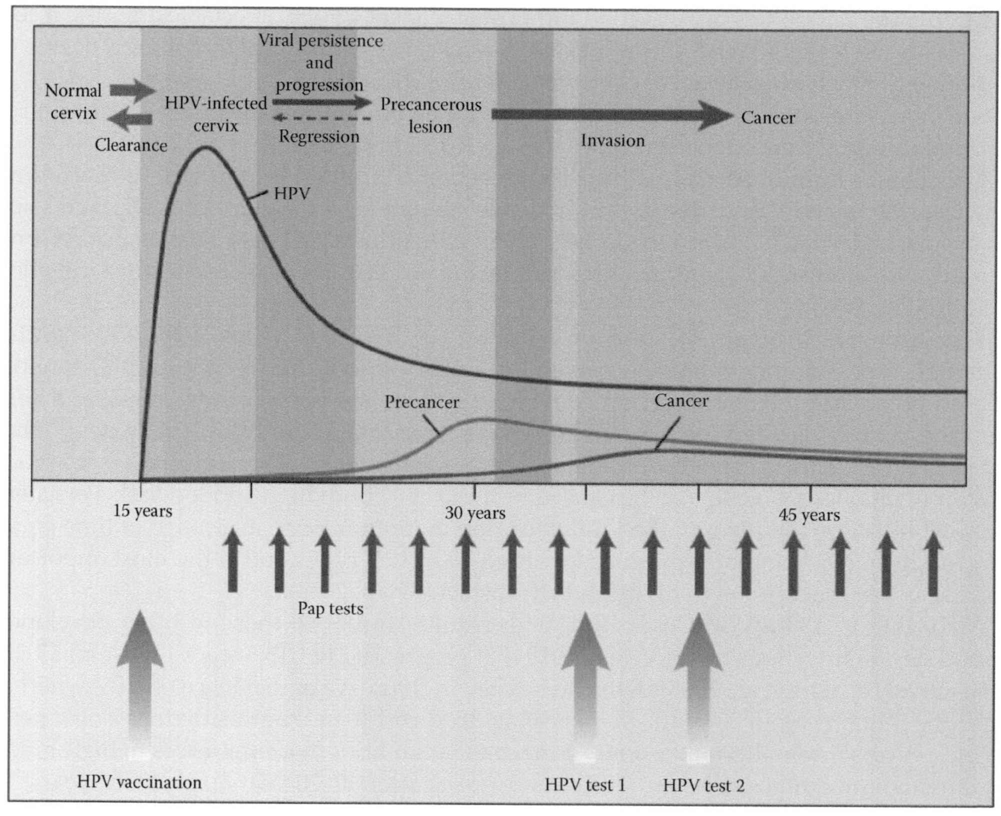

FIGURE 8.1
The natural history of HPV infection and cervical cancer. (From Schiffman, M. et al., *N. Engl. J. Med.*, 353, 2101, 2005.)

are recognized as responsible for the initiation and evolution in invasive tumors. These oncogenes cause the degradation of the tumor suppressor proteins p53 and pRb (retinoblastoma protein) and interfere with the cell cycle regulation (Cuschieri et al., 2004).

Infected epithelial cells activate its defense mechanism; this process occurs during the cell division stage and is controlled by a group of proteins among which p53 and pRB (retinoblastoma protein) are of high importance. Proteins E6 and E7 of HR-HPV interact with the regulatory proteins of these infected cells. The active form of pRb inhibits cell replication by inhibiting DNA replication. The HPV E7 protein binds to the active form of pRb, thereby losing its regulatory function and the cell replication being stimulated (Cuschieri et al., 2004). The cellular p53 has a dual function as regulator, one as a repressor of cell replication and another inducing apoptosis in case of serious injury. The E6 protein of HR-HPV blocks the p53 interacting with its biological function. Moreover, the protein E6–p53 complex induces cytoplasmic degradation of p53 (Molden et al., 2007).

Thus, the interaction of the viral E6 and E7 proteins with p53 and pRb results in the proliferation and cellular immortalization. For this reason, pE6 and pE7 are considered as authentic viral oncogenes. The constant activity of PE6 and PE7 leads to an increasing genomic instability, oncogenic mutation accumulation, additional loss of cellular control, and finally malignant cell development.

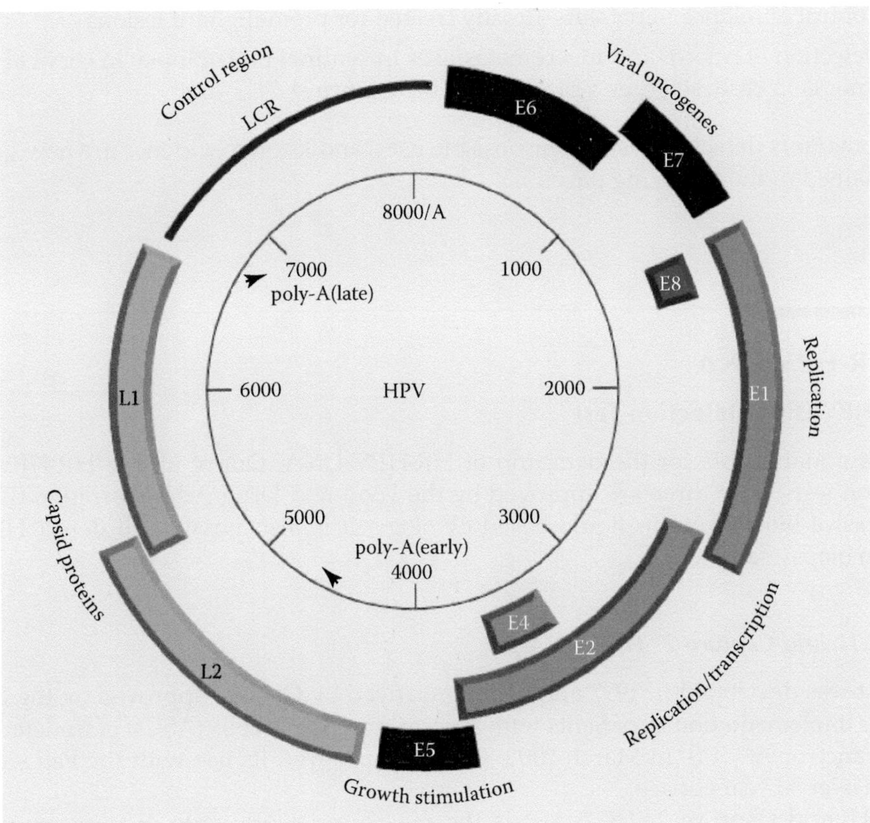

FIGURE 8.2
Genome organization of the papillomavirus: HPV16. (From Lie, A.K. and Kristensen, G., *Expert Rev. Mol. Diagn.*, 8(4), 405, 2008.)

Overexpression of pE6 and pE7 oncoproteins is a need for the development process of carcinogenesis (immortalization–cell proliferation) induced by HR-HPV. During the tumor progression, the viral genomes are integrated into the host chromosomes, which produce a constant level of E6 and E7 proteins, with the stabilization of the mRNA.

Thanks to recent advances in molecular biology, it is possible nowadays identifying and quantifying the presence of E6 and E7 mRNA in affected cells (Ardic et al., 2009).

8.2 Use of Biomarkers in Cervical Cancer

Several screening tests for cervical cancer biomarkers have been designed, which may help in daily clinical practice. The clinical possibilities are

- Primary screening of premalignant lesions
- Triage of abnormal Pap smears

- Control of relapse in patients already treated for premalignant lesions
- Detection of micro- and macrometastases in sentinel node biopsy in cervical carcinoma in early stage, as a predictor of recurrence

The biomarkers detection tests, their possible uses, and known evidence are now going to be explained in the following pages.

8.3 HR-HPV DNA

8.3.1 HPV DNA Detection Test

There are many tests for the detection of HR-HPV DNA. Out of all the HR-HPV DNA detection tests, only three are approved by the Food and Drug Administration (FDA) as noninvasive biomarkers in liquid-based cytology. It is also possible to detect HR-HPV DNA in biopsy samples.

8.3.1.1 Hybrid Capture 2® HPV DNA-HR

The test was developed in 1997 and commercialized by Qiagen, approved by the FDA in 1999 for implementation in patients with atypical squamous cells (ASCs) of undetermined significance or ASCUS. In March 2003, the FDA approved its use with the Pap smear in women over 30 years of age.

The Hybrid Capture 2 (HC2) test is the most used worldwide. It is recommended that other tests should have similar clinical features to HC2 to ensure their clinical validation.

The main problem with the current version of HC2 is its lack of precision due to cross-reactivity with nontarget HPV types. Recent studies have detected a false-positive rate of 5%, in cases where no HR-HPV DNA is detected with polymerase chain reaction (PCR).

8.3.1.2 Cervista®

Approved in March 2009 by the FDA, and commercialized by Hologic, it includes two tests:

- The Cervista® HR-HPV is an in vitro diagnostic test for the qualitative detection of DNA from 14 types of HPV (16, 18, 31, 33, 35.39, 45, 51, 52, 56, 58, 59, 66, and 68) in cervical samples. The test uses a method of multiplying the signal for the detection of specific nucleic acid sequences.
- The limitation of this test is its potential cross-reactivity with other types of HPV, such as 67 and 70 with false-positive results.
- The Cervista® HPV 16/18 only determines the existence of genotypes 16 and 18, which are the higher-risk types of persistence and most frequently associated with cervical cancer.

The limitation of this test is its cross-reactivity with high-risk virus 31 and false negative in cases of low-level infections or sampling errors.

8.3.1.3 cobas 4800® HPV Test

cobas 4800 HPV test (Roche) has a fully automated real-time PCR sample preparation method for amplification and detection (approved by the FDA in April 2011).

There is little literature on analytical or clinical validation of this test. However, the data show that this test meets the requirements of international guidelines to consider itself clinically validated for screening.

8.3.2 Analytical Accuracy and Clinical Use of the Determination of HR-HPV DNA

8.3.2.1 Primary Screening and Preinvasive Lesions

8.3.2.1.1 Primary Screening

In a revision of 15 series from 2000 to 2006 (Puig-Tintoré et al., 2006) comparing the analytical accuracy of cytology and HR-HPV DNA test (most by HC2), it was found that the sensitivity of cytology was substantially lower (61.3%) than that of HR-HPV DNA test (91.1%). The specificity of cytology was 93.5% and that of HR-HPV DNA test was lower (89.3%). The combined value of both techniques showed an improvement in sensitivity of screening (95.7%), with a NPV of 100%, which allow separating the interval between screenings to 5 years if both tests are negative.

The HR-HPV DNA test has been validated as a primary screening test in vaccinated women (Naife population), and in the general population of the Netherlands (Meijer, 2011), cytology is in the background in case of positive test.

8.3.2.1.2 Triage of Abnormal Cytology

In case of abnormal cytology, the performance of HR-HPV DNA test is appropriate in the following cases:

- Initial management of women ≥20 years with ASCUS cytology.
- Initial management of postmenopausal women with LSIL, since less than 50% of menopausal women with LSIL have HPV. Those that are negative to HPV are at minimal risk of developing cancer and do not need colposcopy.

The performance of HR-HPV DNA tests is inappropriate in the initial management of women younger than 20 years with abnormal cytological diagnoses, LSIL in women ≥20 years, or ASC-H (ASCs, cannot exclude HSIL), HSIL, or atypical glandular cells/adenocarcinoma in situ (AGC/AIS) in women of any age.

HR-HPV DNA test should not be repeated in less than 12 months. There are two exceptions:

1. AGC-NOS (atypical glandular cells, not otherwise specified) without injury in the initial management, that is, with negative colposcopy for CIN or AIS.
2. For monitoring women treated for CIN2+, in this case, HR-HPV DNA test must be performed after 6 months of the treatment.

8.3.2.1.3 Posttreatment Control of Preinvasive Lesions

The HR-HPV DNA tests in monitoring patients treated for CIN are very useful to confirm the presence of any residual or recurrent lesions. It is recommended performing an HR-HPV DNA test in the sixth month of follow-up (Puig Tintoré et al., 2006).

The detection of HR-HPV DNA as predictive test of residual or recurrent lesion has a higher sensitivity and specificity, when compared to the use of cytology in the follow-up. In the review of the existing meta-analysis, the sensitivity of the HR-HPV DNA tests to predict treatment failure ranged between 67% and 100%, with a mean of 94.4%. The specificity to predict treatment success ranged between 44% and 100% (KS Cuschieri et al., 2004; Molden et al., 2005; Kraus et al., 2006).

8.3.2.2 Cervical Carcinoma in Early Stages: Sentinel Node

The main method to determine the extent of cervical cancer is laparoscopic surgical staging. Staging studies by image (CT, MRI, PET-CT) have important limitations to determine the true extent of the tumor, not being possible the detection of micrometastases (Mathevet, 2009; Bentivegna et al., 2011). Lymphadenectomy is part of surgical staging of cervical cancer and, in the absence of lymphatic metastases, it has no therapeutic value. The metastatic lymph node involvement is a major independent predictor of survival. The sentinel node is the first lymph node to receive direct lymphatic drainage from the tumor, being predictive for the whole lymphatic chain.

It is very important the correlation between the presence of HR-HPV DNA in the lymph nodes and histopathologically confirmed metastases of early-stage cervical carcinoma. HPV L1 gene fragment in paraffin-embedded tissue specimens of the primary tumor and pelvic lymph nodes from 31 patients with cervical cancer were amplified using HPV-specific PCR primers with general consensus GP5 +/GP6 +. The type of HPV was identified by sequence analysis of the PCR products, and the correlation between the presence of HR-HPV DNA in the lymph node and the clinicopathological indices of cervical carcinoma was analyzed. The positivity rate of HR-HPV DNA in the pelvic lymph nodes was 58.1% in the 31 patients, and in 13 of the patients with confirmed metastases, the detection rate was 84.6% as compared with the rate of 27.8% in the other 18 patients without metastases. The presence of HR-HPV DNA in the lymph node was histologically confirmed associated with metastases. The results of both HPV DNA detection and pathological examination indicated that the obturator, internal iliac and external iliac lymph nodes were more liable to be positive for HPV DNA, accounting for over 90% of the positivity (Sun et al., 2008).

The detection of both HR-HPV DNA by in situ hybridization and CK19 by immunohistochemical method detected lymph node micrometastases in early-stage cervical cancer. As a method of detection on the molecular level, in situ hybridization was more sensitive for the detection of lymph node micrometastases in early-stage cervical cancer. In this study, the group investigated the detection rate and methods of micrometastases in early-stage cervical cancer by detecting the expression of DNA HR-HPV and CK19 in pelvic lymph nodes. A total of 104 lymph nodes with/without pathologically confirmed metastases, from 28 patients with early-stage cervical cancer, were included for the detection of HPV DNA-HR and CK19 expression using in situ hybridization and immunohistochemistry, respectively. The detection rate of HR-HPV DNA in lymph nodes and CK19 in patients with pathologically confirmed lymph node metastases was higher compared to that in lymph nodes in patients without lymph node pathologically confirmed metastases ($P < 0.001$). In all 80 pathologically negative lymph nodes, the positivity rates of HR-HPV DNA detection and CK19 were 45% and 25%, respectively. In 57 lymph nodes in patients without pathologically confirmed lymph node metastases, the positivity rates of HR-HPV DNA detection and CK19 were 43.5% and 24.6%. The detection rates of HR-HPV DNA and CK19 in 15 pathologically confirmed patients without lymph node metastases were 60% and 46.6%, respectively. The detection rates of HR-HPV DNA and CK19 in 104 lymph nodes were 56.7% and 41.3% (KI = 0.46). The results of the two detection methods showed good consistency (Zhang et al., 2012).

8.4 p16-INK4a

The control of the progression of the eukaryotic cell cycle is affected by a complex mechanism of controlled expression and posttranslational molecules modifications (e.g., phosphorylation) of proteins that regulate the cell cycle. p16-INK4a protein plays a crucial role in the regulation of the eukaryotic cell cycle. It is part of the pRb-mediated control of the transition from G1 to S phase and causes cell cycle arrest during the process of cellular differentiation. Therefore, p16-INK4a has an antiproliferative effect when expressed during cell cycle progression. In differentiated epithelial cells, the expression of p16-INK4a protein can normally not be detected by immunocytochemistry. In cases of cervical neoplasia, there is a strong overexpression of p16-INK4a as a result of functional inactivation of the pRb caused by the oncoprotein E7 of HR-HPV (Ishikawa et al., 2006). As E7 is required to establish and maintain the malignant phenotype in precancerous and cancerous lesions associated with HPV, p16-INK4a overexpression is directly linked to the oncogenic activity of the different types of HR-HPV and therefore has been proposed as a surrogate marker of HPV infections (Agoff et al., 2003).

The CINtec® Histology Kit is an immunohistochemistry kit to determine qualitatively the p16-INK4a antigen in tissue sections from biopsies of cervix formalin fixed and paraffin embedded and therefore is an invasive biomarker test, although there is a possibility for determining as a noninvasive marker in liquid-based cytology, together with the determination of the proliferation marker Ki-67, in a dual detection kit.

Its use is indicated in conjunction with slides stained with hematoxylin–eosin prepared from the same sample of cervical tissue, as an aid to increase the diagnostic accuracy and interobserver agreement in the diagnosis of cervical carcinomas and cervical intraepithelial high-grade neoplasms.

Several studies have been published that claim that an overexpression of p16-INK4a has been observed immunohistochemically in a large number of cases of precancerous cervical dysplasia (for 80%–100% of CIN2 lesions and in all CIN3) and invasive cancers. Low-grade intraepithelial lesions (CIN1) show varying levels of overexpression of p16INK4a, typically between 30% and 60% (Regauer and Reich, 2007). The diagnostic interpretation of histological sections from cervical tissue stained with hematoxylin–eosin is associated with a high degree of discordance among pathologists. In various publications (Stoler and Schiffman, 2001), the low level of interobserver agreement and intraobserver agreement on cervical histology has been remarked. Adding staining CINtec® Histology Kit to conventional slides stained with hematoxylin–eosin used for diagnostic procedures, the accuracy of the histomorphological diagnostic procedure is improved. In the interpretation of these results, it should be noted that the p16-INK4a is a cellular protein, which can be expressed at detectable levels in both high-grade dysplastic cervical and cervical cancers, as in cases not associated with cervical dysplasia. A *positive result* is assigned to samples of p16-INK4a-stained slides showing parabasal cell staining layers and basal cells of the squamous epithelium of the cervix, with or without staining the cells of the superficial layers (*diffuse staining pattern*). A *negative result* is assigned to samples of p16INK4a-stained slides showing a negative staining reaction in the squamous epithelium (*negative staining pattern*) or staining of isolated cells or small clusters of cells, for example, a noncontinuous staining not specifically affecting basal and parabasal cells (*focal staining pattern*). The interpretation of slides stained for p16INK4a using CINtec® Histology Kit must be done in conjunction with slides stained with hematoxylin–eosin preparations with the same sample of tissue from the cervix (Figures 8.3 and 8.4).

The clinical performance of the CINtec® Histology Kit has been evaluated in a controlled clinical trial from caliper punch biopsies and conizations collected retrospectively.

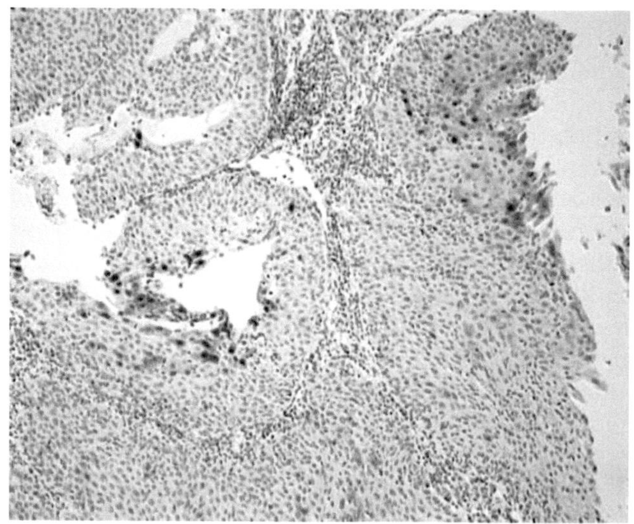

FIGURE 8.3
Metaplasia escamosa madura. CINtec® PLUS histology: Patrón de tinción focal.

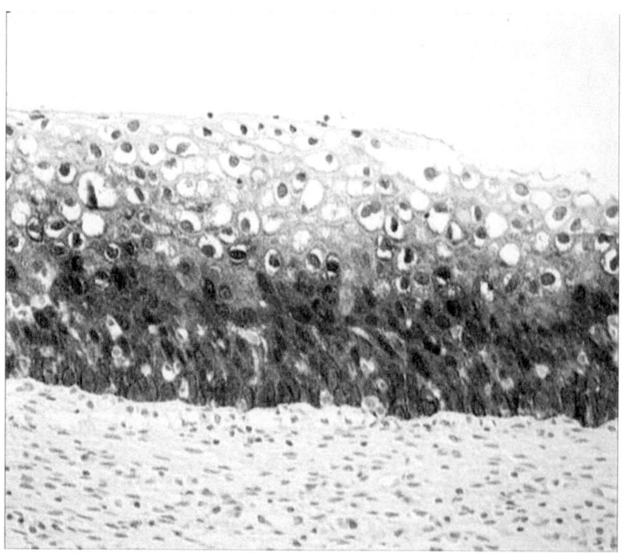

FIGURE 8.4
CINtec® PLUS histology: CIN2.

According to manufacturer's instructions, a total of 500 cervical samples from two European laboratories were used. In the study, pathologists participated in a group of 12 researchers. An improved diagnostic accuracy of CIN2+ by a combined reading of slides stained with hematoxylin–eosin and CINtec® was observed, when compared to slides only with hematoxylin–eosin. The interobserver agreement rates for the detection of CIN2+ were also improved. These data can be checked on the manufacturer's data sheet.

8.5 Cell Proliferation Marker Ki-67

Ki-67 is a proliferation-associated protein that can be detected in the cell nucleus only during proliferation. The cell cycle analysis has shown that the Ki-67 antigen is present at detectable levels in all stages and also in mitosis, whereas resting or inactive cells in the G0 phase show no expression of this antigen (Brown and Gatter, 2002).

The CINtec® PLUS is an immunocytochemical kit for determining simultaneously qualitatively the proteins p16-INK4a and Ki-67 in cervical cytological preparations, a dual test of noninvasive biomarkers. This kit is intended as an aid in identifying women with high-grade intraepithelial lesions, in primary screening and in the subgroup of patients with a cytology result of ASCUS and LSIL or patients with a positive HR-HPV DNA test. In cervical cytologies, p16-INK4a immunostaining is a valuable tool for classifying Pap cytology cases diagnosed as ASCUS or LSIL, with high sensitivity for the detection of underlying CIN2 lesions or greater, similar to the HPV test, but providing a considerably higher specificity (Wentzensen et al., 2007). Furthermore, it has been proposed that p16-INK4a staining cytology is a valuable complementary marker for the classification or triage of women with positive HR-HPV DNA test in cervical cancer screening (Carozzi et al., 2008). It has been demonstrated that all high-grade intraepithelial lesions show overexpression of p16-INK4a (Bergeron et al., 2010). Since a large number of epithelial cells in CIN lesions show proliferation activity, detection of cervical epithelial cell with simultaneous expression of both p16-INK4a and Ki-67 may be interpreted as indicating a transformed state of the cells. Cells with overexpression of p16-INK4a can proliferate actively only if its cell cycle control system is damaged; due to this, the expression of the proliferation marker Ki-67 and p16-INK4a marker within a single cell should exclude each other under normal physiological conditions. Therefore, coexpression of Ki-67 and p16INK4a in certain cells could be considered as an indicator of deregulation of cell cycle control of these cells.

The interpretation of the results of this test is as follows: the procedure of CINtec® PLUS kit generates two reaction products of a different color: one brown precipitates in the place where p16-INK4a antigen is present and a red precipitates in the place where Ki-67 antigen is present. The staining of cells with brown (cytoplasm and/or nucleus) indicates overexpression of p16-INK4a. The staining of cells with red (core) indicates the expression of Ki-67. The cells with both stains show a brown cytoplasmic staining with a core typically deep red. The presence of one or more cervical epithelial cells with the presence of both stains, the brown cytoplasmic and red nucleus immunostaining within the same cell, is interpreted as a positive test result for CINtec® PLUS.

Several studies support the usefulness of this technique when compared to Pap or HR-HPV DNA test. Sensitivity and specificity for detecting CIN2+ are summarized in each table (Tables 8.1 through 8.5).

The data show a high sensitivity and specificity for this test. Therefore, a positive result would indicate that the woman should be referred to colposcopy.

TABLE 8.1

Sensitivity and Specificity for CIN2+ Detection in Primary Screening Using CINtec® PLUS

PALMS (*n* = 27248)	CINtec® PLUS (%)	Papanicolaou (%)
Sensitivity	90	66
Specificity	95	95
Wolfsburg (*n* = 4246)	**CINtec® PLUS (%)**	**Papanicolaou (%)**
Sensitivity	93	65
Specificity	98	99

TABLE 8.2

Sensitivity and Specificity for CIN2+ Detection in Using CINtec® PLUS in LSIL

EEMAPS (*n* = 776)	CINtec® PLUS (%)	VPH-AR (%)
Sensitivity	94	96
Specificity	68	19
PALMS	**CINtec® PLUS (%)**	**VPH-AR (%)**
Sensitivity	85	98
Specificity	54	19

TABLE 8.3

Sensitivity and Specificity for CIN2+ Detection in Using CINtec® PLUS in ASCUS

EEMAPS	CINtec® PLUS (%)	VPH-AR (%)
Sensibility	92	91
Specificity	81	36
PALMS	**CINtec® PLUS (%)**	**VPH-AR (%)**
Sensitivity	94	100
Specificity	78	61

TABLE 8.4

Sensitivity and Specificity for CIN2+ Detection Using CINtec® PLUS in Negative Pap Smear and Positive DNA HR-HPV

Estudio Wolfsburg (>30años)	CINtec® PLUS Sensibilidad (%)	CINtec® PLUS Especificidad (%)
CIN2+	92	85
CIN3+	96	80

TABLE 8.5

Sensitivity and Specificity for CIN2+ Detection Using CINtec® PLUS in PALMS, EEMAPS, and Wolfsburg Trials

	Screening (%)	LSIL (%)	ASCUS (%)	HR-HPV(+) (%)
Sensitivity	90–93	85–94	92–94	92
Specificity	95–98	54–68	78–81	85

8.6 mRNA E6/E7 HPV

Using novel in situ hybridization techniques of mRNA E6 and E7 regions of the virus and subsequent analysis by flow cytometry, it is possible identifying the real cause of development of cervical carcinoma. Besides, this molecular biomarker diagnoses persistent infections by oncogenic viruses in preinvasive lesions with negative results for other tests.

The sensitivity and specificity of HPV E6/E7 mRNA are higher compared to cytology, 92% versus 30%–87%. It has a higher PPV than the determination of HR-HPV DNA, 90% versus 15%–25%. It is a fast and simple application technique, which means lower costs by reducing unnecessary additional tests and treatment.

The future incorporation of this biomarker in histological specimens, such as sentinel lymph node biopsy, will provide additional information to decide treatment regimens and follow-up.

8.6.1 Detection Test E6/E7 HPV mRNA

There are different types of test for detecting E6/E7 mRNA from HR-HPV. The following used liquid-based cytology as samples, so they are noninvasive biomarker tests:

1. The PreTect HPV-Proofer® (Norchip AS, Klokkarstua, Norway). Detects the most frequent 5 genotypes from the material of a liquid-based cytology: 16, 18, 31, 33, and 45.
2. NucliSens EasyQ® HPV (BioMérierux SA, France). Detects the same genotypes as the PreTect HPV-Proofer®.
3. HPV Oncotect E6-E7® (Invirion Diagnostics). Uses the in situ hybridization; cells are not fragmented allowing quantification. Detects all viral genotypes without distinguishing risk category.
4. APTIMA® (Gen Probe). Approved by the FDA on October 2011. It is the only fully automated molecular diagnostic system. It detects 14 HR-HPV genotypes (16, 18, 31, 33, 35, 39, 45, 51, 52, 56, 58, 59, 66, 68) with a liquid-based cytology amplification method using reverse transcriptase (RT) and an RNA polymerase. Among the advantages are as follows: it shows no cross-reactivity with other high-risk virus or with the normal flora or opportunistic organisms that may be present in the cervical outlet. It has the same sensitivity as the HC2® in regard to CIN3 (95%) but APTIMA is more specific than the HC2®.

8.6.2 Analytical Accuracy and Clinical Applicability of HPV E6/E7 mRNA Determination

The PreTect HPV-Proofer®/Easy Q® has favored a higher specificity and a lower sensitivity, while the APTIMA® assay seems to perform more closely to the HR-HPV DNA tests. However, without a complete meta-analysis to pool statistical results, conclusions can only be made based on a descriptive analysis. It has been suggested that the increase in specificity and decrease in sensitivity of the PreTect HPV-Proofer®/Easy Q® are a result of reducing the number of HPV genotypes tested. The PreTect HPV-Proofer®/Easy Q® detects the five higher-risk genotypes compared to the 13 and 14 genotypes tested in the HC2® and APTIMA® tests, respectively. The differences in the genotypes cocktail may influence the test accuracy (Burger et al., 2011) (Figure 8.5).

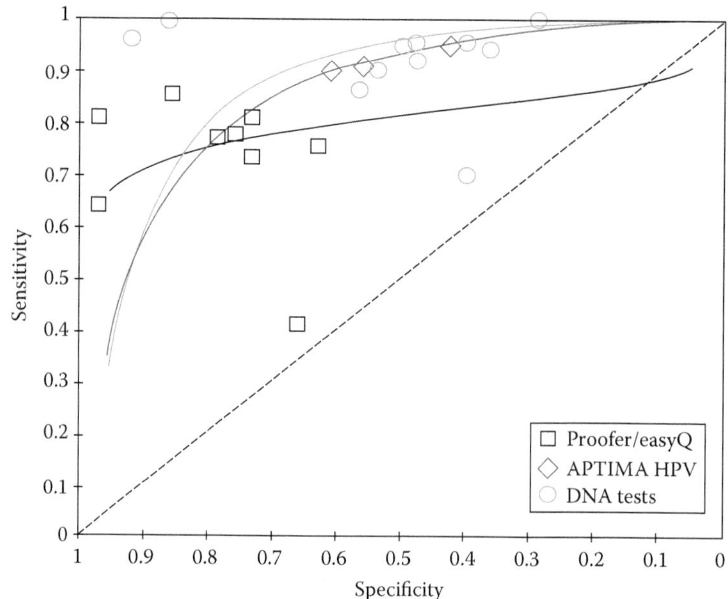

FIGURE 8.5
Summary ROC plot of the APTIMA HPV (diamond) and PreTect HPV-Proofer (square) compared to the DNA HPV test (circle) performance in the same studies. (From Burger, E.A. et al., *Gynecol. Oncol.*, 120(3), 430, 2011.)

Conclusive studies are needed to validate the usefulness of the determination of mRNA E6/E7 clinically. There are already many studies comparing the diagnostic accuracy in relation to other biomarkers. The first two (the PreTect HPV-Proofer® and NucliSens EasyQ® HPV) have the limitation of determining only five of the HR-HPV types, so it should be questioned to what extent this test could replace a more universal test as colposcopy, without losing disease cases.

8.6.2.1 Preinvasive Lesions

The high clinical value of detecting E6/E7 mRNA expression, compared with methods based on HR-HPV DNA, has been reported in several publications (Cuschieri et al., 2004). Hence, new molecular markers are needed to better predict the risk of developing cervical carcinoma and to avoid overtreatment. mRNA testing is one such candidate marker; however, further evaluation regarding its value in primary screening, triage, and follow-up after treatment is still needed. An interesting potential application of mRNA testing is ASCUS/LSIL triage for which HR-HPV DNA testing has poor specificity. Cross-sectional studies have shown that mRNA testing correlates better with the severity of the injury and seems to be more appropriate for risk evaluation than HR-HPV DNA testing (Castle et al., 2007). E6/E7 mRNA testing has the potential to be more cost effective in screening compared to HR-HPV DNA testing, but this has yet to be documented.

Large-scale, population-based studies are required to evaluate the predictive values of mRNA testing in screening and patient management. Preliminary results from ongoing studies with the PreTect HPV-Proofer® indicate that the clinical test sensitivity for detection of CIN2+ may be improved if more high-risk genotypes are included in the kit (Ratman et al., 2007; Trope et al., 2007). It remains to be documented whether the clinical specificity will be weaker if more high-risk genotypes are included.

E6/E7 mRNA testing for high-risk types seems to correlate better with the severity of the injury compared to HR-HPV DNA testing and is a potential marker for the identification of women at risk of cervical carcinoma. Commercial kits for simultaneous genotyping and detection of E6/E7 mRNA from the five most common high-risk HPV types are now available and require further evaluation for primary screening, triage, and follow-up after treatment (Lie and Kristensen, 2008).

Detection of E6/E7 mRNA and the presence of oncogene activity in cervical specimens can be performed by RT-PCR or by nucleic acid sequence–based amplification (NASBA) (Figure 8.6) (Sotlar et al., 2004). So far, few clinical studies have been published; the most important studies are summarized in Table 8.6. The predictive values of HPV mRNA testing in screening have not been investigated in population-based, randomized trials (Lie and Kristensen, 2008).

E6/E7 mRNA levels have been found to increase with injury severity; therefore, the detection of E6/E7 mRNA may be of higher prognostic value and may improve the specificity and PPV compared to HR-HPV DNA testing in screening (Castle et al., 2007; Molden et al., 2007). Additional Norwegian hospital–based and cross-sectional studies have shown that E6/E7 mRNA is positive in 89% of SCC of the cervix and in 77% of high-grade precursor lesions (CIN2/3 or AIS) (Kraus et al., 2006).

8.6.2.2 Cervical Cancer in Early Stage: Sentinel Node

Quantification of intracellular HPV E6/E7 mRNA expression is directly related as a biomarker to the tumor dissemination in early stages of cervical cancer. The test of mRNA HPV E6/E7 serves as the most sensitive available tool for ultrastaging to detect micrometastases in the sentinel node biopsy.

In cervical cancer, the sentinel node procedure is not yet established as a standard procedure, although most of the relevant groups are using it in clinical practice or in the context of translational research (Eiriksson et al., 2012). In the series published, about 1000 patients with cervical cancer in early stage have undergone sentinel node biopsy technique, with detection rates of 90%, 4%–8% false negative rate, and NPV of 97% (Van de Lande et al., 2007; Altgassen et al., 2008; Lécuru et al., 2011; Cibula et al., 2012).

Overall survival for cervical carcinoma at 5 years follow-up is 92% for patients without lymph node involvement and drops to 42% if there are metastatic pelvic lymph nodes. In early stages, local relapses occur in 10%–17% and they usually occur in the first 2 years of follow-up and have a 40% overall survival (Perez et al., 1992; Marchiolé et al., 2005; Peiretti et al., 2012).

Most of the patients affected by early cervical carcinoma have no sentinel node involvement (68%). Between 16% and 21% have positive pelvic lymph nodes, and in 86%, metastases are found in the sentinel nodes (21%–25% macrometastases, 7%–12% micrometastases, and 4%–7% isolated tumor cells) (Lentz et al., 2004; Van Meurs et al., 2009; Juretzka et al., 2004).

The molecular ultrastaging of the sentinel node in gynecological oncology is justified by the importance of detecting lymph node metastases. According to the Philadelphia Consensus, ultrastaging findings in sentinel node in breast cancer are defined as macrometastases (larger than 2 mm), micrometastases (between 2 mm and 0.02 mm), and isolated tumor cells (less than 0.02 mm, including the presence of cytokeratin positive isolated tumor cells) (Schwartz et al., 2002). There is no clear definition of micrometastases in cervical cancers, and detection methods vary from one center to another (Zand et al., 2010). In recent years, most authors are using the definition of the American Joint Committee on Cancer (AJCC) (Cibula et al., 2012).

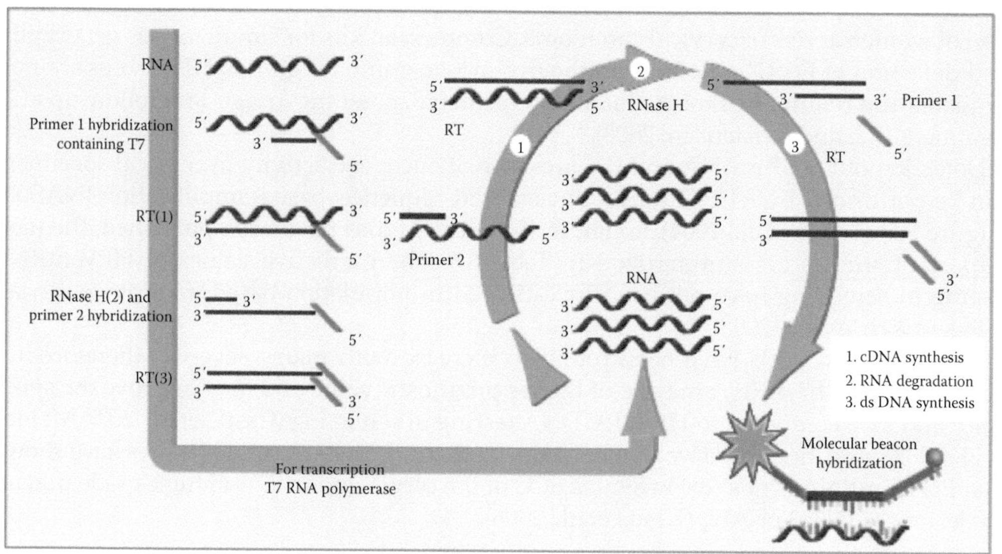

(a)

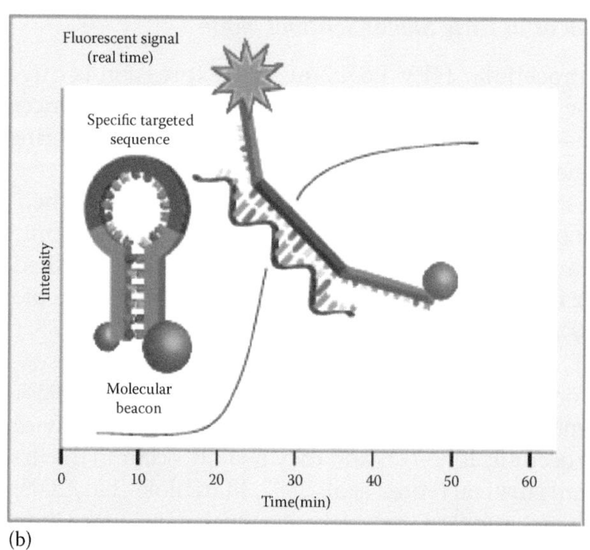

(b)

FIGURE 8.6
Schematic presentation of the NASBA technology including molecular beacons for real-time detection. (a) Two specific primers and three enzymes are required. The reaction is performed at 41°C and is started by the annealing of one primer to the target RNA sequence followed by building of a RNA/DNA hybrid by RT. This hybrid is recognized by Rnase H, which degrades the RNA strand. The other primer anneals to the newly synthesized DNA strand and RT creates a ds DNA molecule with the T7 RNA polymerase which anneals to this sequence and creates single-stranded anti-sense RNAs which in turn are targets for the primers. The reaction repeats itself and within 90 min, more than 1 million new copies are obtained. (Reproduced with permission from Biomerieux.) (b) Molecular beacons are DNA probes with modified ends. Upon binding to complementary RNA transcripts the probe undergoes conformational change and a fluorescence signal is emitted. ds: Double-stranded; RT: Reverse transcriptase. (From Lie, A.K. and Kristensen, G., *Expert Rev. Mol. Diagn.*, 8(4), 405, 2008.)

TABLE 8.6

Cross-Sectional Studies Evaluating Human Papillomavirus mRNA Testing

Study	Population	HPV Methods	Reference Standard	Results
Sotlar et al. (2004)	459 women with histology (109 with CIN 2+)	Consensus and type-specific PCR and RT-PCR	Histology	Increasing prevalence of E6/E7 transcripts with lesions severity (95% of CIN 3 positive)
Cuschieri et al. (2004)	54 women with normal cytology and positive HPV test with 2-year follow-up	PGMY consensus PCR, linear array, and PreTect™ HPV-Proofer	Cytology	RNA testing less sensitive but more specific than DNA testing, indentifies lesions that are more likely to persist and progress
Kraus et al. (2004)	190 cervical biopsies	Consensus and type-specific PCR, PreTect™ HPV-Proofer	Histology	Prevalence of HPV mRNA increased with severity of the lesion; 92% of CIN 3 lesions were positive
Lie et al. (2005)	383 women with positive cytology referred for colposcopy or conization	HC2® and PreTect HPV-Proofer	Histology	All carcinomas and 77% of CIN 2+ lesions were positive by PreTect HPV-Proofer, lower sensitivity and higher specificitycompared with HC II
Molden et al. (2005)	4136 women > 30 years with 2-year follow-up	Consensus and type-specific PCR, PreTect HPV-Proofer	Cytology/histology (n = 23)	4: 4% mRNA positive; 10: 4% DNA positive. 4% had abnormal cytology, CIN 2+ was confirmed in 14 out of 23 HSIL and PreTect HPV-Proofer was positive in 12
Andersson et al (2006)	80 women with positive cytology referred for colposcopy	P16, real-time PCR, PreTect HPV-Proofer	Histology	41% of CIN 2/3 lesions were mRNA positive, independent of viral load but correlated with high expression of p16
Kraus et al. (2006)	204 women with squamous cell carcinoma	In situ hybridization, consensus and type-specific PCR sequencing, PreTect HPV-Proofer	Histology	Overall HPV prevalence 97%, the mRNA test was positive in 92%
Molden et al. (2006)	283 women < 30 years with normal cytology	Consensus and type-specific PCR, PreTect HPV-Proofer	Cytology	32% positive with consensus PCR and 14.5% with PreTect HPV-Proofer
Castle et al. (2007)	540 women selected from screening	PGMY09/11, linear array, Aptima HPV	Histology	mRNA test correlated strongly with severity of the lesion; more than 90% of CIN 3 cases and all carcinomas tested positive

ASCUS: Atypical squamous cells of undetermined significance; CIN: cervical intraepithelial neoplasia; HC2: hybrid capture® 2; HPV: human papillomavirus; HSIL: high-grade squamous intraepithelial lesion; LSIL: low-grade squamous intraepithelial lesion; RT: reverse transcription.

Cibula multicenter study shows that the presence of micrometastases and macrometastases in the sentinel node is associated with a significant reduction in overall survival in cervical cancer. Therefore, the presence of micrometastases would be an independent prognostic factor, more important than the FIGO stage. These patients are included in the same prognostic category as those with macrometastases (Cibula et al., 2012;

Juretzka et al., 2004). Ultrastaging of the selective biopsy of the sentinel node in the management of patients with early-stage cervical cancer may identify a subgroup of patients with micrometastases, which would have been infrastaged by 15% by routine histological methods (Marchioli et al., 2005; Horn et al., 2008).

One of the major limitations in implementing HPV E6/E7 mRNA determination is that the technique does not detect the viral subtypes not included in the different commercial kits. The identification of specific viral subtypes implicated in carcinogenesis in patients with cervical cancer could lead the applicability of the kits that are currently in the market.

In a systematic review of Burger, eight studies have investigated the performance of the PreTect HPV-Proofer®/NucliSENS EasyQ®, two studies investigated the performance of the APTIMA® kit, and one study investigated both mRNA tests on the same patient samples. The review suggests that mRNA diagnostic tests have relevance, but additional studies and economic evaluations must be conducted in order to make a solid clinical conclusion regarding the applicability of HPV mRNA testing (Burger et al., 2011).

In our center, we have experience with the NucliSENS EasyQ® HPV test. It is a test based on mRNA; it directly detects E6/E7 mRNA with high PPV. The sampling is designed for being used on samples obtained with a cervical brush and preserved in a vial ThinPrep containing the PreservCyt solution. We are studying the validation and analysis of E6/E7 mRNA by PCR in tissue samples, surpassing the current application in liquid-based cytology. There are some experimental trials that have implemented the technique in histological sections of anal cancers. The detection of metastases in the sentinel node in cervical cancer and HPV E6/E7 mRNA by PCR may have prognostic value (Fader et al., 2008).

The use of intracellular mRNA HPV E6/E7 expression as a biomarker in cervical cancer leads to a better approach to the patient. It can change the tumor stage, the surgical procedure, and the adjuvant treatment with chemotherapy and radiotherapy. Due to this, the quantification of intracellular E6/E7 mRNA expression could have an impact on morbidity, disease-free survival, and overall survival.

8.7 Cytokeratin 19

Classically, the most used method for the analysis of the sentinel node has been the hematoxylin–eosin in cytological imprint and frozen section. However, conventional analysis shows a low sensitivity (30%) for intraoperative detection of metastases and an estimated false negative rate of 67% (Fader et al., 2008; Diaz et al., 2011). The current translational research lines are focused on the design of improved detection methods through immunohistochemistry and molecular ultrastaging of the sentinel node.

One-step nucleic acid amplification (OSNA®) and pancytokeratin kits like AE1/AE2 have a low specificity and sensitivity detecting the level of mRNA expression in sentinel lymph node in cervical cancer, because the expression of CK19 in these tumors is highly variable. However, the diagnosis would be of higher accuracy than with the conventional analysis (Hibner et al., 2004; Kraus et al., 2006; Yuan et al., 2008).

It would be interesting to compare the accuracy of performing intraoperative diagnosis with hematoxylin–eosin and the postoperative analysis with ultrastaging, detection, and determination of cytokeratins, HR-HPV DNA, or mRNA for the detection of micrometastases.

8.8 SCC

Serum SCC-ag is a member of the ovalbumin family of serine proteinase inhibitors, which can be detected in normal cervical squamous epithelium, columnar epithelium, SCC, and most of adenocarcinomas but barely expressed in normal lymph nodes and endometrium (Looi et al. 2009).

Stenman was the first researcher who detected the expression of SCC cells in peripheral blood tumor as a noninvasive biomarker by RT-PCR in cervical cancer and found that it can be used for staging and evaluating prognosis in epidermoid carcinoma of the uterine cervix (Stenman et al., 1997).

Pretreatment serum SCC levels are high in 28%–88% of patients with squamous cell cervical cancer, and the levels of SCC are related to tumor stage, size, depth of stromal invasion, lymphovascular space status, parametrial involvement, and lymph node status. The clinical relevance of pretreatment serum SCC is still controversial. Some authors report that it has no prognostic value, but others found that it is related to overall survival at univariate analysis, and others report SCC levels as an independent prognostic factor for overall survival (Gaducci et al., 2008).

RT-PCR has been used to accurately measure the levels of gene expression and has become widely used for detecting occult micrometastatic tumor cells in resected lymph node specimens in some malignant diseases as well as in cervical cancer (Van Trappen et al., 2001). The advantages of this technique are the following: the capability to differentiate between baseline levels of gene expression in normal tissue versus altered levels in tumoral tissues; the benefit of a simple, fast, and automated procedure; and the ability to analyze the entire specimen decreasing sampling errors. One of the most common target genes for epithelial carcinoma is the CK19 gene (Gillanders et al., 2004).

In a Chinese study, RT-PCR is used for measuring SCC mRNA levels to detect SLN micrometastases and to determine its effect on disease-free interval, for patients with early-stage cervical cancer. They compared the results with those quantifying CK19 mRNA and found that quantifying SCC mRNA has a higher accuracy than CK19 mRNA in detecting micrometastases in SLNs. The molecular lymphatic metastasis in squamous cell and adenosquamous cervical cancer based on quantification of SCC mRNA is more accurate than that based on histopathology. Some new biotechnology techniques, such as GeneXpert, are capable of doing RNA isolation from lysed tissue, RT, and quantitative PCR all in 30 min, and it gives the potential application of an intraoperative SLN analysis. Then, it would be of great value combining SCC detection with such a fast, accurate intraoperative SLN analysis in cervical cancer because it will allow the surgeon to determine the need of an extent resection during the surgery and a more individualized treatment planning could be designed for these patients. The conclusion showed that SCC is certainly a better marker than CK19 and histopathology for molecular diagnosis of lymph node metastasis in squamous cell and adenosquamous cervical cancer (Song-Hua et al., 2008).

Serial SCC measurements reflect both the tumor response to treatment and the clinical outcome of patients. Increasing SCC levels can precede the clinical diagnosis of recurrent disease in 46%–92% of the cases, with a mean lead time ranging from 2 to 8 months. According to some authors, serum SCC determination during the follow-up does not improve the healing rate of patients who will ultimately develop a recurrence (Gaducci et al., 2008).

8.9 Other Molecular Biomarkers

During the last years, those molecular factors that determine the aggressiveness, local recurrence, metastatic development, and decreased survival of the tumors have started to be discovered. This characterization could select those patients who would benefit from a more aggressive initial treatment.

The main biomarkers identified are as follows:

- Overexpression of angiogenic factors (VEGF, FGF, PDGF)
- Overexpression of c-erb-B2
- 72 kDa metalloproteinase overexpression

There are several studies describing correlations between cell biological invasive markers and survival in cervical cancer patients. In addition to cyclooxygenase-2 (COX-2) and serum SCC-ag levels, there are other markers associated with poor prognosis involved, like the epidermal growth factor receptor (EGFR) and C-erbB-2. Others are related to angiogenesis and hypoxia (like carbonic anhydrase 9 and hypoxia-inducible factor-1α). EGFR and C-erbB-2 are also associated with a poor response to chemoradiation.

In conclusion, EGFR signaling is associated with poor prognosis and response to therapy in cervical cancer patients primarily treated with chemoradiation, whereas markers involved in angiogenesis and hypoxia, COX-2, and serum SCC-ag levels are associated with a poor prognosis (Noordhuis et al., 2011).

8.10 Conclusion and Future Direction

Knowing the causal factors in the development of cervical carcinoma and preinvasive lesions has led to the discovery of several biomarkers. Most of the biomarkers found are in relation to HPV. They have allowed us, as physicians, to make primary prevention strategies such as vaccination against HPV and schemes of secondary prevention through early diagnosis of diseases associated with this virus.

The determination of the HR-HPV DNA is the noninvasive biomarker more used by different protocols. Its application is set for screening or triage, research, and monitoring of abnormal cytology after the treatment of preinvasive lesions.

The implementation of the HPV vaccine around the world is growing yet, but we do not know the limits of it and the real impact on the incidence of cervical cancer and HPV-related tumors. The screening strategies will depend on these events, but it is certain that the role of the HPV biomarkers and specifically HR-HPV DNA test will have an increasing importance.

The p16, Ki-67, and HPV E6/E7 mRNA are noninvasive biomarkers of progression of high-grade intraepithelial lesions, with current clinical application and promising results, although not included in most of international protocols and clinical pathways.

The immunohistochemical and molecular ultrastaging of the sentinel node in cervical cancer by invasive biomarkers as HPV E6/E7 mRNA can detect the presence of micrometastases. The use of intracellular mRNA HPV E6/E7 expression as a biomarker in cervical cancer leads to a better approach to the patient. It can change the tumor stage, the surgical procedure, and the adjuvant treatment with chemotherapy and radiotherapy. Due to this, the quantification of intracellular mRNA HPV E6/E7 expression could have an impact on morbidity, disease-free survival, and overall survival.

One of the major limitations in implementing HPV E6/E7 mRNA determination is that the technique does not detect the viral subtypes not included in the different commercial kits. The identification of specific viral subtypes implicated in carcinogenesis in patients with premalignant or malignant lesions could lead to the applicability of the kits that are currently in the market.

As the role of HR-HPV DNA test is increasingly entrenched and the criteria for their use are clear, more studies on the most modern biomarkers are necessary to get to demonstrate the potential indications in clinical practice, from the screening to the staging of cancer HPV–related tumors.

References

Agoff SN, Lin P, Morihara J, Mao C, Kiviat NB, and Koutsky LA. p16INK4a expression correlates with degree of cervical neoplasia: A comparison with Ki-67 expression and detection of high-risk HPV types. *Modern Pathol* 2003; 16: 665–673.

Altgassen C, Hertel H, Brandstädt A, Köhler C, Dürst M, and Schneider A. Multicenter validation study of the sentinel lymph node concept in cervical cancer: AGO Study Group. *J Clin Oncol* 2008; 26(18): 2943–2951.

Andersson S, Hansson B, Norman I, Gaberi V, Mints M, Hjerpe A, Karlsen F, and Johansson B. Expression of E6/E7 mRNA from 'high risk' human papillomavirus in relation to CIN grade, viral load and p16INK4a. *Int J Oncol* 2006; 29(3): 705–711.

Ardiç N, Oztürk O, Ergünay K, and Sezer O. Investigation of E6/E7 mRNAs of high risk human papilloma virus types by a commercial automatized NASBA assay in cervical swabs. *Mikrobiyoloji bülteni* 2009; 43(3): 463–469.

Barranger E, Cortez A, Uzan S, Callard P, and Darai E. Value of intraoperative imprint cytology of sentinel nodes in patients with cervical cancer. *Gynecol Oncol* 2004; 94: 175–180.

Baseman JG and Koutsky LA. The epidemiology of human papillomavirus infections. *J Clin Virol* 2005; 32(1): S16–S24.

Bentivegna E, Uzan C, Gouy S, Leboulleux S, Duvillard P, Lumbroso J et al. The accuracy of FDG-PET/CT in early-stage cervical and vaginal cancers. *Gynécologie obstétrique fertilit* 2011; 39(4): 193–197.

Bergeron C, Ordi J, Schmidt D, Trunk MJ, Keller T, and Ridder R. Conjunctive p16INK4a testing significantly increases accuracy in diagnosing high-grade cervical intraepithelial neoplasia. *Am J Clin Pathol* 2010; 133: 395–406.

Bosch FX, Diaz M, De Sanjosé S et al. Epidemiología de las infecciones por el virus del papiloma humano (HPV): Riesgo de carcinoma cérvico-uterino y otros tumores ano-genitales. Nuevas opciones preventivas. En: De Sanjosé S and García AM. *4ª Monografía de la Sociedad Española de Epidemiología. Virus del Papiloma Humano y Cáncer: epidemiología y prevención*. Madrid: EMISA, 2006; 31–50.

Bosch FX, Lorincz A, Muñoz M, Meijer CJ, and Shah KV. The causal relation between human papillomavirus and cervical cancer. *J Clin Pathol* 2002; 55: 244–265.

Bosch FX, Manos MM, Muñoz N et al. Prevalence of human papillomavirus in cervical cancer: A worldwide perspective. *J Natl Cancer Inst* 1995; 87: 796–802.

Brown DC and Gatter KC. Ki-67 protein: The immaculate deception? *Histopathology* 2002; 40: 2–11.

Burger EA, Kornør H, Klemp M, Lauvrak V, and Kristiansen IS. HPV mRNA tests for the detection of cervical intraepithelial neoplasia: A systematic review. *Gynecol Oncol* 2011; 120(3): 430–438.

Carozzi F, Confortini M, Dalla Palma P et al. Use of p16INK4a over-expression to increase the specificity of human papillomavirus testing: A nested substudy of the NTCC randomised controlled trial. *Lancet Oncol* 2008; 9: 937–945.

Castle PE, Dockter J, Giachetti C et al. A cross-sectional study of a prototype carcinogenic human papillomavirus E6/E7 messenger RNA assay for detection of cervical precancer and cancer. *Clin Cancer Res* 2007; 13(9): 2599–2605.

Castle PE, Solomon D, Schiffman M, Wheeler CM. HPV type 16 infections and 2-year absolute risk of cervical precancer in women with equivocal or mild cytologic abnormalities. *J Natl Cancer Inst* 2005; 97(14): 1066–1071.

Chow LT and Broker TR. Mechanisms and regulation of papillomavirus DNA replication. En: Saveria Campo MS. *Papillomavirus Research from Natural History to Vaccines and Beyond*. Norwich, U.K.: Caister Academic Press, 2005; 53–71.

Cibula D, Abu-Rustum NR, Dusek L, Zikán M, Zaal a, Sevcik L et al. Prognostic significance of low volume sentinel lymph node disease in early-stage cervical cancer. *Gynecol Oncol* 2012; 124(3): 496–501.

Cuschieri KS, Whitley MJ, and Cubie HA. HPV type specific DNA and RNA persistence-implications for cervical disease progression and monitoring. *J Med Virol* 2004; 73: 65–70.

Cuzick J, Clavel C, Petry KU, Meijer CJLM, Hoyer H, Ratnam S et al. Overview of the European and North American studies on HPV testing in primary cervical cancer screening. *Int J Cancer* 2006; 119: 1095–1101.

de Sanjosé S, Diaz M, Castellsagué X, Clifford G, Bruni L, Muñoz N, Bosch FX. Worldwide prevalence and genotype distribution of cervical human papillomavirus DNA in women with normal cytology: A meta-analysis. *Lancet Infect Dis* 2007; 7(7): 453–459.

De Williers EM, Fauquet C, Broker TR et al. Classification of papillomaviruses. *Virology* 2004; 324: 17–27.

Diaz JP, Gemignani ML, Pandit-Taskar N, Park KJ, Murray MP, Chi DS et al. Sentinel lymph node biopsy in the management of early-stage cervical carcinoma. *Gynecol Oncol* 2011; 120(3): 347–352.

Diestro Tejeda MD, Velasco MS, and Nieto FG. Estado actual de las vacunas frente al virus del papiloma humano (VPH). *Oncología* 2007: 30(2): 42–59.

Eiriksson LR and Covens A. Sentinel lymph node mapping in cervical cancer: The future? *BJOG* 2012; 119(2): 129–133.

Fader AN, Edwards RP, Cost M, Kanbour-Shakir A, Kelley JL, Schwartz B et al. Sentinel lymph node biopsy in early-stage cervical cancer: Utility of intraoperative versus postoperative assessment. *Gynecol Oncol* 2008; 111(1): 13–17.

Ferreccio C, Prado RB, Luzoro AV et al. Population-based prevalence and age distribution of human papillomavirus among women in Santiago, Chile. *Cancer Epidemiol Biomarkers Prev* 2004; 13: 2271–2276.

Font R, Pérez M, Coll C et al. Utilización de modelos longitudinales para estimar el tiempo de regresión/progresión de la infeccion por VPH en una cohorte de mujeres atendidas en centros de planificación familiar en Barcelona, España. *Gac Sanit* 2004; 18(3): 148.

Forslund O, Antonsson A, Edlund K et al. Population-based type-specific prevalence of high-risk human papillomavirus infection in middle-aged Swedish women. *J Med Virol* 2002; 66: 535–541.

Frazer IH, Cox JT, Mayeaux EJ et al. Advances in prevention of cervical cancer and other human papillomavirus-related diseases. *Pediatrics Infect Dis J* 2006; 25: S65–S81.

Gadducci A, Tana R, Cosio S, and Genazzani AR. The serum assay of tumour markers in the prognostic evaluation, treatment monitoring and follow-up of patients with cervical cancer: A review of the literature. *Crit Rev Oncol Hematol* 2008; 66(1): 10–20.

Gillanders WE, Mikhitarian K, Hebert R et al. Molecular detection of micrometastatic breast cancer in histopathology-negative axillary lymph nodes correlates with traditional predictors of prognosis. An interim analysis of a prospective multi-institutional cohort study. *Ann Surg* 2004; 239: 828–840.

Hibner M, Magrina JF, Lefler SR, Cornella JL, Pizarro AR, and Loftus JC. Effects of raloxifene hydrochloride on endometrial cancer cells in vitro. *Gyneco Oncol* 2004; 93(3): 642–646.

Horn L-C, Hentschel B, Fischer U, Peter D, and Bilek K. Detection of micrometastases in pelvic lymph nodes in patients with carcinoma of the cervix uteri using step sectioning: Frequency, topographic distribution and prognostic impact. *Gynecol Oncol* 2008; 111(2): 276–281.

Ishikawa M, Fujii T, Saito M, Nindl I, Ono A, Kubushiro K, Tsukazaki K, Mukai M, and Nozawa S. Overexpression of p16INK4a as an indicator for human papillomavirus oncogenic activity in cervical squamous neoplasia. *Int J Gynecol Cancer* 2006, 16: 347–353.

Juretzka MM, Jensen KC, Longacre TA, Teng NN, and Husain A. Detection of pelvic lymph node micrometastasis in stage IA2-IB2 cervical cancer by immunohistochemical analysis. *Gynecol Oncol* 2004; 93: 107–111.

Khan MJ. The elevated 10-year risk of cervical precancer and cancer in women with HPV type 16 or 18 and the possible utility of type specific HPV testing in clinical practice. *J Natl Cancer Inst* 2005; 97: 1072–1079.

Kjaer SK, Van der Brule AJ, Paull G et al. Type specific persistent of high risk HPV as indicator of high grade cervical squamous intraepithelial lesions in young women: Population based prospective follow up study. *BMJ* 2002; 325: 572.

Kraus I, Molden T, Ernø LE, Skomedal H, Karlsen F, and Hagmar B. Human papillomavirus oncogenic expression in the dysplastic portio; an investigation of biopsies from 190 cervical cones. *Br J Cancer* 2004; 90(7): 1407–1413.

Kraus I, Molden T, Holm R et al. Presence of E6 and E7 mRNA from human papillomavirus types 16, 18, 31, 33, and 45 in the majority of cervical carcinomas. *J Clin Microbiol* 2006; 44(4): 1310–1317.

Lécuru F, Mathevet P, Querleu D, Leblanc E, Morice P, Daraï E, Marret H et al. Bilateral negative sentinel nodes accurately predict absence of lymph node metastasis in early cervical cancer: Results of the SENTICOL study. *J Clin Oncol* 2011; 29(13): 1686–1691.

Lentz SE, Muderspach LI, Felix JC, Ye W, Groshen S, and Amezcua CA. Identification of micrometastases in histologically negative lymph nodes of early-stage cervical cancer patients. *Obstet Gynecol* 2004; 103: 1204–1210.

Lie AK and Kristensen G. Human papillomavirus E6/E7 mRNA testing as a predictive marker for cervical carcinoma. *Expert Rev Mol Diagn* 2008; 8(4): 405–415.

Lie AK, Risberg B, Borge B, Sandstad B, Delabie J, Rimala R, Onsrud M, and Thoresen S. DNA-versus RNA-based methods for human papillomavirus detection in cervical neoplasia. *Gynecol Oncol* 2005; 97(3): 908–915.

Looi ML, Karsani SA, Rahman AM, Mohd Dali AZH, Md Ali SA, Wan Ngah WZ, and Mohd Yusof YA. Plasma proteome analysis of cervical intraepithelial neoplasia and cervical squamous cell carcinoma. *J Biosci* 2009; 34(6): 917–925.

Lowndes CM. Vaccines for cervical cancer. *Epidemiol Infect* 2006; 134(1): 1–12.

Marchiolé P, Buénerd A, Benchaib M, Nezhat K, Dargent D, and Mathevet P. Clinical significance of lymphovascular space involvement and lymph node micrometastases in early-stage cervical cancer: A retrospective case-control surgico-pathological study. *Gynecol Oncol* 2005; 97(3): 727–732.

Mathevet P. Surgical lymph-node evaluation in cervical cancer. *Cancer radiothérapie: journal de la Société française de radiothérapie oncologique* 2009; 13(6–7): 499–502.

Meijer CJL. Changing the primary screening tool of the program in Netherlands. Why and how? *HPV Today* 2011; 24: 4–5.

Molano M, Posso H, Weiderpass E et al. Prevalence and determinants of HPV infection among Colombian women with normal cytology. *Br J Cancer* 2002; 87: 324–333.

Molden T, Kraus I, Karlsen F, Skomedal H, and Hagmar B. Human papillomavirus E6/E7 mRNA expression in women younger than 30 years of age. *Gynecol Oncol* 2006; 100(1): 95–100.

Molden T, Kraus I, Karlsen F, Skomedal H, Nygård JF, and Hagmar B. Comparison of human papillomavirus messenger RNA and DNA detection: A cross-sectional study of 4,136 women >30 years of age with a 2-year follow-up of high-grade squamous intraepithelial lesion. *Cancer Epidemiol Biomarkers Prev* 2005; 14(2): 367–372.

Molden T, Kraus I, Skomedal H, Nordstrom T, and Karlsen F. PreTect HPV-Proofer: Real-time detection and typing of E6/E7 mRNA from carcinogenic human papillomaviruses. *J Virol Methods* 2007; 142(1–2): 204–212.

Noordhuis MG, Eijsink JJ, Roossin kF, deGraeff P, Pras E, Schuuring E, Wisman GB, deBock GH, and vanderZee AG. Prognostic cell biological markers in cervical cancer patients primarily treated with (chemo)radiation: A systematic review. *Int J Radiat Oncol Biol Phys* 2011; 79(2): 325–334.

Opazo MA. Ganglio Centinela en Cancer de Cuello Uterino inicial. *Alasbimn J* 2009; 12(46): AJ46–AJ42.

Oriel JD. Natural history of genital warts. *BR J Vener Dis* 1971; 47: 1–13.

Padilla-Paz LA. Human papillomavirus vaccine: History, immunology, current status, and future prospects. *Clin Obstet Gynecol* 2005; 48(1): 226–240.

Parkin DM. The global health burden of infection-associated cancers in the year 2002. *Int J Cancer* 2006; 118(12): 3030–3044.

Peiretti M, Zapardiel I, Zanagnolo V, Landoni F, Morrow CP, and Maggioni A. Management of recurrent cervical cancer: A review of the literature. *Surg Oncol* 2012; 21(2): 59–66.

Perez CA, Grigsby PW, Nene SM, Camel HM, Galakatos A, Kao MS et al. Effect of tumor size on the prognosis of carcinoma of the uterine cervix treated with irradiation alone. *Cancer* 1992; 69(11): 2796–806.

Puig-Tintoré LM, Cortés X, Castellsague X, Torne A, Ordi J et al. Prevention of cervical cancer: Faced with the vaccination against human papiloma virus 2006, *Prog Obstet Ginecol* 2006; 49(5): 62.

Ratman S, Coutlee F, Bentley J et al. HPV E6/E7 mRNA testing in cervical cancer screening: Preliminary results from a multicenter Canadian study. *Presented at: 24th International Papillomavirus Conference*. Beijing, China, November 3–9, 2007 (Abstract).

Regauer S and Reich O. CK17 and p16 expression patterns distinguish (atypical) immature squamous metaplasia from high-grade cervical intraepithelial neoplasia (CIN III). *Histopathology* 2007; 50: 629–635.

Sakuragi N, Satoh C, Takeda N et al. Incidence and distribution pattern of pelvic and paraaortic lymph node metastasis in patients with stages IB, IIA, and IIB cervical cancer treated with radical hysterectomy. *Cancer* 1999; 85: 1547–1554.

Schiffman M and Castle PE. The promise of global cervical-cancer prevention. *N Engl J Med* 2005; 353: 2101–2104.

Schwartz GF, Giuliano AE, and Veronesi U. Proceedings of the consensus conference on the role of sentinel lymph node biopsy in carcinoma of the breast, April 19–22, 2001, Philadelphia, Pennsylvania. *Cancer* 2002; 94(10): 2542–2551.

Song-Hua Yuan, Xue-Fang Liang, Wei-Hua Jia et al. Cervical cancer using squamous cell carcinoma antigen molecular diagnosis of sentinel lymph node metastases in cervical cancer using squamous cell carcinoma antigen. *Clin Cancer Res* 2008; 14: 5571–5578.

Sotlar K, Stubner A, Diemer D et al. Detection of high-risk human papillomavirus E6 and E7 oncogene transcripts in cervical scrapes by nested RT-polymerase chain reaction. *J Med Virol* 2004; 74(1): 107–116.

Stanley MA. Virus-keratinocyte interactions in the infectious cycle. En: Stern PL and Stanley MA. *HPV and Cervical Cancer.* Oxford: Oxford University Press, 1994; 116–131.

Stanley MA. Human papillomavirus vaccines. *Rev Med Virol* 2006a; 16: 139–149.

Stanley MA. Immune responses to HPV. *Vaccine* 2006b; 1: 16–22.

Stenman J, Lintula S, Hotakainen K et al. Detection of squamous-cell carcinoma antigen expressing tumour cells in blood by reverse transcriptase polymerase chain reaction in cancer of the uterine cervix. *Int J Cancer* 1997; 74: 75–80.

Stoler MH and Schiffman M. Interobserver reproducibility of cervical cytologic and histologic interpretations. *JAMA* 2001; 285: 1500–1505.

Sun Y, Liu GB, and Yu YH. Correlation between human papillomavirus DNA in the lymph nodes and metastasis of early-stage cervical carcinoma. *NanFangYiKeDaXueXueBao* 2008; 28(5): 796–798.

Syrjänen KJ and Syrjánen SM. *Papillomavirus Infections in Human Pathology*. Chichester, U.K.: Wiley & Sons, 2000; 117–141.

Thomas JO, Herrero R, Omigbodun AA et al. Prevalence of papillomavirus infection in women in Ibadan, Nigheria: A population-based study. *Br J Cancer* 2004; 90: 638–645.

Trope A, Sjoborg KD, Eriksen T et al. Comparison of HPV DNA- and RNA-testing in women with cervical neoplasia. *Presented at: 24th International Papillomavirus Conference.* Beijing, China, November 3–9, 2007 (Abstract).

Van de Lande J, Torrenga B, Raijmakers PGHM, Hoekstra OS, van Baal MW, Brölmann HAM et al. Sentinel lymph node detection in early stage uterine cervix carcinoma: A systematic review. *Gynecol Oncol* 2007; 106(3): 604–613.

Van Meurs H, Visser O, Buist MR, Ten Kate FJW, and van der Velden J. Frequency of pelvic lymph node metastases and parametrial involvement in stage IA2 cervical cancer: A population-based study and literature review. *Int J Gynecol Cancer* 2009; 19: 21–26.

VanTrappen PO, Gyselman VG, Lowe DG et al. Molecular quantification and mapping of lymph-node micrometastases in cervical cancer. *Lancet* 2001; 357: 15–20.

Wentzensen N, Bergeron C, Cas F et al. Triage of women with ASCUS and LSIL cytology. Use of qualitative assessment of p16INK4a positive cells to identify patients with high-grade cervical intraepithelial neoplasia. *Cancer Cytopathol* 2007; 111: 58–66.

Woodman CB, Collins S, Winter H et al. Natural history of cervical human papillomavirus infection in young women: A longitudinal cohort study. *Lancet* 2001; 357: 1831–1836.

Yuan S-H, Liang X-F, Jia W-H, Huang J-L, Wei M, Deng L et al. Molecular diagnosis of sentinel lymph node metastases in cervical cancer using squamous cell carcinoma antigen. *Clin Cancer Res* 2008; 14(17): 5571–5578.

Zand B, Euscher ED, Soliman PT, Schmeler KM, Coleman RL, Frumovitz M et al. Rate of para-aortic lymph node micrometastasis in patients with locally advanced cervical cancer. *Gynecol Oncol* 2010: 119 (3): 422–425.

Zhang F, Liu D, Lin B, Hao Y, Zhou D, Qi Y, and Zhang S. Expression of high-risk HPV DNA and CK19 in pelvic lymph nodes in stage Ia-IIa cervical cancer and their clinical value. *Oncol Rep* 2012; 27(6): 1801–1806.

9

Biomarkers of Nucleotide Metabolism in Cervical Cancer

Charles A. Kunos, MD, PhD, Lauren Shunkwiler, BA, and Gina Ferris, BA

CONTENTS

ABSTRACT Each year, more than one-half million women worldwide are diagnosed with cervical cancer. A key to improved treatment results for women with advanced-stage disease is the planned inclusion of inhibitors of ribonucleotide reductase (RNR). Although gaps remain in our knowledge of how best to inhibit RNR during radiochemotherapy treatment of this disease, as yet no other treatment combination can bring the clinical benefit that RNR inhibition–based radiochemotherapy delivers. This chapter discusses RNR structure, mechanism, and pharmacologic inhibition as it pertains to cervical cancer cell radiosensitivity.

9.1 Introduction

Ribonucleotide reductase (RNR) reduces 2′-ribonucleotide diphosphates to their corresponding 2′-deoxyribonucleotide diphosphates (dNDPs). Cells utilize deoxynucleotide triphosphates derived from dNDPs as building blocks for DNA during nuclear and mitochondrial DNA replication and repair. Large quantities of dNDPs are needed in cells duplicating their genome, and the means of regulating RNR for this task are known. Less is known about how cells meet urgent demands for repair of damaged DNA after agents such as ionizing radiation, which alters thousands of bases (e.g., 8-oxoguanine) in intracellular RNA, genomic DNA, and mitochondrial DNA. Add to this about 1000 single-strand breaks and nearly 30 double-strand DNA breaks when cells are exposed to 1 gray (Gy) of ionizing radiation. Demand for dNDPs to repair inflicted damage puts cells in a vital, high-stakes gamble to use quick and short-run scalable pathways of dNDP supply. Cells balance such demand–supply economics by using not only *de novo* RNR enzyme reduction of ribonucleotides but also a complementary deoxynucleoside salvage system (Figure 9.1, Kuo and Kinsella, 1998, Kunos et al., 2009, 2010b, 2011a,b, Kunos and Radivoyevitch, 2011, Kunos, 2012).

When it comes to the radiosensitivity of cervical cancers, disruption of the natural demand–supply economy by increasing dNDP demand (i.e., radiation or cisplatin treatment)

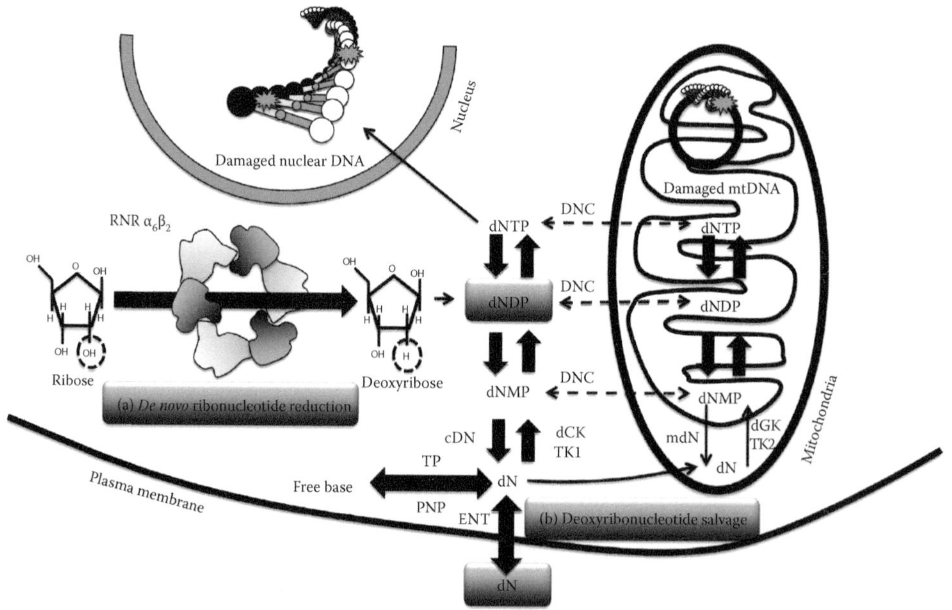

FIGURE 9.1
Diagram of dNDP supply. (a) In one step, RNR reduces a ribonucleotide to a deoxyribonucleotide in a rate-limiting manner. RNR accomplishes this task in its most common form $\alpha_6\beta_2$, representing the union of M1–M2 or M1–M2b. (b) A complementary step involves the recovery of deoxynucleotides. Processing of nucleotide occurs both in the cytosol and in mitochondria through a variety of coordinated enzymes as depicted. Abbreviations include deoxynucleoside (dN), deoxyribonucleotide monophosphate (dNMP), deoxyribonucleotide triphosphate (dNTP), thymidine kinase 1 (TK1) and thymidine kinase 2 (TK2), deoxycytidine kinase (dCK), deoxyguanosine kinase (dGK), cytosolic deoxynucleotidase (cDN), mitochondrial deoxynucleotidase (mdN), deoxynucleotide carrier (DNC), equilibrative nucleoside transporter (ENT), thymidine phosphorylase (TP), purine nucleoside phosphorylase (PNP), and mitochondrial DNA (mtDNA).

while simultaneously confining dNDP supply through pharmacologic inhibition of *de novo* RNR activity (i.e., gemcitabine, hydroxyurea, or triapine treatment) has been tested in clinical trials (Hreshchyshyn et al., 1979, Keys et al., 1999, Morris et al., 1999, Rose et al., 1999, 2007a, Whitney et al., 1999, Eifel et al., 2004, Lanciano et al., 2005, Kunos et al., 2010c, 2011c, Duenas-Gonzalez et al., 2011). Advanced-stage I_{2}–IV_{A} cervical cancers—which deeply invade pelvic tissues rendering them not curable by radical hysterectomy—are aggressive malignancies marked by higher rates of metastases and poorer disease-specific survival than organ-confined cancers. To this point, women with advanced-stage I_{B2}–II_{B} cervical cancer have lower rates of cisplatin radiochemotherapy treatment response (68%) (Candelaria et al., 2006) than women with organ-confined cervical cancer (<6 cm) receiving the same treatment (90%) (Kunos et al., 2010a). Cervical cancers incompletely responding to cisplatin radiochemotherapy foreshadow a very poor overall prognosis, with 50% of women surviving less than 2 years (Schwartz et al., 2009, Kunos et al., 2010a). Worldwide, one-half million women are diagnosed with cervical cancer (Ferlay et al., 2010), and these women have unmet therapeutic needs. In this chapter, current concepts will be explored about how to address these unmet therapeutic needs, banking on the radiosensitivity of cervical cancer.

9.2 Disrupted Nucleotide Metabolism in Cervical Cancers

9.2.1 Nucleotide Production

Human RNR is a tetrameric enzyme that rate limits the extraction of a 2′-hydroxyl from any of the four ribonucleotides to form the matching 2′-deoxyribonucleotide (Kolberg et al., 2004, Hakansson et al., 2006). The larger RNR subunit α (M1) contains three purposeful sites: (1) a redox site of active disulfides that take part in ribonucleotide reduction, (2) a specificity site, and (3) an allosteric site exerting control over specific 2′-deoxyribonucleotide output. The smaller RNR subunit β (M2 or p53R2 [M2b]) contains a dinuclear prosthetic moiety harboring two iron(III) ions stabilizing a tyrosyl radical vital for catalysis (Hakansson et al., 2006). For the α and β subunits to link up, the C-terminus of RNR subunit β is the business end for holoenzyme complex formation (Uhlin and Eklund, 1994). Electron microscopy has determined that human RNR predominantly exists in a $\alpha_6\beta_2$ form (Rofougaran et al., 2006, Fairman et al., 2011), with free interchange among its minimal $\alpha_2\beta_2$ or its higher-order $\alpha_6\beta_6$ forms (Rofougaran et al., 2008). Competitive peptide binding to RNR subunit α, at subsites denoted F_1 for the N-terminal Phe residue and F_7 for the C-terminal Phe residue, inhibits the activity of the enzyme (Xu et al., 2008). Despite some *cross talk* between the M2 and M2b subunits, the absence of a complete tetrameric RNR enzyme results in early embryonic lethality (DeWeese et al., 1998). It turns out that human RNR M2 and M2b are overexpressed in cervical cancers (Kunos et al., 2010c, 2011c, 2012).

Models for the catalytic reduction of 2′-ribonucleotide diphosphates have been investigated in *Escherichia coli* and mice (Stubbe and van der Donk, 1998, Eklund et al., 2001, Reece et al., 2006, Popovic-Bijelic et al., 2011). A thiyl radical in a conserved cysteine residue (C439) initiates substrate reduction by removing a hydrogen from the ribose ring of ribonucleotide diphosphates (Reece et al., 2006). Critical to the initiating step of the reaction is a proton-coupled electron transfer from the M2 or M2b diferric tyrosyl radical (•Y122) through a 35 Å amino acid tunnel to the M1 cysteine (C439) to form the thiyl radical (Reece et al., 2006). Site mutagenesis studies conducted in *E. coli* have identified an amino acid chain of •Y122/W48/Y356 in M2, and then Y731/Y730/C439 in M1 facilitates radical transport (Reece et al., 2006). A disulfide bridge formed between C225 and C462 in the active site of M1 has to be resolved before enzyme activity returns. This bridge is reduced by hydrogen donor proteins, thioredoxin or glutaredoxin. Unlike *E. coli*, the iron(III) ions and tyrosyl radical are labile in mammals, and both must be constantly recycled *in vivo* in a reaction involving iron(II) and oxygen (Mann et al., 1991, Nyholm et al., 1993, Licht et al., 1996, Popovic-Bijelic et al., 2011).

The exquisite and intricate proton-coupled electron transfer can be taken advantage of in anticancer radiochemotherapy strategies. For instance, a substrate analog (e.g., gemcitabine) could block catalysis through covalent intramolecular modification of the subunit α C-terminus (Wang et al., 2009). Alternatively, pharmacologic inactivation of subunit β can be done by one-electron transfer from a drug (e.g., hydroxyurea) to reduce the tyrosyl radical to a normal tyrosine residue (Lassman et al., 1992). A second pharmacologic inactivation could occur with a drug (e.g., triapine) that facilitates release and reduction of iron(III) ions from subunit β. In the presence of oxygen, drug–iron(II) complexes generate reactive oxygen species that reduce the tyrosyl radical to a normal tyrosine residue (Popovic-Bijelic et al., 2011). Further insights into anticancer radiochemotherapy strategies pertinent to cervical cancer are detailed later.

9.2.2 Nucleotide Salvage

Cells may also furnish needed nucleotides by recovering spent deoxyribonucleosides (Kunos and Radivoyevitch, 2011). The rate of salvage depends on the activity of deoxynucleoside kinases—thymidine kinase 1 (TK1) and/or deoxycytidine kinase (dCK) in the cytosol and thymidine kinase 2 (TK2) and deoxyguanosine kinase (dGK) in mitochondria (Figure 9.1). These enzymes phosphorylate deoxyribonucleosides to produce corresponding deoxyribonucleoside monophosphates. TK1 acts in an S-phase-specific manner through a destruction mechanism similar to that of RNR M2. The other three deoxynucleoside kinases act across all other phases of the cell cycle. Deoxynucleoside kinases are variably expressed in human normal and cancer tissues, with TK1 being elevated in cervical cancers (Fujiwaki et al., 2001). After radiation, it is thought that deoxynucleosides enter cells and mitochondria passively by plasma membrane equilibrative nucleoside transporters, and when TK1 and dCK levels spike after radiation, salvaged deoxynucleosides contribute to the repair of radiation-mediated DNA damage (Kunos et al., 2011b).

9.2.3 Effects of Human Papillomavirus in Cervical Cancer

Cervical cancers often are linked to human papillomavirus (HPV), a virus commonly acquired by sexual activity (Munoz et al., 2003, Clifford et al., 2005, Barzon et al., 2010, Lu et al., 2011). Many HPVs induce excessive anogenital squamous cell turnover, with viral DNA from subtypes 16, 18, 31, 35, 39, 45, 51, 52, 56, or 58 found integrated in many human invasive cancers (Clifford et al., 2005). For this chapter, HPV pathophysiology and the manners by which the virus initially steals human host cervical cell machinery to replicate its closed-circular, double-stranded DNA is germane (Hebner and Laimins, 2006). Six early proteins (E1, E2, E4–E7) and two late proteins (L1, L2) direct host cell proteins and enzymes (Hebner and Laimins, 2006). To achieve this goal, HPV-E6 promotes p53 protein degradation. In doing so, the role p53 typically plays in slowing cell transit at a G1/S cell cycle restriction checkpoint is diminished (Scheffner et al., 1990, Werness et al., 1990, Huibregtse et al., 1991). While HPV-E6 disrupts p53 signaling, HPV-E7 eliminates, by a proteasome-dependent degradation, cell cycle barriers put in place by retinoblastoma protein (Gonzalez et al., 2001). Such an HPV-E7 effect allows E2F activation (Huang et al., 1993), turning on S-phase proteins that duplicate DNA. Ultimately, cell cycle checkpoints are superseded and oncogenic phenotypes emerge (Hebner and Laimins, 2006). RNR is intimately involved in 2′-deoxyribonucleotide production in the viral and host DNA replication (Lembo et al., 2006).

9.3 Effects of Radiochemotherapy on Nucleotide Metabolism in Cervical Cancers

DNA is the most well-studied target of radiation-mediated cell death. When DNA damage occurs, the ATM/ATR–CHK2/CHK1-controlled checkpoint responses transiently delay cell cycle progression in G1, S, or G2 phase. This same checkpoint response can invoke prolonged arrests in the G1 phase before subsequent S phase or arrests in the G2 phase before mitosis. Checkpoint delays allow cells to fix damaged DNA. As an example, unrepaired double-strand breaks can result in chromosome regions not being segregated by mitotic spindles. Failure to repair double-strand breaks ultimately results in mitotic catastrophe and cell death.

Radiochemotherapy's capability of sterilizing cervical cancer in this way has been studied in cervical cancer surgical specimens and, perhaps, makes available *in vivo* proof-of-principle evidence of radiochemotherapy effect (Kunos et al., 2010a). Among 464 surgical specimens, a significantly higher proportion (80%) of good responses (i.e., >90% sterilization) was found after radiochemotherapy, as compared to radiation alone (71%, $P < 0.037$). *In vitro* DNA damage studies and qualitative immunohistochemical analyses of RNR subunit expression are now providing compelling molecular evidence that unchecked overexpression of M2 is associated with facile DNA repair, radiation resistance, posttherapy persistence of disease, and shorter cancer-related survival (Kunos et al., 2010b, 2012).

9.3.1 Nucleotide Demand Effects

To efficiently orchestrate the cellular response to dNDP demand that occurs for DNA replication or DNA repair, regulation of RNR activity may be carried out either by adenosine triphosphate (ATP) or by deoxyadenosine triphosphate (dATP) occupying the M1 activity site (Radivoyevitch, 2009). At the activity site, these adaptors of RNR activate (ATP) or deactivate (dATP) the enzyme by altering M1 monomer–dimer–(short-lived tetramer)–hexamer equilibrium (Rofougaran et al., 2006). If the specificity site is empty, ATP-bound, or dATP-bound, RNR reduces cytidine diphosphate (CDP) or uridine diphosphate (UDP). If the specificity site is deoxythymidine triphosphate (dTTP) bound, guanosine diphosphate (GDP) is reduced. If the specificity site is deoxyguanosine triphosphate (dGTP) bound, reduction of adenosine diphosphate (ADP) occurs. It is remarkable how rapidly the feedback cascade of allosteric effectors at an M1 specificity site balances dNDP production (Radivoyevitch, 2009). For instance, in one set of experiments, excess deoxynucleosides provided in cervical cancer cell culture medium suppressed intracellular dCTP concentrations, suggesting inhibition of RNR by dATP binding to its activity site (Kunos et al., 2011b). It is also important to mention that thymidylate synthase supplies the only intracellular source of deoxythymidine monophosphates, and therefore, blockade of thymidylate synthase by 5-fluorouracil (5-FU) also alters RNR activity. Whether a hexamerization site regulates human RNR is debated (Radivoyevitch and Kunos, 2012).

9.3.2 Nucleotide Supply Effects

In a broader sense, the spatial–temporal regulation of M1, M2, and M2b happens by transcriptional regulation and by protein degradation. M1 is long lived and can be detected in low amounts in all phases of the cell cycle (Hakansson et al., 2006). In resting cells or differentiated cells no longer synthesizing DNA, M1 levels slowly decline (Engstrom et al., 1985, Chabes and Thelander, 2000). M2 is short lived, restricted typically to the S phase of the cell cycle, and has a KEN-box sequence identified in late mitosis by the Cdh1•anaphase-promoting complex that leads to protein destruction (Eriksson et al., 1984, Chabes and Thelander, 2000). M2b also appears to be long lived through its lack of a KEN-box, and therefore, it is found in low quantities in all phases of the cell cycle (Hakansson et al., 2006). M2b transcription is p53 dependent (Tanaka et al., 2000, Xue et al., 2003).

There is an emerging recognition that RNR can be effectively inactivated by disrupting M1–M2 or M1–M2b co-association. Currently, there are peptides that competitively bind to the surface of M1 and block M2 or M2B binding (Xu et al., 2008). A bond between the *superintendent* p53 protein and M2b exists, disturbs M1–M2b complex formation by physical interference, and suppresses global RNR activity (Xue et al., 2003). It is alleged that the act of phosphorylating p53 (e.g., after radiation) changes p53 conformation, releases M2b, and permits RNR holoenzyme formation and activity (Xue et al., 2003). Certainly, many phenomena manage immediate supply of demanded dNDPs in cells.

9.3.3 Nucleotide Currency and Economy

Among the mechanisms that cells of the uterine cervix have developed to cope with nucleotide supply and demand requests are differential expression of RNR subunits. Because spontaneous damage in nuclear DNA occurs and mitochondria draw upon nucleotide pools, constitutive low levels of the *regulatory* subunit α (M1) and subunit β' (M2b [p53R2]) are found (Hakansson et al., 2006). Even after ionizing radiation, human cervical cancer cells demonstrated only minor alterations in M1 level (Kuo and Kinsella, 1998). More modest rises in M2b level are detected in cervical cancer cells after ionizing radiation, perhaps attributable to a DNA damage response (Kunos et al., 2009). To look at this from a different vantage, immunohistochemical studies suggest RNR M1 protein levels in uterine cervix cancers rise infrequently after radiochemotherapy (Kunos et al., 2012). RNR M2b immunoreactivity in normal cervix tissue is low, but the majority of uterine cervix cancers show high M2b protein levels (Kunos et al., 2012).

On the other hand, cells use a scalable rise in RNR M2 in an S-phase cell cycle–specific manner to meet dNDP demands when replicating DNA (Eriksson et al., 1984, Engstrom et al., 1985). Dividing cells show a 20-fold rise in RNR M2 level (Hakansson et al., 2006). *In vitro* cervical cancer cells show a 17-fold rise in RNR M2 transcripts and protein levels over 12–18 h after irradiation (Kuo and Kinsella, 1998). It has been suggested that this rise in RNR M2 assists in DNA damage repair (Kunos et al., 2009, 2010b, 2011a,b). Immunohistochemical studies have found that M2 levels are very high in nearly all cases of untreated cervical cancer and remain high after radiochemotherapy (Kunos et al., 2012). Even though data remain scarce, cervical cancers having intense M2 or M2b immunoreactivity had a poor (33%) 5-year estimate for disease-free survival (Kunos et al., 2012).

Analyses of cervical cancer clinical trial data for pretherapy M1, M2, and M2b protein level as a predictor of radiochemotherapy response are forthcoming.

Two of the four classic Rs of radiobiology deal with cellular nucleotide economy—repair and redistribution. A brief discussion of how RNR participates in these two Rs of radiobiology follows.

9.3.3.1 Repair

Reallocating resources to fix radiation-induced DNA damage by error-prone and by error-free processes starts within minutes after radiation damage is detected. Base excision repair, nucleotide excision repair, homologous recombination (error free), and nonhomologous end joining (error prone) mechanisms are recognized means to enact DNA repair. One way to analyze the timely repair of radiation-induced damage is monitoring the formation and resolution of H2AX phosphorylation at Ser-139 (γH2AX). Foci of γH2AX signal mark sites of DNA double-strand breaks (Olive and Banath, 2004). In resting, unirradiated cells, low numbers of γH2AX foci are observed (Figure 9.2). As it turns out, nonlethally irradiated cells generate and

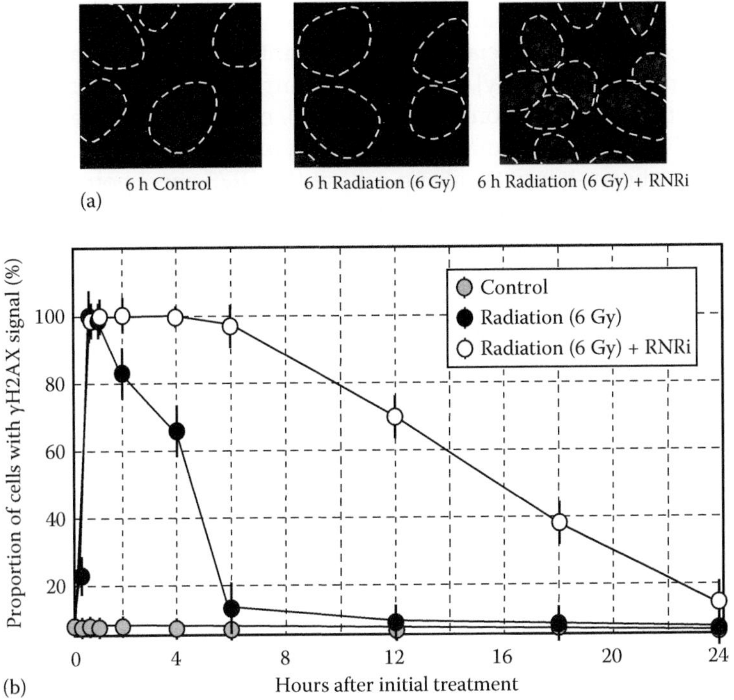

FIGURE 9.2
Repair. (a) CaSki cervical cancer cells underwent sham, radiation (6 Gy), or radiation (6 Gy) plus ribonucleotide reductase inhibitor (RNRi) treatments in a manner described earlier (Kunos et al., 2009). Six hours after the start of the experiment, control cells showed no substantial γH2AX foci. Irradiated cells also had no substantial γH2AX foci. But many γH2AX foci were found when irradiated cells were also treated with an RNRi. Cell nucleus outlines are provided for reference. (b) Manual γH2AX foci counts in three replicates of CaSki cervical cancer cell were done at 0, 30, and 60 min and 2, 4, 6, 12, 18, and 24 h after sham, radiation (6 Gy), or radiation (6 Gy) plus RNRi treatments, as detailed elsewhere (Kunos et al., 2011b). Protracted repair of DNA damage, here marked by unresolved γH2AX foci, occurs after radiation plus RNRi treatment, as compared to radiation alone. For this graph, cell proportion equals the number of cells with >10 γH2AX foci divided by the total number of cells with any visible γH2AX foci. Means (± standard deviations) are indicated.

then resolve γH2AX foci in 3–4 h after radiation exposure (Figure 9.2). During this time, RNR activity rises (Kunos et al., 2009). However, when RNR is blocked by a pharmacologic inhibitor, radiation-induced damage is slowly fixed, such that the γH2AX signal slowly resolves much later than the typical 4 h of repair (Figure 9.2). Inactivated RNR slows recovery from DNA damage and exacerbates radiation-mediated cytotoxicity (Kunos et al., 2009, 2011c).

9.3.3.2 Redistribution

Tumors can be thought of as an unsynchronized population of cells. Those cells residing in S phase of the cell cycle are considered tolerant of radiation death-provoking effects. The reasons for this observation are likely to be many, but it stands to reason that S phase cells having elevated RNR are capable of supplying dNDPs immediately on demand to fix any radiation-induced DNA damage occurring (Gao and Richardson, 2001, Lin et al., 2007).

Radiobiology studies have demonstrated that exponentially growing cervical cancer cells, if not lethally irradiated, stack up in G1/S or G2/M transitions due to checkpoint activation (Kunos et al., 2009, 2011a,c). It is conceivable then that surviving cells after one dose of radiation may redistribute themselves and arrest at more sensitive phases of the cell cycle. Thus, the very next radiation dose, if timed when cells are most susceptible, may be lethal. This effect can be appreciated most poignantly in cervical cancer cells when low-dose-rate radiation (centigray [cGy]/hour) is used during brachytherapy treatment. When exposed to low-dose-rate radiation (e.g., 67 cGy/h), cells arrest at the G2/M checkpoint (Kunos et al., 2011a), which ultimately leads to cytoreduction (Figure 9.3). Meanwhile, inhibiting RNR has been shown to pile up cells at the G1/S checkpoint (Kunos et al., 2009, 2011a,c). Under low-dose-rate conditions, the pharmacologic effect of RNR blockade leads to durable G1/S checkpoint arrest (Kunos et al., 2011a) and greater cell lethality (Figure 9.3). It has been concluded that RNR inhibition impedes DNA damage repair mechanisms that rely on dNDP production and, thus, enhances the radiation sensitivity of cervical cancers by imparting effects on cell cycle phase redistribution.

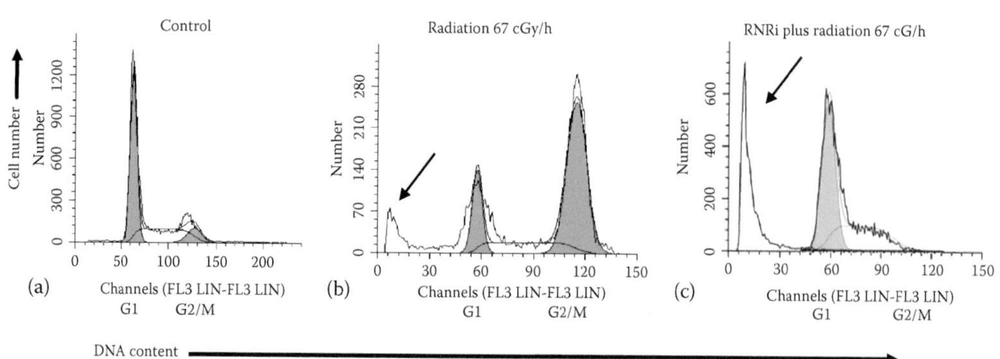

FIGURE 9.3
Redistribution. CaSki cervical cancer cells were treated by sham, radiation (67 cGy/h, 10 Gy), or radiation (67 cGy/h; 10 Gy) plus a RNRi and analyzed for propidium iodide–stained DNA content using a flow cytometer, as described earlier (Kunos et al., 2011a). (a) Control cells reside predominantly in the G1 phase of the cell cycle. (b) Cells exposed to low-dose-rate radiation pile up in the G2/M phase of the cell cycle. Over time, cells incur cumulative radiation damage while arrested in the G2/M phase of the cell cycle and, then, die as indicated by a sub-G1 population (arrow). (c) Cells treated by an RNRi predominantly arrest at the G1/S transition due to an inability to generate *de novo* dNDPs demanded in very high number. Cumulative radiation damage occurring over time when RNR is blocked results in substantial cytotoxicity (sub-G1 phase cells, arrow).

9.4 Therapeutic Mechanisms of Cervical Cancer Treatment

Prominent among the effective radiochemotherapy strategies in cervical cancer management are the RNR inhibitors hydroxyurea, 5-FU, gemcitabine, and triapine (Kunos and Radivoyevitch, 2011, Kunos 2012). Given that the molecular strategies of dNDP supply inhibition share inactivation of RNR, it is striking that these pharmacologic agents lead to a variety of therapeutic responses.

9.4.1 Pharmacologic Inhibition of Ribonucleotide Reductase

Early on, the Gynecologic Oncology Group (GOG-004) assigned, by random assortment, women with advanced-stage cervical cancer to either oral hydroxyurea (80 mg/kg, oral twice weekly) or placebo during pelvic radiation (Hreshchyshyn et al., 1979). Hydroxyurea (HU) irreversibly quenches the M2 or M2b diferric tyrosyl radical (•Y122), essentially making the initiating M1 cysteine (C439) incapable of starting the catalytic reaction (Nyholm et al., 1993). Three-year pelvic disease control and progression-free survival (i.e., free of cancer relapse or death) were improved after radiation–HU, compared to radiation–placebo (Table 9.1, $P < 0.05$). As such, hydroxyurea-mediated block of RNR during radiation became the benchmark by which other radiochemotherapeutic agents would be compared.

The GOG began a series of trials exploring the use of RNR inhibitors in combination with DNA-damaging agents. Up to that time, the more common and consequential component of treatment failure was ineffective sterilization by radiation alone. At that time, a new anticancer DNA-damaging agent was cisplatin (Bonomi et al., 1985). Cisplatin actively engages cells in DNA adduct repair for up to 24 h, eliciting constant nucleotide payouts from RNR (Olive and Banath, 2009). To elucidate this effect, the GOG conducted a randomized trial (GOG-0043) of three cisplatin dose schedules in 496 women for persistent pelvic or extrapelvic cervical cancer disease response. Most (93%) women had undergone pelvic radiation at a point in time prior to receiving any cisplatin infusions. On trial, regimen 1 was cisplatin 50 mg/m^2 every 21 days; regimen 2 was cisplatin 100 mg/m^2 every 21 days; and regimen 3 was cisplatin 20 mg/m^2 daily for 5 consecutive days. These regimens recurred for a total maximum cisplatin dose of 400 mg/m^2, providing there was no evidence of tumor progression. Among 444 evaluable patients, best overall response rates were 21% for regimen 1, 31% for regimen 2, and 25% for regimen 3 ($P = 0.015$). With an understanding of cisplatin's cytoreductive properties, ability to synchronize cells in radiosensitive phases of the cell cycle, and contribution to DNA damage that taxing nucleotide supply, investigators initiated clinical trials of single-drug and multiple-drug cisplatin combinations with radiation for the treatment of cervical cancer.

Therefore, in one of the first group wide clinical trials, GOG-085 evaluated whether a radiation–cisplatin–5-FU combination was superior to a radiation–hydroxyurea combination (Whitney et al., 1999). This approach introduced the hybrid concept of dual DNA damaging agents (i.e., radiation, cisplatin) and RNR inhibition by a nucleoside analog (i.e., 5-FU) versus radical elimination (i.e., hydroxyurea). So in this randomized clinical trial, women underwent radiation and hydroxyurea (80 mg/kg, oral twice weekly) or underwent radiation, cisplatin (bolus 50 mg/m^2 4 h before radiation, days 1 and 29), and 5-FU (protracted infusion 1000 mg/m^2/day, days 2–5 and 30–33). After this, it was found that a radiation–cisplatin–5-FU combination improved disease control (Table 9.1) and progression-free survival ($P = 0.033$). Correspondingly, the Radiation Therapy Oncology Group (RTOG-9001) found comparable outcomes (Morris et al., 1999, Eifel et al., 2004). RTOG-9001 allocated

TABLE 9.1

Cervical Cancer Clinical Trials Incorporating Ribonucleotide Reductase Inhibition

Citation	Years of Study	No. of Patients	FIGO Stages	DNA Damage Agent(s)	dNTP Supply Inhibitor	No. of Pelvic Relapses by 3 Years	No. of Extrapelvic Relapses by 3 Years	3-Year Progression-Free Survival Estimate
Hreshchyshyn et al. (1979)	1970–1976	47	III_B–IV_A	Radiation	Hydroxyurea	15 (32%)	NR	25%
		43		Radiation	None	22 (51%)	NR	15%
Whitney et al. (1999)	1986–1990	191	II_B–IV_A	Radiation	Hydroxyurea	58 (30%)	40 (21%)	52%
		177		Radiation + cisplatin	5-FU	44 (25%)	31 (18%)	60%
Morris et al. (1999)	1990–1997	193	I_{B2}–IV_A	Radiation (extended)	None	68 (35%)	64 (33%)	50%
Eifel et al. (2004)		195		Radiation + cisplatin	5-FU	39 (20%)	27 (14%)	70%
Rose et al. (1999)	1992–1997	177	II_B–IV_B	Radiation	Hydroxyurea	60 (34%)	NR	40%
Rose et al. (2007)		176		Radiation + cisplatin	None	Radiation	None	62%
		173		Radiation + cisplatin	5-FU Hydroxyurea	36 (21%)	NR	62%
Keys et al. (1999)	1992–1997	186	I_{B2}	Radiation	None	44 (24%)	25 (13%)	64%
		183		Radiation + cisplatin	None	19 (10%)	19 (10%)	78%
Lanciano et al. (2005)	1997–2000	159	II_B–IV_A	Radiation	5-FU	22 (14%)[a]	46 (29%)[a]	54%
		157		Radiation + cisplatin		25 (16%)[a]	28 (18%)[a]	60%
Duenas-Gonzalez et al. (2011)	2002–2004	256	II_B–IV_A	Radiation + cisplatin	None	42 (16%)	42 (16%)	65%
		259		Radiation + cisplatin	Gemcitabine	29 (11%)	21 (8%)[b]	74%
Kunos et al. (2010c)	2006–2008	10	I_{B2}–IV_B	Radiation + cisplatin	Triapine	0 (0%)	1 (10%)	88%
Kunos et al. (2011c)	2009–2011	25	I_{B2}–IV_B	Radiation + cisplatin	Triapine	1 (4%)	4 (16%)	NR

Note: FIGO, The International Federation of Gynecology and Obstetrics.

[a] Four-year cumulative incidence rate for the pelvis alone and extrapelvic (abdominal, para-aortic, the bone, liver, and lung).

[b] Women received adjuvant cisplatin (50 mg/m^2) day 1 and gemcitabine 1 gm/m^2 day 1 + day 8.

women randomly to extended-field radiation alone or to four-field pelvic radiation, cisplatin (bolus 75 mg/m^2 within 16 h after radiation, days 1, 22, and 42), and 5-FU (protracted infusion 1000 mg/m^2/day, days 2–5, 23–26, and 43–46). Gains in pelvic disease control, extrapelvic disease control (Table 9.1), and 3-year progression-free survival ($P = 0.0003$) were recorded for the radiation–cisplatin–5-FU combination in opposition to radiation alone.

Shortly thereafter, GOG-120 randomly allotted women with advanced-stage cervical cancer to one of three cisplatin-based radiochemotherapy treatments (Rose et al., 1999). Regimen 1 was daily pelvic radiation and once weekly cisplatin (bolus 40 mg/m^2) followed by brachytherapy. Regimen 2 was the same radiation but day 1 and day 29 cisplatin (bolus 50 mg/m^2) and 96 h infusion 5-FU (4000 mg maximum) plus oral hydroxyurea (twice weekly, 2000 mg/m^2). Regimen 3 was the same radiation and twice weekly oral hydroxyurea (3000 mg/m^2). After this, 3-year pelvic disease control and extrapelvic disease control were found to be superior with regimens 1 and 2 (Table 9.1). It was discovered that the addition of two RNR inhibitors, 5-FU and hydroxyurea, resulted in no gain in clinical benefit over the weekly cisplatin regimen (Table 9.1). Long-term data corroborate a gain in progression-free survival for regimen 1 ($P < 0.01$) and for regimen 2 ($P < 0.01$), as compared to regimen 3 (Rose et al., 2007a). It has become commonplace to administer weekly cisplatin in radiochemotherapy practice due to its technically favorable administration schedule (Kunos et al., 2008). To back up these results, GOG-0165 randomized advanced-stage cervical cancer patients to weekly cisplatin (bolus 40 mg/m^2) versus 5-FU (protracted venous infusion 225 mg/m^2/day, day 1–5 of 5 weekly cycles) (Lanciano et al., 2005). Cisplatin–radiation was deemed more effective than 5-FU–radiation (Table 9.1).

Interrupting RNR at its diferric tyrosyl radical (•Y122) has been met with the most clinical success in cervical cancer management (Kunos et al., 2010c, 2011c). A more potent RNR inhibitor 3-aminopyridine-2-carboxaldehyde thiosemicarbazone (3-AP, triapine) creates a molecular intermediate (Fe^{2+}-3-AP) that collapses the tyrosyl free radical through a local reactive oxygen species (Popovic-Bijelic et al., 2011). 3-AP's cell death–provoking effect may be a result of RNR being unable to create on-the-spot deoxynucleotides needed to fix DNA damage (Kunos et al., 2009, 2010b). A phase I clinical trial was done in 10 women with advanced-stage cervical cancer and involved 3-AP (25 mg/m^2, three times weekly) plus once weekly cisplatin (40 mg/m^2) during daily radiation (Kunos et al., 2010c). Median survivor follow-up is now 38 months, and progression-free survival is 88% at 3 years (Table 9.1). A phase II study of 3-AP–cisplatin radiochemotherapy in 25 additional women with cervical and vaginal cancers has been resulted (Table 9.1). 3-AP radiochemotherapy achieved complete clinical responses in 24 (96%) of 25 women (median follow-up 20 months, range 2–35 months). Twenty-three (96%) of 24 women had 3-month posttherapy positron emission and computed tomography scans that recorded metabolic activity in the cervix or vagina equal or less than that of the cardiac blood pool, suggesting complete metabolic responses. The most frequent, reversible 3-AP radiochemotherapy-related adverse events included fatigue, nausea, diarrhea, and electrolyte abnormalities. Based on these outstanding results, a randomized phase II study of 3-AP–cisplatin radiation versus cisplatin radiation is beginning in the United States under the auspices of the National Cancer Institute–Cancer Therapy Evaluation Program (NCI protocol #9434).

9.4.2 Nucleoside Analogs

To be pharmacologically useful, nucleoside analogs such as cytarabine, fludarabine, and gemcitabine require activation by dCK in the salvage pathway of deoxynucleosides (Perez-Perez et al., 2005). The most clinically successful of nucleoside analogs in cervical cancer management is gemcitabine. Gemcitabine annihilates the catalytic site of M1 through a covalent bond when it masquerades as a CDP analog; this inactivates the RNR α_2 dimer (Wang et al., 2009). A phase II clinical study of radiation, cisplatin (40 mg/m^2), and gemcitabine (125 mg/m^2) resulted a 78% complete response rate (Duenas-Gonzalez et al., 2005). In phase III testing (Duenas-Gonzalez et al., 2011), regimen 1 consisted of once weekly cisplatin (bolus 40 mg/m^2) plus gemcitabine (bolus 125 mg/m^2) during pelvic radiation. This was followed by two adjuvant 21-day cycles of cisplatin (50 mg/m^2, day 1) plus gemcitabine (1000 mg/m^2, days 1 and 8). Regimen 2 involved once weekly cisplatin (bolus 40 mg/m^2) and the same radiation. A hazard for cervical cancer disease relapse or death was lowered by 32% when gemcitabine was included (Table 9.1, $P = 0.023$). And yet controversy exists (Thomas, 2011). It has been stated that gemcitabine may have been effective with radiochemotherapy because it cured more patients upfront from its radiosensitizing effect. Or else, gains from gemcitabine may have been successful because it delayed scoring of disease recurrences from an adjuvant lead-time bias effect. Either interpretation can be concluded from the data reported. In a GOG gemcitabine radiochemotherapy trial (GOG-9912), the radiation–cisplatin–gemcitabine combination was not tolerated (Rose et al., 2007b). Further study is needed.

9.4.3 Pharmacologic Inhibition of Nucleoside Salvage

Pharmacologic inhibitors of nucleoside salvage pathway enzymes have not been studied extensively. To be pharmacologically useful, drugs such as cytarabine, fludarabine, and gemcitabine must be activated by dCK (Perez-Perez et al., 2005). Ionizing radiation has been shown to enhance TK1 expression (Boothman et al., 1994). Oncologic phenotypes may manifest altered levels and activities of nucleoside salvage proteins and enzymes (Weinberg et al., 1981). These findings do point to the future importance of targeting the nucleoside salvage pathway as an anticancer strategy in cervical cancer management.

9.5 Future Ribonucleotide Reductase Inhibitor Clinical Development in Cervical Cancer Management

The past decade has seen women with advanced-stage cervical cancer profit from RNR inhibitor therapies. Stakeholders, both patient and physician, need to advocate for oral or transdermal radiosensitizing RNR inhibitors that can be added safely to radiation therapy so that care can be delivered in both resource-rich and resource-poor nations. Optimal radiochemotherapy logistics, patient preexistent morbidity, and treatment-related toxicity modulate enthusiasm for RNR inhibitors in the clinic. Improvements in cervical cancer care margins will likely embrace cytoreductive therapies that generate damaged DNA combined with biological agents that slow or halt its repair.

References

Barzon L, Militello V, Pagni S, Franchin E, Dal Bello F, Mengoli C et al. 2010. Distribution of human papillomavirus types in the anogenital tract of females and males. *J Med Virol.* 82(8):1424–1430.

Bonomi P, Blessing JA, Stehman FB, DiSaia PJ, Walton L, Major FJ. 1985. Randomized trial of three cisplatin dose schedules in squamous-cell carcinoma of the cervix: A Gynecologic Oncology Group study. *J Clin Oncol.* 3(8):1079–1085.

Boothman D, Davis T, Sahijdak W. 1994. Enhanced expression of thymidine kinase in human cells following ionizing radiation. *Int J Radiat Oncol Biol Phys.* 30:391–398.

Candelaria M, Chanona-Vilchis J, Cetina L, Flores-Estrada D, López-Graniel C, González-Enciso A et al. 2006. Prognostic significance of pathological response after neoadjuvant chemotherapy or chemoradiation for locally advanced cervical carcinoma. *Int Semin Surg Oncol.* 3:3.1–3.8.

Chabes A, Thelander L. 2000. Controlled protein degradation regulates ribonucleotide reductase activity in proliferating mammalian cells during the normal cell cycle and in response to DNA damage and replication blocks. *J Biol Chem.* 275(23):17747–17753.

Clifford GM, Gallus S, Herrero R, Munoz N, Snijders PJF, Vaccarella S et al. 2005. Worldwide distribution of human papillomavirus types in cytologically normal women in the International Agency for Research on Cancer HPV prevalence surveys: A pooled analysis. *Lancet.* 366(9490):991–998.

DeWeese T, Shipman J, Larrier N, Buckley N, Kidd L, Groopman J et al. 1998. Mouse embryonic stem cells carrying one or two defective Msh2 alleles respond abnormally to oxidative stress inflicted by low-level radiation. *Proc Natl Acad Sci USA.* 95:11915–11920.

Duenas-Gonzalez A, Cetina-Perez L, Lopez-Graniel C, Gonzalez-Enciso A, Gomez-Gonzalez E, Rivera-Ruby L et al. 2005. Pathologic response and toxicity assessment of chemoradiotherapy with cisplatin versus cisplatin plus gemcitabine in cervical cancer: A randomized phase II study. *Int J Radiat Oncol Biol Phys.* 61(3):817–823.

Duenas-Gonzalez A, Zarba J, Patel F, Alcedo J, Beslija F, Casanova L et al. 2011. A phase III, open-label, randomized study comparing concurrent gemcitabine plus cisplatin and radiation followed by adjuvant gemcitabine and cisplatin versus concurrent cisplatin and radiation in patients with stage IIB to IVA carcinoma of the cervix. *J Clin Oncol.* 29(13):1678–1685.

Eifel PJ, Winter K, Morris M, Levenback C, Grigsby PW, Cooper J et al. 2004. Pelvic irradiation with concurrent chemotherapy versus pelvic and para-aortic irradiation for high-risk cervical cancer: An update of radiation therapy oncology group trial (RTOG) 90-01. *J Clin Oncol.* 22(5):872–880.

Eklund H, Uhlin U, Farnegardh M, Logan DT, Nordlund P. 2001. Structure and function of the radical enzyme ribonucleotide reductase. *Prog Biophys Mol Biol.* 77(3):177–268.

Engstrom Y, Erriksson S, Jildevik I, Skog S, Thelander L, Tribukait B. 1985. Cell cycle-dependent expression of mammalian ribonucleotide reductase. Differential regulation of the two subunits. *J Biol Chem.* 26:9114–9116.

Eriksson S, Graslund A, Skog S, Thelander L. 1984. Cell cycle-dependent regulation of mammalian ribonucleotide reductase. The S phase-correlated increase in subunit M2 is regulated by de novo protein synthesis. *J Biol Chem.* 259:11695–11700.

Fairman J, Wijerathna S, Ahmad M, Xu H, Nakano R, Jha S et al. 2011. Structural basis for allosteric regulation of human ribonucleotide reductase by nucleotide-induced oligomerization. *Nat Struct Mol Biol.* 18(3):316–322.

Ferlay J, Shin H, Bray F, Forman D, Mathers C, Parkin D. 2010. GLOBOCAN 2008 cervical cancer incidence and mortality worldwide. Lyon, France: International Agency for Research on Cancer. [cited May 25, 2012]. Available from: http://globocan.iarc.fr/factsheets/cancers/cervix.asp.

Fujiwaki R, Hata K, Moriyama M, Iwanari O, Katabuchi H et al. 2001. Clinical value of thymidine kinase in patients with cervical carcinoma. *Oncology.* 61:47–54.

Gao J, Richardson D. 2001. The potential of iron chelators of the pyridoxal isonicotinoyl hydrazone class as effective antiproliferative agents, IV: The mechanisms involved in inhibiting cell-cycle progression. *Blood.* 98(3):842–850.

Gonzalez S, Stremlau M, He X, Baile J, Münger K. 2001. Degradation of the retinoblastoma tumor suppressor by the human papillomavirus type 16 E7 oncoprotein is important for functional inactivation and is separable from proteasomal degradation of E7. *J Virol.* 75(16):7583–7591.

Hakansson P, Hofer A, Thelander L. 2006. Regulation of mammalian ribonucleotide reduction and dNTP pools after DNA damage and in resting cells. *J Biol Chem.* 281(12):7834–7841.

Hebner C, Laimins L. 2006. Human papillomaviruses: Basic mechanisms of pathogenesis and oncogenicity. *Rev Med Virol.* 16:83–97.

Hreshchyshyn MM, Aron BS, Boronow RC, Franklin EW, 3rd, Shingleton HM, Blessing JA. 1979. Hydroxyurea or placebo combined with radiation to treat stages IIIB and IV cervical cancer confined to the pelvis. *Int J Radiat Oncol Biol Phys.* 5(3):317–322.

Huang P, Patrick D, Edwards G, Goodhart P, Huber H, Miles L et al. 1993. Protein domains governing interactions between E2F, the retinoblastoma gene product, and human papillomavirus type 16 E7 protein. *Mol Cell Biol.* 13(2):953–960.

Huibregtse J, Scheffner M, Howley P. 1991. A cellular protein mediates association of p53 with the E6 oncoprotein of human papillomavirus types 16 or 18. *EMBO J.* 10(13):4129–4135.

Keys HM, Bundy BN, Stehman FB, Muderspach LI, Chafe WE, Suggs CL, 3rd et al. 1999. Cisplatin, radiation, and adjuvant hysterectomy compared with radiation and adjuvant hysterectomy for bulky stage IB cervical carcinoma. *N Engl J Med.* 340(15):1154–1161.

Kolberg M, Strand KR, Graff P, Andersson KK. 2004. Structure, function, and mechanism of ribonucleotide reductases. *Biochimica et Biophysica Acta.* 1699(1–2):1–34.

Kunos C. 2012. Therapeutic mechanisms of treatment in cervical and vaginal cancer. *Oncol Hematol Rev.* 8(1):55–60.

Kunos C, Ali S, Abdul-Karim F, Stehman F, Waggoner S. 2010a. Posttherapy residual disease associates with long-term survival after chemoradiation for bulky stage 1_B cervical carcinoma: A Gynecologic Oncology Group study. *Am J Obstet Gynecol.* 203(4):351.e1–351.e8.

Kunos C, Chiu S, Pink J, Kinsella T. 2009. Modulating radiation resistance by inhibiting ribonucleotide reductase in cancers with virally or mutationally silenced p53 protein. *Radiation Res.* 172(6):666–676.

Kunos C, Colussi V, Pink J, Radivoyevitch T, Oleinick N. 2011a. Radiosensitization of human cervical cancer cells by inhibiting ribonucleotide reductase: Enhanced radiation response at low dose rates. *Int J Radiat Oncol Biol Phys.* 80(4):1198–1204.

Kunos C, Ferris G, Pyatka N, Pink J, Radivoyevitch T. 2011b. Deoxynucleoside salvage facilitates DNA repair during ribonucleotide reductase blockade in human cervical cancers. *Radiat Res.* 176(4):425–433.

Kunos C, Gibbons H, Simpkins F, Waggoner S. 2008. Chemotherapy administration during pelvic radiation for cervical cancer patients aged ≥55 years in the SEER-Medicare population. *J Oncol.* 2008:1–7.

Kunos C, Radivoyevitch T. 2011. Molecular strategies of deoxynucleotide triphosphate supply inhibition used in the treatment of gynecologic malignancies. *Gynecol Obstetric.* S4:001 doi:10.4172/2161-0932.S4-001.

Kunos C, Radivoyevitch T, Kresak A, Dawson D, Jacobberger J, Yang B et al. 2012. Elevated ribonucleotide reductase levels associate with suppressed radiochemotherapy response in human cervical cancers. *Int J Gynecol Cancer.* 22(9):1463–1469. doi: 10.1097/IGC.0b013e318270577f.

Kunos C, Radivoyevitch T, Pink J, Chiu S, Stefan T, Jacobberger J et al. 2010b. Ribonucleotide reductase inhibition enhances chemoradiosensitivity of human cervical cancers. *Radiation Res.* 174(5):574–581.

Kunos C, Waggoner S, Von Gruenigen V, Eldermire E, Pink J, Dowlati A et al. 2010c. Phase I trial of intravenous 3-aminopyridine-2-carboxaldehyde thiosemicarbazone (3-AP, NSC #663249) in combination with pelvic radiation therapy and weekly cisplatin chemotherapy for locally advanced cervical cancer. *Clin Cancer Res.* 16(4):1298–1306.

Kunos C, Waggoner S, Zanotti K, DeBernardo R, Heugel A, Fusco N et al. 2011c. Phase 2 trial of pelvic radiation, weekly cisplatin, and 3-aminopyridine-2-carboxaldehyde thiosemicarbazone (3-AP, NSC #663249) for locally advanced cervical and vaginal cancer. *J Clin Oncol.* 29(Suppl):Abstract #5034.

Kuo M-L, Kinsella T. 1998. Expression of ribonucleotide reductase after ionizing radiation in human cervical carcinoma cells. *Cancer Res.* 58:2245–2252.

Lanciano R, Calkins A, Bundy BN, Parham G, Lucci JA, 3rd, Moore DH et al. 2005. Randomized comparison of weekly cisplatin or protracted venous infusion of fluorouracil in combination with pelvic radiation in advanced cervix cancer: A gynecologic oncology group study. *J Clin Oncol.* 23(33):8289–8295.

Lassman G, Thelander L, Graslund A. 1992. EPR stopped-flow studies of the reaction of the tyrosyl radical of protein R2 from ribonucleotide reductase with hydroxyurea. *Biochem Biophys Res Commun.* 188:879–887.

Lembo D, Donalisio M, Cornaglia M, Azzimonti B, Demurtas A, Landolfo S. 2006. Effect of high-risk human papillomavirus oncoproteins on p53R2 gene expression after DNA damage. *Virus Res.* 122(1–2):189–193.

Licht S, Gerfen G, Stubbe J. 1996. Thiyl radicals in ribonucleotide reductases. *Science.* 271:477–481.

Lin Z, Belcourt M, Carbone R, Eaton J, Penketh P, Shadel G et al. 2007. Excess ribonucleotide reductase R2 subunits coordinate the S phase checkpoint to facilitate DNA damage repair and recovery from replication stress. *Biochem Pharmacol.* 73:760–772.

Lu B, Viscidi R, Lee J, Wu Y, Villa L, Lazcano-Ponce E et al. 2011. Human papillomavirus (HPV) 6, 11, 16, and 18 seroprevalence is associated with sexual practice and age: Results from the multinational HPV Infection in Men Study (HIM Study). *Cancer Epidemiol Biomarkers Prev.* 20(5):990–1002.

Mann G, Graslund A, Ochiai E, Ingemarson R, Thelander L. 1991. Purification and characterization of recombinant mouse and herpes simplex virus ribonucleotide reductase R2 subunit. *Biochemistry* 30:1939–1947.

Morris M, Eifel PJ, Lu J, Grigsby PW, Levenback C, Stevens RE et al. 1999. Pelvic radiation with concurrent chemotherapy compared with pelvic and para-aortic radiation for high-risk cervical cancer. *N Engl J Med.* 340(15):1137–1143.

Munoz N, Bosch FX, de Sanjose S, Herrero R, Castellsague X, Shah KV et al. 2003. Epidemiologic classification of human papillomavirus types associated with cervical cancer. *N Engl J Med.* 348(6):518–527.

Nyholm S, Thelander L, Graslund A. 1993. Reduction and loss of the iron center in the reaction of the small subunit of mouse ribonucleotide reductase with hydroxyurea. *Biochemistry* 32(43):11569–11574.

Olive P, Banath J. 2004. Phosphorylation of histone H2AX as a measure of radiosensitivity. *Int J Radiat Oncol Biol Phys.* 58(2):331–335.

Olive P, Banath J. 2009. Kinetics of H2AX phosphorylation after exposure to cisplatin. *Cytometry B Clin Cytom.* 76(2):79–90.

Perez-Perez M-J, Hernandez A-I, Priego E-M, Rodriguez-Barrios F, Gago F, Camarasa M-J et al. 2005. Mitochondrial thymidine kinase inhibitors. *Cur Top Med Chem.* 5:1205–1219.

Popovic-Bijelic A, Kowol C, Lind M, Luo J, Himo F, Enyedy E et al. 2011. Ribonucleotide reductase inhibition by metal complexes of Triapine (3-aminopyridine-2-carboxaldehyde thiosemicarbazone): A combined experimental and theoretical study. *J Inorg Biochem.* 105(11):1422–1431.

Radivoyevitch T. 2009. Automated mass action model space generation and analysis methods for two-reactant combinatorially complex equilibriums: An analysis of ATP-induced ribonucleotide reductase R1 hexamerization data. *Biol Direct.* 4:50.1–50.19.

Radivoyevitch T, Kunos C. 2012. On model ensemble analyses of nonmonotonic data. *Nucleosides Nucleotides Nucleic Acids.* 31(2):147–156.

Reece S, Hodgkiss J, Stubbe J, Nocera D. 2006. Proton-coupled electron transfer: The mechanistic underpinning for radical transport and catalysis in biology. *Phil Trans R Soc B.* 361:1351–1364.

Rofougaran R, Crona M, Vodnala M, Sjoberg B, Hofer A. 2008. Oligomerization status directs overall activity regulation of the *Escherichia coli* class Ia ribonucleotide reductase. *J Biol Chem.* 283(51):35310–35318.

Rofougaran R, Vodnala M, Hofer A. 2006. Enzymatically active mammalian ribonucleotide reductase exists primarily as an $alpha_6beta_2$ octamer. *J Biol Chem.* 281(38):27705–27711.

Rose P, Ali S, Watkins E, Thigpen J, Deppe G, Clark-Pearson D et al. 2007a. Long-term follow-up of a randomized trial comparing concurrent single agent cisplatin, cisplatin-based combination chemotherapy, or hydroxyurea during pelvic irradiation for locally advanced cervical cancer: A Gynecologic Oncology Group study. *J Clin Oncol.* 25(19):2804–2810.

Rose P, Bundy BN, Watkins EB, Thigpen JT, Deppe G, Maiman MA et al. 1999. Concurrent cisplatin-based radiotherapy and chemotherapy for locally advanced cervical cancer. *N Engl J Med.* 340(15):1144–1153.

Rose P, DeGeest K, McMeekin S, Fusco N. 2007b. A phase I study of gemcitabine followed by cisplatin concurrent with whole pelvic radiation therapy in locally advanced cervical cancer: A Gynecologic Oncology Group study. *Gynecol Oncol.* 107:274–279.

Scheffner M, Werness B, Huibregtse J, Levine A, Howley P. 1990. The E6 oncoprotein encoded by human papillomavirus types 16 and 18 promotes the degradation of p53. *Cell.* 63(6):1129–1136.

Schwartz J, Grigsby P, Dehdashti F, Delbeke D. 2009. The role of ^{18}F-FDG PET in assessing therapy response in cancer of the cervix and ovaries. *J Nucl Med.* 50(5 Suppl):64S–73S.

Stubbe J, van der Donk J. 1998. Protein radicals in enzyme catalysis. *Chem Rev.* 98:705–762.

Tanaka H, Arakawa H, Yamaguchi T, Shiraishi K, Fukuda S, Matsui K et al. 2000. A ribonucleotide reductase gene involved in a p53-dependent cell-cycle checkpoint for DNA damage. *Nature.* 404(6773):42–49.

Thomas G. 2011. Are we making progress in curing advanced cervical cancer? *J Clin Oncol.* 29(13):1654–1656.

Uhlin U, Eklund H. 1994. Structure of ribonucleotide reductase protein R1. *Nature.* 345:593–598.

Wang J, Lohman G, Stubbe J. 2009. Mechanism of inactivation of human ribonucleotide reductase with p53R2 by gemcitabine 5′-diphosphate. *Biochemistry* 48(49):11612–11621.

Weinberg G, Ullman D, Martin Jr. D. 1981. Mutator phenotypes in mammalian cell mutants with distinct biochemical defects and abnormal deoxyribonucleoside triphosphate pools. *Proc Natl Acad Sci USA.* 78(4):2447–2451.

Werness B, Levine A, Howley P. 1990. Association of human papillomavirus type 16 and 18 E6 proteins with p53. *Science.* 248(4951):76–79.

Whitney CW, Sause W, Bundy BN, Malfetano JH, Hannigan EV, Fowler WC, Jr. et al. 1999. Randomized comparison of fluorouracil plus cisplatin versus hydroxyurea as an adjunct to radiation therapy in stage IIB-IVA carcinoma of the cervix with negative para-aortic lymph nodes: A Gynecologic Oncology Group and Southwest Oncology Group study. *J Clin Oncol.* 17(5):1339–1348.

Xu H, Fairman J, Wijerathna S, Kreischer N, LaMacchia J, Helmbrecht E et al. 2008. The structural basis for peptidomimetic inhibition of eukaryotic ribonucleotide reductase: A conformationally flexible pharmacophore. *J Med Chem.* 51(15):4653–4659.

Xue L, Zhou B, Liu X, Qiu W, Jin Z, Yen Y. 2003. Wild-type p53 regulates human ribonucleotide reductase by protein-protein interaction with p53R2 as well as hRRM2 subunits. *Cancer Res.* 63(5):980–986.

Section IV

Ovarian Cancer

10

Noninvasive Early Biomarkers in Ovarian Cancer

Sharon A. O'Toole, MSc, PhD, Eugen Ancuta, MSc, MD, PhD, Ream Langhe, MB CHB, MSc, Dolores J. Cahill, PhD, Mairead Murphy, PhD, Cara Martin, MSc, PhD, Lynda McEvoy, PhD, Cathy Spillane, PhD, Orla Sheils, MA, PhD, Emmanuel Petricoin, PhD, Lance Liotta, MD, PhD, and John J. O'Leary, MD, MB, BCh, BAO, BSc, MSc, DPhil

CONTENTS

ABSTRACT One of the major challenges in cancer research is the identification of stable biomarkers, which can be routinely measured noninvasively in easily accessible samples. Ovarian cancer is one such disease that would benefit from improved diagnostic markers.

Ovarian cancer is the leading cause of death from gynecological malignancy in the western world. The vast majority of patients present with advanced-stage disease, and this is due to the lack of a reliable screening test and the absence of symptoms. Improved early detection of ovarian cancer is likely to have substantial effects on overall ovarian cancer survival and quality of life, since the disease demonstrates excellent survival with currently available therapies when diagnosed at an early stage. One way to facilitate early detection of ovarian cancer is through screening, but currently available diagnostic tools, including ovarian cancer biomarkers and clinical imaging, lack sufficient specificity and sensitivity for implementation in a population-based screening program.

This chapter reviews currently available noninvasive biomarkers for the early detection of ovarian cancer and provides an outlook on the potential improvements in these noninvasive diagnostic tools that may lead to improved diagnosis of ovarian cancer. The utility of novel technologies to identify noninvasive biomarkers in ovarian cancer will be discussed, such as microRNA (miRNA) detection, autoantibody (AAb) profiling, and circulating tumor cell (CTC) enumeration.

The ability to sensitively and specifically predict the presence of early disease and its status, stage, and associated therapeutic efficacy has the potential to revolutionize ovarian cancer detection and treatment and to greatly improve the quality of life and survival rates of ovarian cancer patients.

10.1 Introduction: Ovarian Cancer Background

Ovarian cancer is the leading cause of death from gynecological malignancy in the western world. The worldwide distribution of incidence and mortality is depicted in Figures 10.1 and 10.2 (Globocan, 2008; http://globocan.iarc.fr). Ovarian cancer has remained the most challenging of gynecological malignancies for two reasons. First, early-stage disease cannot be detected easily. Second, standard chemotherapy often fails and patients develop chemoresistant disease.

Incidence of disease rises dramatically after onset of menopause. Genetic alterations in the breast cancer susceptibility 1 (*BRCA1*) and 2 (*BRCA2*) genes are associated with an increased lifetime risk for ovarian cancer (Hensley et al., 2002). Ovarian cancer risk tends to be reduced by factors that interrupt ovulation (Sueblinvong and Carney, 2009).

The vast majority of ovarian cancers are epithelial tumors that are then subdivided into a number of histological categories that differ in many respects including epidemiology,

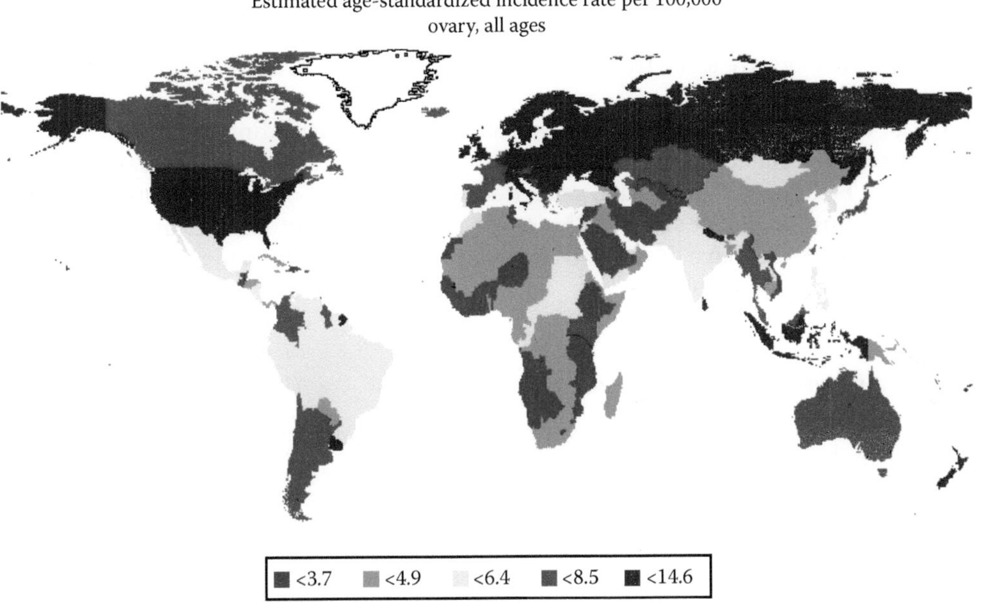

FIGURE 10.1
Estimated age standardized worldwide incidence rate of ovarian cancer. (From Ferlay, J. et al., GLOBOCAN 2008, Cancer Incidence and Mortality Worldwide: IARC CancerBase No. 10 [Internet]. Lyon, France: International Agency for Research on Cancer, 2010.)

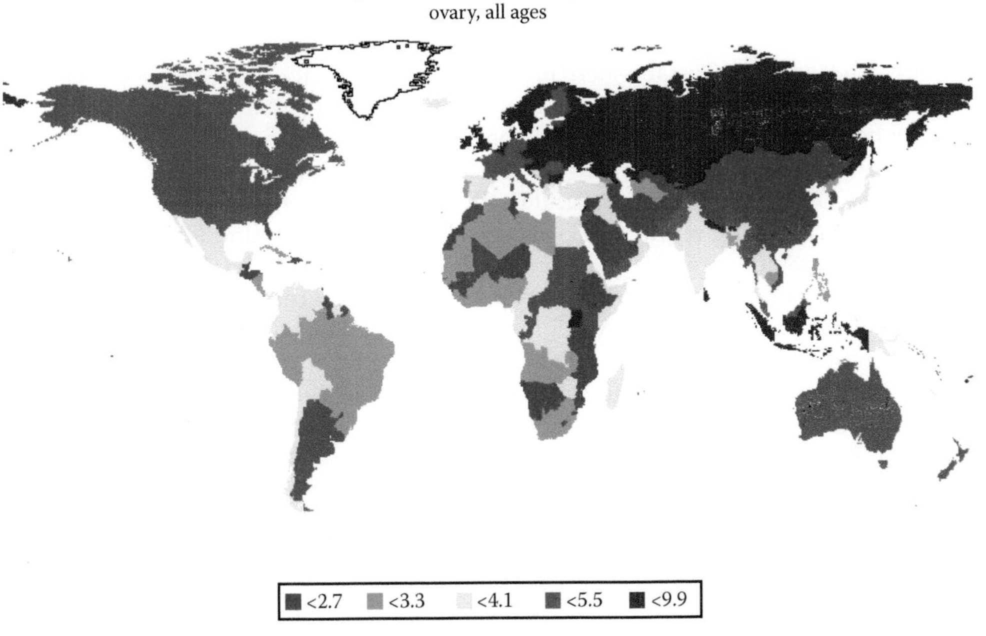

FIGURE 10.2
Estimated age standardized worldwide mortality rate of ovarian cancer. (From Ferlay, J. et al., GLOBOCAN 2008, Cancer Incidence and Mortality Worldwide: IARC CancerBase No. 10 [Internet]. Lyon, France: International Agency for Research on Cancer, 2010.)

genetics, responsiveness to chemotherapy, and expression of tumor markers (Bast et al., 2009). Generally, epithelial ovarian tumors can be categorized into type I and type II (Bell, 2005). Type I tumors are slow growing, while type II tumors are of high grade and rapidly metastasize.

Schorge et al. (2010) describe a number of hypotheses regarding ovarian cancer etiology that can be related to the risk factors identified, for example, incessant ovulation. Generally, it is thought that ovarian cancer occurs as a result of transformation of the surface epithelium (Landen et al., 2008); however, more recent studies of ovarian cancer have postulated that it may have developed in the fallopian tube and metastasized (Crum et al., 2007; Kurman and Shih, 2010).

10.1.1 Symptoms and Treatment of Ovarian Cancer

The symptoms of ovarian cancer are nonspecific and often occur when the disease is already spread throughout the abdominal cavity. Early-stage ovarian cancer has up to a 90% 5-year overall survival rate, whereas late-stage cancers have less than a 30% 5-year survival rate.

The accepted standard of care treatment is debulking surgery and carboplatin/paclitaxel chemotherapy. While many women respond well to chemotherapy, the disease usually recurs and patients develop chemoresistant disease. New targeted biological agents, particularly those involved in antiangiogenesis (e.g., bevacizumab) and those targeting the poly (ADP-ribose) polymerase (PARP) enzyme, hold the most promise for improving the outcome of ovarian cancer.

10.1.2 Current Diagnostic Approaches

Currently, there are no established national ovarian cancer screening programs in place. Current detection strategies include ultrasound (US) and cancer antigen-125 (CA-125); however, both have their drawbacks resulting in the lack of a reliable, sensitive screening test for ovarian cancer. Recently, the Prostate, Lung, Colorectal and Ovarian (PLCO) Cancer Screening Trial in the United States reported no mortality benefit for annual screening with CA-125 and transvaginal ultrasound (TVUS) (Buys et al., 2011). However, results are awaited from the UK Collaborative Trial of Ovarian Cancer Screening (UKCTOCS) (http://www.ukctocs.org.uk/) trial that will be reported in 2014 on the effectiveness of US and CA-125 for screening. The trial uses a calculation called the *risk of ovarian cancer algorithm* (ROCA). Rather than just looking at the results of a single CA-125 test, they look for changes in CA-125 over time to try to predict the woman's risk of having the disease (Menon et al., 2012). In contrast, PLCO used a single cutoff for CA-125.

Other markers used routinely include CA 19-9 (a monosialoganglioside antigen widely used in gastrointestinal adenocarcinoma diagnostics) that is elevated in 68%–83% of mucinous ovarian cancers but in only 28%–29% of nonmucinous types, providing a differential diagnostic tool for nonmucinous versus mucinous subtypes. Serum CA 15-3, CA 72-4, and CEA levels are often measured as they can be elevated in, respectively, 50%–56%, 63%–71%, and 25%–50%, of ovarian cancer patients (Kobayashi et al., 2012). These markers assist in the management of tumors that do not express CA-125 and may assist in distinguishing tumors of non-ovarian origin. Details on the most common currently used noninvasive biomarkers are listed in Table 10.1.

TABLE 10.1

Noninvasive Diagnostic Markers for Ovarian Cancer

Marker	Source	Details	Marker Type	Sensitivity (%)	Specificity (%)	Reference
CA-125	Serum	Cell surface glycoprotein	Protein	89	72	Moss et al. (2005)
HE4 (ROMA)	Serum	HE4 used in conjunction with CA-125	Protein	83 94.3	90 75	Wu et al. (2012) Moore et al. (2010)
OVA1	Serum	CA-125 II, transthyretin (prealbumin), apolipoprotein A1, b2-microglobulin, and transferrin	Protein	93	43	Abraham (2010), Muller (2010)
RMI	Serum, imaging, and menopausal status	US, menopausal status, and CA125	Protein and imaging and menopausal status	71–88 84.6	74–97 75	 Moore et al. (2010)
US	Imaging	Morphologic (grayscale) US	Imaging	88–100	39–87	Webb (2007)
FDG–PET	Imaging		Imaging	92	60	Fenchel et al. (2002)
FDG–PET, MRI, and US	Imaging	Combination of three imaging modalities	Imaging	92	85	Fenchel et al. (2002)

10.2 Invasive and Noninvasive Diagnostic Biomarkers

The National Institutes of Health defines a biomarker as "a characteristic that is objectively measured and evaluated as an indicator of normal biological processes, pathogenic processes, or pharmacologic responses to a therapeutic intervention" (Biomarkers Definitions Working Group, 2001). The ability to diagnose or treat a disease by measuring a biological molecule from a noninvasive source, such as blood or urine, has a significant advantage over traditional pathological techniques because direct access to diseased tissue is not required. Invasive procedures particularly in obtaining ovarian tissue carry significant risk for the patient and also involve a more prolonged hospital visit, specialist consultants, and significantly higher costs.

While bodily fluids are one of the more attractive noninvasive procedures for biomarker discovery, they also have disadvantages in the degree of heterogeneity seen between patients, and as mentioned earlier, there are many ovarian cancer subtypes. Blood is a complex body fluid with fluid and cellular components and this complexity can influence biomarker discovery. The manner in which blood is collected and stored can, for some assay formats, also have an impact on the results. The large dynamic range of proteins in the blood, serum, plasma, or other body fluids can also add to the complexity (Anderson and Anderson, 2002). Imaging is also a popular choice for noninvasive cancer diagnostics, but it has not proven sensitive enough to date; however, the evolution of molecular imaging holds a lot of promise in this area.

10.3 Brief Description on Invasive Biomarkers

Recent research publications about invasive and noninvasive biomarkers for ovarian cancer are widely available, focusing on their role in diagnosis, clinical prognosis, treatment efficacy, and monitoring (Coticchia et al., 2008; Suh et al., 2010). To date, a large panel of putative invasive biomarkers are described in ovarian cancer, the most important being listed in Table 10.2 (Suh et al., 2010).

According to their role in specific diagnosis, ovarian cancer biomarkers can be classified as (1) *stage nonspecific biomarkers* including hK6 and hK7, hepatocyte nuclear factor (HNF)-1β, and Wilms' tumor 1 (WT-1), (2) *early tumor stage* including CBK, and (3) *later tumor stage biomarkers* such as thymidine phosphorylase (TP), chloride intracellular channel 4 (CLIC4), and vascular smooth muscle cell growth-promoting factor (VSGP/F)-spondin (Suh et al., 2010). Moreover, in relation to their prognostic value, candidate invasive biomarkers for ovarian cancer can be subdivided as (a) *favorable-prognostic biomarkers* such as PR, hK11, and 13 and (b) *unfavorable-prognostic biomarkers* consisting of integrins, WT-1, CD24, M-CAM, c-Ets1, β III tubulin, extracellular matrix metalloproteinase inducer (EMMPRIN), granulin–epithelin precursor (GEP), p-glycoprotein, and topoisomerase II (Suh et al., 2010). Several reports on prognostic biomarkers focus on global prognostic value as well as on specific subtypes and different stages of ovarian cancer reflected in survival analysis.

Some of the interesting biomarkers are discussed in more detail later. VSGP/F-spondin is overexpressed in patients with advanced ovarian cancer (Pyle-Chenault et al., 2005) and is implicated in exonal guidance and differentiation of nerve cells (Attur et al., 2009). Its role in disease progression monitoring, treatment efficacy, and prognosis remains uncertain

TABLE 10.2

List of Invasive Biomarkers for Ovarian Cancer Diagnosis and Prognosis

Ovarian Cancer Invasive Biomarkers
Kallikreins: hK6, 7, 11, 13
HNF-1β
WT-1
CKB (creatine kinase, brain)
TP[a]
CLIC4
VSGP/F-spondin
PR (progesterone receptor)
Integrins: $\alpha_5\beta_6$ integrin, α-V integrin
B III tubulin
CD24
C-Ets1
EMMPRIN
GEP
Indoleamine 2,3-dioxygenase
M-CAM
p-glycoprotein
Topoisomerase II
ATP7B

[a] Biomarkers identified in both tissue and serum.

(Suh et al., 2010). TP is used to detect late-stage ovarian cancer; the level and activity significantly correlate with malignant and advanced-stage tumors as well as with high-grade disease (Miszczak-Zaborska et al., 2004). Based on its role in pathological cancer pathways (tumor growth, neoangiogenesis, and metastasis), TP not only has diagnostic value but also has potential as a prognostic and efficacy biomarker (Bronckaers et al., 2009). CLIC4 may have a dual role in the diagnosis and prognosis of advanced-stage ovarian tumors. Increased cellular expression and mislocalization in subcellular compartments are commonly reported (Suh et al., 2007). Kallikreins present with both diagnostic and prognostic function in ovarian cancer and are discussed in more detail later. Although overexpression of hK8, hK11, and hK13 is considered *protective* being associated with better survival and reduced risk of recurrence (Borgoño et al., 2003, 2006; Scorilas et al., 2004; McIntosh et al., 2007), hK6, hK7, and hK10 are well-known indicators of advanced ovarian cancer and progressive disease (Hoffman et al., 2002; Luo et al., 2003; Psyrri et al., 2008). Moreover, a combination of different members of the kallikrein family and other non-kallikrein markers offer prognostic potential in ovarian cancer (Shan et al., 2007). WT-1 is a specific diagnostic and a prognostic invasive biomarker for the serous subtype of ovarian carcinoma (Hwang et al., 2004). HNF-1β expression is upregulated in patients with clear cell ovarian carcinoma as a specific diagnostic marker, being also detected in peritoneal fluid (Tsuchiya et al., 2003; Kato et al., 2007).

The search for novel biomarkers in tissue and ascites material continues using technologies such as whole-genome analysis, transcription profiling, microRNA (miRNA) profiling, and proteomic profiling. The ultimate goal is to translate these biomarkers into early diagnostic markers.

10.4 Noninvasive Biomarkers for Ovarian Cancer Diagnosis

10.4.1 FDA-Approved Biomarkers of Ovarian Cancer

10.4.1.1 CA-125

To date, CA-125 is the most widely used biomarker for ovarian cancer. CA-125 is a cell surface glycoprotein that is encoded by the MUC16 gene. The protein has a single transmembrane domain and provides a protective mucosal barrier against foreign particles and infectious agents on the surface of epithelial cells on the surface of the female reproductive tract (Singh et al., 2008). The CA-125 antigen can be secreted into the circulation following phosphorylation by epidermal growth factor (Verheijen et al., 1999). Its serum levels are elevated in 90% of patients with late-stage ovarian cancer, yet CA-125 levels are only elevated in approximately 50% of early-stage ovarian cancers, thus limiting its use for early diagnosis. An additional limitation of CA-125 is its elevation in a variety of cancers other than ovarian such as pancreatic, breast, and lung cancer and in noncancerous conditions such as endometriosis, fibroids, pelvic inflammatory disease, benign cysts, pregnancy, and liver disease (Nossov et al., 2008). The sensitivity and specificity for CA-125 are 89% and 72%, respectively (Moss et al., 2005); it is raised in approximately only 50% of early-stage epithelial ovarian cancers (EOCs) and in 75%–90% of patients with advanced disease (Moss et al., 2005; Gupta and Lis, 2009). CA-125 screening combined with TVUS increases sensitivity and specificity to 89.4% and 99.8%, respectively (Menon et al., 2009).

10.4.1.2 HE4

Human epididymis protein 4 (HE4) is a low-molecular-weight glycoprotein that is expressed predominantly in epithelial cells of the epididymis and other tissues throughout the body including the breast and the female genital tract (Drapkin et al., 2005; Holcomb et al., 2011). HE4 is encoded by the WFDC2 gene and contains two whey acid proteins and a four-disulfide core made up of eight cysteine residues (Gao et al., 2011). HE4 was initially predicted to be a protease inhibitor involved in the process of sperm maturation (Kirchhoff, 1998; Bingle et al., 2002; Clauss et al., 2005); however, the physiological functions of HE4 have, as yet, not been fully identified. It has been reported to be overexpressed in early and recurrent ovarian, pulmonary, and endometrial cancers, breast adenocarcinomas, and mesotheliomas and less frequently in renal, gastrointestinal, and transitional cell carcinomas (Bingle et al., 2002; Drapkin et al., 2005; Galgano et al., 2006; Anastasi et al., 2010).

10.4.1.2.1 Serum/Plasma HE4

The diagnostic and prognostic potential of serum/plasma HE4 levels has been examined in numerous ovarian cancer studies. HE4 has been detected at high concentrations in the serum of patients with ovarian cancer, particularly women with serous and endometrioid adenocarcinoma, and furthermore, it was found to be increased in more than half of the ovarian cancers, which do not express CA-125 (Drapkin et al., 2005; Bouchard et al., 2006; Moore et al., 2008; Van Gorp et al., 2011; Kalapotharakos et al., 2012). In addition, HE4 is not overexpressed as often in endometriosis or in many benign gynecological diseases (Hellstrom et al., 2003; Moore et al., 2012).

HE4 has been approved by the Food and Drug Administration (FDA) for monitoring recurrence and progression in patients with EOC (Andersen et al., 2010; Montagnana et al., 2011) and more recently as part in the multi-assay algorithm Risk of Ovarian Malignancy Algorithm (ROMA™) to aid the estimate of the risk of malignancy in premenopausal and postmenopausal women presenting with an adnexal mass who will undergo surgical intervention (Moore et al., 2009, 2011). Several studies showed that HE4 could predict the recurrence of the disease earlier than CA-125 (Anastasi et al., 2010; Schummer et al., 2012). In addition, HE4 has been reported recently as a novel biomarker that has the highest sensitivity either alone or in combination with CA-125 for detecting ovarian cancer particularly in the early stages (Moore et al., 2008). Moreover, HE4 was shown to have a higher specificity and comparable sensitivity to CA-125 (HE4 sensitivity 88.9% and specificity 91.8% compared to CA-125 sensitivity 83.3% and specificity 59.5%) for detection of ovarian cancer in premenopausal women with adnexal masses, thus reducing the number of unnecessary surgeries for benign disease (Holcomb et al., 2011).

High preoperative HE4 measurements were found to be associated with advanced-stage disease and poor prognosis in patients with ovarian cancer (Paek et al., 2011; Kalapotharakos et al., 2012; Kong et al., 2012), and HE4 is a marker for aggressiveness of the disease and a predictor of overall survival (Trudel et al., 2012). High levels of preoperative HE4 have been suggested in a retrospective study to be correlated with shorter progression-free survival in multivariate analysis (Paek et al., 2011). Another study found that increasing levels of HE4 before initiating first-line chemotherapy were associated with poor prognosis in EOC (Steffensen et al., 2011). Therefore, serum HE4 may be useful as an independent prognostic marker in patients with ovarian cancer.

A meta-analysis, which reviewed nine studies involving 1807 women, showed that the pooled sensitivity and specificity for HE4 for the diagnosis of ovarian cancer (where the control group was healthy women) were 83% and 90%, respectively. When the control group was made up of women with benign disease, the pooled sensitivity and specificity for HE4 were 74% and 90%, respectively (Wu et al., 2012).

HE4 has also been assessed in a multi-analyte assay, named the Risk of Ovarian Malignancy Algorithm (ROMA™), to predict malignancy and facilitate further management planning in women who present with ovarian masses (Moore et al., 2009, 2011). This assay combines the result of HE4 and CA-125 as well as the menopausal status into a numerical score. ROMA has been validated for the following combinations: HE4 enzyme immunoassay (EIA) + CA-125 EIA, HE4 EIA + CA-125 Architect, HE4 Architect + CA-125 Architect, and HE4 Elecsys + CA-125 Elecsys. At 75% specificity, ROMA has demonstrated 93%–94% sensitivity with a negative predictive value of 93%–98%. ROMA has been shown to be more sensitive (94%) than the risk of malignancy index (RMI) (75%) at 75% specificity (Moore et al., 2011). A recent meta-analysis found that ROMA had a higher sensitivity to predict advanced EOC than early-stage EOC and was more accurate in postmenopausal women compared to premenopausal women (Li et al., 2012). Furthermore, ROMA is less specific, but more sensitive, than HE4, and both ROMA and HE4 are more specific than CA-125 for EOC prediction (Li et al., 2012), but CA-125 had better diagnostic accuracy. ROMA has potential in the clinic in distinguishing EOC from benign pelvic mass (Chan et al., 2012; Li et al., 2012), but further work needs to be done especially in assessing its potential in early-stage disease.

10.4.1.2.2 Urinary HE4

Measuring HE4 in urine can provide a less invasive way of detecting and monitoring ovarian cancer. Hellstrom et al. (2010) detected HE4 in urine at a specificity of 94.4%. The area under the curve (AUC) for early cases was 0.969, while for late cases, the AUC was 0.964 (Hellstrom et al., 2010). In a limited study, this mode of ovarian cancer diagnosis has been investigated as a point-of-care device and shows promising results (Wang et al., 2011).

10.4.1.3 OVA1

OVA1 (Vermillion, Quest Diagnostics) is the first FDA-approved blood test that assists the clinician to determine if an ovarian adnexal mass is malignant or benign prior to planned surgery. The test is FDA approved for women older than 18 years of age with an ovarian adnexal mass for which surgery is planned and who are not yet referred to gynecological oncologists, as an aid to further assess the likelihood that malignancy is present when the physician's independent clinical and radiological evaluation does not indicate malignancy. The test is not approved as a screening or stand-alone diagnostic test. The test measures the levels of five different proteins in patient serum, CA-125-II, transthyretin (prealbumin), apolipoprotein A1, beta-2-microglobulin, and transferrin (ova-1.com). The levels of these proteins are interpreted by proprietary software to determine a single numerical OVA1 score. The software algorithm determines a score based on menopausal status, differentiating patients either into a low- or high-risk group (Rein et al., 2011). The software generates a score between 0 and 10, 0 indicating high probability of a benign growth and 10 indicating high probability of malignancy. This test is used to determine which patients are at highest risk of malignancy and, hence, are most suitable to be referred to a gynecological oncologist. Surgery performed by a gynecological oncologist on malignant ovarian adnexal mass results in improved patient survival compared with surgery performed by less specialized surgeons (Engelen et al., 2006). OVA1 is claimed to have a sensitivity of 92.5% and a specificity of 42.8%, with a positive predictive value (PPV) of 42.3% and a negative predictive value of 92.7% (Muller, 2010). However, OVA1 has not been tested in screening patients for early-stage disease (Rein et al., 2011). There are also limitations to the use of this test due to assay interference as a result of triglyceride levels and rheumatoid factor levels (Muller, 2010).

10.4.2 Proteomics

The discovery of new biomarkers in biofluids such as blood, urine, and saliva can help to develop more sensitive and specific diagnostic and prognostic tests that will permit the early detection and treatment of patients with ovarian cancers, early detection of recurrence, treatment monitoring, and discrimination of benign pelvic masses. Proteomics, together with the innovative high-throughput technologies, might be a highly promising way to identify new biomarkers for both detection and tailoring therapy. Some new recent advances in proteomics combined with upfront sample enrichment nanotechnologies are producing powerful biomarker discovery workflows that are able to detect proteins at ultralow levels of detection (Fredolini et al., 2010). These new proteomic pipelines provide an accelerated opportunity to extend beyond the initial broad-scale profiling efforts that indicated an untapped biomarker archive was present for early-stage ovarian cancer detection (Petricoin et al., 2002). As the proteomic field is rapidly advancing in the technical analytical precision, sensitivity, and accuracy of the tools and platforms used as the engines for biomarker discovery and measurement, significant challenges remain (Liotta and Petricoin, 2012) for facile biomarker discovery efforts. Such impediments include sample processing and biobanking issues, biofluid collection methodologies, lack of biological tie-in of the marker to disease pathophysiology that result in overall slow rates of rigorous validation in large clinical trials. Despite these roadblocks, the field has produced a series of candidate biomarkers that appear to be very promising and that together may represent future panels of assays that could demonstrate the high sensitivity and specificity required for clinical implementation in the ovarian cancer field. Some of the interesting biomarkers in this area are discussed in more detail in the following.

10.4.2.1 Osteopontin

Ye et al. (2006) identified osteopontin fragments in urine as a marker for ovarian cancer. The marker provides an example of the information content of low-molecular-weight proteins/peptides in urine and their posttranslational modifications. Ye et al. collected urine samples preoperatively from postmenopausal women with ovarian cancer and benign conditions, and from nonsurgical controls, these were analyzed by surface-enhanced laser desorption/ionization mass spectrometry and 2D gel electrophoresis. Selected proteins from mass profiles were purified by chromatography and followed by liquid chromatography–tandem mass spectrometry sequence analysis. Specific antibodies were generated for further characterization, including immunoprecipitation and glycosylation. Enzyme-linked immunosorbent assays (ELISAs) were employed for preliminary validation in patients of 128 ovarian cancer, 52 benign conditions, 44 other cancers, and 188 healthy controls. A protein ($m/z \sim 17{,}400$) with higher peak intensities in cancer patients than in benign conditions and controls was identified and subsequently defined as eosinophil-derived neurotoxin (EDN). A glycosylated form of EDN was specifically elevated in ovarian cancer patients. A cluster of COOH-terminal osteopontin was identified from 2D gels of urine from cancer patients. Modified forms of EDN and osteopontin fragments were elevated in early-stage ovarian cancers, and a combination of both resulted to 93% specificity and 72% sensitivity.

Specific elevated posttranslationally modified urinary EDN and osteopontin COOH-terminal fragments in ovarian cancer might lead to potential noninvasive screening tests for early diagnosis. Urine is a promising noninvasive body fluid for measurement novel biomarkers.

10.4.2.2 Kallikreins

Kallikrein-related peptidases are secreted serine proteases that exert stimulatory or inhibitory effects on tumor progression. A recent study by Bandiera et al. (2009) demonstrated that kallikrein-related peptidase 5 (KLK5) is elevated in the serum of patients with ovarian carcinoma. Bandiera et al. examined KLK5 levels and antibody (IgG and IgM) response to KLK5 in the serum of 50 healthy women, 50 patients with benign pelvic masses, 17 patients with ovarian borderline tumors, and 50 patients with ovarian carcinomas, using ELISA. At 95% specificity for healthy controls, 52% of patients with ovarian carcinoma showed high serum KLK5 (sKLK5) levels, whereas patients with benign pathological lesions or borderline tumors showed low or undetectable sKLK5 levels. sKLK5 levels were positively associated with ovarian cancer stage categories (International Federation of Gynecologists and Obstetricians [FIGO]), implying a possible role of sKLK5 in ovarian cancer progression. Elevated levels of KLK5-specific antibodies were noted in 20% of patients with benign masses, 26% of patients with borderline tumors, and 36% of patients with ovarian carcinomas when compared with healthy controls. The authors reported that KLK5 antibodies were also found in patients with undetectable sKLK5 levels. Based on this study, KLK5 is a potential new biomarker that could be used in combination with other biomarkers for ovarian cancer detection. The existence of KLK5 antibodies in ovarian cancer suggests that KLK5 might represent a possible target for immune-based therapies. Kallikreins are a subgroup of serine proteases with diverse physiological functions. The human kallikrein gene family has now been fully characterized and includes 15 members tandemly located on chromosome 19q13.4. Strong experimental evidence supports a link between kallikreins and endocrine malignancies and, especially, ovarian cancer (Yousef and Diamandis, 2002). Three new kallikreins have been shown to be potential diagnostic and prognostic markers for ovarian cancer. Many other kallikreins are also differentially expressed in ovarian cancer, and preliminary reports underline their possible prognostic value. The mechanism by which kallikreins could be involved in ovarian cancer pathology is not known. A likely link could be their regulation through the steroid hormone receptor pathway.

10.4.2.3 Mesothelin

Mesothelin (MSLN) is a 40 kDa glycosylphosphatidylinositol-linked glycoprotein. In normal tissues, the expression of MSLN has subsequently been shown to be largely restricted to mesothelial cells, although immunoreactivity has also been reported in epithelial cells of the trachea, tonsil, fallopian tube, and kidney. MSLN has been shown to be overexpressed in pancreatic carcinomas, gastric carcinoma, and ovarian carcinoma cell lines. MSLN is overexpressed in ovarian cancer tissues with a poor clinical outcome and has been previously identified to activate phosphoinositide 3-kinase (PI3K)/Akt signalling and inhibit paclitaxel-induced apoptosis. Chang et al. (2012) investigated the correlation between MSLN and matrix metalloproteinase (MMP)-7 in the progression of ovarian cancer and the mechanism of MSLN in enhancing ovarian cancer invasion. The expression of MSLN correlated with MMP-7 expression in human ovarian cancer tissues. Overexpressing MSLN or ovarian cancer cells treated with MSLN showed enhanced migration and invasion of cancer cells through the induction of MMP-7. MSLN regulated the expression of MMP-7 through the extracellular-signal-regulated kinase (ERK) 1/2, Akt, and c-Jun N-terminal kinase (JNK) pathways. The expression of MMP-7 and the migrating ability of MSLN-treated ovarian cancer cells were suppressed by ERK1/2- or JNK-specific inhibitors or a decoy AP-1 (activator protein 1) oligonucleotide in in vitro experiments, whereas in vivo animal experiments also demonstrated that mice treated with mitogen-activated protein kinase (MAPK)/ERK- or JNK-specific inhibitors have decreased intratumor MMP-7 expression, delayed tumor growth, and extended the survival of mice. MSLN enhances ovarian cancer invasion by MMP-7 expression through the MAPK/ERK and JNK signal transduction pathways. Blocking the MSLN-related pathway could be a potential strategy for inhibiting the growth of ovarian cancer.

It has been also recently reported (Luborsky et al., 2011) that women with prematurely reduced ovarian function, such as with *ovulatory dysfunction*, *ovarian failure*, and unexplained infertility, have significantly more MSLN antibodies (59%, 44%, and 25%, respectively) compared with a control group. This is in contrast to women with endometriosis who did not have the MSLN antibodies, although they are also at higher risk of ovarian cancer. The results of this study support the suggestion that infertility in women is linked to increased risk of ovarian cancer, which also has similar characteristics in women who have an autoimmune disease of the ovary. The study involved 109 women with infertility, 28 women with ovarian cancer, 24 women with benign ovarian tumors (BOTs) or cysts, and 152 healthy women. Among those categorized as infertile, they were 25 women with the risk of premature ovarian failure, 23 women with endometriosis, 17 women with ovulatory dysfunction, and 44 women with unexplained infertility. Overall, compared with healthy women, the MSLN antigen levels in infertility women and those with ovarian cancer and BOTs or cysts are higher.

10.4.2.4 Matrix Metalloproteinases

Recent reports (Kamat et al., 2006; Zhang et al., 2011) describe that increased expression of MMP-2, MMP-9, and the urokinase-type plasminogen activator (uPA) is associated with progression from benign to advanced ovarian cancer. Proteases have been linked to the malignant phenotype of cancer. Gelatinolytic activity and protein expression of MMP-2 and MMP-9 were analyzed in tissue extracts of 19 cystadenomas and 18 low malignant potential (LMP) tumors, as well as 41 primary tumors of advanced ovarian cancer stage International Federation of Gynecology and Obstetrics IIIc/IV and their corresponding omentum metastases by quantitative gelatin zymography and Western blot. In the same tissue extracts, antigen levels of uPA and its inhibitor PAI-1 were determined by ELISA. Protein expression of pro-MMP-2 (72 kDa) and pro-MMP-9 (92 kDa) and antigen levels of uPA and PAI-1 were low in BOTs but increased significantly from LMP tumors to advanced ovarian cancers. The highest values of all of the proteolytic factors were detected in omentum metastases. Active MMP-2 enzyme (62 kDa) was detected only in ovarian cancer (66%) and corresponding metastases (93%) but never in benign or LMP tumors. The activation rate of MMP-2 to its active isoform was higher in the metastases. Comparing both proteolytic systems, higher PAI-1 concentrations were consistently found in cancers with high pro-MMP-9 expression. These data indicate that members of the plasminogen activator system, as well as the metalloproteinases MMP-2/MMP-9, increase with growing malignant potential of ovarian tumors. Zhang et al. (2011) reported significantly higher serum levels of MMP-9 in malignant ovarian cancer patients compared to benign and normal controls. Elevated MMP-9 correlated with FIGO staging, tumor grade, and peritoneal metastasis. In addition, Laios et al. (2013) have reported a similar finding and have also shown that chemosensitivity can be restored when resistant ovarian cancer cells are treated with an MMP-9 inhibitor. These findings are of particular relevance to the development of protease inhibitors as new therapeutic approaches in ovarian cancer.

10.4.3 Molecular Approaches

Many of the molecular approaches to date including comparative genomic hybridization and transcription profiling have been performed on tumor tissue and are briefly discussed in the previous invasive biomarkers section. However, some molecular approaches have shown promise in the noninvasive diagnosis of ovarian cancer using blood, serum, plasma, urine, and saliva as sources of genetic material.

10.4.3.1 Transcriptome

10.4.3.1.1 Blood

Whole-blood RNA expression profiles offer potential, but it is not possible to discriminate the signature from the blood components versus the tumor cells; unless the CTCs are isolated directly, this is discussed in more detail later. Studies examining whole-blood RNA expression profiles have interrogated genes that are differentially expressed in patients to determine prognosis as opposed to diagnosis but may offer potential in the preoperative setting in relation to tumor biology and optimization of treatment. A signature of genes involved in metastasis, invasion, and inflammation was found to be significantly downregulated in native unstimulated blood leukocytes from ovarian cancer patients with a poor prognosis (Isaksson et al., 2012).

10.4.3.1.2 Saliva

A recent study has examined the potential of using transcriptome analysis of saliva to detect ovarian cancer. A panel of five biomarkers (AGPAT1, B2M, BASP2, IER3, and IL1B) had the potential to discriminate ovarian cancer patients from healthy controls in a study of 56 women with a sensitivity of 85.7% and a specificity of 91.4% (Lee et al., 2012). This approach offers potential and warrants validation in a large trial.

10.4.3.2 microRNAs

miRNAs are endogenous noncoding RNA sequences of about 22 nucleotides (Lagos-Quintana et al., 2001). miRNAs inhibit gene expression by inducing degradation or repressing translation of mRNAs when the nucleotide sequences of miRNAs are entirely or partially complementary to the 3′-untranslated regions (UTR) of targeted mRNAs (Miska, 2005; Esquela-Kerscher and Slack, 2006). Several studies report that miRNAs are aberrantly expressed in human cancer (Calin and Croce, 2006; Esquela-Kerscher and Slack, 2006), which indicate that such miRNAs may function as oncogenes or tumor suppressor genes (Calin et al., 2002; Takamizawa et al., 2004; Chan et al., 2005; He et al., 2005; Iorio et al., 2005; Lu et al., 2005; Zhang et al., 2006). An accumulating body of evidence shows that expression patterns of miRNAs might be beneficial in the diagnosis of cancer and prediction of outcome (Dahiya and Morin, 2010).

miRNAs have been interrogated in many ovarian cancer studies and have demonstrated prognostic capabilities, but many of these studies involved analysis of tumor tissue (Flavin et al., 2008; Merritt et al., 2008). Other studies showed that the deregulated miRNAs seen in ovarian cancer are associated with histological type, tumor stage/grade, BRCA mutated/epigenetically changed, primary or recurrent tumors, and survival (Iorio et al., 2007; Laios et al., 2008; Nam et al., 2008; Zhang et al., 2008; Eitan et al., 2009; Gallagher et al., 2009; Lee et al., 2009; Wyman et al., 2009; van Jaarsveld et al., 2010).

Recent studies have demonstrated that miRNAs are circulating freely in the serum and other body fluids in a highly stable, cell-free form (Chen et al., 2008; Chim et al., 2008; Gilad et al., 2008; Hunter et al., 2008; Lawrie et al., 2008; Mitchell et al., 2008; Taylor and Gercel-Taylor, 2008). In addition, miRNAs have been shown to be released into the circulation from tumor cells (Mitchell et al., 2008). Profiles of miRNAs in serum and plasma were found to be changed in cancer and other diseases compared to normal healthy controls (Chen et al., 2008; Lawrie et al., 2008; Mitchell et al., 2008; Taylor and Gercel-Taylor, 2008). This indicates the feasibility of using miRNAs as novel noninvasive diagnostic and prognostic biomarker. The first study that reported miRNAs in the serum was in 2008 and showed that the serum level of miR-21 was associated with relapse-free survival in patients diagnosed with diffuse large B-cell lymphoma (Lawrie et al., 2008).

The feasibility of profiling miRNAs from the serum of ovarian cancer patients was described in one study (Resnick et al., 2009). In this study, three overexpressed miRNAs were identified as potential oncomirs: miR-21, miR-92, and miR-93, with miR-92 being the most consistent overexpressed miRNA in the serum. High expression levels of miR-93 were associated with shorter progression-free and overall survival in ovarian cancer patients. Furthermore, miR-127, miR-155, and miR-99b were underexpressed in the serum of ovarian cancer patients (Resnick et al., 2009). Interestingly, miR-127 was identified previously as a potent tumor suppressor in ovarian cell lines (Zhang et al., 2008), which supports the underexpression seen in this study.

Overexpressed miRNAs were also identified from tumor-releasing exosomes of patients with ovarian cancer. These structures are endosome-derived organelles that are actively secreted through an exocytosis pathway (Iero et al., 2008). One study showed that the level of circulating tumor-derived exosomes in the serum of women with invasive ovarian cancer was higher than their level in women with benign ovarian disease and normal controls. In addition to that, the level of the exosomes was significantly greater in women with advanced disease. These results suggest that profiling of miRNAs from circulating tumor exosomes could be used as a potential diagnostic marker for screening of asymptomatic women and monitoring of the disease recurrence (Taylor and Gercel-Taylor, 2008).

Profiling of whole-blood miRNAs in ovarian cancer patients was examined in one study; however, the pattern of profiling was not sensitive enough to be used for screening or monitoring of progression of ovarian cancer (Hausler et al., 2010). Profiling of peripheral blood miRNA could be combined with other serum biomarkers such as CA-125 and TVUS to improve the overall screening of ovarian cancer (Hausler et al., 2010).

In addition to miRNAs, small nucleolar RNAs (snoRNA) that guide chemical modifications of other RNAs have received attention recently. Liao et al. (2010) have described how differential expression of snoRNA species may be detected in plasma samples from patients with non-small-cell lung cancer. This approach holds much promise for application in the ovarian cancer field as distinct repertoires of snoRNAs are ascribed to particular ovarian neoplasms.

10.4.4 Metabolomics

In the search for more sensitive and specific biomarkers for cancer, metabolomics has offered great promise as a noninvasive diagnostic method for diagnosis (Griffin and Shockcor, 2004).

10.4.4.1 Blood

In ovarian cancer, Zhang et al. (2012) have used metabolomics to discriminate between EOC and BOT. They confirmed four metabolomic biomarkers (L-tryptophan, LysoPC(18:3), LysoPC(14:0), and 2-piperidinone) as having discriminatory ability. Recently, Chen et al. (2011) developed an ultra-performance liquid chromatographic–tandem mass spectrometry analytical method according to FDA guidance to obtain reproducible, sensitive, and abundant metabolic information for ovarian cancer. 27-Nor-5β-cholestane-3, 7, 12, 24, 25 pentol glucuronide (CPG) was verified as a potential biomarker for EOC. Furthermore, CPG was proven to have an elevated concentration level in ovarian cancer tissues compared with BOT tissues.

10.4.4.2 Urine

Slupsky et al. (2010) have successfully used urine metabolite analysis for detecting early-stage breast and ovarian cancer. They discovered differences in 67 metabolite concentrations measured in urine from a cohort of apparently healthy female subjects compared to subjects with ovarian cancer. The urinary metabolite changes revealed many metabolites decreased in relative concentration with a cancer (both EOC and breast cancer) phenotype when compared with healthy samples.

10.4.5 Autoantibody Profiling

Autoantibody (AAb) profiling of ovarian cancer patient serum to identify biomarkers has received a lot of interest, and recently, a number of studies have interrogated the AAb profile associated with ovarian cancer (Hudson et al., 2007; Gagnon et al., 2008; Taylor et al., 2009; Gnjatic et al., 2010; Murphy et al., 2012a). The method by which the tumor-associated AAb response is generated is an area of increasing interest and has recently been reviewed (Murphy et al., 2012b). There is a known humoral immune response to malignancy (a proposed model of generation is outlined in Figure 10.3). Autoantibodies as biomarker entities have advantages over other markers as they are present in the serum, preventing more invasive biopsy procedures, and the AAb can remain for months and even years. Antibodies are also stable entities with a long half-life ($t½$ = 21 days). A further advantage in terms of bioassay development is that as the serum autoantibodies bind the protein biomarker, even if a panel of different proteins are used in the assay, only one labeled secondary antibody, which detects the Fc region of the primary antibody (e.g., anti-human IgG), is required for detection (Murphy et al., 2012b). In terms of ovarian cancer, histotype, grading, and staging are the most important parameters relating to the AAb profile. The serous papillary histotype has a strong correlation with the presence of p53 AAbs (Murphy et al., 2012a).

The best-characterized autoantigen/AAb relationship is the tumor suppressor protein p53. AAbs to p53 have been identified in the serum of patients with many different cancers (Soussi, 2000) and are also found in approximately 25% of ovarian cancer patients

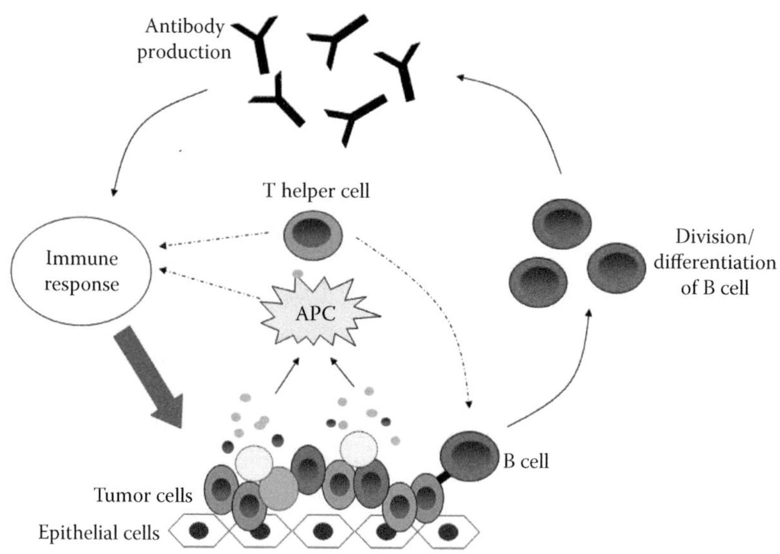

FIGURE 10.3
Model proposing the generation of circulating autoantibodies in cancer patients. At the site of tumor development, tissue damage leads to the release of proteins and cellular debris. The antigen-presenting cells (APCs) then present these proteins to the immune response, ultimately resulting in B-cell proliferation and antibody production.

(Vogl et al., 2000; Li et al., 2008; Murphy et al., 2012a). There is a high association of p53 mutation with type II tumors, meaning that anti-p53 autoantibodies are predominantly associated with high-grade ovarian cancers (Tsai-Turton et al., 2009). Up to 80% of type II tumors exhibit mutated p53; however, it is still unclear, and there is ongoing investigation into why just a subset (20%–40%) of these cases generate anti-p53 antibodies (Piura and Piura, 2009).

AAbs to MSLN have relatively recently been characterized and are being interrogated for their usefulness in the clinic. Some studies have identified AAbs to MSLN to be OC specific (Ho et al., 2005); however, other studies have also identified MSLN AAbs in healthy women (Hellstrom et al., 2008).

AAbs to NY-ESO-1 have been identified in many studies that have interrogated the AAb profile of ovarian cancer patients (Stockert et al., 1998; Odunsi et al., 2003; Milne et al., 2008; Piura and Piura, 2009). Similarly to p53 AAbs, AAbs to NY-ESO-1 have been suggested to be associated with type II tumors (Lu et al., 2011). However, AAbs to NY-ESO-1 have also been identified in other cancers, such as melanoma (Stockert et al., 1998) and breast cancer (Piura and Piura, 2010).

AAbs to HSP-90 have been implicated in the pathogenesis of autoimmune diseases (Faulds et al., 1995; Hayem et al., 1999) and also in malignancies such as osteocarcinoma (Trieb et al., 2000) and ovarian cancer (Vidal et al., 2004). Vidal et al. (2004) have postulated that AAbs to HSP 90 are tumor associated and stage specific. Anti-HSP 90 autoantibodies of the IgA class have also been linked to ovarian cancer (Korneeva et al., 2000).

AAbs to survivin have also been identified in two studies of ovarian cancer patient sera; however, these antibodies are not specific to OC (Taylor et al., 2009). AAbs to survivin are not specific to ovarian cancer; however, they may be of use in an AAb biomarker panel, perhaps in ovarian cancer staging.

Although AAbs identify a great hope for cancer diagnosis, including early diagnosis, for example, the EarlyCDT-Lung™, a test offered by Oncimmune (USA), may aid in the early detection of lung cancer in high-risk populations (Chapman et al., 2012). However, AAb diagnostic tests for cancers, including ovarian, have yet to be fully translated in the clinic/materialize in the hands of clinicians.

10.4.6 Circulating DNA and Epigenetic Changes

Cell-free tumor DNA can exist in the circulation of a patient with cancer that can carry information on mutations and tumor burden. Individual mutations have been assessed, but recently, a method for tagged-amplicon deep sequencing (TAm-Seq) has been developed and used to identify mutations in ovarian cancer patients. Mutations were identified in *TP53* in circulating DNA from 46 plasma samples of advanced ovarian cancer patients. This low-cost, high-throughput method offers potential for future diagnostics and personalized medicine approaches (Forshew et al., 2012).

As sequencing technologies develop, this area will become a hot topic for the future. Shotgun DNA sequencing has also shown promise in the area of ovarian cancer diagnostics (Chan et al., 2013) by obtaining a noninvasive, genome-wide view of cancer-associated copy number variations and mutations in DNA in plasma. These technologies require further validation, and while costly at present, sequencing costs continue to fall as the technology develops.

Various epigenetic changes including CpG island methylation and histone modification have been identified in ovarian cancer. These aberrations are associated with distinct disease subtypes and may be both present and detectable in circulating serum of ovarian cancer patients. Several epigenetic changes have shown promise for their diagnostic, prognostic, and predictive capacity but still need further validation (Seeber and van Diest, 2012).

10.4.7 Circulating Tumor Cells

Hematogenous dissemination of tumor cells, referred to as CTCs, from a primary tumor, is a necessary step for the establishment of metastases at secondary sites in the body. CTCs circulate in the peripheral blood of cancer patients and are extremely rare in healthy people; thus, their detection and isolation can provide significant clinical insight into disease diagnosis and prognosis. Indeed, CTCs have been demonstrated to be of predictive and prognostic value among patients with prostate, breast, and colorectal cancer (Allard et al., 2004; Cristofanilli et al., 2004; Paterlini-Brechot and Benali, 2007; de Bono et al., 2008). These findings have led to speculation that CTCs may hold potential as novel diagnostic and prognostic biomarkers for other solid tumors, including ovarian cancer.

While distant metastasis is a late complication of ovarian cancer and historically ovarian cancer was thought to spread primarily by direct extension into the abdominal cavity, multiple studies have established the presence of tumorlike epithelial cells in the peripheral blood of ovarian cancer patients (Marth et al., 2002; Judson et al., 2003; Wimberger et al., 2007; Fan et al., 2009; Aktas et al., 2011; Poveda et al., 2011; Obermayr et al., 2013). However, although there is a strong consensus in the literature that CTCs are present in a subset of women with ovarian malignancy, no clear consensus has been reached on the clinical relevance of these CTCs. Initial studies seemed to indicate that there was no prognostic value in the detection of CTCs in the peripheral blood of ovarian cancer patients (Marth et al., 2002; Judson et al., 2003; Wimberger et al., 2007). However, more recent studies have

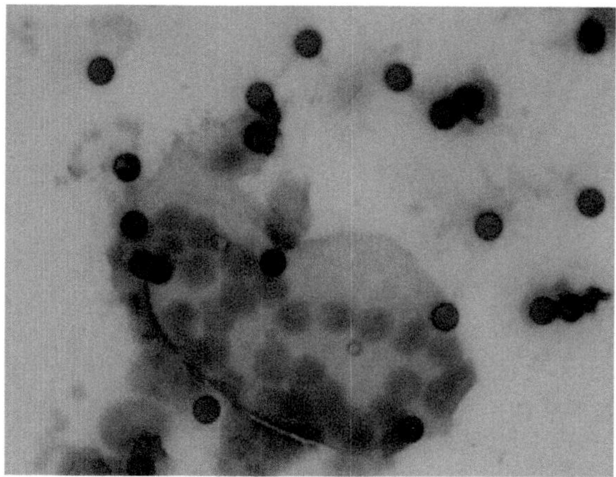

FIGURE 10.4
Capture of CTCs from an ovarian cancer patient using the ScreenCell device.

suggested that CTC positivity (Fan et al., 2009; Aktas et al., 2011) or elevated levels of CTCs (Poveda et al., 2011) can significantly correlate with disease-free survival. The discrepancies observed within the literature are probably due to differing study design, study population, sample size, and follow-up periods.

In addition to a growing body of evidence of the prognostic utility of CTCs in ovarian malignancies, a recent study by Obermayr et al. (2013) demonstrated the potential of CTCs to inform treatment regimes. This study described a novel panel of ovarian CTC markers, which were used to interrogate the peripheral blood of ovarian cancer patient for the presence of CTCs. Overall in this study, CTCs were detected in 24.5% of baseline samples and 20.4% of follow-up samples; of the 68 CTC positive samples, 69% were identified by the overexpression of cyclophilin C (PPIC). Moreover, the detection of PPIC-positive CTCs in patients 6 months after completion of adjuvant chemotherapy was observed to be significantly overrepresented in platinum-resistant patients and also predicative of poor outcome. This demonstrates that enumeration and characterization of CTCs may offer an improved method for early detection of aggressive disease coupled with assessment of treatment efficacy and/or information on treatment regime.

Several technologies have been used for isolation of CTCs from patients (Yu et al., 2011), and one promising technology is the ScreenCell device (Desitter et al., 2011) that is a simple and innovative noninvasive technology for isolating circulating rare cells from whole blood. It provides easy access to fixed or live CTCs and circulating tumor microemboli, allowing a full range access to phenotypical, genotypical, and functional characterization of these cells. An example of CTCs isolated from an ovarian cancer patient with this device is shown in Figure 10.4.

10.5 Imaging

Imaging plays an integral role in the diagnosis and management of ovarian cancer patients; examples of imaging technologies are displayed in Figure 10.5. Ovarian masses or cysts are commonly detected by noninvasive imaging in patients with pelvic symptoms

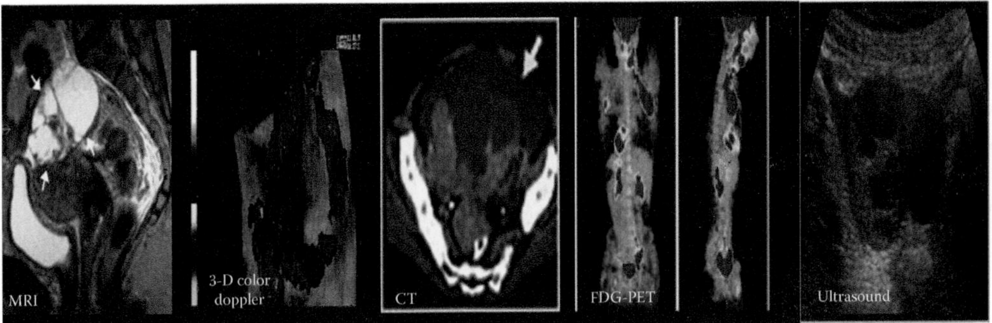

FIGURE 10.5
Different imaging methodologies used in ovarian cancer diagnosis and monitoring: MRI, 3D color Doppler, CT, FDG–PET, and US. The arrows in CT and MRI point to presumed tumor. The color Doppler shows blood flow, red for arterial and blue for venous. In the FDG–PET image, the red is activity; presumed tumor. The US shows what appears to be a normal right ovary and queries pelvic fluid/mass on the left.

or in patients being screened for ovarian cancer. The majority of these masses are benign, particularly in premenopausal women. Thin-walled, unilocular, cystic structures smaller than 5 cm in diameter are likely to be benign and can be followed with imaging. However, cysts may be very complex in appearance, and differentiation from ovarian malignancy may not be possible using standard imaging techniques alone, resulting in patients undergoing surgical exploration. The mainstay of ovarian imaging is grayscale TVUS. Structural features of ovarian cysts (size, septae, and solid projections) may be correlated with likelihood of malignancy. The presence of ascites or peritoneal nodules is also suggestive of malignancy. While there are many benefits to US, the main limitations include cost and difficulty in tracking progression and location of the tumor, given that it is felt the majority of ovarian cancers spread rapidly (Rein et al., 2011). TVS augmented by color Doppler mapping of vessel distribution has recently been shown to improve the detection of adnexal malignancies when compared to grayscale imaging (Guerriero et al., 2002). Computed axial tomography (CAT) is of limited value in assessing ovarian masses but will detect metastatic disease. It is most widely used for disease staging, selection of patients for cytoreductive surgery, assessment of treatment response, and the detection of recurrence. Preoperative computed tomography (CT) is also important in identifying unusual disease patterns that may suggest non-ovarian origin. Magnetic resonance imaging (MRI) provides structural information (Okamoto et al., 2007) and is of value in further characterizing masses that are indeterminate on US or where clinical circumstances dictate. Evaluating different MRI sequences allows recognition of blood products, fat, and fibrous tissues and, therefore, enables accurate diagnosis of benign lesions such as endometriomas, ovarian dermoids, and fibromas that can appear complex on US. MRI has been shown to be as accurate as CT in the evaluation of disease extent in advanced ovarian cancer (Tempany et al., 2000); however, it is not widely used as a staging tool due to its expense and limited availability. ^{18}Fluorodeoxyglucose–positron-emission tomography (FDG–PET) scanning has emerged as a useful technique in the management of ovarian tumors (Picchio et al., 2003; Yoshida et al., 2004). FDG–PET does not play a significant additional role in diagnosis; however, the role of combined PET/CT modality has recently begun to be reexplored for initial disease staging, particularly because PET/CT scans pick up small unsuspected lesions and, thereby, provide a better disease assessment of the whole body in a single examination. Castellucci et al. (2007) have shown that the PPV (100%) and accuracy (92%) of FDG–PET imaging for malignant ovarian disease were higher than the PPV (80%) and accuracy (80%)

of TVUS. Fenchel et al. (2002) evaluated the utility of FDG–PET in the characterization of asymptomatic adnexal masses in a series of 101 preoperative patients and showed a sensitivity of 58% and specificity of 76%. This was compared with MRI and US, and the overall sensitivities and specificities are outlined in Table 10.1. When FDG–PET is analyzed jointly with US and MRI findings, the three modalities had a sensitivity of 92% and specificity of 85%. However, this is similar to using US and MRI together, and there is no reported advantage in adding FDG–PET for characterization of adnexal lesions.

10.6 Genetic Testing and Ethnic Group Markers for Ovarian Cancer

As previously alluded, mutations in the *BRCA1* and *BRCA2* genes are associated with an increased lifetime risk for the development of ovarian cancer (Hensley et al., 2002). These mutations are present in about 10%–15% of ovarian cancer patients. Ovarian cancer risk differs by gene, with *BRCA1* associated with a 36%–63% lifetime risk and *BRCA2* mutation carriers having a 10%–27% lifetime risk (Anglian Breast Cancer Study Group, 2000; Chen and Parmigiani, 2007). Prophylactic salpingo-oophorectomy significantly reduces cancer risk and mortality in these women (Rebbeck et al., 2002; Domchek et al., 2006).

People of Ashkenazi Jewish heritage are more likely to harbor mutations in the *BRCA* genes than the general population. Three common mutations have been identified in Ashkenazi Jewish *BRCA1/2* mutation carriers: c.68_69delAG (185delAG or 187delAG) and c.5266dupC (5382insC or 5385insC) in *BRCA1* and c.5946delT (6174delT) in *BRCA2* (Struewing et al., 1995; Neuhausen et al., 1996; Oddoux et al., 1996). The high frequency of these mutations has led to the development of panel testing for the three common Jewish mutations.

10.7 Innovative Technologies in Ovarian Cancer Diagnosis

The development of point-of-care devices that have revolutionized the medical world has also entered the field of ovarian cancer diagnosis with point-of-care devices being developed for CA-125 (Raamanathan et al., 2012; Wang et al., 2012) and HE4 (Wang et al., 2011). Technologies range from bio-nano-chip systems to 3D electrochemical devices to microchip ELISA-based detection modules that employ a portable detection system, that is, a cell phone/charge-coupled device. Such technologies have the potential to influence survival outcome from ovarian cancer by allowing access to rapid, low-cost screening tools. In addition, the ability to multiplex and perform highly sensitive assays is crucial for future validation of biomarker panels, and many of these emerging technologies offer this potential.

10.8 Recommended Tests/Panels in Combination with/without Imaging for Early Diagnosis

Any test panel or algorithm for ovarian cancer diagnosis involves CA-125 and has been developed to increase the accuracy of CA-125. The RMI uses US, menopausal status, and CA-125 and has been utilized in the United Kingdom for two decades, providing sensitivity that has ranged from 71% to 88% and specificity from 74% to 97% for identifying patients with malignant disease. The ROMA has been used in combination with CA-125 to increase sensitivity. Although not routinely used in the clinic, ROMA has recently been approved by the FDA for ovarian cancer diagnosis in patients presenting with a pelvic mass. This algorithm combines serum levels of CA-125 and HE4 along with menopausal status in a logistic regression model to identify a patient as low risk or high risk for having ovarian carcinoma. The OVA1 panel described earlier also utilizes CA-125. CA-125 screening combined with TVU increases sensitivity and specificity to 89.4% and 99.8%, respectively (Menon et al., 2009). The UKCTOCS trial uses a calculation called the *ROCA*. Rather than just looking at the results of a single CA-125 test, they look for changes in CA-125 over time, to try to predict the woman's risk of having the disease. This is used in conjunction with US and takes into account age-specific risk. Results are awaited from this trial that will be reported in 2014.

10.9 Advantages and Challenges in Developing Molecular Biomarkers for Early Detection

The advantages of developing early detection markers for ovarian cancer are clear from the statistics, as diagnosis when the disease is confined to the ovary (stage I) can result in greater than 90% cure (Engel et al., 2002). As mentioned earlier, the challenges in achieving this are numerous, as early-stage disease may have no symptoms or nonspecific symptoms, which is why ovarian cancer is often referred to as the *silent killer*. Early-stage diagnosis that accounts for about 25% of cases is often an incidental finding and often is identified when the patient is undergoing routine examination or being investigated for a nongynecological condition. In addition, effective screening tools are currently not available, in particular for early-stage disease. Owing to the rather low incidence of the disease in the general population, potential screening tests must provide very high specificity to avoid unnecessary interventions in false-positive cases (Bast, 2003). Another major challenge for researchers in this area is the lack of availability of blood samples from early-stage cancer patients which is necessary for the validation of any potential early diagnostic marker. Biobanks from the ovarian cancer and other cancer screening trials have assisted in overcoming this challenge, but such samples may be limited, may not have ethical approval to be used in other studies, and are very precious indicating the need for well-curated biobanks on an international scale.

10.10 Market Players in Ovarian Cancer

The past year has seen major changes in the global ovarian cancer therapeutics market that is expected to achieve threefold growth by 2020, reaching $2352 m (http://www.reportlinker.com/p0843058-summary/Ovarian-Cancer-Therapeutics-Global-Drug-Forecasts-and-Treatment-Analysis.html [February 2012]). This high growth rate is expected due to the strength of the pipeline candidates, which are anticipated to change the treatment paradigm of ovarian cancer when launched. Bevacizumab (Avastin), a VEGF inhibitor, is leading the way in new biological drugs for ovarian cancer, and ongoing randomized trials will help identify which patients should receive bevacizumab in first-line rather than in the relapsed setting, the optimal duration of bevacizumab therapy, and how it should be combined with alternative treatment strategies. The major players in the therapeutic market include F. Hoffmann-La Roche Ltd., GlaxoSmithKline plc, Amgen Inc., AstraZeneca PLC, and Boehringer Ingelheim GmbH. The key classes of mechanism of action include microtubule stabilizers, vascular endothelial growth factor receptor (VEGFR) inhibitors, immunomodulators, folate receptor inhibitors, PARP inhibitors, topoisomerase inhibitors, interleukins, mammalian target of rapamycin (mTOR) inhibitors, and PI3K inhibitors.

The diagnostic arena has also seen some advances; Vermillion Inc., a molecular diagnostics company, developed OVA1, with support from Quest Diagnostics. OVA1 is only available through Quest Diagnostics. Abbott, Fujirebio, and F. Hoffmann La Roche Ltd., all play

TABLE 10.3

Summary of Patents Granted for Ovarian Cancer Diagnosis from 2011 to 2012

Patent No	Title	Date	Marker	Technology
US8187889	Protein markers for the diagnosis and prognosis of ovarian and breast cancer	May 29, 2012	Truncated forms of cytosolic serine hydroxymethyl transferase (cSHMT), T-box transcription factor 3 (Tbx3) and utrophin	2D gel electrophoresis and MALDI TOF mass spectrometry
US8088390	Methods for the early diagnosis of ovarian cancer	January 3, 2012	Stratum corneum chymotryptic enzyme	mRNA (tissue)
US 8030060	Gene signature for diagnosis and prognosis of breast cancer and ovarian cancer	October 4, 2011	28 gene signature for prognosis in ovarian cancer	mRNA (tissue)
US 7985843	Compositions and methods for the therapy and diagnosis of ovarian cancer	July 26, 2011	Antibody- or antigen-binding fragment	Immunoassay
US 7935531	Methods for the early diagnosis of ovarian cancer	May 3, 2011	Hepsin protease	PCR (tissue)
US 792818	Antigen polypeptide for the diagnosis and/or treatment of ovarian cancer	April 19, 2011	OVTA	ELISA
US 7906635	Nucleotide and amino acid sequences and assays and methods of use thereof for diagnosis of ovarian cancer	March 15, 2011	Novel nucleotide and amino acid sequences	Sequencing
US 7795211	Methods for the early diagnosis of ovarian cancer	September 14, 2010	Hepsin	PCR (tissue)
US 7785841	Methods for the early diagnosis of ovarian cancer	August 31, 2010	PUMP-1 protease (matrix metalloprotease 7)	PCR and immunohistochemistry (tissue)

major roles in ovarian cancer diagnostics, and with FDA approval for HE4 and ROMA, this area will grow in the future. Molecular diagnostics is a rapidly advancing area of research and medicine, with new technologies and applications being continually added that will transform the ovarian cancer diagnostic and therapeutic markets in the years ahead.

10.11 Patents for Ovarian Cancer Diagnosis

A patent search on http://www.patentlens.net/for ovarian cancer diagnosis reveals 192 entries, either granted or applied for. These vary in technology with some of the recent patents focusing on miRNA profiles and proteomics. Others focus on combined panels for breast and ovarian cancer and consist of mRNA gene signature profiles. Many of the patents contain work performed on tissue specimens, so these may not be suitable for non-invasive diagnosis. A list of granted patents from 2010 to 2012 is given in Table 10.3.

10.12 Concluding Remarks and Future Perspective

While the future looks bright for ovarian cancer treatment with the introduction of new drugs, the diagnosis of ovarian cancer clearly needs more research to identify novel epidemiologic, genetic, or blood-based markers of ovarian cancer risk. A combination of improved imaging techniques, potentially incorporating molecular markers, may improve diagnostic capability. As ovarian cancer is quite a heterogenous disease, it is likely that one single biomarker will not be sufficient for diagnosis, but a panel of biomarkers may be more appropriate. In the emerging era of personalized medicine, these biomarkers may also be useful in determining the most suitable treatment for ovarian cancer patients. As regards screening, the medical and scientific field awaits the results of the UKCTOCS trial that are due in 2014. This will determine if screening for ovarian cancer using US and CA125 can improve the overall mortality from this disease. In conclusion, research must continue to develop a reliable and sensitive diagnostic test for ovarian cancer.

This review was inspired by research gratefully funded by the Ovarian Cancer Charity, the Emer Casey Foundation (www.emercaseyfoundation.com).

References

Abraham, J. 2010. OVA1 test for preoperative assessment of ovarian cancer. *Community Translations* 7:249–250.

Aktas, B. Kasimir-Bauer, S. Heubner, M. Kimmig, R. Wimberger, P. 2011. Molecular profiling and prognostic relevance of circulating tumor cells in the blood of ovarian cancer patients at primary diagnosis and after platinum-based chemotherapy. *International Journal of Gynecological Cancer* 21:822–830.

Allard, WJ. Matera, J. Miller, MC. Repollet, M. Connelly, MC. Rao, C. Tibbe, AG. Uhr, JW. Terstappen, LW. 2004. Tumor cells circulate in the peripheral blood of all major carcinomas but not in healthy subjects or patients with non-malignant diseases. *Clinical Cancer Research* 10:6897–6904.

Anastasi, E. Marchei, GG. Viggiani, V. Gennarini, G. Frati, L. Reale, MG. 2010. HE4: A new potential early biomarker for the recurrence of ovarian cancer. *Tumour Biology* 31:113–119.

Andersen, MR. Goff, BA. Lowe, KA. Scholler, N. Bergan, L. Drescher, CW. Paley, P. Urban, N. 2010. Use of a symptom index, CA125, and HE4 to predict ovarian cancer. *Gynecologic Oncology* 116:378–383.

Anderson, NL. Anderson, NG. 2002. The human plasma proteome: History, character, and diagnostic prospects. *Molecular Cell Proteomics* 1:845–867.

Anglian Breast Cancer Study Group. 2000. Prevalence and penetrance of BRCA1 and BRCA2 mutations in a population-based series of breast cancer cases. *British Journal of Cancer* 83:1301–1308.

Attur, MG. Palmer, GD. Al-Mussawir, HE. Dave, M. Teixeira, CC. Rifkin, DB. Appleton, CT. Beier, F. Abramson, SB. 2009. F-spondin, a neuroregulatory protein, is up-regulated in osteoarthritis and regulates cartilage metabolism via TGF-beta activation. *FASEB Journal* 23:79–89.

Bandiera, E. Zanotti, L. Bignotti, E. Romani, C. Tassi, R. Todeschini, P. Tognon, G. et al. 2009. Human kallikrein 5: An interesting novel biomarker in ovarian cancer patients that elicits humoral response. *International Journal of Gynecological Cancer* 19:1015–1021.

Bast, RC Jr. 2003. Status of tumor markers in ovarian cancer screening. *Journal of Clinical Oncology* 21:200s–205s.

Bast, RC Jr. Hennessy, B. Mills, GB. 2009. The biology of ovarian cancer: New opportunities for translation. *Nature Reviews Cancer* 9:415–428.

Bell, DA. 2005. Origins and molecular pathology of ovarian cancer. *Modern Pathology* 18 Suppl 2:S19–S32.

Bingle, L. Singleton, V. Bingle, CD. 2002. The putative ovarian tumour marker gene HE4 (WFDC2) is expressed in normal tissues and undergoes complex alternative splicing to yield multiple protein isoforms. *Oncogene* 21:2768–2773.

Biomarkers Definitions Working Group. 2001. Biomarkers and surrogate endpoints: Preferred definitions and conceptual framework. *Clinical Pharmacology and Therapeutics* 69:89–95.

Borgoño, CA. Fracchioli, S. Yousef, GM. Rigault de la Longrais, IA. Luo, LY. Soosaipillai, A. Puopolo, M. et al. 2003. Favorable prognostic value of tissue human kallikrein 11 (hK11) in patients with ovarian carcinoma. *International Journal of Cancer* 106:605–610.

Borgoño, CA. Kishi, T. Scorilas, A. Harbeck, N. Dorn, J. Schmalfeldt, B. Schmitt, M. Diamandis, EP. 2006. Human kallikrein 8 protein is a favorable prognostic marker in ovarian cancer. *Clinical Cancer Research* 12:1487–1493.

Bouchard, D. Morisset, D. Bourbonnais, Y. Tremblay, GM. 2006. Proteins with whey-acidic-protein motifs and cancer. *The Lancet Oncology* 7:167–174.

Bronckaers, A. Gago, F. Balzarini, J. Liekens, S. 2009. The dual role of thymidine phosphorylase in cancer development and chemotherapy. *Medicinal Research Reviews* 29:903–953.

Buys, SS. Partridge, E. Black, A. Johnson, CC. Lamerato, L. Isaacs, C. Reding, DJ. et al. 2011. Effect of screening on ovarian cancer mortality: The Prostate, Lung, Colorectal and Ovarian (PLCO) Cancer Screening Randomized Controlled Trial. *JAMA* 305:2295–2303.

Calin, GA. Croce, CM. 2006. MicroRNA signatures in human cancers. *Nature Reviews Cancer* 6:857–866.

Calin, GA. Dumitru, CD. Shimizu, M. Bichi, R. Zupo, S. Noch, E. Aldler, H. et al. 2002. Frequent deletions and down-regulation of micro- RNA genes miR15 and miR16 at 13q14 in chronic lymphocytic leukemia. *Proceedings of the Academy of Sciences of the United States of America* 99:15524–15529.

Castellucci, P. Perrone, AM. Picchio, M. Ghi, T. Farsad, M. Nanni, C. Messa, C. et al. 2007. Diagnostic accuracy of 18F-FDG PET/CT in characterizing ovarian lesions and staging ovarian cancer: Correlation with transvaginal ultrasonography, computed tomography, and histology. *Nuclear Medicine Communications* 28:589–595.

Chan, JA. Krichevsky, AM. Kosik, KS. 2005. MicroRNA-21 is an antiapoptotic factor in human glioblastoma cells. *Cancer Research* 65:6029–6033.

Chan, KC. Jiang, P. Zheng, YW. Liao, GJ. Sun, H. Wong, J. Siu, SS. et al. 2013. Cancer genome scanning in plasma: Detection of tumor-associated copy number aberrations, single-nucleotide variants, and tumoral heterogeneity by massively parallel sequencing. *Clinical Chemistry* 59:211–224.

Chan, KK. Chen, CA. Nam, JH. Ochiai, K. Wilailak, S. Choon, AT. Sabaratnam, S. et al. 2012. The use of HE4 in the prediction of ovarian cancer in Asian women with a pelvic mass. *Gynecologic Oncology* (In Press) doi 10.1016/j.ygyno.2012.09.034.

Chang, MC. Chen, CA. Chen, PJ. Chiang, YC. Chen, YL. Mao, TL. Lin, HW. Lin Chiang, WH. Cheng, WF. 2012. Mesothelin enhances invasion of ovarian cancer by inducing MMP-7 through MAPK/ERK and JNK pathways. *Biochemical Journal* 442:293–302.

Chapman, CJ. Healey, GF. Murray, A. Boyle, P. Robertson, C. Peek, LJ. Allen, J. et al. 2012. EarlyCDT®-Lung test: Improved clinical utility through additional autoantibody assays. *Tumour Biology* 33:1319–1326.

Chen, J. Zhang, X. Cao, R. Lu, X. Zhao, S. Fekete, A. Huang, Q. et al. 2011. Serum 27-nor-5β-cholestane-3,7,12,24,25 pentol glucuronide discovered by metabolomics as potential diagnostic biomarker for epithelium ovarian cancer. *Journal of Proteome Research* 10:2625–2632.

Chen, S. Parmigiani, G. 2007. Meta-analysis of BRCA1 and BRCA2 penetrance. *Journal of Clinical Oncology* 25:1329–1333.

Chen, X. Ba, Y. Ma, L. Cai, X. Yin, Y. Wang, K. Guo, J. et al. 2008. Characterization of microRNAs in serum: A novel class of biomarkers for diagnosis of cancer and other diseases. *Cell Research* 18:997–1006.

Chim, SS. Shing, TK. Hung, EC. Leung, TY. Lau, TK. Chiu, RW. Lo, YM. 2008. Detection and characterization of placental microRNAs in maternal plasma. *Clinical Chemistry* 54:482–490.

Clauss, A. Lilja, H. Lundwall, A. 2005. The evolution of a genetic locus encoding small serine proteinase inhibitors. *Biochemical and Biophysical Research Communications* 333:383–389.

Coticchia, CM. Yang, J. Moses, MA. 2008. Ovarian cancer biomarkers: Current options and future promise. *Journal of the National Comprehensive Cancer Network* 6:795–802.

Cristofanilli, M. Budd, GT. Ellis, MJ. Stopeck, A. Matera, J. Miller, MC. Reuben, JM. et al. 2004. Circulating tumor cells, disease progression, and survival in metastatic breast cancer. *The New England Journal of Medicine* 351:781–791.

Crum, CP. Drapkin, R. Miron, A. Ince, TA. Muto, M. Kindelberger, DW. Lee, Y. 2007. The distal fallopian tube: A new model for pelvic serous carcinogenesis. *Current Opinion in Obstetrics & Gynecology* 19:3–9.

Dahiya, N. Morin, PJ. 2010. MicroRNAs in ovarian carcinomas. *Endocrine-Related Cancer* 17:F77–F89.

de Bono, JS. Scher, HI. Montgomery, RB. Parker, C. Miller, MC. Tissing, H. Doyle, GV. Terstappen, LW. Pienta, KJ. Raghavan, D. 2008. Circulating tumor cells predict survival benefit from treatment in metastatic castration-resistant prostate cancer. *Clinical Cancer Research* 14:6302–6309.

Desitter, I. Guerrouahen, BS. Benali-Furet, N. Wechsler, J. Jänne, PA. Kuang, Y. Yanagita, M. et al. 2011. A new device for rapid isolation by size and characterization of rare circulating tumor cells. *Anticancer Research* 31:427–441.

Domchek, SM. Friebel, TM. Neuhausen, SL. Wagner, T. Evans, G. Isaacs, C. Garber, JE. et al. 2006. Mortality after bilateral salpingo-oophorectomy in BRCA1 and BRCA2 mutation carriers: A prospective cohort study. *The Lancet Oncology* 7:223–229.

Drapkin, R. von Horsten, HH. Lin, Y. Mok, SC. Crum, CP. Welsh, WR. Hecht, JL. 2005. Human epididymis protein 4 (HE4) is a secreted glycoprotein that is overexpressed by serous and endometrioid ovarian carcinomas. *Cancer Research* 65:2162–2169.

Eitan, R. Kushnir, M. Lithwick-Yanai, G. David, MB. Hoshen, M. Glezerman, M. Hod, M. Sabah, G. Rosenwald, S. Levavi, H. 2009. Tumor microRNA expression patterns associated with resistance to platinum based chemotherapy and survival in ovarian cancer patients. *Gynecologic Oncology* 114:253–259.

Engel, J. Eckel, R. Schubert-Fritschle, G. Kerr, J. Kuhn, W. Diebold, J. Kimmig, R. Rehbock, J. Hölzel, D. 2002. Moderate progress for ovarian cancer in the last 20 years: Prolongation of survival, but no improvement in the cure rate. *European Journal of Cancer* 38:2435–2445.

Engelen, MJ. Kos, HE. Willemse, PH. Aalders, JG. de Vries, EG. Schaapveld, M. Otter, R. van der Zee, AG. 2006. Surgery by consultant gynecologic oncologists improves survival in patients with ovarian carcinoma. *Cancer* 106:589–598.

Esquela-Kerscher, A. Slack, FJ. 2006. Oncomirs—microRNAs with a role in cancer. *Nature Reviews. Cancer* 6:259–269.

Fan, T. Zhao, Q. Chen, JJ. Chen, WT. Pearl, ML. 2009. Clinical significance of circulating tumor cells detected by an invasion assay in peripheral blood of patients with ovarian cancer. *Gynecologic Oncology* 112:185–191.

Faulds, G. Conroy, S. Madaio, M. Isenberg, D. Latchman, D. 1995. Increased levels of antibodies to heat shock proteins with increasing age in Mrl/Mp-lpr/lpr mice. *British Journal of Rheumatology* 34:610–615.

Fenchel, S. Grab, D. Nuessle, K. Kotzerke, J. Rieber, A. Kreienberg, R. Brambs, HJ. Reske, SN. 2002. Asymptomatic adnexal masses: Correlation of FDG PET and histopathologic findings. *Radiology* 223:780–788.

Flavin, RJ. Smyth, PC. Finn, SP. Laios, A. O'Toole, SA. Barrett, C. Ring, M. et al. 2008. Altered eIF6 and Dicer expression is associated with clinicopathological features in ovarian serous carcinoma patients. *Modern Pathology* 21:676–684.

Forshew, T. Murtaza, M. Parkinson, C. Gale, D. Tsui, DW. Kaper, F. Dawson, SJ. et al. 2012. Noninvasive identification and monitoring of cancer mutations by targeted deep sequencing of plasma DNA. *Science Translational Medicine* 4:136ra68.

Fredolini, C. Meani, F. Luchini, A. Zhou, W. Russo, P. Ross, M. Patanarut, A. et al. 2010. Investigation of the ovarian and prostate cancer peptidome for candidate early detection markers using a novel nanoparticle biomarker capture technology. *American Association of Pharmaceutical Scientists Journal* 12:504–518.

Gagnon, A. Kim, JH. Schorge, JO. Ye, B. Liu, B. Hasselblatt, K. Welch, WR. Bandera, CA. Mok, SC. 2008. Use of a combination of approaches to identify and validate relevant tumor-associated antigens and their corresponding autoantibodies in ovarian cancer patients. *Clinical Cancer Research* 14:764–771.

Galgano, MT. Hampton, GM. Frierson, HF Jr. 2006. Comprehensive analysis of HE4 expression in normal and malignant human tissues. *Modern Pathology* 19:847–853.

Gallagher, MF. Flavin, RJ. Elbaruni, SA. McInerney, JK. Smyth, PC. Salley, YM. Vencken, SF. et al. 2009. Regulation of microRNA biosynthesis and expression in 2102Ep embryonal carcinoma stem cells is mirrored in ovarian serous adenocarcinoma patients. *Journal of Ovarian Research* 2:19.

Gao, L. Cheng, HY. Dong, L. Ye, X. Liu, YN. Chang, XH. Cheng, YX. Chen, J. Ma, RQ. Cui, H. 2011. The role of HE4 in ovarian cancer: Inhibiting tumour cell proliferation and metastasis. *The Journal of International Medical Research* 39:1645–1660.

Gilad, S. Meiri, E. Yogev, Y. Benjamin, S. Lebanony, D. Yerushalmi, N. Benjamin, H. et al. 2008. Serum microRNAs are promising novel biomarkers. *PLoS One* 3:e3148.

Gnjatic, S. Ritter, E. Buchler, MW. Giese, NA. Brors, B. Frei, C. Murray, A. et al. 2010. Seromic profiling of ovarian and pancreatic cancer. *Proceedings of the National Academy of Sciences of the United States of America* 107:5088–5093.

Griffin, JL. Shockcor, JP. 2004. Metabolic profiles of cancer cells. *Nature Reviews Cancer* 4:551–561.

Guerriero, S. Alcazar, JL. Coccia, ME. Ajossa, S. Scarselli, G. Boi, M. Gerada, M. Melis, GB. 2002. Complex pelvic mass as a target of evaluation of vessel distribution by color Doppler sonography for the diagnosis of adnexal malignancies: Results of a multicenter European study. *Journal of Ultrasound in Medicine* 21:1105–1111.

Gupta, D. Lis, CG. 2009. Role of CA125 in predicting ovarian cancer survival—A review of the epidemiological literature. *Journal of Ovarian Research* 2:13.

Hausler, SF. Keller, A. Chandran, PA. Ziegler, K. Zipp, K. Heuer, S. Krockenberger, M. et al. 2010. Whole blood-derived miRNA profiles as potential new tools for ovarian cancer screening. *British Journal of Cancer* 103:693–700.

Hayem, G. De Bandt, M. Palazzo, E. Roux, S. Combe, B. Eliaou, JF. Sany, J. Kahn, MF. Meyer, O. 1999. Anti-heat shock protein 70 kDa and 90 kDa antibodies in serum of patients with rheumatoid arthritis. *Annals of the Rheumatic Diseases* 58:291–296.

He, H. Jazdzewski, K. Li, W. Liyanarachchi, S. Nagy, R. Volinia, S. Calin, GA. et al. 2005. The role of microRNA genes in papillary thyroid carcinoma. *Proceedings of the National Academy of Sciences of the United States of America* 102:19075–19080.

Hellstrom, I. Friedman, E. Verch, T. Yang, Y. Korach, J. Jaffar, J. Swisher, E. et al. 2008. Anti-mesothelin antibodies and circulating mesothelin relate to the clinical state in ovarian cancer patients. *Cancer Epidemiology, Biomarkers & Prevention* 17:1520–1526.

Hellstrom, I. Heagerty, PJ. Swisher, EM. Liu, P. Jaffar, J. Agnew, K. Hellstrom, KE. 2010. Detection of the HE4 protein in urine as a biomarker for ovarian neoplasms. *Cancer Letters* 296:43–48.

Hellström, I. Raycraft, J. Hayden-Ledbetter, M. Ledbetter, JA. Schummer, M. McIntosh, M. Drescher, C. Urban, N. Hellström, KE. 2003. The HE4 (WFDC2) protein is a biomarker for ovarian carcinoma. *Cancer Research* 63:3695–3700.

Hensley, M. Alektiar, D. Chi, D. 2002. Ovarian and fallopian-tube cancer. In: Barakat, R. Bevers, M. Gershenson, D. Hoskins, W. editors. *Handbook of Gynecologic Oncology*. London, U.K.: Martin Dunitz.

Ho, M. Hassan, R. Zhang, J. Wang, QC. Onda, M. Bera, T. Pastan, I. 2005. Humoral immune response to mesothelin in mesothelioma and ovarian cancer patients. *Clinical Cancer Research* 11:3814–3820.

Hoffman, BR. Katsaros, D. Scorilas, A. Diamandis, P. Fracchioli, S. Rigault de la Longrais, IA. Colgan, T. et al. 2002. Immunofluorometric quantification and histochemical localisation of kallikrein 6 protein in ovarian cancer tissue: A new independent unfavourable prognostic biomarker. *British Journal of Cancer* 87:763–771.

Holcomb, K. Vucetic, Z. Miller, MC. Knapp, RC. 2011. Human epididymis protein 4 offers superior specificity in the differentiation of benign and malignant adnexal masses in premenopausal women. *American Journal of Obstetrics and Gynecology* 205:358 e1–e6.

Hudson, ME. Pozdnyakova, I. Haines, K. Mor, G. Snyder, M. 2007. Identification of differentially expressed proteins in ovarian cancer using high-density protein microarrays. *Proceedings of the National Academy of Sciences of the United States of America* 104:17494–17499.

Hunter, MP. Ismail, N. Zhang, X. Aguda, BD. Lee, EJ. Yu, L. Xiao, T. et al. 2008. Detection of microRNA expression in human peripheral blood microvesicles. *PLoS One* 3:e3694.

Hwang, H. Quenneville, L. Yaziji, H. Gown, AM. 2004. Wilms tumor gene product: Sensitive and contextually specific marker of serous carcinomas of ovarian surface epithelial origin. *Applied Immunohistochemistry & Molecular Morphology* 12:122–126.

Iero, M. Valenti, R. Huber, V. Filipazzi, P. Parmiani, G. Fais, S. Rivoltini, L. 2008. Tumour-released exosomes and their implications in cancer immunity. *Cell Death and Differentiation* 15:80–88.

Iorio, MV. Ferracin, M. Liu, CG. Veronese, A. Spizzo, R. Sabbioni, S. Magri, E. et al. 2005. MicroRNA gene expression deregulation in human breast cancer. *Cancer Research* 65:7065–7070.

Iorio, MV. Visone, R. Di Leva, G. Donati, V. Petrocca, F. Casalini, P. Taccioli, C. et al. 2007. MicroRNA signatures in human ovarian cancer. *Cancer Research* 67:8699–8707.

Isaksson, HS. Sorbe, B. Nilsson, TK. 2012. Whole blood RNA expression profiles in ovarian cancer patients with or without residual tumors after primary cytoreductive surgery. *Oncology Reports* 27:1331–1335.

Judson, PL. Geller, MA. Bliss, RL. Boente, MP. Downs, LS. Argenta, PA. Carson, LF. 2003. Preoperative detection of peripherally circulating cancer cells and its prognostic significance in ovarian cancer. *Gynecologic Oncology* 91:389–394.

Kalapotharakos, G. Asciutto, C. Henic, E. Casslen, B. Borgfeldt, C. 2012. High preoperative blood levels of HE4 predicts poor prognosis in patients with ovarian cancer. *Journal of Ovarian Research* 5:20.

Kamat, AA. Fletcher, M. Gruman, LM. Mueller, P. Lopez, A. Landen, CN Jr. Han, L. Gershenson, DM. Sood, AK. 2006. The clinical relevance of stromal matrix metalloproteinase expression in ovarian cancer. *Clinical Cancer Research* 12:1707–1714.

Kato, N. Toukairin, M. Asanuma, I. Motoyama, T. 2007. Immunocytochemistry for hepatocyte nuclear factor-1b (HNF-1b): A marker for ovarian clear cell carcinoma. *Diagnostic Cytopathology* 35:193–197.

Kirchhoff, C. 1998. Molecular characterization of epididymal proteins. *Reviews of Reproduction* 3:86–95.

Kobayashi, E. Ueda, Y. Matsuzaki, S. Yokoyama, T. Kimura, T. Yoshino, K. Fujita, M. Kimura, T. Enomoto, T. 2012. Biomarkers for screening, diagnosis, and monitoring of ovarian cancer. *Cancer Epidemiology, Biomarkers & Prevention* 21:1902–1912.

Kong, SY. Han, MH. Yoo, HJ. Hwang, JH. Lim, MC. Seo, SS. Yoo, CW. Kim, JH. Park, SY. Kang, S. 2012. Serum HE4 level is an independent prognostic factor in epithelial ovarian cancer. *Annals of Surgical Oncology* 19:1707–1712.

Korneeva, I. Bongiovanni, AM. Girotra, M. Caputo, TA. Witkin, SS. 2000. IgA antibodies to the 27-kDa heat-shock protein in the genital tracts of women with gynecologic cancers. *International Journal of Cancer* 87:824–828.

Kurman, RJ. Shih, IeM. 2010. The origin and pathogenesis of epithelial ovarian cancer: A proposed unifying theory. *The American Journal of Surgical Pathology* 34:433–443.

Lagos-Quintana, M. Rauhut, R. Lendeckel, W. Tuschl, T. 2001. Identification of novel genes coding for small expressed RNAs. *Science* 294:853–858.

Laios, A. Mohamed, BM. Kelly, L. Flavin, R. Finn, S. McEvoy, L. Gallagher, M. et al. 2013. Pre-treatment of platinum resistant ovarian cancer cells with an MMP-9/MMP-2 inhibitor prior to cisplatin enhances cytotoxicity as determined by high content screening. *International Journal of Molecular Sciences* 14:2085–2103.

Laios, A. O'Toole, S. Flavin, R. Martin, C. Kelly, L. Ring, M. Finn, SP. et al. 2008. Potential role of miR-9 and miR-223 in recurrent ovarian cancer. *Molecular Cancer* 7:35.

Landen, CN. Birrer, MJ. Sood, AK. 2008. Early events in the pathogenesis of epithelial ovarian cancer. *Journal of Clinical Oncology* 26: 995–1005.

Lawrie, CH. Gal, S. Dunlop, HM. Pushkaran, B. Liggins, AP. Pulford, K. Banham, AH. et al. 2008. Detection of elevated levels of tumour-associated microRNAs in serum of patients with diffuse large B-cell lymphoma. *British Journal of Haematology* 141:672–675.

Lee, CH. Subramanian, S. Beck, AH. Espinosa, I. Senz, J. Zhu, SX. Huntsman, D. van de Rijn, M. Gilks, CB. 2009. MicroRNA profiling of BRCA1/2 mutation-carrying and non-mutation-carrying high-grade serous carcinomas of ovary. *PLoS One* 4:e7314.

Lee, YH. Kim, JH. Zhou, H. Kim, BW. Wong, DT. 2012. Salivary transcriptomic biomarkers for detection of ovarian cancer: For serous papillary adenocarcinoma. *Journal of Molecular Medicine* 90:427–434.

Li, F. Tie, R. Chang, K. Wang, F. Deng, S. Lu, W. Yu, L. Chen, M. 2012. Does risk for ovarian malignancy algorithm excel human epididymis protein 4 and CA125 in predicting epithelial ovarian cancer: A meta-analysis. *BMC Cancer* 12:258.

Li, L. Wang, K. Dai, L. Wang, P. Peng, XX. Zhang, JY. 2008. Detection of autoantibodies to multiple tumor-associated antigens in the immunodiagnosis of ovarian cancer. *Molecular Medicine Reports* 1:589–594.

Liao, J. Yu, L. Mei, Y. Guarnera, M. Shen, J. Li, R. Liu, Z. Jiang, F. 2010. Small nucleolar RNA signatures as biomarkers for non-small-cell lung cancer. *Molecular Cancer* 9:198.

Liotta, LA. Petricoin, EF 3rd. 2012. Omics and cancer biomarkers: Link to the biological truth or bear the consequences. *Cancer Epidemiology, Biomarkers & Prevention* 21:1229–1235.

Lu, D. Kuhn, E. Bristow, RE. Giuntoli, RL 2nd. Kjaer, SK. Shih, IeM. Roden, RB. 2011. Comparison of candidate serologic markers for type I and type II ovarian cancer. *Gynecologic Oncology* 122:560–566.

Lu, J. Getz, G. Miska, EA. Alvarez-Saavedra, E. Lamb, J. Peck, D. Sweet-Cordero, A. et al. 2005. MicroRNA expression profiles classify human cancers. *Nature* 435:834–838.

Luborsky, JL. Yu, Y. Edassery, SL. Jaffar, J. Yip, YY. Liu, P. Hellstrom, KE. Hellstrom, I. 2011. Autoantibodies to mesothelin in infertility. *Cancer Epidemiology, Biomarkers & Prevention* 20:1970–1978.

Luo, LY. Katsaros, D. Scorilas, A. Fracchioli, S. Bellino, R. van Gramberen, M. de Bruijn, H. et al. 2003. The serum concentration of human kallikrein 10 represents a novel biomarker for ovarian cancer diagnosis and prognosis. *Cancer Research* 63:807–811.

Marth, C. Kisic, J. Kaern, J. Trope, C. Fodstad, O. 2002. Circulating tumor cells in the peripheral blood and bone marrow of patients with ovarian carcinoma do not predict prognosis. *Cancer* 94:707–712.

McIntosh, MW. Liu, Y. Drescher, C. Urban, N. Diamandis, EP. 2007. Validation and characterization of human kallikrein 11 as a serum marker for diagnosis of ovarian carcinoma. *Clinical Cancer Research* 13:4422–4428.

Menon, U. Gentry-Maharaj, A. Hallett, R. Ryan, A. Burnell, M. Sharma, A. Lewis, S. et al. 2009. Sensitivity and specificity of multimodal and ultrasound screening for ovarian cancer, and stage distribution of detected cancers: Results of the prevalence screen of the UK collaborative trial of ovarian cancer screening (UKCTOCS). *The Lancet Oncology* 10:327–340.

Menon, U. Kalsi, J. Jacobs, I. 2012. The UKCTOCS experience—Reasons for hope? *International Journal of Gynecological Cancer* 22:S18–S20.

Merritt, WM. Lin, YG. Han, LY. Kamat, AA. Spannuth, WA. Schmandt, R. Urbauer, D. et al. 2008. Dicer, Drosha, and outcomes in patients with ovarian cancer. *The New England Journal of Medicine* 359:2641–2650.

Milne, K. Barnes, RO. Girardin, A. Mawer, MA. Nesslinger, NJ. Ng, A. Nielsen, JS. et al. 2008. Tumor-infiltrating T cells correlate with NY-ESO-1-specific autoantibodies in ovarian cancer. *PLoS One* 3:e3409.

Miska, EA. 2005. How microRNAs control cell division, differentiation and death. *Current Opinion in Genetics & Development* 15:563–568.

Miszczak-Zaborska, E. WójcikKrowiranda, K. Kubiak, R. Bieńkiewicz, A. Bartkowiak, J. 2004. The activity of thymidine phosphorylase as a new ovarian tumor marker. *Gynecologic Oncology* 94:86–92.

Mitchell, PS. Parkin, RK. Kroh, EM. Fritz, BR. Wyman, SK. Pogosova-Agadjanyan, EL. Peterson, A. et al. 2008. Circulating microRNAs as stable blood-based markers for cancer detection. *Proceedings of the National Academy of Sciences of the United States of America* 105:10513–10518.

Montagnana, M. Danese, E. Giudici, S. Franchi, M. Guidi, GC. Plebani, M. Lippi, G. 2011. HE4 in ovarian cancer: From discovery to clinical application. *Advances in Clinical Chemistry* 55:1–20.

Moore, RG. Brown, AK. Miller, MC. Skates, S. Allard, WJ. Verch, T. Steinhoff, M. et al. 2008. The use of multiple novel tumor biomarkers for the detection of ovarian carcinoma in patients with a pelvic mass. *Gynecologic Oncology* 108:402–408.

Moore, RG. Jabre-Raughley, M. Brown, AK. Robison, KM. Miller, MC. Allard WJ, Kurman, RJ et al. 2010. Comparison of a novel multiple marker assay vs the Risk of Malignancy Index for the prediction of epithelial ovarian cancer in patients with a pelvic mass. *American Journal of Obstetrics and Gynecology* 203:228.e1–228.e6.

Moore, RG. McMeekin, DS. Brown, AK. DiSilvestro, P. Miller, MC. Allard, WJ. Gajewski, W. Kurman, R. Bast, RCJr, Skates, SJ. 2009. A novel multiple marker bioassay utilizing HE4 and CA125 for the prediction of ovarian cancer in patients with a pelvic mass. *Gynecologic Oncology* 112:40–46.

Moore, RG. Miller, MC. Disilvestro, P. Landrum, LM. Gajewski, W. Ball, JJ. Skates, SJ. 2011. Evaluation of the diagnostic accuracy of the risk of ovarian malignancy algorithm in women with a pelvic mass. *Obstetrics Gynecology* 118:280–288.

Moore, RG. Miller, MC. Steinhoff, MM. Skates, SJ. Lu, KH. Lambert-Messerlian, G. Bast, RC Jr. 2012. Serum HE4 levels are less frequently elevated than CA125 in women with benign gynecologic disorders. *American Journal of Obstetrics and Gynecology* 206:351.e1–351.e8.

Moss, EL. Hollingworth, J. Reynolds, TM. 2005. The role of CA125 in clinical practice. *Journal of Clinical Pathology* 58:308–312.

Muller, CY. 2010. Doctor, should I get this new ovarian cancer test-ova1? *Obstetrics and Gynecology* 116:246–247.

Murphy, MA. O'Connell, DJ. O'Kane, SL. O'Brien, JK. O'Toole, S. Martin, C. Sheils, O. O'Leary, JJ. Cahill, DJ. 2012a. Epitope presentation is an important determinant of the utility of antigens identified from protein arrays in the development of autoantibody diagnostic assays. *Journal of Proteomics* 75:4668–4675.

Murphy, MA. O'Leary, JJ. Cahill, DJ. 2012b. Assessment of the humoral immune response to cancer. *Journal of Proteomics* 7515:4573–4579.

Nam, EJ. Yoon, H. Kim, SW. Kim, H. Kim, YT. Kim, JH. Kim, JW. Kim, S. 2008. MicroRNA expression profiles in serous ovarian carcinoma. *Clinical Cancer Research* 14:2690–2695.

Neuhausen, SL. Mazoyer, S. Friedman, L. Stratton, M. Offit, K. Caligo, A. Tomlinson, G. et al. 1996. Haplotype and phenotype analysis of six recurrent BRCA1 mutations in 61 families: Results of an international study. *American Journal of Human Genetics* 58:271–280.

Nossov, V. Amneus, M. Su, F. Lang, J. Janco, JM. Reddy, ST. Farias-Eisner, R. 2008. The early detection of ovarian cancer: From traditional methods to proteomics. Can we really do better than serum CA-125? *American Journal of Obstetrics and Gynecology* 199:215–223.

Obermayr, E. Castillo-Tong, DC. Pils, D. Speiser, P. Braicu, I. Van Gorp, T. Mahner, S. Sehouli, J. Vergote, I. Zeillinger, R. 2013. Molecular characterization of circulating tumor cells in patients with ovarian cancer improves their prognostic significance—A study of the OVCAD consortium. *Gynecologic Oncology* 128:15–21.

Oddoux, C. Struewing, JP. Clayton, CM. Neuhausen, S. Brody, LC. Kaback, M. Haas, B. et al. 1996. The carrier frequency of the BRCA2 6174delT mutation among Ashkenazi Jewish individuals is approximately 1%. *Nature Genetics* 14:188–190.

Odunsi, K. Jungbluth, AA. Stockert, E. Qian, F. Gnjatic, S. Tammela, J. Intengan, M. et al. 2003. NY-ESO-1 and LAGE-1 cancer-testis antigens are potential targets for immunotherapy in epithelial ovarian cancer. *Cancer Research* 63:6076–6083.

Okamoto, Y. Tanaka, YO. Tsunoda, H. Yoshikawa, H. Minami, M. 2007. Malignant or borderline mucinous cystic neoplasms have a larger number of loculi than mucinous cystadenoma: A retrospective study with MR. *Journal of Magnetic Resonance Imaging* 26:94–99.

Paek, J. Lee, S-H. Yim, G-W. Lee, M. Kim, Y-J. Nam, E-J. 2011. Prognostic significance of human epididymis protein 4 in epithelial ovarian cancer. *European Journal of Obstetrics, Gynecology, and Reproductive Biology* 158:338–342.

Paterlini-Brechot, P. Benali, NL. 2007. Circulating tumor cells (CTC) detection: Clinical impact and future directions. *Cancer Letters* 253:180–204.

Petricoin, EF. Ardekani, AM. Hitt, BA. Levine, PJ. Fusaro, VA. Steinberg, SM. Mills, GB. et al. 2002. Use of proteomic patterns in serum to identify ovarian cancer. *Lancet* 359:572–577.

Picchio, M. Sironi, S. Messa, C. Mangili, G. Landoni, C. Gianolli, L. Zangheri, B. et al. 2003. Advanced ovarian carcinoma: Usefulness of [(18)F]FDG-PET in combination with CT for lesion detection after primary treatment. *The Quarterly Journal of Nuclear Medicine* 47:77–84.

Piura, B. Piura, E. 2009. Autoantibodies to tumor-associated antigens in epithelial ovarian carcinoma. *Journal of Oncology* 2009:581939.

Piura, E. Piura, B. 2010. Autoantibodies to tumor-associated antigens in breast carcinoma. *Journal of Oncology* 2010:264926.

Poveda, A. Kaye, SB. McCormack, R. Wang, S. Parekh, T. Ricci, D. Lebedinsky, CA. Tercero, JC. Zintl, P. Monk, BJ. 2011. Circulating tumor cells predict progression free survival and overall survival in patients with relapsed/recurrent advanced ovarian cancer. *Gynecologic Oncology* 122:567–572.

Psyrri, A. Kountourakis, P. Scorilas, A. Markakis, S. Camp, R. Kowalski, D. Diamandis, EP. Dimopoulos, MA. 2008. Human tissue kallikrein 7, a novel biomarker for advanced ovarian carcinoma using a novel in situ quantitative method of protein expression. *Annals of Oncology* 19:1271–1277.

Pyle-Chenault, RA. Stolk, JA. Molesh, DA. Boyle-Harlan, D. McNeill, PD. Repasky, EA. Jiang, Z. Fanger, GR. Xu, J. 2005. VSGP/F-spondin: A new ovarian cancer marker. *Tumour Biology* 26:245–257.

Raamanathan, A. Simmons, GW. Christodoulides, N. Floriano, PN. Furmaga, WB. Redding, SW. Lu, KH. Bast, RC Jr. McDevitt, JT. 2012. Programmable bio-nano-chip systems for serum CA125 quantification: Toward ovarian cancer diagnostics at the point-of-care. *Cancer Prevention Research* 5:706–716.

Rebbeck, TR. Lynch, HT. Neuhausen, SL. Narod, SA. Van't Veer, L. Garber, JE. Evans, G. et al. 2002. Prevention and observation of surgical end points study group. Prophylactic oophorectomy in carriers of BRCA1 or BRCA2 mutations. *The New England Journal of Medicine* 346:1616–1622.

Rein, BJD. Gupta, S. Dada, R. Safi, J. Michener, C. Agarwal, A. 2011. Potential markers for detection and monitoring of ovarian cancer. *Journal of Oncology* 2011:475983.

Resnick, KE. Alder, H. Hagan, JP. Richardson, DL. Croce, CM. Cohn, DE. 2009. The detection of differentially expressed microRNAs from the serum of ovarian cancer patients using a novel real-time PCR platform. *Gynecologic Oncology* 112:55–59.

Schorge, JO. Modesitt, SC. Coleman, RL. Cohn, DE. Kauff, ND. Duska, LR. Herzog, TJ. 2010. SGO White Paper on ovarian cancer: Etiology, screening and surveillance. *Gynecologic Oncology* 119:7–17.

Schummer, M. Drescher, C. Forrest, R. Gough, S. Thorpe, J. Hellstrom, I. Hellstrom, KE. Urban, N. 2012. Evaluation of ovarian cancer remission markers HE4, MMP7 and Mesothelin by comparison to the established marker CA125. *Gynecologic Oncology* 125:65–69.

Scorilas, A. Borgoño, CA. Harbeck, N. Dorn, J. Schmalfeldt, B. Schmitt, M. Diamandis, EP. 2004. Human kallikrein 13 protein in ovarian cancer cytosols: A new favorable prognostic marker. *Journal of Clinical Oncology* 22:678–685.

Seeber, LM. van Diest, PJ. 2012. Epigenetics in ovarian cancer. *Methods in Molecular Biology* 863:253–269.

Shan, SJ. Scorilas, A. Katsaros, D. Diamandis, EP. 2007. Transcriptional upregulation of human tissue kallikrein 6 in ovarian cancer: Clinical and mechanistic aspects. *British Journal of Cancer* 96:362–372.

Singh, AP. Senapati, S. Ponnusamy, MP. Jain, M. Lele, SM. Davis, JS. Remmenga, S. Batra, SK. 2008. Clinical potential of mucins in diagnosis, prognosis, and therapy of ovarian cancer. *The Lancet Oncology* 9:1076–1085.

Slupsky, CM. Steed, H. Wells, TH. Dabbs, K. Schepansky, A. Capstick, V. Faught, W. Sawyer, MB. 2010. Urine metabolite analysis offers potential early diagnosis of ovarian and breast cancers. *Clinical Cancer Research* 16:5835–5841.

Soussi, T. 2000. p53 Antibodies in the sera of patients with various types of cancer: A review. *Cancer Research* 60:1777–1788.

Steffensen, KD. Waldstrom, M. Brandslund, I. Jakobsen, A. 2011. Prognostic impact of prechemotherapy serum levels of HER2, CA125, and HE4 in ovarian cancer patients. *International Journal of Gynecological Cancer* 21:1040–1047.

Stockert, E. Jager, E. Chen, YT. Scanlan, MJ. Gout, I. Karbach, J. Arand, M. Knuth, A. Old, LJ. 1998. A survey of the humoral immune response of cancer patients to a panel of human tumor antigens. *The Journal of Experimental Medicine* 187:1349–1354.

Struewing, JP. Abeliovich, D. Peretz, T. Vishay, N. Kaback, MM. Collins, FS. Brody, LC. 1995. The carrier frequency of the BRCA1 185delAG mutation is approximately 1 percent in Ashkenazi Jewish individuals. *Nature Genetics* 11:198–200.

Sueblinvong, T. Carney, ME. 2009. Current understanding of risk factors for ovarian cancer. *Current Treatment Options in Oncology* 10:67–81.

Suh, KS. Crutchley, JM. Koochek, A. Ryscavage, A. Bhat, K. Tanaka, T. Oshima, A. Fitzgerald, P. Yuspa, SH. 2007. Reciprocal modifications of CLIC4 in tumor epithelium and stroma mark malignant progression of multiple human cancers. *Clinical Cancer Research* 13:121–131.

Suh, KS. Park, WS. Castro, A. Patel, H. Blake, P., Liang, M. Goy, A. 2010. Ovarian cancer biomarkers for molecular biosensors and translational medicine. *Expert Review of Molecular Diagnostics* 10:1069–1083.

Takamizawa, J. Konishi, H. Yanagisawa, K. Tomida, S. Osada, H. Endoh, H. Harano, T. et al. 2004. Reduced expression of the let-7 microRNAs in human lung cancers in association with shortened postoperative survival. *Cancer Research* 64:3753–3756.

Taylor, DD. Gercel-Taylor, C. 2008. MicroRNA signatures of tumor-derived exosomes as diagnostic biomarkers of ovarian cancer. *Gynecologic Oncology* 110:13–21.

Taylor, DD. Gercel-Taylor, C. Parker, LP. 2009. Patient-derived tumor reactive antibodies as diagnostic markers for ovarian cancer. *Gynecologic Oncology* 115:112–120.

Tempany, CM. Zou, KH. Silverman, SG. Brown, DL. Kurtz, AB. McNeil, BJ. 2000. Staging of advanced ovarian cancer: Comparison of imaging modalities—Report from the Radiological Diagnostic Oncology Group. *Radiology* 215:761–767.

Trieb, K. Gerth, R. Holzer, G. Grohs, JG. Berger, P. Kotz, R. 2000. Antibodies to heat shock protein 90 in osteosarcoma patients correlate with response to neoadjuvant chemotherapy. *British Journal of Cancer* 82:85–87.

Trudel, D. Tetu, B. Gregoire, J. Plante, M. Renaud, M-C. Bachvarov, D. Douville, P. Bairati, I. 2012. Human epididymis protein 4 (HE4) and ovarian cancer prognosis. *Gynecologic Oncology* 127:511–515.

Tsai-Turton, M. Santillan, A. Lu, D. Bristow, RE. Chan, KC. Shih, IeM. Roden, RB. 2009. p53 autoantibodies, cytokine levels and ovarian carcinogenesis. *Gynecologic Oncology* 114:12–17.

Tsuchiya, A. Sakamoto, M. Yasuda, J. Chuma, M. Ohta, T. Ohki, M. Yasugi, T. Taketani, Y. Hirohashi, S. 2003. Expression profiling in ovarian clear cell carcinoma: Identification of hepatocyte nuclear factor-1 beta as a molecular marker and a possible molecular target for therapy of ovarian clear cell carcinoma. *The American Journal of Pathology* 163:2503–2512.

Van Gorp, T. Cadron, I. Despierre, E. 2011. HE4 and CA125 as a diagnostic test in ovarian cancer: Prospective validation of the Risk of Ovarian Malignancy Algorithm. *British Journal of Cancer* 104:863–870.

Van Jaarsveld, MT. Helleman, J. Berns, EM. Wiemer, EA. 2010. MicroRNAs in ovarian cancer biology and therapy resistance. *The International Journal of Biochemistry & Cell Biology* 42:1282–1290.

Verheijen, RH. von Mensdorff-Pouilly, S. van Kamp, GJ. Kenemans, P. 1999. CA 125: Fundamental and clinical aspects. *Seminars in Cancer Biology* 9:117–124.

Vidal, CI. Mintz, PJ. Lu, K. Ellis, LM. Manenti, L. Giavazzi, R. Gershenson, DM. et al. 2004. An HSP90-mimic peptide revealed by fingerprinting the pool of antibodies from ovarian cancer patients. *Oncogene* 23:8859–8867.

Vogl, FD. Frey, M. Kreienberg, R. Runnebaum, IB. 2000. Autoimmunity against p53 predicts invasive cancer with poor survival in patients with an ovarian mass. *British Journal of Cancer* 83:1338–1343.

Wang, P. Ge, L. Yan, M. Song, X. Ge, S. Yu, J. 2012. Paper-based three-dimensional electrochemical immunodevice based on multi-walled carbon nanotubes functionalized paper for sensitive point-of-care testing. *Biosensors & Bioelectronics* 32:238–243.

Wang, S. Zhao, X. Khimji, I. Akbar, R. Qiu, W. Edwards, D. Cramer, DW. Ye, B. Demirci, U. 2011. Integration of cell phone imaging with microchip ELISA to detect ovarian cancer HE4 biomarker in urine at the point-of-care. *Lab on a Chip* 11:3411–3418.

Webb, J. 2007. Ultrasound in ovarian carcinoma. In: Reznek, RH, ed. *Cancer of the Ovary*. Cambridge: Cambridge University Press, pp. 94–111.

Wimberger, P. Heubner, M. Otterbach, F. Fehm, T. Kimmig, R. Kasimir-Bauer, S. 2007. Influence of platinum-based chemotherapy on disseminated tumor cells in blood and bone marrow of patients with ovarian cancer. *Gynecologic Oncology* 107:331–338.

Wu, L. Dai, ZY. Qian, YH. Shi, Y. Liu, FJ. Yang, C. 2012. Diagnostic value of serum human epididymis protein 4 (HE4) in ovarian carcinoma: A systematic review and meta-analysis. *International Journal of Gynecological Cancer* 22:1106–1112.

Wyman, SK. Parkin, RK. Mitchell, PS. Fritz, BR. O'Briant, K. Godwin, AK. Urban, N. Drescher, CW. Knudsen, BS. Tewari, M. 2009. Repertoire of microRNAs in epithelial ovarian cancer as determined by next generation sequencing of small RNA cDNA libraries. *PLoS One* 4:e5311.

Ye, B. Skates, S. Mok, SC. Horick, NK. Rosenberg, HF. Vitonis, A. Edwards, D. et al. 2006. Proteomic-based discovery and characterization of glycosylated eosinophil-derived neurotoxin and COOH-terminal osteopontin fragments for ovarian cancer in urine. *Clinical Cancer Research* 12:432–441.

Yoshida, Y. Kurokawa, T. Kawahara, K. Tsuchida, T. Okazawa, H. Fujibayashi, Y. Yonekura, Y. Kotsuji, F. 2004. Incremental benefits of FDG positron emission tomography over CT alone for the preoperative staging of ovarian cancer. *American Journal of Roentgenology* 182:227–233.

Yousef, GM. Diamandis, EP. 2002. Kallikreins, steroid hormones and ovarian cancer: Is there a link? *Minerva Endocrinology* 27:157–166.

Yu, M. Stott, S. Toner, M. Maheswaran, S. Haber, DA. 2011. Circulating tumor cells: Approaches to isolation and characterization. *The Journal of Cell Biology* 192:373–382.

Zhang, L. Huang, J. Yang, N. Greshock, J. Megraw, MS. Giannakakis, A. Liang, S. et al. 2006. MicroRNAs exhibit high frequency genomic alterations in human cancer. *Proceedings of the National Academy of Sciences of the United States of America* 103:9136–9141.

Zhang, L. Volinia, S. Bonome, T. Calin, GA. Greshock, J. Yang, N. Liu, CG. et al. 2008. Genomic and epigenetic alterations deregulate microRNA expression in human epithelial ovarian cancer. *Proceedings of the National Academy of Sciences of the United States of America* 105:7004–7009.

Zhang, T. Wu, X. Yin, M. Fan, L. Zhang, H. Zhao, F. Zhang, W. et al. 2012. Discrimination between malignant and benign ovarian tumors by plasma metabolomic profiling using ultra performance liquid chromatography/mass spectrometry. *Clinica Chimica Acta* 413:861–868.

Zhang, W. Yang, HC. Wang, Q. Yang, ZJ. Chen, H. Wang, SM. Pan, ZM. Tang, BJ. Li, QQ. Li, L. 2011. Clinical value of combined detection of serum matrix metalloproteinase-9, heparanase, and cathepsin for determining ovarian cancer invasion and metastasis. *Anticancer Research* 31:3423–3428.

11

Biomarkers in Ovarian Endometrioid Carcinoma

Murat Oznur, MD, PhD, Serap Memik, MS, Mehmet Gunduz, MD, PhD, and Esra Gunduz, DMD, PhD

CONTENTS

ABSTRACT Among cancer diseases, after breast cancer, gynecologic cancer is the second most prevalent cause of mortality and morbidity in women. In the United States, ovarian cancer is the second most common gynecologic cancer after endometrial cancer. Because of its nonspecific symptoms and absence of reliable biomarkers, its diagnosis frequently occurs at advanced disease stages. The presence of drug-resistant histological types limits the long-term cure rates and makes ovarian cancer the most lethal gynecologic malignancy. In ovarian cancers, early detection is rare, and when it is detected, it has pelvic spread. It is mostly sporadic but also has familial cancer syndromes. As a genetic approach to ovarian carcinogenesis, it is a complex, multistep polychromosomal process. Different cytogenetic events lead to cancer initiation, growth, and progression. Each histological subtype of ovarian cancer is characterized by distinct histogenetic events and chromosomal abnormalities. The promotion of protooncogenes or the *silencing* of tumor suppression genes might be the initial pathogenesis of ovarian carcinoma. This chapter focuses on the techniques that are being used or proposed for early prognosis and diagnosis of ovarian carcinomas. Some pathways have been described to be the cause of ovarian endometrioid carcinoma. The ovarian carcinomas including endometrioid subtypes may represent distinctive pathways of tumorigenesis and disease development. This distinction could potentially be reflected in the levels of tumor-produced factors that enter into the circulation and serve as biomarkers of malignant growth. To compose an investigation panel combined with one or more biomarkers or alone, there are a lot of suspected biomarkers that have been studied for the early detection or the differential diagnosis of both ovarian and its subtypes.

11.1 Introduction

11.1.1 Why Is It Important?

After heart diseases, cancer is the second most prevalent cause of death in developed countries. Among cancer diseases, after breast cancer, gynecologic cancer is the second most prevalent cause of mortality and morbidity in women. Although it differs from one country to another, the prevalence of gynecologic cancers in eastern countries is on the order of endometrial, ovarian, and cervical cancers (Ucar and Bekar 2010).

11.1.2 Epidemiology

Ovarian cancer is the second most common gynecologic cancer after endometrial cancer. The prevalence of ovarian cancer could change according to different geographic regions. Especially in European countries such as Scandinavian countries and the United Kingdom, Canada, and North America, its incidence is higher. In the United States, the incidence of ovarian cancer is 33 cases per 100,000 women aged 50 years or older. Internationally, the incidence is 3.1 cases per 100,000 women in Japan and 21 cases per 100,000 women in Sweden (Figure 11.1) (GLOBOCAN 2008 (IARC)). The variety of environment and lifestyle may be the reason of this diversity. Ovarian cancer in women generates 4% of all cancers and causes 6% of cancer deaths. It is predicted that there are 192,000 cases all over the world (Ucar and Bekar 2010). The American Cancer Society estimated that there would be 21,880 new cases of ovarian cancer in 2010 and 13,850 deaths from the disease ("American Cancer Society, Cancer Facts and Figures 2009"). Ovarian cancer is more common among white women the United States.

11.1.3 Types of Ovarian Cancer

Ovarian cancers begin with the dedifferentiation of the cells overlying the ovary. These cells can be incorporated into the ovary during ovulation to proliferate. Ovarian cancer typically spreads to the peritoneal surfaces and omentum. Spreading of ovarian carcinoma could be actualized by the way of local extension, lymphatic invasion, intraperitoneal implantation, hematogenous dissemination, and transdiaphragmatic passage. Intraperitoneal dissemination is the most common and recognized characteristic of ovarian cancer. Malignant cells can implant anywhere in the peritoneal cavity but are more likely to implant in sites of stasis along the peritoneal fluid circulation. These mechanisms of dissemination represent the rationale to conduct surgical staging, debulking surgery, and intraperitoneal administration of chemotherapy.

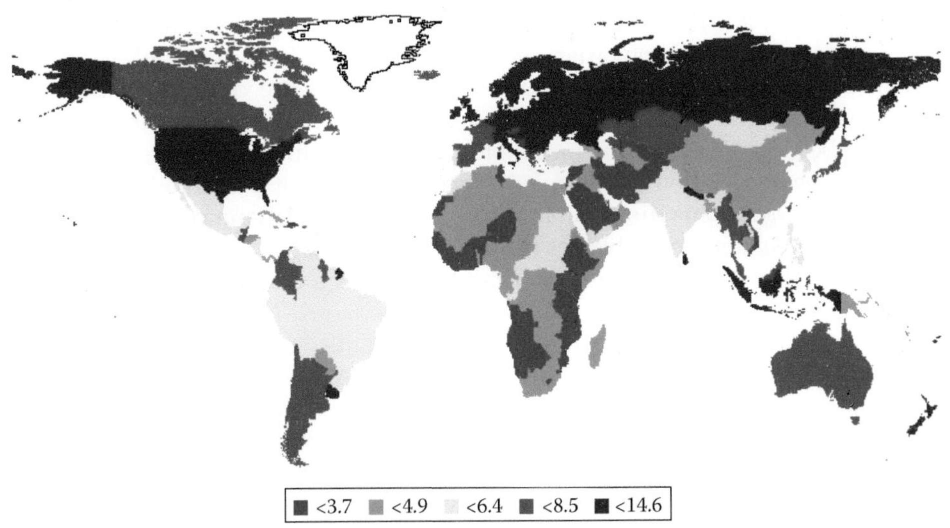

FIGURE 11.1
Reported ovarian cancer rates per 100,000 women (age standardized): The age-standardized incidence rates of ovarian cancer in year 2008 are shown. The highest incidence rates (>8 per 100,000) are reported in North America, Europe, and North Asia, and the lowest rates (<5 per 100,000) are reported in Africa, the Middle East, and China. (Data from GLOBOCAN 2008 (IARC) International Agency for Research on Cancer, World Health Organization.)

In contrast, hematogenous spread is clinically unusual early on in the disease process, although it is not infrequent in patients with advanced disease (Green et al. 2012).

According to histological specifications, ovarian cancers are heterogeneous. In histological classification, *epithelial ovarian carcinomas* are the most common form of ovarian cancers (Bunz 2008; Lalwani et al. 2011). This subtype of cancers develops from ovary's surface cells. It includes papillary serous cystadenocarcinoma, borderline adenocarcinoma, adenocarcinoma that is not otherwise specified, endometrioid tumor, serous cystadenocarcinoma, papillary, mucinous cystadenocarcinoma, clear-cell ovarian tumor, mucinous adenocarcinoma, and cystadenocarcinoma (Kosary 2007). These ovarian carcinoma subtypes may represent distinctive pathways of tumorigenesis and disease development. This distinction could potentially be reflected in the levels of tumor-produced factors that enter into the circulation and serve as biomarkers of malignant growth (Nolen et al. 2009).

11.1.4 Diagnosis and Treatment

Diagnosis of ovarian cancer starts with a physical examination, including a pelvic examination. Transvaginal ultrasound and CA-125, a blood test (sometimes other markers), can be supplementary. The diagnosis must be confirmed with surgery to inspect the abdominal cavity and which biopsies could be taken.

As ovarian cancer has nonspecific symptoms, that is, symptoms that are vague, often occur only after the cancer has spread, and can be misdiagnosed as being caused by other benign conditions, and it has no reliable biomarkers, its diagnosis frequently occurs at advanced disease stages. The presence of drug-resistant histological types limits the long-term cure rates and makes ovarian cancer the most lethal gynecologic malignancy (Lalwani et al. 2011; Morrison et al. 2012). In ovarian cancers, early detection is rare, and when it is detected, it has pelvic spread. It is mostly sporadic but has got familial cancer syndromes. With the emerging evidence that major ovarian carcinoma subtypes, including high-grade serous, clear cell, endometrioid, mucinous, and low-grade serous are distinct disease entities, subtype-specific diagnosis is important for the management of ovarian carcinoma. These subtypes can be identified based on morphological criteria differing with respect to genetic risk factors, precursor lesions, molecular alterations, stage at presentation, and clinical behavior. In addition to this differential diagnosis, there are differences in chemosensitivity among ovarian carcinoma subtypes (Kalloger et al. 2011).

Similar to other epithelial cancers, ovarian cancer has a distinctive pattern of spread, including intravascularly as well as through lymphatics. More frequently, however, ovarian cancer spreads over the peritoneal surface. While spreading by this way it produces nodules on the serosal and parietal peritoneum. At stage I, when cancer is limited to the ovaries, nearly 90% of patients can be cured with currently available treatment. Unfortunately at stages III–IV, when the disease spreads from the pelvis, less than 30% of patients survive in the long term. Detection of preclinical disease at an earlier stage in a larger fraction of patients might improve survival (Bast 2004).

Conventional treatment for ovarian cancer is to remove the uterus, ovaries, omentum, and lymph nodes in the pelvis and abdomen by surgery. Surgery is performed to remove as much of the cancer as possible and to stage the disease by assessing the spread of the cancer. As a treatment, surgery alone does not cure the disease since most women will have a widespread disease. Hence, chemotherapy, before or after the surgery, is necessary as a further treatment (Morrison et al. 2012).

In a common thought, ovarian carcinomas more frequently arise from surface epithelial cells. Patients suffer from the disease resulting in death because of the increasing recurrence rate in spite of actual therapy, including surgery and chemotherapy. Cancer researchers obviously look for new markers to use for oncological diagnosis and therapy that are specific to cancer stem cell (Oktem et al. 2012). In conclusion, there has been a call for subtype-specific clinical trials to identify more effective therapies for those cancers. In an effort to improve diagnostic accuracy, current studies are ongoing to determine whether an immunohistochemical panel of molecular markers could reproduce consensus subtype assignment (Kalloger et al. 2011).

TABLE 11.1

Five-Year Survival Rates for Epithelial Ovarian Carcinoma by *FIGO Stage*

Stage IA	87%
Stage IB	71%
Stage IC	79%
Stage IIA	67%
Stage IIB	55%
Stage IIC	57%
Stage IIIA	41%
Stage IIIB	25%
Stage IIIC	23%
Stage IV	11%
Overall survival rate	**46%**

Source: Green, A.E. et al., Ovarian cancer. Medscape Reference: Drugs, Diseases and Procedures, http://emedicine.medscape.com/article/255771-overview#a0104, medline, Updated: Sep 26, 2012.

11.1.5 Prognosis

Although the 5-year survival rate for ovarian cancer has improved significantly in the past 30 years, the prognosis for ovarian cancer remains poor overall, with a 46% 5-year survival rate (Table 11.1). The prognosis of ovarian cancer is closely related to the stage at diagnosis as determined according to the staging system developed by the International Federation of Gynecology and Obstetrics (FIGO) (look staging Table 11.1). Approximately 20%, 5%, 58%, and 17% of women present with stages I, II, III, and IV, respectively (Woodward et al. 2007; Chan et al. 2008).

11.2 Ovarian Endometrioid Carcinoma

Among epithelial ovarian carcinomas, endometrioid and serous subtypes account for the majority of malignant ovarian tumors (>75%) (Seidman and Kurman 2003). OEC is the second most common subtype of ovarian cancers (10%–20% of cases). It affects women during the fifth and sixth decades of life and is frequently associated with endometriosis (up to 42% of cases are associated with ipsilateral ovarian or pelvic endometriosis). In patients with hereditary nonpolyposis colorectal cancer (HNPCC) syndrome, it is the most common histological subtype of ovarian cancer (Lalwani et al. 2011).

Ovarian endometrioid carcinomas (OECs) are thought to arise through transformation of ovarian endometriosis. It is a common and typically benign disorder that is defined as the occurrence of ectopic endometrial tissue found aberrantly as part of the ovary (Madore et al. 2010).

Endometrioid carcinomas of the ovarian tumors are solid masses with predominant cystic forms. Ovarian endometrioid cells often resemble endometrial cells. These cells are characterized by the presence of epithelial elements, stromal elements, or a combination of both, mimicking the structure of endometrium. This evokes the endometriosis, which results in *retrograde menstruation*. Actually, this disease has been well documented in the literature to be associated with endometrioid ovarian cancer in 30%–40% of patients (Keita et al. 2011).

11.3 Different Noninvasive Molecular Biomarkers Currently Used and under Development for OEC

11.3.1 Genetic Biomarkers

As a genetic approach to ovarian carcinogenesis, it is a complex, multistep polychromosomal process. Different cytogenetic events lead to cancer initiation, growth, and progression. Each histological subtype of ovarian cancer is characterized by distinct histogenetic events and chromosomal abnormalities. The promotion of protooncogenes or the *silencing* of tumor suppression genes might be the initial pathogenesis of ovarian carcinoma (Lalwani et al. 2011).

Some pathways have been described to be the cause of OEC. A hypothetic model of the pathogenesis of malignant transformation of endometriosis has recently been described and explains the different oncologic mechanisms for different histological subtypes.

As possible causes of malignant transformation of endometriosis, epithelial hyperplasia and carcinogenesis under the influence of unopposed estrogen stimulation have been proposed for OEC (Mandai et al. 2009).

With recent advances in the field of histopathology and cytogenetic, Lalwani et al. (2011) have researched several studies regarding the pathophysiological features and natural history of ovarian cancer. In their review, they have shown that high- or low-grade serous, endometrioid, and clear-cell carcinomas are characterized by mutations involving the TP53, K-ras/BRAF, CTNNB1, and PIK3CA genes. They have mentioned the mutations of CTNNB1, PTEN, and PIK3CA at low-grade tumors and the mutations of TP53, BRCA1, and PIK3CA at high-grade tumors of OEC (Lalwani et al. 2011).

Recent advances in molecular techniques have introduced some molecular events that lead to ovarian carcinoma development. Yet, there is no molecular marker available that is generally accepted as a prognostic indicator. Besides the controversies (Zorn et al. 2009), studies are in progress. The mutation frequency of β-catenin in OEC ranges from 16% to 54%, and it is accepted as a molecular alteration in endometrioid carcinomas. Deregulation of β-catenin has been described to be caused by oncogenic mutation of the β-catenin gene (CTNNB1), mutations in the APC gene, or alterations of the Wnt signal transduction pathway. To assess the expression of β-catenin in endometrioid ovarian carcinoma, Rosen et al. (2010) have studied a total of 49 patients with primary OEC. They have reported that they had observed a low membranous expression of β-catenin and a high mitotic count, which were significantly associated with poor prognosis and early recurrence of OEC (Rosen et al. 2010).

The transcription factor Wilms' tumor-1 (WT1) is differentially expressed in epithelia and is considered to be a putative biomarker in epithelial ovarian carcinomas. Nuclear WT1 protein is observed in tubal and ovarian surface epithelia, but it is not expressed in endometrial epithelium. Although the majority of serous carcinomas exhibit nuclear WT1 protein aberrations, it is limited in OECs (0%–30% of the cases). So, WT1's efficacy as a biomarker is controversial.

Besides WT1, there are several genetic aberrations being investigated in epithelial ovarian carcinomas. The most well-documented mutations consist of the mutations of the TP53 gene, aberrant activation of β-catenin (CTNNB1) protein signaling, and loss of heterozygosity for the PTEN. As the gene mutation analyses are not perfectly concordant, it is unclear whether these aberrations are histotype specific. So, the controversy goes on to define the molecular characteristics of OEC and to address the aberrations with the current histopathological classification system (Madore et al. 2010).

Lowery et al. (2012) have reviewed and researched the subtypes of ovarian cancer. They have succeeded, although the studies based on population consistently identified endometriosis as a significant risk factor for the development of clear-cell and endometrioid cancers, yet there are no specific steps involved in the molecular pathogenesis of these cancers. They have reported that mutations in the KRAS, BRAF, PTEN, and β-catenin genes have a low frequency, but the ARID1A, a candidate tumor suppressor gene that encodes a member of the SWI/SNF family, is thought to be mutated in a significant portion of clear-cell and endometrioid ovarian cancers. They have also reported that while growth factor-A receptor type 2 mutations have been found just in clear-cell cancers, microsatellite instability is seen in both clear-cell and endometrioid ovarian cancers. In this review, Lowery has considered the biological interactions between inflammatory mediators, hormonal status, and intrinsic immunological variations as the factors of theories that are caused for malignancies. Additionally, they have validated the loss of immunohistochemically detectable BAF250a, the encoded protein that has got a strong and frequent correlation between mutation of the ARID1A gene. They have considered the finding of loss of BAF250a in atypical endometriosis adjacent suggesting to being an early event in the development of many of these cancers. They have advised researchers to determine whether this somatic event was associated with clinical features or epidemiological risk factors (Lowery et al. 2012).

Similar to current studies (Guan et al. 2011; Wiegand et al. 2011; Lowery et al. 2012), which have recently described the mutation of the ARID1A gene and loss of the corresponding protein BAF250a as a frequent event in clear-cell and endometrioid carcinomas of the ovary, Wiegand et al. (2011) have determined whether BAF250a loss is common in other malignancies. To determine this, immunohistochemistry for BAF250a was performed on tissue microarrays in more than 3000 cancers (including carcinomas of breast, lung, thyroid, endometrium, kidney, stomach, oral cavity, cervix, pancreas, colon, and rectum). Besides these malignancies, they have also researched endometrial stromal sarcomas, gastrointestinal stromal tumors, sex cord–stromal tumors, and major types of lymphomas. As a result, they reported that although they have found BAF250a loss in endometrial carcinomas at a frequent rate, it was infrequent in other types of malignancies and it might be considered as an early event in carcinogenesis. Since BAF250a loss is seen at similar rates in endometrial carcinomas and in ovarian carcinomas of clear-cell and endometrioid type, though it is uncommon in other malignancies, they have concluded that loss of BAF250a is a particular feature of carcinomas arising from endometrial glandular epithelium (Wiegand et al. 2011).

11.3.2 mRNA Studies

Inflammation is part of both physiological and pathological processes of epithelial remodeling of ovary and the endometrium. In this process, being a pro-inflammatory mediator, interleukin (IL)-1 is particularly involved in the modulation of a variety of ovary and endometrial functions. The ovary that has got cyclic ovulation function contains a complete IL-1 system. So, in this process, IL-1 appears as a key mediator of inflammation-associated ovulation process. In this gynecological site, IL-1 is produced locally in the endometrium, suggesting its potential role in the implantation and inflammatory-like processes. In addition, IL-1 also plays a role in epithelial ovarian carcinoma and in endometrial tumors. Since aberrant production of IL-1 by ectopic cells may promote a neoplastic transformation in the ovary, Keita et al. (2011) have examined whether expression of IL-1RI and IL-1RII at level of protein and mRNA was altered in endometrioid carcinoma cells in comparison with endometrial cells, clear cells, serous and mucinous ovarian cancer cells. They examined whether the alteration of IL-1Rs expression may provide molecular evidence for defective control of IL-1 as a key player in ovarian endometrioid carcinogenesis. They have analyzed the IL1-Rs expression at the levels of the protein and mRNA using immunofluorescent and real-time polymerase chain reaction methods, respectively. As a result, they have reported that endometrioid cells exhibit a specific decrease in IL-1RII expression, whereas IL-1RI was constantly expressed in all studied cell subtypes (Keita et al. 2011).

11.3.3 Microsatellite Instability/Loss of Heterozygosity Studies

Some counterparts of OEC arise from the uterine endometrium, so they have some similar somatic mutations. When compared with uterine EC, the OEC has a similar frequency of β-catenin (CTNNB1) mutations (38%–50% of cases) but a lower rate of microsatellite instability (up to 19%) and PTEN mutations (occur between exons 3 and 8) (20%). The mutations of CTNNB1, which have been described in exon 3 (codons 32, 33, 37, and 41), involve the phosphorylation sequence for glycogen synthase kinase 3-β. In a way these mutations likely represent early genetic events in the pathogenesis of OEC. Gilks and Prat (2009) also noted that PTEN mutations and 10q23 loss of heterozygosity are seen in endometriosis associated with OECs, which represent early oncologic events (Gilks and Prat 2009).

Mutations in a number of genes, including K-ras, BRAF, PTEN, and CTNNB1 (β-catenin) but especially involving the CTNNB1 and PTEN genes and microsatellite instability, are commonly seen in low-grade early-stage OECs, which originate from borderline tumors or endometriosis with a good prognosis. Among these mutations, K-ras activation and PTEN dysfunction are specific for OECs. Besides, p53 mutations or overexpression, which is seen in high-grade OECs patients, shows poor prognosis (Kobayashi 2009).

11.3.4 Proteomics Studies

All the authorities suggested that the different histological subtypes, including clear cell, endometrioid, mucinous, and serous subtype, of ovarian carcinoma have distinct clinical histories and characteristics. Every researcher aimed to determine specific biomarker, but most of the studies have not performed comprehensive analyses based on subtype specificity. Toyoma et al. (2012), using tissue specimens from 39 patients of ovarian carcinoma of the different histological subtypes, have performed 2D gel electrophoresis–based differential proteomic analysis. By using a 34 additional test sample, they have validated these candidates by Western blotting. They have observed the expression pattern consistent with the screening. They have reported 77 protein spots to be up- or downregulated in a subtype-specific manner. They have pointed out the aberrations of annexin-A4 (ANXA4), phosphoserine aminotransferase (PSAT1), cellular retinoic acid–binding protein 2 (CRABP2), and serpin B5 (SPB5) as the most significant differences that were observed (Toyama et al. 2012).

11.3.5 Genomic Stability Studies

Aurora kinase A (AURKA), a serine/threonine kinase, has been shown to regulate the cell cycle checkpoint and maintain genomic integrity. It is overexpressed in various carcinomas. Being a tumor suppressor gene, BRCA2 has an important role in maintaining genomic stability. Yang et al. (2011), in their recent study, have suggested that AURKA regulates genomic instability and tumorigenesis through cell cycle dysregulation and suppression of BRCA2 expression. In that study, they determined AURKA and BRCA2 expression in endometrioid ovarian carcinoma and correlated them with clinicopathological characteristics and patient survival. They performed immunohistochemical staining in 51 primary endometrioid ovarian carcinoma tumor samples and then analyzed the associations between AURKA and BRCA2 expression and clinical factors and observed the expressions of AURKA and BRCA2 as 48% and 29% of the samples, respectively. In conclusion, they have reported that they have also observed a negative regulatory loop exists between AURKA and BRCA2 expression in the OEC. They added that while their results about AURKA expression were unfavorable and BRCA2 was a favorable prognostic factor in the OEC, combination of these two markers might give a better prediction for the prognosis of patients with endometrioid ovarian carcinoma than individual marker alone (Yang et al. 2011).

11.3.6 Phosphorylated Genes Studies

Amsterdam et al. (2011) have examined the possibility that the localization of phosphorylated ERK1 and ERK2 (pERK1/2) can serve as a marker for the development of benign and borderline tumors as well as carcinoma of the ovary by an immunohistochemical method on ovarian paraffin sections, obtained from women aged 41–83 years. They have reported that they have found a very intensive labeling in 77.3% cells of endometrioid ovarian carcinomas. According to the results, they have suggested that since nuclear pERK1/2 could be mitogenic, it could serve as a reliable marker for the progression of ovarian cancer. It was interesting for them to observe the intense labeling of pERK1/2 being confined to the peripheral areas of OEC. As a conclusion, they have reported that immunohistochemical staining of normal and ovarian tumor cells with anti-pERK1/2 is a reliable marker for early detection of the cancer, which might assist in the early diagnosis and prognosis of this lethal disease (Amsterdam 2011).

11.3.7 Microarray Studies

Carbonic anhydrase IX (CAIX) is a strictly membranous expressed metalloenzyme involved in cell adhesion, pH homeostasis, and cancer progression. Choschzick et al. (2011) have analyzed tissue microarray of 205 well-characterized primary ovarian carcinomas to assess the role of CAIX in primary ovarian cancer by immunohistochemistry using a four-step scoring system. They have observed high levels of CAIX expression to be related to mucinous and endometrioid phenotype of ovarian carcinomas while there was no association between CAIX overexpression and tumor stage, grading, and mitotic count of ovarian carcinomas. In conclusion, they have reported that CAIX was overexpressed in a main proportion of mucinous and endometrioid ovarian carcinomas and related to poor patient outcome (Choschzick et al. 2011).

11.3.8 Circulating Antigen as a Biomarker: CA-125

Serum CA-125 levels could be used clinically for patients with endometrial cancer as it has been presented as a circulating antigen in patients with epithelial ovarian cancer. Higher serum CA-125 levels correlate with stage or histopathological factors and the clinical utility of serum CA-125 measurements could be useful in predicting extrauterine disease. At present, CA-125 appears to be a significant independent predictor of extrauterine spread of disease and has been shown to be a better predictor of disease than depth of invasion or grade. Yildiz et al. (2012) have studied 147 women with pathologically proven endometrial carcinoma to evaluate whether a preoperative serum CA-125 level in patients with endometrial carcinoma could provide additional information in determining the stage of disease and which cutoff value was optimal in this respect. They have also examined the associations of preoperative CA-125 levels with the tumor stage, histological type and grade, and the lymph node positivity. They have compared the levels of 20 and 35 IU/mL of serum tumor marker CA-125 to determine the values of the cutoff point. In conclusion, they have reported that high CA-125 levels significantly correlated with advanced stage and lymph node metastases (Yildiz et al. 2012).

Besides the aforementioned study, there are some other approaches for serum CA-125 levels. Elevated CA-125 levels could be detected in only half of patients of ovarian cancers with stages I–II. As it is not satisfactory for identification of ovarian cancers, more sensitive and specific biomarkers or biomarker panels are needed. For this purpose Nosov et al. (2009) have analyzed protein profiles using surface enhanced laser desorption and ionization time-of-flight mass spectroscopy and identified three differentially expressed serum proteins for the detection of ovarian cancer: apolipoprotein A-1 (ApoA-1), transthyretin (TTR), and transferrin (TF) combined with CA-125. The objectives of their study were to assess the effectiveness of the panel in the detection of early-stage serous and endometrioid ovarian cancers. As a result, they have reported that when combined with CA-125, a panel of four serum biomarkers effectively detected early-stage ovarian cancers with the highest reported overall sensitivity of 96% and among them the highest sensitivity was seen for the detection of endometrioid subtype of early-stage carcinomas (98%) (Nosov et al. 2009).

All the studies about biomarkers in OECs (3.1–3.8) are summarized in Table 11.2.

TABLE 11.2

Summary of Biomarkers in Ovarian Endometrioid Carcinoma

Group and Study	Comment
Genetic biomarkers	
Lalwani et al. (2011)	
• CTNNB1, PTEN, PIK3CA mutations	• At low-grade tumors
• TP53, BRCA1, PIK3CA mutations	• At high-grade tumors
Rosen et al. (2010)	
Low membranous expression of β-catenin and a high mitotic count	Poor prognosis and early recurrence risk
Madore et al. (2010)	Efficacy as a biomarker is controversial
WT1 protein aberrations, mutations of TP53, aberrant activation of β-catenin (CTNNB1), and loss of heterozygosity for the PTEN	It is unclear whether these aberrations are histotype specific
Lowery et al. (2012)	
The loss of BAF250a protein correlated with mutation of the ARID1A gene	Early event in the development of cancers
Wiegand et al. (2011)	
Loss of BAF250a	Early event in carcinogenesis
mRNA studies	
Keita et al. (2011)	
Pro-inflammatory mediator, interleukin (IL)-1	Specific decrease in IL-1RII expression
Microsatellite instability/loss of heterozygosity studies	
Gilks and Prat (2009)	
PTEN mutations and 10q23 loss of heterozygosity	Represent early oncologic events
Kobayashi (2009)	
CTNNB1 and PTEN mutations and microsatellite instability	In low-grade early-stage tumors
Proteomics studies	
Toyoma et al. (2012)	
Aberrations of annexin-A4 (ANXA4), phosphoserine aminotransferase (PSAT1), cellular retinoic acid–binding protein 2 (CRABP2), and serpin B5 (SPB5)	Among 77 protein up- or downregulated, the most significant difference was observed for these aberrations
Genomic stability studies	
Yang et al. (2011)	
AURKA, BRCA2 expressions, and the association between them	AURKA unfavorable and BRCA2 favorable but combination might give better prediction
Phosphorylated genes studies	
Amsterdam et al. (2011)	
Phosphorylated ERK1 and ERK2 (pERK1/2)	Reliable marker for early detection
Microarray studies	
Choschzick et al. (2011)	
Carbonic anhydrase IX (CAIX)	Overexpression is related to poor outcome
Circulating antigen as a biomarker: CA-125	
Yildiz et al. (2012)	
Serum CA-125 levels	Significantly correlated with advanced stage and lymph node metastases
Nosov et al. (2009)	
Apolipoprotein A-1 (ApoA-1), transthyretin (TTR), and transferrin (TF) combined with CA-125	A panel of four serum biomarkers effectively detected early stage

11.4 Conclusion and Future Direction

As a conclusion there has been a call for subtype-specific clinical trials, to identify more effective therapies for those cancers. In an effort to improve diagnostic accuracy, current studies are going on to set out to determine if an immunohistochemical panel of molecular markers could reproduce consensus subtype assignment (Kalloger et al. 2011).

The goal of molecular studies is to determine disease heterogeneity. Although there are some advances about molecular and epidemiological etiology of ovarian cancer, survival of the disease is still poor. No effective strategy has been identified yet for early detection of this cancer (Lowery et al. 2012).

In ovarian cancers, the mechanisms of transformation of normal cell lines to malignancy have not been completely elucidated yet. So mutations in several oncogenes and tumor suppressor genes are still suspicious molecular targets for identification of this cancer (Lowery et al. 2012). Understanding the mechanisms of the development of ovarian cancer and elucidating its pathogenesis and pathophysiology are intrinsic to prevent the disease and to search for effective therapies.

As a genetic approach to ovarian carcinogenesis, it is a complex, multistep polychromosomal process. Different cytogenetic events lead to cancer initiation, growth, and progression. Each histological subtype of ovarian cancer is characterized by distinct histogenetic events and chromosomal abnormalities. The promotion of protooncogenes or the *silencing* of tumor suppression genes might be the initial pathogenesis of ovarian carcinoma (Lalwani et al. 2011). Early detection of ovarian cancer could have a major impact on the disease. Two-stage strategies are likely to be most effective. Multiple serum markers will be needed for an optimal initial stage besides other medical screening strategies.

The studies that have the notion to detect the ovarian cancer subtypes on a molecular basis and that have the aim to develop candidate subtype-specific biomarkers that can help to define the basis of tumor histology at a molecular level are needed. For effective screening of ovarian cancer, some biological studies are needed. Several studies have documented that most ovarian cancers must be clonal. Multiple genetic changes are required for the transformation of ovarian surface epithelial cells to ovarian cancer. Substantial heterogeneity has been observed in the pattern of alterations in oncogenes and tumor suppressor genes among ovarian cancers. New and more studies will be needed to detect ovarian cancers at an early stage.

Gene expression array analysis, proteomics, and lipomics are being utilized to identify markers that can be used in combination with current markers. The sequential use of multiple markers and other medical screening techniques could provide a cost-effective strategy to detect a disease of intermediate prevalence. With the success of current strategies, ovarian cancer screening will develop. A better understanding of human genetics should identify individuals at increased risk, facilitating cost-effective screening. In the future, with the advances of technology, detecting cancer diseases at an early stage will almost certainly accelerate.

References

American Cancer Society, Cancer Facts and Figures 2009. Available at http://www.cancer.org/downloads/STT/500809 web.pdf. Accessed January 25, 2010.

Amsterdam, A., E. Shezen, C. Raanan, L. Schreiber, D. Prus, Y. Slilat, A. ben-arie, and R. Seger. 2011. Nuclear localization of phosphorylated ERK1 and ERK2 as markers for the progression of ovarian cancer. *Int J Oncol* 39:649–656, doi: 10.3892/ijo.2011.1090.

Bast, R.C. Jr. 2004. Early detection of ovarian cancer: New technologies in pursuit of a disease that is neither common nor rare. *Trans Am Clin Climatol Assoc* 115:233–248.

Bunz, F. (ed.) 2008. Chapter 6 Genetic alternations in common cancers: Ovarian cancer. *Principles of Cancer Genetics,* pp. 242–243. Springer Science.

Chan, J.K., D. Teoh, J.M. Hu, J.Y. Shin, K. Osann, and D.S. Kapp. 2008. Do clear cell ovarian carcinomas have poorer prognosis compared to other epithelial cell types? A study of 1411 clear cell ovarian cancers. *Gynecol Oncol* June 2008 109(3):370–376.

Choschzick, M., E. Oosterwijk, V. Müller, L. Woelber, R. Simon, H. Moch, and P. Tennstedt. 2011. Overexpression of carbonic anhydrase IX (CAIX) is an independent unfavorable prognostic marker in endometrioid ovarian cancer. *Virchows Archiv* 459 (2):193–200. doi: 10.1007/s00428-011-1105-y.

Gilks, C.B. and J. Prat. 2009. Ovarian carcinoma pathology and genetics: Recent advances. *Hum Pathol* 40(9):1213–1223. doi: 10.1016/j.humpath.2009.04.017.

GLOBOCAN 2008 (IARC), International Agency for Research on Cancer, World Health Organization. http://globocan.iarc.fr.

Green A.E., A.A. Garcia, and S. Ahmed. 2012. Ovarian cancer. *Medscape Reference: Drugs, Diseases and Procedures,* http://emedicine.medscape.com/article/255771-overview#a0104, medline, Updated: September 26, 2012.

Guan, B., T.-L. Mao, P.K. Panuganti, E. Kuhn, R.J. Kurman, D. Maeda, E. Chen, Y.-M. Jeng, T.-L. Wang, and I.-M. Shih. 2011. Mutation and loss of expression of ARID1A in uterine low-grade endometrioid carcinoma. *Am J Surg Pathol* 35(5):625–632.

Kalloger, S.E., M. Köbel, S. Leung, E. Mehl, D. Gao, K.M. Marcon, C. Chow, B.A. Clarke, D.G. Huntsman, and C.B. Gilks. 2011. Calculator for ovarian carcinoma subtype prediction. *Mod Pathol* 24(4):512–521.

Keita, M., Y. AinMelk, M. Pelmus, P. Bessette, and A. Aris. 2011. Endometrioid ovarian cancer and endometriotic cells exhibit the same alteration in the expression of interleukin-1 receptor II: To a link between endometriosis and endometrioid ovarian cancer. *J Obstet Gynaecol Res* 37(2):99–107. doi: 10.1111/j.1447-0756.2010.01320.x.

Kobayashi, H. 2009. Ovarian cancer in endometriosis: Epidemiology, natural history, and clinical diagnosis. *Int J Clin Oncol* 14(5):378–382. doi: 10.1007/s10147-009-0931-2.

Kosary, C.L. 2007. Chapter 16: Cancers of the ovary. *SEER Survival Monograph: Cancer Survival Among Adults: US SEER Program, 1988–2001, Patient and Tumor Characteristics,* pp. 133–144. no. SEER Program. NIH Pub. No. 07-6215. National Cancer Institute.

Lalwani, N., S.R. Prasad, R. Vikram, A.K. Shanbhogue, P.C. Huettner, and N. Fasih. 2011. Histologic, molecular, and cytogenetic features of ovarian cancers: Implications for diagnosis and treatment. *Radiographics* 31(3):625–646. doi: 10.1148/rg.313105066.

Lowery, W.J., J.M. Schildkraut, L. Akushevich, R. Bentley, J.R. Marks, D. Huntsman, and A. Berchuck. 2012. Loss of ARID1A-associated protein expression is a frequent event in clear cell and endometrioid ovarian cancers. *Int J Gynecol Cancer* 22(1):9–14.

Madore, J., F. Ren, A. Filali-Mouhim, L. Sanchez, M. Kobel, P.N. Tonin, D. Huntsman, D.M. Provencher, and A.M. Mes-Masson. 2010. Characterization of the molecular differences between ovarian endometrioid carcinoma and ovarian serous carcinoma. *J Pathol* 220(3):392–400. doi: 10.1002/path.2659.

Mandai, M., K. Yamaguchi, N. Matsumura, T. Baba, and I. Konishi. 2009. Ovarian cancer in endometriosis: Molecular biology, pathology, and clinical management. *Int J Clin Oncol* 14(5):383–391. doi: 10.1007/s10147-009-0935-y.

Morrison, J., K. Haldar, S. Kehoe, and T.A. Lawrie. 2012. Chemotherapy versus surgery for initial treatment in advanced ovarian epithelial cancer. *Cochrane Gynaecological Cancer Group Copyright © 2012 The Cochrane Collaboration.* John Wiley & Sons, Ltd. Published online: August 15, 2012; assessed as up-to-date: June 21, 2012. doi: 10.1002/14651858.CD005343.pub3.

Nolen, B., A. Marrangoni, L. Velikokhatnaya, D. Prosser, M. Winans, E. Gorelik, and A. Lokshin. 2009. A serum based analysis of ovarian epithelial tumorigenesis. *Gynecol Oncol* 112(1):47–54. doi: 10.1016/j.ygyno.2008.09.043.

Nosov, V., F. Su, M. Amneus, M. Birrer, T. Robins, J. Kotlerman, S. Reddy, and R. Farias-Eisner. 2009. Validation of serum biomarkers for detection of early-stage ovarian cancer. *Am J Obstet Gynecol* 200(6):639 e1–e5. doi: 10.1016/j.ajog.2008.12.042.

Oktem, G., M. Sanci, A. Bilir, Y. Yildirim, S.D. Kececi, S. Ayla, and S. Inan. 2012. Cancer stem cell and embryonic development-associated molecules contribute to prognostic significance in ovarian cancer. *Int J Gynecol Cancer* 22(1):23–29.

Rosen, D.G., Z. Zhang, B. Chang, X. Wang, E. Lin, and J. Liu. 2010. Low membranous expression of beta-catenin and high mitotic count predict poor prognosis in endometrioid carcinoma of the ovary. *Mod Pathol* 23(1):113–122.

Seidman, J.D. and Kurman, R.J. 2003. Pathology of ovarian carcinoma. *Hematol Oncol Clin North Am* 17(4):909–925, vii.

Toyama, A., A. Suzuki, T. Shimada, C. Aoki, Y. Aoki, Y. Umino, Y. Nakamura, D. Aoki, and T. A. Sato. 2012. Proteomic characterization of ovarian cancers identifying annexin-A4, phosphoserine aminotransferase, cellular retinoic acid-binding protein 2, and serpin B5 as histology-specific biomarkers. *Cancer Sci* 103(4):747–755. doi: 10.1111/j.1349-7006.2012.02224.x.

Ucar, T. and M. Bekar 2010. Türkiye'de ve Dünyada Jinekolojik Kanserler. *Türk Jinekolojik Onkoloji Dergisi.* no. Haziran 2010, Cilt 13, (Sayı 3,):Sayfa 55–60.

Wiegand, K.C., A.F. Lee, O.M. Al-Agha, C. Chow, S.E. Kalloger, D.W. Scott, C. Steidl, S.M. Wiseman, R.D. Gascoyne, B. Gilks, and D.G. Huntsman. 2011. Loss of BAF250a (ARID1A) is frequent in high-grade endometrial carcinomas. *J Pathol* 224(3):328–333.

Woodward, E.R., H.V. Sleightholme, A.M. Considine, S. Williamson, J.M. McHugo, and D.G. Cruger. 2007. Annual surveillance by CA125 and transvaginal ultrasound for ovarian cancer in both high-risk and population risk women is ineffective. *BJOG* December 2007 114(12):1500–1509.

Yang, F., X. Guo, G. Yang, D.G. Rosen, and J. Liu. 2011. AURKA and BRCA2 expression highly correlate with prognosis of endometrioid ovarian carcinoma. *Mod Pathol* 24(6):836–845. doi: 10.1038/modpathol.2011.44.

Yildiz, A., H. Yetimalar, B. Kasap, C. Aydin, S. Tatar, F. Soylu, and F.S. Yildiz. 2012. Preoperative serum CA 125 level in the prediction of the stage of disease in endometrial carcinoma. *Eur J Obstet Gynecol Reprod Biol* 16(2):191–195. doi: 10.1016/j.ejogrb.2012.05.038.

Zorn, K.K., C. Tian, W.P. McGuire, W.J. Hoskins, M. Markman, F.M. Muggia, P.G. Rose, R.F. Ozols, D. Spriggs, and D.K. Armstrong. 2009. The prognostic value of pretreatment CA 125 in patients with advanced ovarian carcinoma: A Gynecologic Oncology Group study. *ACS–Cance,* 115(5):1028–1035.

12

MUC16/CA125: A Candidate Tumor Marker for Diagnosis and Therapy in Ovarian Cancer

Houda Bouanene, PhD, and Jemni Ben Chibani, PhD

CONTENTS

ABSTRACT MUC16 (CA125) protein is a high-molecular-weight mucin overexpressed in the majority of epithelial ovarian cancers (EOCs) but not in the epithelium of normal ovaries suggesting a central role in EOC pathogenesis. Several lines of evidence point toward the involvement of MUC16 in many physiological mechanisms such as adhesion, migration, and invasion. The isolation, composition, structure, molecular characteristics, and functional relevance of MUC16/CA125 and its constituents are discussed in relation to recent advancements as an exciting target for a specific cancer immunotherapy. MUC16-based therapeutic cancer vaccines are currently under clinical investigation. More detailed knowledge of the protein and oligosaccharide structures of MUC16/CA125 will be important in identifying specific role(s) in health and disease. Throughout this review, we have emphasized biochemical and immunological properties of MUC16 that make this tumor-associated antigen a novel, attractive, and tangible target for tumor immunotherapy.

12.1 Introduction

Epithelial ovarian cancer (EOC) has the highest mortality rate of the cancers unique to women. Membrane mucins have several functions in epithelial cells, including cytoprotection, extravasation during metastases, and maintenance of luminal structure and signal transduction [1]. Despite the achievements of high response rates with surgery followed by chemotherapy [2,3], 75% of women ultimately die of complications associated with disease progression. Although studies show that the survival of early-stage disease is significantly higher than those with advanced cancers, approximately 20%–30% of these patients will die of their disease [4–6]. The molecular mechanisms underlying the metastatic process of this cancer are not well understood. One family of cell-associated and secreted glycoproteins, the mucin glycoproteins, has been implicated in events leading to metastasis of several epithelial cancers [7]. Recently, mucins have attracted interest as potential targets for immunotherapy of cancers of several organs, including the ovaries. MUC16 mucin with its special properties and complex biochemical structure and fascinating function may well be a candidate for developing immunotherapy/vaccines for ovarian cancer. This review focuses on the role and regulation of MUC16/CA125 by emphasizing the biochemical and immunological properties of MUC16 that make this tumor-associated antigen a novel, attractive, and tangible target for tumor immunotherapy.

12.1.1 General Properties of *Mucins*

Mucins are macromolecules laying the cells in contact with the external environment. Human mucins contribute to mucociliary defense, an innate immune defense system that protects the airways against pathogens and environmental toxins [8]. Mucins are the main components of mucus and are synthesized and secreted by specialized cells of the epithelium (goblet cells, cells of mucous glands) or non-mucin-secreting cells. Human mucin genes show common features: large size of their mRNAs, large nucleotide tandem repeat (TR), and complex expression at both tissular and cellular level [9]. Mucins are highly glycosylated macromolecules (≥50% carbohydrate, wt/wt). Mucin protein backbones are characterized by numerous TRs that contain proline and are high in serine and/or threonine residues, the sites of O-glycosylation [8]. Currently, there are 20 known mucins that have been structurally and functionally divided into two distinct classes: secreted mucins and membrane-bound mucins [10]. The first one is made of the five, large, secreted, gel-forming mucins MUC6, MUC2, MUC5AC, MUC5B, and MUC19 that form oligomeric structures. The other family is made of membrane-tethered mucins. Like secreted mucins, membrane-bound mucins are made of at least a mucin-like domain, that is, a large portion made of TRs enriched in proline residues and in hydroxy amino acids that carry the *O*-glycans. The membrane-bound mucins may be subdivided into two distinct groups: small mucins and large mucins [11]. In the airways, secreted mucins (e.g., MUC5AC and MUC5B) are the key for mucociliary clearance, and transmembrane mucins (e.g., MUC1 and MUC4) contribute to glycocalyx barrier function [8,12].

12.1.2 Mucin Expression in Normal and Cancerous Ovarian Tissues

Mucin genes are independently regulated and their expression is organ and cell type specific [13]. The secreted and transmembrane mucins that constitute the mucous barrier are largely unrecognized as effectors of carcinogenesis. However, both types of mucins are intimately involved in inflammation and cancer [14]. Aberrations in expression of mucin glycoproteins have been observed during malignant transformation of human ovarian epithelium [1]. EOCs expressed several mucins including MUC1, MUC2,

MUC4, and MUC5AC; MUC3 and MUC5B were rarely expressed [7]. MUC1 is one of the early hallmarks of tumorigenesis and is overexpressed and underglycosylated on almost all human epithelial cell adenocarcinomas [15]. It is expressed on the surface of ovarian cancer cells [16]. A high expression of MUC1 may contribute to a poor prognosis in ovarian carcinoma [1]. The underglycosylated MUC1 epitopes are expressed by all histotypes of primary ovarian adenocarcinomas, by the vast majority of metastatic lesions, and by possible ovarian cancer precursor lesions, but not by normal ovarian tissue [17]. MUC2 is a secretory mucin that is normally expressed mainly in the colon and rectum. MUC2 expression also has been used in the differential diagnosis of ovarian tumors [18]. To date, several mucins have been identified to be involved in ovarian cancer of which the most undisputed one is MUC16. This mucin is expressed at the apical surface of coelomic epithelia and its derivatives including epithelial cells in the Mullerian duct, fallopian tube, endometrium, endocervix, and mesothelial cells lining the peritoneal and pleural cavities [19–21]. MUC16 has been shown to provide a protective barrier for the epithelial surface from bacterial adherence [22] and mechanical injury [23]. Furthermore, MUC16 in the endometrium of the uterus has been shown to prevent the attachment of trophoblast during nonreceptive status [24]. However, for each tissue, specific and unique molecule appears to be implicated in a different manner. It is conceivable that this molecule may have different properties in each either in normal or in pathological conditions.

12.2 Molecular Biology and Biochemical Structure of MUC16

Although hampered by the complexity of the molecule from both the proteomic and glycomic perspectives and the difficulties inherent in working with a molecule of its size and repetitive nature, numerous studies provided structural and molecular analysis of MUC16/CA125. Elucidation of the molecular nature of CA125 may help to explore its potential as a diagnostic marker. A deep knowledge of the CA125 molecule is required to examine whether some of its biochemical characteristics, like glycosylation, could allow the distinction of CA125 from normal and tumor origins and, therefore, be useful in developing new ovarian cancer markers.

The antigen CA125/MUC16 was first recognized by the murine monoclonal antibody OC125 by Bast et al. [25]. The identity of the moieties with which OC125 reacts must await the outcome of further biochemical analyses. The cancer antigen CA125 has been defined as a marker primarily for ovarian carcinoma [26]. In 2001, O'Brien et al. [27] and Yin and Lloyd [28] provided tools for further studies by elucidating the feature of CA125 through the cloning of the corresponding gene. These studies highlighted the main characteristics of this tumor marker that are as follows: CA125 is encoded by the gene MUC16 that corresponds to an extracellular superstructure dominated by repeat sequences. The previously mentioned research groups revealed that CA125 is a membrane protein with some splice variants sharing the same intracellular and transmembrane regions. The primary structure of CA125 elucidated that it represents a giant mucin-like glycoprotein with an average molecular weight between 2.5 and 5 million Da [27]. These findings make a genomic insight into the CA125, the main tumor marker routinely used in the management of ovarian cancer. The MUC16 has been mapped to the chromosome 19 p13.3. It has been reported to show that CA125 molecule is composed of a glycosylated N-terminal domain that has been proposed to be made up of 13,000 amino acids, a large glycosylated TR domain (of 156 amino acids each), and a cytoplasmic domain, and there is a typically high content of proline, serine, and threonine [28]. The CA125 extracellular domain consists of the sea urchin sperm protein, enterokinase, and agrin (SEA) domains repeated 7, 12, or 60 times, according to the variant. SEA domains consist of about 120 residues, of which about 80 residues are highly conserved and were first identified in SEA [29]. Accumulated experimental evidence has shown that CA125 resides on a molecule of very complex architecture in terms of both protein backbone and oligosaccharide structures [27,30]. Based on these results, intense researches on MUC16 began. Owing to the technical problems associated with deglycosylation of mucins, the biochemical characterization of the protein backbone and the linked glycans has been fraught with difficulties [30].

The interest in functional proteomics has motivated a number of approaches toward systems-wide analysis of posttranslational modifications. Unfortunately, the proteomic analysis of mucin-type O-linked glycosylation, such as CA125/MUC16, has been difficult due to the complexity and microheterogeneity of *O*-linked glycans and lack of general reagents for efficient enrichment and recovery [31]. The identification of MUC16 with proteomics is difficult due to its large size and the presence of the dense O-glycosylation. The core protein is extremely large and highly substituted with oligosaccharides, which only allow access to a highly restricted portion of the protein and block the use of these parts of the molecule for protein identification. The problem is primarily due to the difficulty in removing *O*-glycans while keeping both the protein and glycans intact. In contrast to N-glycosylation, there is no single enzyme capable of complete O-deglycosylation, so chemical methods must be employed.

As with all other glycoproteins, the carbohydrate components were not generally analyzed in the context of their sequence location, principally due to the experimental difficulty in identifying and isolating glycopeptides containing specific glycosylation sites. Instead, carbohydrate has been released by endoglycosidases, hydrazinolysis, or reductive elimination, thereby losing the sequence context of the glycan structures. A number of rigorous biophysical analyses were used for the identification of N- and O-linked glycopeptides of MUC16/CA125 and provided an exhaustive analysis of CA125 glycans derived from epithelial ovarian tumor cells. Complete structural analysis of the CA125 molecule requires sequencing of its oligosaccharides and localization of its glycosylation sites [30]. These efforts yield the major core structures identified in glycans isolated from MUC16 indicating that the *N*-linked glycans are primarily high-mannose and bisecting-type *N*-linked glycans including Man5-Man9GlcNAc2. As for O-glycosylation, the oligosaccharides linked to CA125 present unusual features such as the expression of branched core 1 antennae (Galβ1–3GalNAc) in the core type 2 glycan (Galβ1–3GlcNAcβ(1-6)GalNAc) [30]. Several subspecies of CA125 were described [32]; however, it is not known whether any of the CA125 subspecies is linked to specific physical conditions. Based on the newly available tools, rapid advances began to clarify the role of MUC16 and the pathways by which this tumor marker with its glycans are tightly involved in the development and dissemination of ovarian cancer. An understanding of the signal and recognitive properties of CA125–oligosaccharide epitopes is an initial step that may have significant biomedical implications in creating a strategy to modify the carbohydrate-dependent interactions of CA125. A deeper knowledge of the CA125 molecule is required to examine whether some of its biochemical characteristics, like glycosylation, could allow the distinction of CA125 from normal and tumor origins. Since the carbohydrate side chains modulate the interaction of the protein with its environment, influencing its solubility, activity, and biologic fate and getting insights and understanding of altered glycosylation of CA125 will offer a brand-new vision in modifying cancer behavior and treating this lethal disease in the future. In this context, it is important to note that the binding patterns of both *N*- and *O*-linked glycan-reactive lectins indicated distinct differences in carbohydrate composition between CA125 antigen isolated from amniotic fluid and human ovarian carcinoma (OVCAR-3) cell line [33]. In other physiological conditions, the CA125 shows heterogeneous structure, existing in different glycoisoforms with subtle differences in the profile of molecular forms in comparison to placental tissue-derived and cancer-derived CA125 antigen [34]. Thus, the glycan structure is determined not only by the nature of the protein it is bound to but also by the tissue or cell where it is made [35].

12.3 Regulation of CA125/MUC16 at the Molecular Level and Biological Role in Tumorigenesis

It is known that CA125 antigen can vary widely in molecular mass, depending on the biological source of the antigen and the physiological condition in which it is expressed [36]. Clearly, there are a number of major modifications affecting the CA125; principal among these are the gene expression [37], the posttranslational modifications mainly the glycosylation, and the morphology that reflects the biochemical properties that are different under diverse physiological conditions [38,39].

12.3.1 Overexpression of MUC16 in Ovarian Cancer Tissue

Interestingly and yet unexplained, the level of MUC16 expression is dramatically changed during ovarian cancer transformation. This alteration can be achieved transcriptionally through tissue-specific or cell type–specific promoters that lead to the production of mRNA species that diverge in the 5′-untranslated region [40]. The most recent mRNA sequence available for CA125 (AF414442) exceeds 66 kb and resolves to 84 exons spanning over 130 kb of genomic DNA. The CA125 mRNA was first characterized as a 5.8 kb transcript [28] before 5′ additions extended the sequence to its present form [27,41].

A previous study has shown that MUC16 mRNA is overexpressed in ovarian cancer tissues compared with nonmalignant or benign tissue, but how CA125 production is regulated at the mRNA level is unclear [37]. The altered expression of MUC16 supports the gene's potential role, at least in part, in the pathogenesis of ovarian cancer and possibly in other types of cancer. For a better understanding of changes in gene expression during ovarian tumorigenesis and the identification of specific tumor markers that may lead to novel strategies for diagnosis and therapy for this disease, Rangel et al. identified five novel serial analysis of gene expression (SAGE) tags specifically expressed in ovarian cancer; among them was HOST1 that was found to be identical to the gene encoding ovarian marker CA125 (MUC16) [42]. The overexpression of MUC16 in ovarian cancer tissue was not disturbed alone; it was accompanied by a heterogeneous level of some sialyltransferases as a consequence of oncogenic transformation of the ovary. A change in sialyltransferase activity in the disease may alter MUC16 glycosylation [37] and, thus, the physical character of the mucin's extracellular domain. The high level of MUC16 overexpression in ovarian cancer and its role as an oncogene make it an ideal molecular target for novel therapies.

12.3.2 Phenotypic Consequences of the Glycosylation of CA125

Mucin has been difficult to characterize, owing to its large molecular weight, polydispersity, and high degree of glycosylation. The large size of mucin has, on the other hand, turned out to be of great advantage in imaging the molecule directly [43]. Earlier transmission electron micrographic studies by Fiebrig et al. [44] revealed long fibers approximately 400 nm long in pig gastric mucin (PGM). More recent atomic force microscopy (AFM) studies of ocular mucin [45] show individual fibers with a broad distribution of contour lengths. Round et al. [46] correlated the conformations with differing amounts of glycosylation by imaging different fractions obtained on a CsCl gradient. Thereby, there is an attractiveness and inescapable logic to this type of approach that would provide, after more than 20 years of investigation, sufficient data on MUC16 changes during ovarian carcinogenesis. An understanding of the basic structure, viscoelastic properties, and interactions of mucin glycoproteins is of considerable current interest to biomedical applications. These physical properties are of direct relevance to the physiological functions of mucins, in particular MUC16, in normal and diseased states.

An earlier study was done to shed light on heterogeneity in the structure of MUC16. This study provides the first evidence for a potential functional link between CA125 and its structure. Noticeable differences were observed between hCA125 (CA125 isolated from healthy women) and cCA125 (CA125 isolated from patients with EOC) [38]. This distinctness is probably related to the carbohydrate composition of both *N*- and *O*-glycans, which might influence the observed ferning pattern [47]. However, whether the spider arborescence of cCA125 antigen is a result of ovarian cancer or a cause remains unknown. The aggregation of mucin is of particular importance; it causes conformational as well as configurational changes in the glycoprotein, thus perturbing the location of carbohydrate domains [33]. The issue of structural heterogeneity of CA125 antigen was also addressed by comparing ferning morphology of pregnancy- and cancer-derived molecules (pCA125 and cCA125, respectively). The picture that emerges is that of a macromolecule with a complex organization with a sponge-like appearance for pCA125 and more compact structure for cCA125. The observed specificities of each antigen may be relevant for relating biochemical properties of CA125 antigen with its morphology [48]. In the same context, Milutinovic et al. reported that CA125 antigen isolated from amniotic fluid and OVCAR-3 cell line was found to be heterogeneous in respect to the existence of multiple glycoforms, with *O*-linked glycan chains predominating [39]. So, different glycosylation patterns and possible variations in the production of CA125 glycoprotein in reproductive and related tissues have been presumed [47,48]. In relation to this, the observed pronounced microheterogeneity of CA125–oligosaccharide chains that also differ in normal and pathological conditions might be of special importance from both basic and biomedical aspects [48]. Data on glycosylation of CA125 point to the existence of glycosylation differences [47]. Taken together, these results show that CA125 may have important roles in ovarian cancer pathogenesis and early diagnosis.

12.3.3 Role of MUC16

Alterations in mucin structures in cancer have many biological and pathological consequences, because potential ligands responsible for interactions between cancer cells and their microenvironment are changed. This influences the growth and survival of the cell, its ability to invade and metastasize, and its interactions with lectins and cell surface receptors or cells of the immune system [49]. Notably, the findings that certain transmembrane mucins induce transformation and promote tumor progression have provided the experimental basis for demonstrating that inhibitors of their function are effective as antitumor agents in preclinical models [14]. One of these mucins, MUC16, has particularly important functions in ovarian tumorigenesis. CA125 antigen encoded by MUC16, known as the hallmark of serous epithelial ovarian carcinoma, is far from being fully explored regarding the diagnostic potential of its glycans [50,51]. Due to the extraordinary size and structure of MUC16, it could be hypothesized that this molecule displays multiple functions not only in ovarian cancer but also in other MUC16+ cancers of epithelial origin, for example, breast cancer [52]. MUC16 has proven to be useful as serum tumor marker to monitor the response to treatment in patients with ovarian carcinoma [53]. It is expressed by various tissues, notably the conjunctiva and the lachrymal glands, where it can play a protective role against bacterial infection [22]. Despite the prognostic relevance in ovarian cancer, the physiological role of MUC16 in tumor progression and metastasis remained elusive. Some roles of MUC16 in ovarian cancer have been recently elucidated. So far, glycosylation analysis has pointed to extreme heterogeneity, that is, the existence of many different molecular glycoforms of CA125. The biological meaning of this heterogeneity is not yet understood, and due to the structural complexity, more experiments are needed to gain complete insight into all existing forms and for their complete characterization. However, the accumulated experimental evidence indicates that the structural properties of this tumor marker may be more relevant in distinguishing between benign and malignant conditions than the measurement of its concentrations alone [54].

The role of MUC16 in ovarian cancer is gradually emerging. Recent advances in molecular biology have enabled researchers to better comprehend MUC16 mechanisms by which this tumor marker interacts with other molecules, with the intention of creating new strategies for ovarian cancer prevention and therapy. This is essential for improved understanding of clinical implications of MUC16 in ovarian cancer and for future therapeutic applications. Worth molecular investigations on MUC16 have resulted in much medicinally relevant information, allowing us to trace new routes in ovarian cancer research concerning clinical manipulation.

The biological properties of MUC16 and its altered expression and posttranslational modifications confer an important role to MUC16 in tumor progression and metastasis. Notably, the knockdown of MUC16 expression in NIH:OVCAR-3 cells has no influence on ovarian tumor cell proliferation rate. Notably, the knockdown of MUC16 expression in NIH:OVCAR-3 cells has neither influence on ovarian tumor cell proliferation rate nor on increasing spontaneous apoptosis [55]. Whereas in SCID mice the knockdown of MUC16 impairs ovarian cancer cells from forming tumors [56]. Contrariwise to ovarian cancer cells, the knockdown of MUC16 in breast cancer cells resulted in significant decrease in the rate of cell growth, tumorigenicity, and increased apoptosis [57].

On the one hand, MUC16 is tightly associated with various biologically active, defensive molecules and serves as a major protective barrier against pathogens [58]. On the other hand, both cell surface MUC16 (csMUC16) and shed MUC16 (sMUC16) protect ovarian tumor cells from immune attack, and thereby it has an immunosuppressive role and it is important in tumor cell metastasis by promoting tumor growth [59]. sMUC16 is an inhibitor of the cytolytic antitumor responses of natural killer (NK) cells [60], while csMUC16 acts as an antiadhesive molecule and prevents the formation of the immunological synapse between ovarian cancer cells and NK cells [61].

It is interesting to note that csMUC16 can facilitate cell adhesion by interacting with a suitable binding partner such as mesothelin or Siglec-9 [59]. Evidence for a strong relationship between csMUC16 and peritoneal invasiveness has been reinforced based largely on studies showing the binding of MUC16 to the peritoneal surfaces by serving as a ligand of mesothelin [62–64]. MUC16 has been demonstrated to mediate cell adhesion by binding to other cell surface glycoproteins such as galectin-1 and mesothelin [62–65]. The binding of MUC16 to mesothelin is of particular interest because this interaction implicates a role for MUC16 in dissemination of ovarian cancer cells to the peritoneal cavity [62]. The accumulated data point to a scenario where expression of MUC16 by ovarian tumor cells promotes their metastasis via several mechanisms. Via its interaction with mesothelin, MUC16 has been previously demonstrated to be involved not only in ovarian cancer metastasis but also in the metastasis of solid tumors to the central nervous system [66]. A better understanding of the molecular structure of regulatory regions as well as mechanisms governing MUC16 expression is also mandatory if one wants to assign its direct roles in carcinogenesis and better understand its influence on the biological properties of the tumor cell. Studies aiming at deciphering the signaling pathways will allow identification of potential therapeutic targets.

MUC16 is cleaved and shed into the bloodstream and has been the focus of active research as a biomarker in the serum for a variety of tumor types [67]. With respect to its preeminent place as an ovarian tumor marker, much of the work carried out to date on CA125/MUC16 has focused on its potential implication in the development and dissemination of ovarian cancer. However, MUC16 has shown to be one molecule with multiple functions in cancer and other diseases. Expression of CA125/MUC16 in normal tissues and in different pathological and physiological conditions implies a wide biological role for CA125/MUC16 [68]. Numerous studies suggest roles for MUC16 in endometriosis, secretion, and other tissue-specific functions such as in the upper respiratory tract [23,69–71]. MUC16 has also an important role in promoting proliferation in breast cancer cells [52–57]. Besides, MUC16 has immunosuppressive properties that allow the immune evasion of ovarian cancer cells from the host immune system and in fetal tolerance from maternal immune rejection during early pregnancy [23,72,73].

These observations together imply that MUC16 is a multifunctional molecule owing to its high complicated structure and different biochemical and immunological properties. Thereby, the findings that MUC16 induces transformation and promotes tumor progression have provided the experimental basis for demonstrating that inhibitors of their function are effective as antitumor agents in preclinical models [74]. Targeted therapies with anti-CA125 antibodies conjugated to cytotoxic drugs are currently under study in animal models. Biologic and immunologic therapies seem to augment what can be accomplished with optimal chemotherapy and thus could provide an incremental improvement in patient management [75]. Immunotherapy with a conventional mouse monoclonal antibody specific for CA125 shows intriguing results, in which human anti–mouse antibody responses correlated significantly with a considerable survival benefit of patients with advanced-stage ovarian cancer [76]. Furthermore, vaccination with a suitable anti-idiotypic antibody offers an effective way to induce specific immunity against a primarily nonimmunogenic tumor antigen such as CA125 and is associated with a positive impact on the survival of patients with recurrent ovarian cancer with few side effects [77]. In a recent study, a novel human immunotherapeutic agent highly specific for MUC16 with potential for treating ovarian cancer and other MUC16-expressing tumors was described [78]. Of special interest, another study that considers MUC16/CA125 as a driver of transformation designed a target-based high-content screen to identify and classify compounds that exhibit differential effect on MUC16-expressing cells [79]. Therefore, as proposed by Felder et al., the modulation of MUC16 expression may serve as a useful strategy to control the progression of ovarian cancer via immunologic therapy [56]. Notably, the development of novel monoclonal antibodies against the proximal (carboxy-terminal) portions of MUC16 may be useful for the characterization of MUC16 biology and allow for future studies in targeted therapy and diagnostics [80].

The MUC16 domains are the critical contributors to the biophysical properties of this tumor marker. Tumorigenicity is mediated by interaction of the cytoplasmic tail with intracellular signaling molecules [22]. The amino domain, also known as the *N*-terminus, is of particular interest in MUC16, as it is where the heavy glycosylation occurs in the Golgi apparatus during posttranslational modification. This domain is heavily glycosylated and has many side chains of simple sugars. Because of this extended heavily glycosylated conformation, MUC16, as a member of membrane-associated mucins, may have antiadhesive properties, provide a protective barrier for the cell membrane, and prevent cell–cell and cell–protein interactions [81–83]. MUC16-expressing tumors adhere to NK cells, downregulate CD16, and suppress NK response, which may promote immune evasion [23,60–72]. CA125/MUC16 selectively modulates the sensitivity of EOC cells to genotoxic agents [40]. The unusual features of the oligosaccharides linked to CA125 suggest a role for CA125 in cell-mediated immune response [30]. There is evidence that CA125 attenuates complement lysis of antibody-sensitized cells [84]. In vivo data suggest that MUC16 drives a more aggressive phenotype in ovarian cancer, including increased growth, invasion, and dissemination [85]. Finally, efforts have been undertaken to develop anti-CA125 antibodies specific for the cell-associated form of the antigen, which is of particular interest for targeted therapy [86].

12.3.4 Clinical Applications of MUC16–CA125 (Apart from Ovarian Cancers)

Limitations of the diagnostic usefulness of CA125 include its elevation in nongynecologic conditions such as hepatitis and pancreatitis [87] as well as a variety of benign disease conditions. The levels of serum CA125 in hepatitis cirrhosis patients were correlated with lesion of liver and ascites degree [88]. Raised CA125 levels are sometimes found in patients with benign gynecologic conditions, such as menstruation, endometriosis, and pelvic inflammatory disease. Pregnancy should be ruled out when increased CA125 levels are found in women during the childbearing years [87]. Breast, lung [89], pancreatic [90], and gastric cancers [91] are common causes of elevated CA125 values. Concentrations of CA125 have also been widely investigated in endometrial cancers and were found to be a useful prognostic tool [92]. Preoperative serum CA125 levels were considered to be an adjunct method of monitoring patients with uterine papillary serous carcinoma and may be important for management planning, prognostication, and counseling in these women [93]. CA125 is used routinely for the screening, diagnosis, and stratification of some cancer diseases, but recently, the role of this tumor marker has also been explored in the context of patients with heart failure. CA125 has emerged as a potential biomarker in heart failure by showing correlations with clinical, hemodynamic, and echocardiographic parameters indicative of the severity of the disease [94]. As for the non-sMUC16, currently, one of the most widely used applications of MUC16/CA125 is in the follow-up of patients with diagnosed disease in most of the digestive tract adenocarcinomas [95]. CA125 may also have a role as a beneficial parameter in the determination of pulmonary tuberculosis activity and the evaluation of response to treatment [96]. Serum CA125 is a useful index in the diagnosis of ultrasonographically detected ascites in patients with nephrotic syndrome [97]. Measurement of CA125 level, especially the level in pleural effusion, not only provides useful information for distinctive diagnosis of different kinds of lung diseases but also is a good target in the evaluation of disease extent and effect of treatments in patients with different kinds of lung diseases [98]. Finally, the reliability of salivary CA125 testing makes it a feasible adjunctive diagnostic tool for the detection of oral squamous cell carcinoma [99]. After reading this chapter, readers should be aware of the expanding role of the tumor marker CA125 that is presently available in the routine clinical laboratory and clinical applications that are currently in widespread use.

12.3.5 Concluding Remarks

MUC16's functions are beginning to be elucidated in EOC cells with a considerable potential importance in the biology and treatment of ovarian malignancies, whereas the normal function of MUC16 is for the most part unknown because of the complexity of its post-translational modifications, and in particular of its glycosylations, which necessitates more effort to explore possible links between specific subspecies of MUC16 and specific physical conditions. As for the development of new diagnostic assays, it should be based on particular properties of those oligosaccharide chains, which are different in normal and pathological conditions. The analysis of glycomics and carbohydrate-blocking and carbohydrate-based vaccines is still in its infancy. With the rapid growth of this field of medicinal glycoscience, treatment based on MUC16 carbohydrate could be promising. The development of new molecular biology techniques will allow researchers to determine the biological role of MUC16 in the process of ovarian tumor progression and response to therapy.

References

1. Feng H, Ghazizadeh M, Konishi H, and Araki T. Expression of MUC1 and MUC2 mucin gene products in human ovarian carcinomas. *Jpn J Clin Oncol* 2002; 32: 525–529.
2. Eisenkop SM, Spirtos NM, Friedman RL, Lin WC, Pisani AL, and Perticucci S. Relative influences of tumor volume before surgery and the cytoreductive outcome on survival for patients with advanced ovarian cancer: A prospective study. *Gynecol Oncol* 2003; 90: 390–396.
3. Ozols RF, Bundy BN, Greer BE, Fowler JM, Clarke-Pearson D, Burger RA, Mannel RS, DeGeest K, Hartenbach EM, and Baergen R. Phase III trial of carboplatin and paclitaxel compared with cisplatin and paclitaxel in patients with optimally resected stage III ovarian cancer: A Gynecologic Oncology Group study. *J Clin Oncol* 2003; 21: 3194–3200.
4. Averette HE, Janicek MF, and Menck HR. The National Cancer Data Base report on ovarian cancer. American College of Surgeons Commission on Cancer and the American Cancer Society. *Cancer* 1995; 76: 1096–1103.
5. Heintz AP, Odicino F, Maisonneuve P, Beller U, Benedet JL, Creasman WT, Ngan HY, and Pecorelli S. Carcinoma of the ovary. *Int J Gynaecol Obstet* 2003; 83: 135–166.
6. Kosary CL. FIGO stage, histology, histologic grade, age and race as prognostic factors in determining survival for cancers of the female gynecological system: An analysis of 1973–87 SEER cases of cancers of the endometrium, cervix, ovary, vulva, and vagina. *Semin Surg Oncol* 1994; 10: 31–46.
7. Giuntoli RL, Rodriguez GC, Whitaker RS, Dodge R, and Voynow JA. Mucin gene expression in ovarian cancers. *Cancer Res* 1998; 58: 5546–5550.
8. Rose MC and Voynow JA. Respiratory tract mucin genes and mucin glycoproteins in health and disease. *Physiol Rev* 2006; 86: 245–278.
9. Porchet N and Aubert JP. Les gènes MUC Mucin or not mucin? That is the question. *Med Sci* 2004; 20: 569–574.

10. Chauhan SC, Deepak Kumar D, and Jaggi M. Mucins in ovarian cancer diagnosis and therapy. *J Ovarian Res* 2009; 2: 21.
11. Desseyn JL, Tetaert D, and Gouyer V. Architecture of the large membrane-bound mucins. *Gene* 2008; 410: 215–222.
12. Thornton DJ, Rousseau K, and McGuckin MA. Structure and function of the polymeric mucins in airways mucus. *Annu Rev Physiol* 2008; 70: 459–486.
13. Ho SB, Niehans GA, Lyftogt C, Yan PS, Cherwitz DL, Gum ET, Dahiya R, and Kim YS. Heterogeneity of mucin gene expression in normal and neoplastic tissues. *Cancer Res* 1993; 53: 641–651.
14. Kufe DW. Mucins in cancer: Function, prognosis and therapy. *Nat Rev Cancer* 2009; 9: 874–885.
15. Moore A, Medarova Z, Potthast A, and Dai G. In vivo targeting of underglycosylated MUC-1 tumor antigen using a multimodal imaging probe. *Cancer Res* 2004; 64: 1821–1827.
16. Obermair A, Schmid BC, Packer LM, Leodolter S, Birner P, Ward BG, Crandon AJ, McGuckin MA, and Zeillinger R. Expression of MUC1 splice variants in benign and malignant ovarian tumours. *Int J Cancer* 2002; 100: 166–171.
17. Van Elssen CH, Frings PW, Bot FJ, Vande Vijver KK, Huls MB, Meek B, Hupperets P, Germeraad WT, and Bos GM. Expression of aberrantly glycosylated Mucin-1 in ovarian cancer. *Histopathology* 2010; 57: 597–606.
18. Lau SK, Weiss LM, and Chu PG. Differential expression of MUC1, MUC2, and MUC5AC in carcinomas of various sites: An immunohistochemical study. *Am J Clin Pathol* 2004; 122: 61–69.
19. Kabawat SE, Bast RC Jr., Bhan AK, Welch WR, Knapp RC, and Colvin RB. Tissue distribution of a coelomic-epithelium-related antigen recognized by the monoclonal antibody OC125. *Int J Gynecol Pathol* 1983; 2: 275–285.
20. Nouwen EJ, Pollet DE, Eerdekens MW, Hendrix PG, Briers TW, and De Broe ME. Immunohistochemical localization of placental alkaline phosphatase, carcinoembryonic antigen, and cancer antigen 125 in normal and neoplastic human lung. *Cancer Res* 1986; 46: 866–876.
21. Nouwen EJ, Hendrix PG, Dauwe S, Eerdekens MW, and De Broe ME. Tumor markers in the human ovary and its neoplasms. A comparative immunohistochemical study. *Am J Pathol* 1987; 126: 230–242.
22. Blalock TD, Spurr-Michaud SJ, Tisdale AS, Heimer SR, Gilmore MS, Ramesh V, and Gipson IK. Functions of MUC16 in corneal epithelial cells. *Invest Ophthalmol Vis Sci* 2007; 48: 4509–4518.
23. Hardardottir H, Parmley TH 2nd, Quirk JG Jr., Sanders MM, Miller FC, and O'Brien TJ. Distribution of CA125 in embryonic tissues and adult derivatives of the fetal periderm. *Am J Obstet Gynecol* 1990; 163: 1925–1931.
24. Gipson IK, Blalock T, Tisdale A, Spurr-Michaud S, Allcorn S, Stavreus-Evers A, and Gemzell K. MUC16 is lost from the uterodome (pinopode) surface of the receptive human endometrium: In vitro evidence that MUC16 is a barrier to trophoblast adherence. *Biol Reprod* 2008; 78: 134–142.
25. Bast RC Jr., Feeney M, Lazarus H, Nadler LM, Colvin RB, and Knapp RC. Reactivity of a monoclonal antibody with a human ovarian carcinoma. *J Clin Invest* 1981; 68: 1311–1337.
26. Davis HM, Zurawski VR Jr., Bast RC Jr., and Klug TL. Characterization of the CA 125 antigen associated with human epithelial ovarian carcinomas. *Cancer Res* 1986; 46: 6143–6148.
27. O'Brien TJ, Beard JB, Underwood LJ, Dennis RA, Santin AD, and York L. The CA125 Gene: An extracellular superstructure dominated by repeat sequences. *Tumour Biol* 2001; 22: 348–366.
28. Yin BWT and Lloyd KO. Molecular cloning of the CA125 ovarian cancer antigen. Identification as a new mucin, MUC16. *J Biol Chem* 2001; 276: 27371–27375.
29. Maeda T, Inoue M, Koshiba S, Yabuki T, Aoki M, Nunokawa E, Seki E et al. Solution structure of the SEA domain from the murine homologue of ovarian cancer antigen CA125 (MUC16). *J Biol Chem* 2004; 279: 13174–13182.
30. KuiWong N, Easton RL, Panico M, Sutton-Smith M, Morrison JC, Lattanzio FA, Morris HR, Clark GF, Dell A, and Patankar MS. Characterization of the oligosaccharides associated with the human ovarian tumor marker CA125. *J Biol Chem* 2003; 278: 28619–28634.
31. Hang HC and Bertozzi CR. The chemistry and biology of mucin-type O-linked glycosylation. *Bioorg Med Chem* 2005; 13: 5021–5034.

32. Nustad K, Lebedin Y, Lloyd KO, Shigemasa K, de Bruijn HW, Jansson B, Nilsson O, Olsen KH, O'Brien TJ, and ISOBMTD-1Workshop. Epitopes on CA125 from cervical mucus and ascites fluid and characterization of six new antibodies. Third report from the ISOBM TD-1 workshop. *Tumour Biol* 2002; 23: 303–314.
33. Jankovic MM and Milutinovic BS. Glycoforms of CA125 antigen as a possible cancer marker. *Cancer Biomark* 2008; 4: 35–42.
34. Milutinovic B and Jankovic M. Analysis of the protein and glycan parts of CA125 antigen from human amniotic fluid. *Arch Biol Sci* 2007; 59: 97–103.
35. Marchal I, Golfier G, Dugas O, and Majed M. Bioinformatics in glycobiology. *Biochimie* 2003; 85: 75–81.
36. Kobayashi H, Ida W, Fujii T, Terao T, and Kawashima Y. Heterogeneity of CA125 antigens released from human endometrial heterotopic epithelium and ovarian cancer. *Nippon Sanka Fujinka Gakkai Zasshi* 1992; 44: 571–576.
37. Bouanène H, Sahrawi W, Mokni M, Fatma LB, Bouriga A, Limen HB, Khairi H, AhmedS B, and Miled A. Correlation of heterogeneous Expression of sialyltransferases and MUC16 in ovarian tumor tissues. *Onkologie* 2011; 34: 165–169.
38. Bouanène H, Saibi W, Mokni M, Sriha B, Ben Fatma L, Ben Limem H, Ben Ahmed S, Gargouri A, and Miled A. Biochemical and morphological differences between CA125 isolated from healthy women and patients with epithelial ovarian cancer from Tunisian population. *Pathol Oncol Res* 2012; 18: 325–330.
39. Jankovic MM and Milutinovic BS. Pregnancy-associated CA125 antigen as mucin: Evaluation of ferning morphology. *Mol Hum Reprod* 2007; 13: 405–408.
40. Boivin M, Lane D, Piché A, and Rancourt C. CA125 (MUC16) tumor antigen selectively modulates the sensitivity of ovarian cancer cells to genotoxic drug-induced apoptosis. *Gynecol Oncol* 2009; 115: 407–413.
41. O'Brien TJ, Beard JB, Underwood LJ, and Shigemasa K. The CA 125 gene: A newly discovered extension of the glycosylated N-terminal domain doubles the size of this extracellular superstructure. *Tumor Biol* 2002; 23: 154–169.
42. Rangel LB, Sherman-Baust CA, Wernyj RP, Schwartz DR, Cho KR, and Morin PJ. Characterization of novel human ovarian cancer-specific transcripts (HOSTs) identified by serial analysis of gene expression. *Oncogene* 2003; 22: 7225–7232.
43. Bansil R and Turner BS. Mucin structure, aggregation, physiological functions and biomedical applications. *Curr Opin Colloid Interface Sci* 2006; 11: 164–170.
44. Fiebrig I, Harding S, Rowe A, Hyman S, and Davis S. Transmission electron microscopy studies on pig gastric mucin and its interactions with chitosan. *Carbohydr Polym* 1995; 28: 239–244.
45. Round A, Berry M, McMaster T, Stoll S, Gowers D, Corfield AP, and Miles MJ. Heterogeneity and persistence length in human ocular mucins. *Biophys J* 2002; 83: 1661–1670.
46. Round A, Berry M, McMaster T, Corfield A, and Miles M. Glycopolymer charge density determines conformation in human ocular mucin gene products: An atomic force microscope study. *J Struct Biol* 2004; 145: 246–253.
47. Jankovic MM and Tapuskovic BT. Molecular forms and microheterogeneity of the pregnancy-associated CA125 antigen. *Hum Rep* 2005; 20: 2632–2638.
48. Shrivastava HY, Sreeram KJ, and Nair BU. Aggregation of mucin by chromium(III) complexes as revealed by electrokinetic and rheological studies: Influence on the tryptic and O-glycanase digestion of mucin. *J Biomol Struct Dyn* 2004; 21: 671–680.
49. Brockhausen I. Mucin-type O-glycans in human colon and breast cancer: Glycodynamics and functions. *EMBO Rep* 2006; 7: 599–604.
50. Jankovic M. Cancer antigen 125: Biochemical properties and diagnostic significance. *Jugoslov Med Biohem* 2001; 20: 201–206.
51. Jankovic M and Milutinovic B. Pregnancy-associated ca125 antigen as mucin: Evaluation of ferning morphology. *Mol Hum Reprod* 2007; 13: 405–408.
52. Reinartz S, Failer S, Schuell T, and Wagner U. CA125 (MUC16) gene silencing suppresses growth properties of ovarian and breast cancer cells. *Eur J Cancer* 2012; 48: 1558–1569.

53. Duffy MJ, Bonfrer JM, Kulpa J, Rustin GJ, Soletormos G, Torre GC, Tuxen MK, and Zwirner M. CA125 in ovarian cancer: European Group on Tumor Markers guidelines for clinical use. *Int J Gynecol Cancer* 2005; 15: 679–691.
54. Jankovic M, Kosanoviv M, and Milutinovic B. Glycans as a target in the detection of reproductive tract cancers. *JMB* 2008; 27: 17–29.
55. Thériault C, Pinard M, Comamala M, Migneault M, Beaudin J, Matte I, Boivin M, Piché A, and Rancourt C. MUC16 (CA125) regulates epithelial ovarian cancer cell growth, tumorigenesis and metastasis. *Gynecol Oncol* 2011; 121: 434–443.
56. Felder M, Connor J, Rakhmilevich A, Qu X, Kapur A, Manish S, and Patankar MS. The mucin MUC16 protects ovarian cancer cells from innate immune responses. *Cancer Res* 2012; 72(8 Suppl), abstract no. 319. doi:1538-7445.AM2012–319.
57. Lakshmanan I, Ponnusamy MP, Das S, Chakraborty S, Haridas D, Mukhopadhyay P, Lele SM, and Batra SK. MUC16 induced rapid G2/M transition via interactions with JAK2 for increased proliferation and anti-apoptosis in breast cancer cells. *Oncogene* 2012; 31: 805–817.
58. Kim KC. Role of epithelial mucins during airway infection. *Pulm Pharmacol Ther* 2012; 25: 415–419.
59. Belisle JA, Horibata S, Jennifer GA, Petrie S, Kapur A, André S, Gabius HJ et al. Identification of Siglec-9 as the receptor for MUC16 on human NK cells, B cells, and monocytes. *Mol Cancer* 2010; 9: 118.
60. Patankar MS, Yu J, Morrison JC, Belisle JA, Lattanzio FA, Deng Y, Wong NK, Morris HR, Dell A, and Clark GF. Potent suppression of natural killer cell response mediated by the ovarian tumor marker CA125. *Gynecol Oncol* 2005; 99: 704–713.
61. Gubbels JA, Felder M, Horibata S, Belisle JA, Kapur A, Holden H, Petrie S et al. MUC16 provides immune protection by inhibiting synapse formation between NK and ovarian tumor cells. *Mol Cancer* 2010; 9: 11.
62. Rump A, Morikawa Y, Tanaka M, Minami S, Umesaki N, Takeuchi M, and Miyajima A. Binding of ovarian cancer antigen CA125/MUC16 to mesothelin mediates cell adhesion. *J Biol Chem* 2004; 279: 9190–9198.
63. Gubbels JA, Belisle J, Onda M, Rancourt C, Migneault M, Ho M, Bera TK et al. Mesothelin-MUC16 binding is a high affinity, N-glycan dependent interaction that facilitates peritoneal metastasis of ovarian tumors. *Mol Cancer* 2006; 5: 50.
64. Bergan L, Gross JA, Nevin B, Urban N, and Scholler N. Development and in vitro validation of anti-mesothelin biobodies that prevent CA125/Mesothelin-dependent cell attachment. *Cancer Lett* 2007; 255: 263–274.
65. Seelenmeyer C, Wegehingel S, Lechner J, and Nickel W. The cancer antigen CA125 represents a novel counter receptor for galectin-1. *J Cell Sci* 2003; 116: 1305–1318.
66. Johnson MD, Vito F, and Xu H. MUC16 expression and risk of adenocarcinoma metastases to peritoneum, pleura, leptomeninges, and brain. *Appl Immunohistochem Mol Morphol* 2010; 18: 250–253.
67. O'Brien TJ, Tanimoto H, Konishi I, and Gee M. More than 15 years of CA 125: What is known about the antigen, its structure and its function. *Int J Biol Markers* 1998; 13: 188–195.
68. Bast RC Jr., Xu FJ, Yu YH, Barnhill S, Zhang Z, and Mills GB. CA125: The past and the future. *Int J Biol Markers* 1998; 13: 179–187.
69. Gaetje R, Winnekendonk DW, Scharl A, and Kaufmann M. Ovarian cancer antigen CA 125 enhances the invasiveness of the endometriotic cell line EEC145. *J Soc Gynecol Investig* 1990; 6: 278–281.
70. Jäger K, Wu G, Sel S, Garreis F, Bräuer L, and Paulsen FP. MUC16 in the lacrimal apparatus. *Histochem Cell Biol* 2007; 127: 433–438.
71. Davies JR, Kirkham S, Svitacheva N, Thornton DJ, and Carlstedt I. MUC16 is produced in tracheal surface epithelium and submucosal glands and is present in secretions from normal human airway and cultured bronchial epithelial cells. *Int J Biochem Cell Biol* 2007; 39: 1943–1954.
72. Belisle JA, Gubbels JA, Raphael CA, Migneault M, Rancourt C, Connor JP, and Patankar MS. Peritoneal natural killer cells from epithelial ovarian cancer patients show an altered phenotype and bind to the tumour marker MUC16 (CA125). *Immunology* 2007; 122: 418–429.

73. Mc Donnel AC, Van Kirk EA, Austin KJ, Hansen TR, Belden EL, and Murdoch WJ. Expression of CA-125 by progestational bovine endometrium: Prospective regulation and function. *Reproduction* 2003; 126: 615–620.
74. Junutula JR, Raab H, Clark S, Bhakta S, Leipold DD, Weir S, Chen Y et al. Site-specific conjugation of a cytotoxic drug to an antibody improves the therapeutic index. *Nat Biotechnol* 2008; 26: 925–932.
75. Berek JS, Schultes BC, and Nicodemus CF. Biologic and immunologic therapies for ovarian cancer. *J Clin Oncol* 2003; 21: 168s–174s.
76. Gordon AN, Schultes BC, Gallion H, Edwards R, Whiteside TL, Cermak JM, and Nicodemus CF. CA125- and tumor-specific T-cell responses correlate with prolonged survival in oregovomab-treated recurrent ovarian cancer patients. *Gynecol Oncol* 2004; 94: 340–351.
77. Wagner U, Köhler S, Reinartz S, Giffels P, Huober J, Renke K, Schlebusch H et al. Immunological consolidation of ovarian carcinoma recurrences with monoclonal anti-idiotype antibody ACA125: Immune responses and survival in palliative treatment. *Clin Cancer Res* 2001; 7: 1154–1162.
78. Xiang X, Feng M, Felder M, Connor JP, Man YG, Patankar MS, and Ho M. HN125: A Novel immunoadhesin targeting MUC16 with potential for cancer therapy. *J Cancer* 2011; 2: 280–291.
79. Rao TD, Rosales N, and Spriggs DR. Dual-fluorescence isogenic high-content screening for MUC16/CA125 selective agents. *Mol Cancer Ther* 2011; 10: 1939–1948.
80. DharmaRao T, Park KJ, Smith-Jones P, Iasonos A, Linkov I, Soslow RA, and Spriggs DR. Novel monoclonal antibodies against the proximal (carboxy-terminal) portions of MUC16. *Appl Immunohistochem Mol Morphol* 2010; 18: 462–472.
81. Ligtenberg MJ, Buijs F, Vos HL, and Hilkens J. Suppression of cellular aggregation by high levels of episialin. *Cancer Res* 1992; 52: 2318–2324.
82. Carraway KL, Fregien N, Carraway KL, 3rd, and Carraway CA. Tumor sialomucin complexes as tumor antigens and modulators of cellular interactions and proliferation. *J Cell Sci* 1992; 103: 299–307.
83. Komatsu M, Carraway CA, Fregien NL, and Carraway KL. Reversible disruption of cell-matrix and cell-cell interactions by overexpression of sialomucin complex. *J Biol Chem* 1997; 272: 33245–33254.
84. Murdoch WJ, Van Kirk EA, and Smedts AM. Complement-inhibiting effect of ovarian cancer antigen CA-125. *Cancer Lett* 2006; 236: 54–57.
85. Manson RG, Thapi D, Ma X, Rosales N, and Spriggs D. MUC16/CA125 specific targeting of critical signaling kinases in ovarian cancer. *J Clin Oncol (Meeting Abstracts)* 2009; 27: 15S e22112.
86. Singleton J, Guillen DE, Scully MS, Xue J, Moffet J, Chen C, Patel SR et al. Characterization of antibodies to CA 125 that bind preferentially to the cell-associated form of the antigen. *Tumour Biol* 2006; 27: 122–132.
87. Gadducci A, Cosio S, Carpi A, Nicolini A, and Genazzani AR. Serum tumor markers in the management of ovarian, endometrial and cervical cancer. *Biomed Pharmacother* 2004; 58: 24–38.
88. Xu J, Liu J, Guo JX, Ma HB, Zhao J, Liu AX, Xu WN, Li BA, and Mao YL. Evaluation on clinical value of serum CA-125 level in hepatitis cirrhosis. *Zhonghua Shi Yan He Lin Chuang Bing Du Xue Za Zhi.* 2010; 24: 334–336.
89. Sjövall K, Nilsson B, and Einhorn N. The significance of serum CA 125 elevation in malignant and nonmalignant diseases. *Gynecol Oncol* 2002; 85: 175–178.
90. Haglund C. Tumour marker antigen CA125 in pancreatic cancer: A comparison with CA19-9 and CEA. *Br J Cancer* 1986; 54: 897–901.
91. Emoto S, Ishigami H, Yamashita H, Yamaguchi H, Kaisaki S, and Kitayama J. Clinical significance of CA125 and CA72-4 in gastric cancer with peritoneal dissemination. *Gastric Cancer* 2012; 15: 154–161.
92. Chen YL, Huang CY, Chien TY, Huang SH, Wu CJ, and Ho CM. Value of pre-operative serum CA125 level for prediction of prognosis in patients with endometrial cancer. *Aust N Z J Obstet Gynaecol* 2011; 51: 397–402.

93. Olawaiye AB, Rauh-Hain JA, Withiam-Leitch M, Rueda B, Goodman A, and del Carmen MG. Utility of pre-operative serum CA-125 in the management of uterine papillary serous carcinoma. *Gynecol Oncol* 2008; 110: 293–298.
94. Vizzardi E, D'Aloia A, Curnis A, and Dei Cas L. Carbohydrate antigen 125: A new biomarker in heart failure. *Cardiol Rev* 2013; 21: 23–26.
95. Streppel MM, Vincent A, Mukherjee R, Campbell NR, Chen SH, Konstantopoulos K, Goggins MG, Van Seuningen I, Maitra A, and Montgomery EA. Mucin 16 (cancer antigen 125) expression in human tissues and cell lines and correlation with clinical outcome in adenocarcinomas of the pancreas, esophagus, stomach, and colon. *Hum Pathol* 2012; 43: 1755–1763.
96. Sahin F and Yildiz P. Serum CA-125: Biomarker of pulmonary tuberculosis activity and evaluation of response to treatment. *Clin Invest Med* 2012; 35: E223–E228.
97. Peng T, Guo L, Xia Q, and Yang X. Clinical significance of serum CA125 in nephrotic syndrome. *Clin Lab* 2012; 58: 113–115.
98. Tomita Y. Clinical evaluation and tissue distribution of CA125 in patients with pleural effusion. *Igaku Kenkyu* 1989; 59: 90–96.
99. Balan JJ, Rao RS, Premalatha B, and Patil S. Analysis of tumor marker CA 125 in saliva of normal and oral squamous cell carcinoma patients: A comparative study. *J Contemp Dent Pract* 2012; 13: 671–675.

13

Role of HE4 in the Management of Ovarian Cancer

Daniel Abehsera, MD, PhD, Javier De Santiago, MD, PhD, and Ignacio Zapardiel, MD, PhD

CONTENTS

ABSTRACT In 2008, ovarian cancer was the seventh most common cancer in women worldwide, and incidence rates were highest in developed countries. Survival from ovarian cancer is related to the stage at diagnosis; 5-year survival is over 90% for the minority of women with stage I disease. This drops to about 75%–80% for regional disease and 25% for those with distant metastases. The potential benefit of screening is its ability to identify ovarian cancer at a more localized and curable stage, leading to reduced mortality from the disease. Interest in early detection as a method of reducing mortality has grown with the discovery of serum tumor markers associated with ovarian malignancies and with improved diagnostic accuracy of pelvic ultrasonography. Intensive research is ongoing to identify additional markers and a cost-effective screening strategy. Measurement of the serum concentration of the cancer antigen (CA) 125 glycoprotein antigen is the most widely studied biochemical method of screening for ovarian cancer. Serum CA125 values are elevated in approximately 50% of women with early-stage disease and in over 80% of women with advanced ovarian cancer. Human epididymis protein 4 (HE4) appears to have a similar sensitivity to CA125 when comparing serum from ovarian cancer cases to healthy controls and a higher sensitivity when comparing ovarian cancer cases to benign gynecological disease. HE4 addition in combination with CA125 appears to be an effective tool for early detection of recurrence or monitoring response to treatment.

13.1 Introduction

Ovarian tumors are quite frequent. Most are benign and usually occur in young women, while the evil are more often in elderly patients. Among gynecological cancers, ovarian cancer is the third in frequency after cervical and endometrial cancer. However, it has a higher mortality rate because of the difficulty of making an early diagnosis. Worldwide in 2008, ovarian cancer was the seventh most common cancer in women, and incidence rates were highest in developed countries (Jemal et al., 2011). In fact, ovarian cancer is the leading cause of death from gynecological malignancy in the United States. Approximately 22,280 cases are expected to be diagnosed in the United States in 2012 with an expected 15,500 deaths attributable to ovarian cancer (Siegel et al., 2012). The incidence of ovarian cancer increases with age; the highest proportion of cases are diagnosed in women 50–59 years of age. It has a high mortality rate due to the difficulty of making an early diagnosis. In fact, the lethality of ovarian cancer is primarily attributable to the advanced stage of the disease at the time of initial diagnosis. Approximately 70% of patients present with disease that has spread beyond the ovaries (Jemal et al., 2004). Despite advances in cytotoxic therapies, only 30% of patients with advanced-stage ovarian cancer survive 5 years after initial diagnosis (Naora and Montell, 2006). The fact that usually the diagnosis of the disease is in advanced stages of the same, which carries a high mortality, necessitates the search for a diagnostic strategy that enables detection of ovarian cancer at an early stage of the disease.

The interest in early detection as a mechanism to achieve the reduction in mortality has increased with the discovery of serum tumor markers associated with malignant ovarian tumors (especially cancer antigen [CA] 125) and with a more precise diagnosis of pelvic ultrasound. The research is focused on identifying additional markers and to establish a cost-effective screening strategy. Clinical trials are underway to determine whether screening with blood tests and/or ultrasound examinations successively reduces ovarian cancer mortality. Until we have those results, there is a consensus that women with ovarian cancer risk should or should not undergo this screening. Human epididymis protein 4 (HE4) appears to have a similar sensitivity to CA125 when comparing serum from ovarian cancer cases to healthy controls and a higher sensitivity when comparing ovarian cancer cases to benign gynecological disease. HE4 addition in combination with CA125 appears to be an effective tool for early detection of recurrence or monitoring response to treatment.

13.2 Human Epididymis Protein 4

HE4 is a putative serum tumor marker for ovarian cancer, which was first identified as a transcript exclusively expressed in distal epididymis (Kirchhoff, 1991). HE4 is also referred to as WFDC2 because it contains two whey acidic protein (WAP) domains and four-disulphide core comprising eight cysteine residues. The HE4 gene is part of a family of protease inhibitors that function in protective immunity and is expressed primarily in the reproductive tract and upper airways and can be detected in the sera of patients (Hellstrom et al., 2003; Drapkin et al., 2005; Bingle et al., 2006; Bouchard et al., 2006).

In addition to the male reproductive system, HE4 is expressed in a variety of normal human tissues, including regions of the respiratory tract and nasopharynx, as well as in a number of tumor cell lines (Bingle et al., 2002); and not expressed in normal ovarian surface epithelium (Drapkin et al., 2005). In malignant neoplasms, a tumor-restricted pattern of upregulation makes HE4 a potential biomarker for various solid tumors such as ovarian cancer (Drapkin et al., 2005; Hellstrom et al., 2010; Lamy et al., 2010), pulmonary adenocarcinoma (Bingle et al., 2006; Yamashita et al., 2011), endometrial cancer (Moore et al., 2008), mesothelioma (Hegmans et al., 2009), and breast cancer (Galgano et al., 2006).

As the same way as other tumor markers, HE4 levels are influenced by the age of the patient as well as by cigarette smoking. Bolstad et al. (2012) studied HE4 reference limits and natural variation in a Nordic reference population. The study showed that age is the main determinant of HE4 in healthy subjects, corresponding to 2% higher HE4 levels at 30 years (compared to 20 years), 9% at 40 years, 20% at 50 years, 37% at 60 years, 63% at 70 years, and 101% at 80 years. HE4 levels are 29% higher in smokers than in nonsmokers. In a similar study with serum samples from 1101 healthy women and 67 pregnant women analyzed, it was observed that serum levels of HE4 are decreased in pregnancy and increased with age (Moore et al., 2012). In addition, it has been demonstrated that serum HE4 concentration is not dependent on menstrual cycle or hormonal treatment among endometriosis patients and healthy premenopausal women; therefore, the HE4 measurement in healthy premenopausal women as well as in women with endometriosis can be carried out at any phase of the menstrual cycle, and irrespective of hormonal medication, extending the benefits of HE4 use in clinical practice (Hallamaa et al., 2012).

The role of HE4 in the epithelial ovarian cancer is not clearly established. Various studies suggest that HE4 plays a key role in ovarian cancer cell adhesion and motility (Gao et al., 2011; Lu et al., 2012).

13.3 Use of HE4 for Diagnosis between Benign and Malignant Ovarian Tumors

Schummer et al. (1999) showed that HE4 gene was overexpressed mainly in patients with ovarian carcinomas. They used the comparative hybridization of cDNA arrays to discover genes with potential for the diagnosis of ovarian cancer. An array of 21,500 unknown ovarian cDNAs was hybridized with labeled first-strand cDNA from 10 ovarian tumors and 6 normal tissues. One hundred and thirty-four clones were overexpressed in at least 5 of the 10 tumors. These cDNAs were sequenced and compared to public sequence databases. One of these, the gene HE4, was found to be expressed primarily in some ovarian cancers.

Several studies reported preferential expression of HE4 in epithelial ovarian carcinomas, mainly in cases of serous and endometrioid epithelial carcinomas (Schwartz et al., 2002; Schaner et al., 2003). Drapkin et al. (2005) concluded that 93% of serous and 100% of endometrioid epithelial ovarian cancer expressed HE4, whereas only 50% and 0% of clear-cell carcinomas and mucinous tumors were positive, respectively. Although adenocarcinomas of the lung, and occasional breast, transitional cell endometrial and pancreatic carcinomas had moderate or high HE4 expression, ovarian serous carcinomas showed, on average, the highest expression (Galgano et al., 2006). These observations led to the proposal that, due to its small size and secreted nature, HE4 might be a good candidate serum marker for this type of cancer (Montagnana et al., 2011).

Accurately discriminating patients with ovarian cancer from benign pelvic lesions is crucial for appropriate treatment planning and patients' outcome. It is of great benefit to patients at high risk of having ovarian cancer to be treated by gynecologic oncologists. Gynecologic oncologists who have specialty training are more competent to give proper surgical management including complete surgical staging or optimal cytoreductive surgery to patients with ovarian cancer. For these reasons, it is imperative to determine the possibility of having ovarian cancer for patients presenting with a pelvic mass (Figure 13.1). Tumor markers play an important role in the differential diagnosis of patients with a pelvic mass. Serum CA125 has been routinely tested for predicting the presence of ovarian cancer in clinical practice. Its insufficiency in sensitivity and specificity prompts development and evaluation of many novel tumor markers. HE4 is one of the most promising biomarkers for ovarian cancer diagnosis. Recent studies (Moore et al., 2008; Huhtinen et al., 2009; Nolen et al., 2010; Moore et al., 2012; Zheng and Gao, 2012) have evaluated HE4 as a single marker or in combination with CA125 and other biomarkers for the discrimination of epithelial ovarian cancer from benign pelvic disease. All authors found significantly higher HE4 serum level in epithelial ovarian cancer than in benign controls and combined HE4 and CA125 had better ability to discriminate epithelial ovarian cancer from benign disease than either HE4 or CA125 alone.

Specifically, Huhtinen et al. (2009) showed that serum HE4 was not increased in patients with endometriosis compared with healthy controls and that adding HE4 to CA125 testing provides a more accurate tool for distinguishing patients with ovarian cancer from

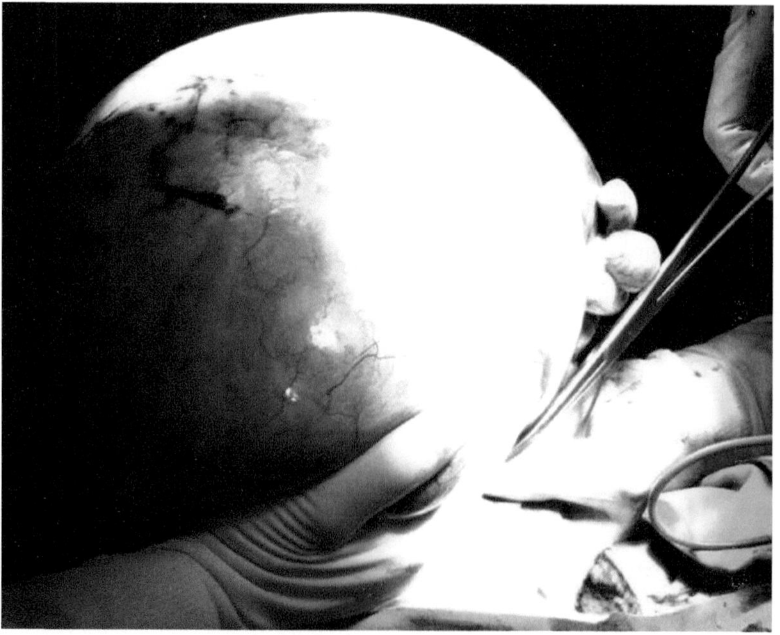

FIGURE 13.1
Giant serous tumor of the ovary. The patient presented for pelvic discomfort and increasing abdominal girth.

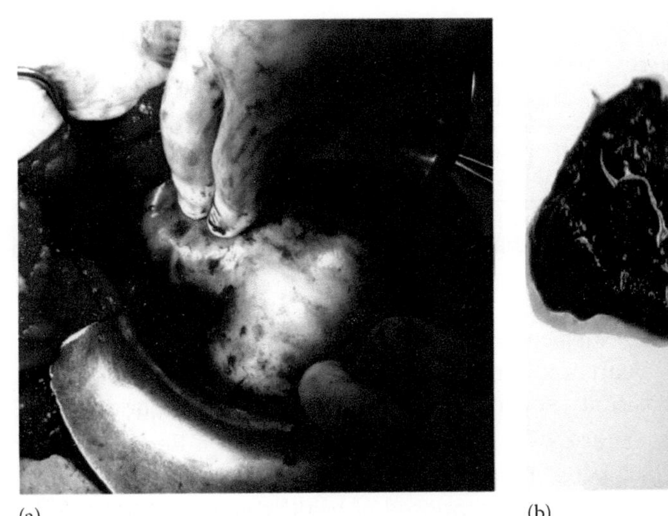
(a)

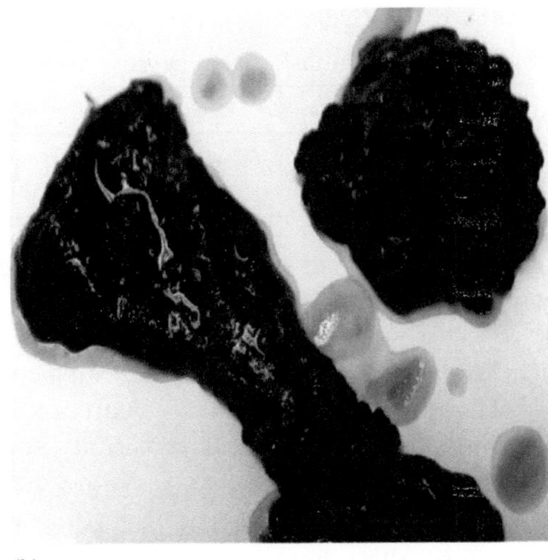
(b)

FIGURE 13.2
Laparotomy in a patient of 35 years that showed a left adnexal tumor with elevation of the tumor marker CA125 (CA125 335 UI/mL [normal < 35]). (a) The tumor visualized by ultrasound corresponded to a twisted tuboovarian abscess. (b) After excision, the piece showed abundant areas of hemorrhage and necrosis.

those with ovarian endometriotic cysts. Zheng et al. reached similar conclusions, adding further that the measure of HE4 is a useful tool for the differential diagnosis between epithelial ovarian cancer and the pelvic inflammatory disease (Zheng and Gao, 2012) (Figure 13.2).

The largest of all studies, evaluating HE4 and CA125 for diagnosis between benign and malignant ovarian tumors, is presented by Moore et al. communicating data about 1042 women with benign disease. HE4 levels were less often elevated than CA125 statistically significant. A marked difference was observed in patients with endometriosis in which HE4 was elevated in 3% of patients and CA125 in 67%. Serous ovarian tumors were associated with elevated levels of HE4 in 8% of patients and CA125 in 20%; uterine fibroids in 8% versus 26%; dermoids in 1% versus 21%; and inflammatory disease in 10% versus 37%. They find these differences particularly in premenopausal patients (Moore et al., 2012).

However, a slight superiority of CA125 has been reported in the differential diagnosis of epithelial ovarian carcinoma by stage of disease. For stage I ovarian carcinoma, HE4 as a single marker was superior to CA125, which was the best single marker in stages II–IV (Lenhard et al., 2011). The United States Food and Drug Administration recently approved the use of serum HE4 for monitoring ovarian cancer patients in order to detect recurrence in a timely manner (Kim et al., 2011).

Most studies on HE4 were performed on Caucasian population. Kim et al. report on comparison of diagnostic utility of CA125 and HE4 in Korean women. In premenopausal women, HE4 was superior to CA125 in distinguishing epithelial ovarian cancer from benign ovarian mass, while the opposite was true for postmenopausal patients. The diagnostic performance of the combination of HE4 and CA125 was in most cases higher than CA125 alone; and the Risk of Ovarian Malignancy Algorithm (ROMA) index allowed the patient classification into the high- or low-risk groups with 88% sensitivity and 94% specificity (Kim et al., 2011).

TABLE 13.1

Meta-Analyses Published that Discuss the Diagnostic Role of HE4 in Epithelial Ovarian Cancer

	Subjects	Sensitivity	Specificity	Area under the ROC Curve (%)
Yu et al.	2607	80% (CI 77%–82%)	91% (CI 90%–92%)	94
Wu et al.	1807	83% (CI 77%–88%)	90% (CI 87%–92%)	88

Two meta-analyses have been published that discuss the diagnostic role of HE4 in epithelial ovarian cancer (Table 13.1):

1. Yu et al. (2012) included 2607 subjects in this meta-analysis and concluded that HE4 is better than CA125 as an auxiliary indicator for the diagnosis of ovarian cancer in terms of better sensitivity, specificity, likelihood ratio positive, and likelihood ratio negative.
2. Wu et al. (2012) included 1807 subjects in this meta-analysis and got the following results: when the control group was composed of healthy women, the pooled sensitivity and specificity for HE4 in diagnosing ovarian cancer were 83% and 90%, respectively. When the control group was composed of women with benign disease, the pooled sensitivity and specificity for HE4 were 74% and 90%.

13.4 Use of HE4 in Algorithms for the Screening of Ovarian Cancer

13.4.1 Risk of Ovarian Malignancy Algorithm

The Risk of Ovarian Malignancy Algorithm (ROMA) is a predictive index developed and validated from two separate pilot studies that basically take into account the serum concentrations of both biomarkers (CA125 and HE4) and the pre- or postmenopausal status (Moore et al., 2008, 2009). Moore et al. conducted a prospective multicenter double-blind trial to validate a predictive model using the dual-marker combination of HE4 and CA125 to assess epithelial ovarian cancer risk in women presenting with a pelvic mass. A total of 129 epithelial ovarian cancer, 22 tumors of low malignant potential, and 352 benign samples were consecutively assessed. The predictive algorithm was performed to determine sensitivity with specificity set at 75%. The logistic regression model included coefficients for the natural log of both HE4 and CA125 values and based on menopausal status. However, to date, it has been validated only by using Fujirebio EIA HE4 in conjunction with Abbott ARCHITECT CA125 assay or CanAg CA125 EIA, with two specific cutoff values and not in conjunction with other second-generation CA125 immunoassays. This model showed a sensitivity of 92% in postmenopausal women, 76% in premenopausal women, and 89% in combined pre- and postmenopausal women. These findings led to the conclusion that this dual-marker combination might represent the most effective tool in the stratification of women at high and low risk for epithelial ovarian cancer. In all patients affected by pelvic mass, we observed that the diagnostic performance of ROMA was no better than HE4 alone since the area under the ROC curve of HE4 in the postmenopausal women was slightly higher versus ROMA and almost identical in premenopausal subjects. These findings led Montagnana et al. (2011) to conclude that measurement of CA125 for the estimation of the ROMA predictive index might be unnecessary because HE4 alone provided the best assessment of risk.

Two commercial immunoassays for HE4 have been compared, and the diagnostic accuracy of HE4, CA125, and the combinatory ROMA algorithm for epithelial ovarian cancer has been evaluated. The ARCHITECT CMIA HE4 assay was compared with the Fujirebio EIA HE4, and the risk for epithelial ovarian cancer by the combinatory ROMA algorithm was assessed with both HE4 assays. The two HE4 assays showed a good correlation and a similar clinical value, with a greater precision for CMIA (Ruggeri et al., 2011).

Bandiera et al. (2011) analyzed the diagnostic and prognostic value of serum HE4 and ROMA algorithm in epithelial ovarian cancer. They tested preoperative serum samples of 419 women (140 healthy controls, 131 ovarian benign cysts, 34 endometriosis, and 114 epithelial ovarian cancers) for CA125 and HE4 using fully automated methods (Abbott ARCHITECT) and validated cutoff values. They obtained the following results:

- For the discrimination of benign masses from epithelial ovarian cancer in premenopausal women: the sensitivity and specificity were 92.3% and 59.4% for CA125, 84.6% and 94.2% for HE4, and 84.6% and 81.2% for ROMA.
- For the discrimination of benign masses from epithelial ovarian cancer in postmenopausal women: the sensitivity and specificity were 94.3% and 82.3% for CA125, 78.2% and 99.0% for HE4, and 93.1% and 84.4% for ROMA.
- In patients with epithelial ovarian cancer, elevated CA125, HE4, and ROMA levels were associated with advanced Federation of Gynecologists and Obstetricians (FIGO) stage, suboptimal debulking, ascites, positive cytology, lymph node involvement, and advanced age.
- Elevated HE4 and ROMA, but not CA125, were associated with undifferentiated tumors.
- In multivariable analysis, elevated HE4 and ROMA were independent prognostic factors for shorter overall, disease-free, and progression-free survival.

They concluded that multicenter studies are needed to draw firm conclusions about the applicability of HE4 and ROMA in clinical practice.

With the objective of validating the ROMA algorithm in an independent prospective study, Van Gorp et al. studied 389 patients with a pelvic mass who were scheduled to have surgery. Preoperative serum levels of HE4 and CA125 were measured, and the performance of each of the markers, as well as that of ROMA, was analyzed. When all malignant tumors were included, ROMA and HE4 did not perform significantly better than CA125 alone. Using a cutoff for ROMA of 12.5% for premenopausal patients, the test had a sensitivity of 67.5% and a specificity of 87.9%. With a cutoff of 14.4% for postmenopausal patients, the test had a sensitivity of 90.8% and a specificity of 66.3%. For epithelial ovarian cancer versus benign disease, the area under the ROC curve of ROMA increased to 0.913 and for invasive epithelial ovarian cancer versus benign disease to 0.957. These authors concluded that the measurement of HE4 serum levels does not contribute to the diagnosis of ovarian cancer (Van Gorp et al., 2011).

Molina et al. evaluated HE4 in comparison with CA125 and the ROMA algorithm in healthy women and in patients with benign and malignant gynecological diseases. They studied 285 patients and concluded that the ROMA algorithm might be further improved if it is used only in patients with normal HE4 and abnormal CA125 serum levels. The ROMA algorithm in HE4 positive had a similar sensitivity and only increases the specificity by 3.2% compared to HE4 alone (Molina et al., 2011).

Li et al. (2012) published a meta-analysis with data of 7792 tests retrieved from 11 studies. The overall estimates of ROMA for epithelial ovarian cancer predicting were sensitivity

(0.89, 95% CI 0.84–0.93), specificity (0.83, 95% CI 0.77–0.88), and area under the ROC curve (0.93, 95% CI 0.90–0.95). Comparison of epithelial ovarian cancer predictive value between HE4 and CA125 found, specificity: HE4 (0.93, 95% CI 0.87–0.96), CA125 (0.84, 95% CI 0.76–0.90); area under the ROC curve: CA125 (0.88, 95% CI 0.85–0.91), HE4 (0.82, 95% CI 0.78–0.85). Comparison of ovarian cancer predictive value between HE4 and CA125 found, area under the ROC curve: CA125 (0.89, 95% CI 0.85–0.91) and HE4 (0.79, 95% CI 0.76–0.83). Comparison among the three tests for epithelial ovarian cancer prediction found, sensitivity: ROMA (0.86, 95% CI 0.81–0.91) and HE4 (0.80, 95% CI 0.73–0.85); specificity: HE4 (0.94, 95% CI 0.90–0.96), ROMA (0.84, 95% CI 0.79–0.88), and CA125 (0.78, 95% CI 0.73–0.83).

13.4.2 Comparison between Different Algorithms for the Screening of Ovarian Cancer

The risk malignancy index (RMI): In case of a suspicious pelvic mass or symptoms, a serum CA125 test is requested and the patient is referred to an abdominal and vaginal ultrasound. Based on menopausal status, ultrasound findings, and serum CA125 level, the RMI is calculated. If RMI is ≥200, the patient enters the national cancer fast track guidelines. RMI is presently the most accurate tool for stratifying patients into high- and low-risk groups. Two prospective multicenter studies including 1159 and 548 patients, respectively, showed for RMI a sensitivity of 92% and 81% and a specificity of 82% and 85%, respectively, at a cutoff value of 200 (Van den Akker, 2010; Håkansson et al., 2012). Four studies have been published to date comparing the ROMA algorithm with RMI (Table 13.2):

1. Moore et al. (2010) applied both algorithm diagnoses in 457 patients, with the following results: at a set specificity of 75%, ROMA had a sensitivity of 94.3% and RMI had a sensitivity of 84.6% for distinguishing benign status from epithelial ovarian cancer. In patients with stage I and II disease, ROMA achieved a sensitivity of 85.3% compared with 64.7% for RMI.
2. Jacob et al. (2011) applied the marker HE4 with CA125 individually, in combination, within the RMI and the ROMA algorithm, in 160 patients, with the following results: Both markers showed similar diagnostic performance in the detection of epithelial ovarian cancer, but HE4 was not elevated in endometriosis. Comparison of nonmalignant diagnoses versus early-stage ovarian and tubal cancers revealed that HE4 and ROMA displayed the best diagnostic performance. While RMI detects peritoneal cancer better than all other models, there is no other detection benefit from RMI compared to HE4 alone or included in ROMA.

TABLE 13.2

Studies that Compare the Ability to Differentiate between Benign and Malignant, Using ROMA Algorithm and the RMI

	Patients	ROMA (Sensitivity/Specificity)	RMI (Sensitivity/Specificity)
Moore et al.	457	94.3%/75%	84.6%/75%
Jacob et al.	160	89.6%/87.3%	75.7%/98.6%
Anton et al.	128	74.1%/75.8%	63%/92.4%
Karlsen et al.	1218	94.4%/76.5%	94.4%/81.5%

3. Anton et al. (2012) applied the marker HE4 with CA125 individually, in combination, within the RMI and the ROMA algorithm, in 128 patients, with the following results: The sensitivities associated with the ability of CA125, HE4, ROMA, or RMI to distinguish between malignant versus benign ovarian masses were 70.4%, 79.6%, 74.1%, and 63%, respectively. Among carcinomas, the sensitivities of CA125, HE4, ROMA (pre- and postmenopausal), and RMI were 93.5%, 87.1%, 80%, 95.2%, and 87.1%, respectively. The most accurate numerical values were obtained with RMI, although the four parameters were shown to be statistically equivalent.
4. Karlsen et al. (2012) applied the marker HE4 with CA125 individually, in combination, within the RMI and the ROMA algorithm, in 1218 patients, with the following results: differentiating between OC and benign disease the specificity was 62.2 (CA125), 63.2 (HE4), 76.5 (ROMA), and 81.5 (RMI) at a set sensitivity of 94.4.

OVA 1 is a test approved by the FDA for the evaluation and diagnosis of ovarian cancer. OVA 1 is a value derived from the combination of five biomarkers: transthyretin, apolipoprotein-A1, beta-2-microglobulin, transferrin, and CA125 combined with software that assesses the possibility of malignancy in women with ovarian mass in which surgical intervention is planned. Macuks et al. (2012) applied the ROMA and the OVA 1 test in 238 patients with ovarian tumors and to establish a new ovarian cancer risk assessment algorithm in conjunction with ultrasound score and menopausal status. Results show that mean serum concentrations of CA125, HE4, and beta-2-microglobulin were upregulated, but apolipoprotein A1, transferrin, and transthyretin were downregulated among ovarian cancer patients. When only one biomarker was introduced in the logistic regression analysis, together with ultrasonographic score and menopausal status, HE4 was more accurate than CA125 in ovarian cancer diagnostic, but when both biomarkers were included in the logistic regression analyses, ovarian cancer diagnostic accuracy was increased.

13.5 HE4 and Ovarian Cancer Prognosis

Prognostication is an essential step in the management of cancer patients. Some prognostic factors related to the patient, the tumor, and the environment are well recognized in ovarian cancer. In particular, stage, histology, grade, and residual disease are the main clinical prognostic factors that are taken into account for the primary treatment of women with OC (Crawford et al., 2005; Winter et al., 2007). The biological characteristics of ovarian cancer may help predict the patient's prognosis and her response to medical and surgical therapies. The identification of pretreatment serologic biomarkers is a promising avenue to better determine the expected course and outcome of ovarian cancer and to reduce the burden of this disease. Preliminary studies have found an association with relapse or survival with, for example, the decline in CA125 from pre- to postoperative levels and the expression of nuclear maspin in ovarian cancer cells (Solomon et al., 2006; Zivanovic et al., 2009).

Preoperative serum level of HE4 is a biomarker strongly associated with standard prognostic factors of ovarian cancer. It is observed as an important shift of the HE4 median values between early and advanced FIGO stages (Bandiera et al., 2011; Escudero et al., 2011; Paek et al., 2011; Van Gorp et al., 2011; Trudel et al., 2012). Several studies consistently reported variations of HE4 levels according to histological types, with higher levels in serous tumors (Huhtinen et al., 2009; Escudero et al., 2011; Van Gorp et al., 2011; Trudel et al., 2012). It is also observed that women with moderately or poorly differentiated carcinoma had higher levels of HE4 than those with well-differentiated carcinoma (Van Gorp et al., 2011; Trudel et al., 2012). The associations between preoperative HE4 levels and standard prognostic factors associated with a worse prognosis show that preoperative HE4 is an indicator of OC aggressiveness.

In women with the highest levels of HE4, there is a significantly increased risk of death (Bandiera et al., 2011; Trudel et al., 2012). In addition, the association between preoperative HE4 levels and mortality was greater than the observed association between preoperative CA125 levels and mortality. This suggests that HE4 might be a more promising biomarker for prognosis than CA125 (Trudel et al., 2012).

The studies that have assessed the prognostic effect of preoperative serum HE4 levels on ovarian cancer progression reported an independent effect of preoperative serum levels of HE4 (Bandiera et al., 2011; Paek et al., 2011; Kong et al., 2012; Trudel et al., 2012).

13.6 Role of HE4 in Monitoring Ovarian Cancer

The vast majority of ovarian epithelial cancer patients will relapse within 2–5 years (Cannistra, 2004). It has become standard clinical practice to include CA125 testing in patient surveillance. Elevation in CA125 often precedes clinical evidence of relapse by imaging or physical exam (Rustin et al., 2001). HE4 has received approval by the Food and Drug Administration as a recurrence monitoring marker. Limited information suggests that rising HE4 could detect a recurrence earlier than CA125 (Allard et al., 2008; Havrilesky et al., 2008; Anastasi et al., 2010; Schummer, 2012).

Other studies suggested that HE4 collected at different times during the management of women with OC could also have a prognostic significance. An exploratory study conducted among 23 women in remission showed that serum levels of HE4 collected about 3–5 months after the end of first-line chemotherapy were associated with biopsy-proven disease recurrence (Han et al., 2011). In another study, it has been reported that higher levels of HE4 collected after surgery but just before first-line chemotherapy were associated with progression (Steffensen et al., 2011).

13.7 Patents with Ovarian Cancer

The complex pathophysiology of cancer requires multiple, sensitive and specific biomarkers for both early diagnosis and therapeutic monitoring improvement. It is now obvious that the lack of a single diagnostic marker, as already proven in many types of cancers, makes it likely for a panel of biomarkers to be capable of improving the sensitivity and specificity of a single biomarker. Biomarker discovery using novel technology can improve prognostic upgrading and can pinpoint new molecular targets for innovative therapy. Although many molecular markers have been identified, the general opinion is that a set of tests investigating soluble and/or tissue-related markers would be more appropriate for diagnosis, prognosis, and therapy monitoring in cancer. One of the important goals of oncology is to develop biomarkers that can be identified through simple, less invasive methods proving the potential to identify cancer risk, the possibility to improve early diagnostic, and display utility in accurate grading and treatment monitoring. The proteome is the mirror of all the cellular changes that take place in time due to the initiation of a pathological status. In this context, although individual validated biomarkers are important in several types of cancers, panels of several biomarkers (e.g., three to five) can enhance the individual biomarker. The hope relies in the patterns of multiple biomarkers, protein signatures that have increased cancer specificity. The number of validated biomarkers in human cancer is still small, and extended studies are being performed in an attempt to validate new biomarkers and/or to generate panels of classical biomarkers, in order to identify early and precisely the development of a neoplastic process. Although the rate of introducing new biomarkers in clinical practice is extremely low and single markers are suitable in some cases, there is an unanimous consensus that multiple (three to five) markers used as a single marker or in combination with others in panels perform better in terms of sensitivity and specificity in early diagnosis (Neagu et al., 2011).

In the last decade, several patents disclosing methods and biomarkers useful for the early diagnosis of ovarian cancer have been published (Table 13.3). In Tables 13.4 through 13.8, a brief description of the latest five patents published in this field between 2009 and 2010 is provided (Tables 13.4 through 13.8) (Veneroni et al., 2011).

TABLE 13.3

Performance of Biomarkers in Samples from Ovarian Cancer Patients

Biomarkers	Population	Sensitivity (%)	Specificity (%)
CA125/IL-6/IL-8/VEGF/EGF	44 early-stage cancers 37 benign, 45 controls	84	95
CA125/IL-6/G-CSF/VEGF/EGF	44 early-stage cancers 37 benign, 45 controls	86.5	93
Leptin/prolactin/ostepontin/IGF2	100 cancers, 106 controls	95	94
Leptin/prolactin/ostepontin/IGF2/MIF/A125	Training set: 113 cancers, 181 controls Test set: 43 cancers, 181 controls	95.3	99.4
CA125/HE4/glycudelin/PLAUR/MUCI/PA1-1	200 cancers (133 stage I/II), 396 healthy controls	80.5	96.5
CA125	143 cancers, 124 benign, 344 controls	78	98
HE4		68–82	98
Mesothelin		31–44	98
CA125/CA19-9/EGFR/CRP/myoglobin/APOA1/APOC3/MIP1A/IL-6/IL-18/tenascin C	115 cancers, 93 benign 24 controls, 13 nonovarian cancers	91.3	88.5

Source: Veneroni, R. et al., *Recent Pat. Biomark.*, 1, 1, 2011.

TABLE 13.4

Panel 50 of Biomarkers Identified in the Patent WO2009145815

Group I (Upregulated in Sample Test vs. Control Sample) 31
CSE1 chromosome segregation 1-like, casein kinasel, v-Crk sarcoma virus CT10 oncogene homolog, topoisomerase (DNA) II alpha, c-src tyrosine kinase, catechol-*O*-methyltransferase, WAS protein family-member 1, erythrocyte membrane protein band 4.9 (dematin), potassium large conductance calcium-activated cannel-subfamily M, alpha member 1-, nuclear receptor coactivator 3, TEA domain family member 1-SV40 transcriptional enhancer factor-, peroxisome biogenesis factor 1, translin-associated factor X, G protein-coupled receptor 51, solute carrier family 9 (sodium/hydrogen exchanger)- isoform 1 (antiporter, NA+/H+ amiloride sensitive)-, integrin-alpha 2 (CD49B alpha 2 subunit of VLA-2 receptor), MCM6 minichromosome maintenance deficient 6, syntaxin 6, KH domain containing-RNA building signal transduction associated 1, dystrophia myotinica-ptotein kinase, eukaryotic translation initiation factor 4 gamma 1, Rho GDP dissociation inhibitor (GDI) beta, endothelin receptor type A, synaptophysin, transcription factor 3-E2A immunoglobulin enhancer binding factors E12/E47 fibranectin 3, RA5 p21 protein activator (GTPase activating protein) 1, SW/SNF related matrix associated actin dependent regulator of chromatin-subfamily a member2-, syntaxin binding protein 5 (tomosyn), Ras-GTPase-activating protein SH3-domain-binding protein, glutamate receptor (ionotropic *N*-methyl D-aspartate 2B).
Group II (Downregulated in Sample Test vs. Control Sample) 19
Sinapsin II, sortilin-related receptor-L (DLR class) A repeats-containing-, excision repair cross-complementing roden repair deficiency complementation group 2, signal transducer and activator of transcription 6 interleukin-4 induced, tripartite motif-containing 3, protein kinase C-theta, syntaxin 8, glutamateammonia ligase (glutamine synthase), protein kinase C beta 1, chromosome condensation 1, DEAH (Asp-Glu-Ala-His) box polipeptide 16, ribosomal protein L22, caveolin 1 caveolae protein 22 kDa, retinoblastoma-like 2 (p130), cyclin-dependent kinase inhibitor 1A (p21, Cip1), protein tyrosine phosphatase receptor-type Z polipeptide 1, general transcription factor II-i, adaptor-related protein complex 2 alpha 1 subunit, linker for activation of T cells.

Source: Veneroni, R. et al., *Recent Pat. Biomark.*, 1, 1, 2011.

TABLE 13.5

Panel of Biomarkers Identified in the Patent US20097605003

CA125, CA125 II, CA15-3, CA19-9, CA72-4, CA195, CEA, 110 kDa Component of the Extracellular Domain of the Epidermal Growth Factor Receptor (p110EGFR), Creatine Kinase B (CKB), Dianon NB 70/K, Galactosyltransferase, Haptoglobin, HE4, Kallikrein 6 and 10 (NES-1). LASA, HER-2/neu, Lysophosphatidic Acid (LPA), Macrophage Colony Stimulating Factor (M-CSF, CSF-1), Osteopontin, Placental Alkaline Phosphate (PLAP), Prostasin, Sialyl TN, Tissue Kallikreins, Tissue Peptide Antigen (TPA), Tumor Associated Trypsin Inhibitors (TATI), Urinary Gonadotropin Peptide.

Source: Veneroni, R. et al., *Recent Pat. Biomark.*, 1, 1, 2011.

TABLE 13.6

Panel of Biomarkers Identified in the Patent US20100055690

(A) 13 Biomarkers
Hepcidin, Inter-alpha (globulin) inhibitor H4 (plasma Kallikrein-sensitive glycoprotein) (ITIH4), Connective tissue-activating peptide (CTAPIII), Transthyretin (TTR), Transferrin (TFR), Beta-2 microglobin (B2M), Apoplipoprotein A1 (ApoA1), CRP *N*-terminal fragment, ApoA1-ApoAII dimer, Platelet Factor 4-*N*-terminal truncation, m/z value 3897.378 protein, identified as a fragment of protein C inhibitor, m/z value 7900.679 protein, identified as an sodium adduct of platelet factor 4 and Truncated serum amyloid.
(B) 7 Biomarkers
Hepcidin, Inter-alpha (globulin) inhibitor H4 (plasma Kallikrein-sensitive glycoprotein) (ITIH4), Connective tissue-activating peptide (CTAPIII), Transthyretin (TTR), Transferrin (TFR), Beta-2 microglobin (B2M), Apoplipoprotein A1 (ApoA1).

Source: Veneroni, R. et al., *Recent Pat. Biomark.*, 1, 1, 2011.

TABLE 13.7

Panel of 42 Biomarkers Identified in the Patent WO2010042525

Alphal-Antitrypsin, alpha2-Antiplasmin, alpha2-HS-Glycoprotein, ADAMS, AR5B, BAFF Receptor, C2, C5, C6, C9, Cadherin-5, Coagulation Factor Xa, Contactin-1, Contactin-4, ERBB1, Growth Hormone Receptor, Flat-1, FIGF, HSP90α, IL-12 Rβ2, IL-13 Rαl. IL-18 Rβ, Kallikrein 6, Kallistatin, LY9, MCP-3, MIP-5, MMP-7, MRC2, NRP1, PCI, Prekallikrein, Properdin, RBP, RGM-C, SAP, SCFsR, SLPI, sL-Selectin, Thrombin/Prothrombin, TIMP-2, Troponin T.

Source: Veneroni, R. et al., *Recent Pat. Biomark.*, 1, 1, 2011.

TABLE 13.8

Panel of 52 Biomarkers Identified in the Patent US20100081151

Group I (36 Proteins Overexpressed Twofold)
1.953 kDa, 2.065 kDa, 2.216 kDa, 2.928 kDa, 2.937 kDa, 3.143 kDa, 3.423 kDa, 3.427 kDa, 3.423 kDa, 3.427 kDa, 4.144 kDa, 4.375 kDa, 4.456 kDa, 4.629 kDa, 5.064 kDa, 7.550 kDa, 7.657 kDa, 7.756 kDa, 8.117 kDa, 10.874 kDa, 16.850 kDa, 18.559 kDa, 18.912 kDa, 18.98 kDa, 19.186 kDa, 22.959 kDa, 29.19 kDa, 29.512 kDa, 30.103 kDa, 33.217 kDa, 36.296 kDa, 42.401 kDa, 53.11 kDa (al-AT), 53.531 kDa, 83.689 kDa, or 84.133 kDa.
Group II (16 Proteins Underexpressed Twofold)
6.884 kDa, 6.931 kDa, 12.785 kDa (transthyretin), 13.797 kDa (transthyretin), 20.989 kDa, 27.595 kDa, 27.977 kDa (apolipoprotein Al), 40.067 kDa, 54.605 kDa, 78.9 kDa (transferrin), 79.909 kDa, 90.834 kDa, 91.878 kDa, 92.935 kDa, 105.778 kDa, or 106.624 kDa (IgG).

Source: Veneroni, R. et al., *Recent Pat. Biomark.*, 1, 1, 2011.

13.8 Conclusions

1. HE4 is helpful in distinguishing epithelial ovarian cancer from benign pelvic mass.
2. ROMA is a promising predictor of epithelial ovarian cancer to replace CA125, but its utilization requires further exploration.
3. ROMA performs equally well as the ultrasound depending RMI and might be valuable as a first-line biomarker for selecting high-risk patients for referral to a tertiary center and further diagnostics.
4. HE4 is a promising biomarker for prognosis in patients with epithelial ovarian cancer.

References

Allard J, Somers E, Theil R et al. 2008. Use of a novel biomarker HE4 for monitoring patients with epithelial ovarian cancer. *J Clin Oncol (Meeting Abstracts)*. 26:5535.

Anastasi E, Marchei GG, Viggiani V et al. 2010. HE4: A new potential early biomarker for the recurrence of ovarian cancer. *Tumour Biol*. 31:113–119.

Anton C, Carvalho FM, Oliveira EI et al. 2012. A comparison of CA125, HE4, risk ovarian malignancy algorithm (ROMA), and risk malignancy index (RMI) for the classification of ovarian masses. *Clinics (Sao Paulo)*. 67(5):437–441.

Bandiera E, Romani C, Specchia C et al. 2011. Serum human epididymis protein 4 and risk for ovarian malignancy algorithm as new diagnostic and prognostic tools for epithelial ovarian cancer management. *Cancer Epidemiol Biomarkers Prev.* 20(12):2496–2506.

Bingle L, Cross SS, High AS et al. 2006. WFDC2 (HE4): A potential role in the innate immunity of the oral cavity and respiratory tract and the development of adenocarcinomas of the lung. *Respir Res.* 7:61.

Bingle L, Singleton V, Bingle CD. 2002. The putative ovarian tumour marker gene HE4 (WFDC2), is expressed in normal tissues and undergoes complex alternative splicing to yield multiple protein isoforms. *Oncogene.* 21(17):2768–2773.

Bolstad N, Øijordsbakken M, Nustad K et al. 2012. Human epididymis protein 4 reference limits and natural variation in a Nordic reference population. *Tumour Biol.* 33(1):141–148.

Bouchard D, Morisset D, Bourbonnais Y et al. 2006. Proteins with whey-acidic-protein motifs and cancer. *Lancet Oncol.* 7(2):167–174.

Cannistra SA. 2004. Cancer of the ovary. *N Engl J Med.* 351:2519–2529.

Crawford SC, Vasey PA, Paul J et al. 2005. Does aggressive surgery only benefit patients with less advanced ovarian cancer? Results from an international comparison within the SCOTROC-1 Trial. *J Clin Oncol.* 23(34):8802.

Drapkin R, von Horsten HH, Lin Y et al. 2005. Human epididymis protein 4 (HE4) is a secreted glycoprotein that is overexpressed by serous and endometrioid ovarian carcinomas. *Cancer Res.* 65(6):2162–2169.

Escudero JM, Auge JM, Filella X et al. 2011. Comparison of serum human epididymis protein 4 with cancer antigen 125 as a tumor marker in patients with malignant and nonmalignant diseases. *Clin Chem.* 57(11):1534–1544.

Galgano MT, Hampton GM, Frierson HF Jr. 2006. Comprehensive analysis of HE4 expression in normal and malignant human tissues. *Mod Pathol.* 19(6):847–853.

Gao L, Cheng HY, Dong L et al. 2011. The role of HE4 in ovarian cancer: Inhibiting tumour cell proliferation and metastasis. *J Int Med Res.* 39(5):1645–1660.

Håkansson F, Høgdall EV, Nedergaard L et al. 2012. Risk of malignancy index used as a diagnostic tool in a tertiary centre for patients with a pelvic mass. *Acta Obstet Gynecol Scand.* 91(4):496–502.

Hallamaa M, Suvitie P, Huhtinen K et al. 2012. Serum HE4 concentration is not dependent on menstrual cycle or hormonal treatment among endometriosis patients and healthy premenopausal women. *Gynecol Oncol.* 125(3):667–672.

Han JJ, Yu M, Houston N et al. 2011. Progranulin is a potential prognostic biomarker in advanced epithelial ovarian cancers. *Gynecol Oncol.* 120(1):5–10.

Havrilesky LJ, Whitehead CM, Rubatt JM et al. 2008. Evaluation of biomarker panels for early stage ovarian cancer detection and monitoring for disease recurrence. *Gynecol Oncol.* 110:374–382.

Hegmans JP, Veltman JD, Fung ET et al. 2009. Protein profiling of pleural effusions to identify malignant pleural mesothelioma using SELDI-TOF MS. *Technol Cancer Res Treat.* 8(5):323–332.

Hellstrom I, Heagerty PJ, Swisher EM et al. 2010. Detection of the HE4 protein in urine as a biomarker for ovarian neoplasms. *Cancer Lett.* 296(1):43–48.

Hellstrom I, Raycraft J, Hayden-Ledbetter M et al. 2003. The HE4 (WFDC2) protein is a biomarker for ovarian carcinoma. *Cancer Res* 63(13):3695–3700.

Huhtinen K, Suvitie P, Hiissa J et al. 2009. Serum HE4 concentration differentiates malignant ovarian tumours from ovarian endometriotic cysts. *Br J Cancer.* 100(8):1315–1319.

Jacob F, Meier M, Caduff R et al. 2011. No benefit from combining HE4 and CA125 as ovarian tumor markers in a clinical setting. *Gynecol Oncol.* 121(3):487–491.

Jemal A, Bray F, Center MM et al. 2011. Global cancer statistics. *CA Cancer J Clin.* 61(2):69.

Jemal A, Tiwari RC, Murray T et al. 2004. *CA Cancer J Clin.* 54(1):8–29.

Karlsen MA, Sandhu N, Høgdall C et al. 2012. Evaluation of HE4, CA125, risk of ovarian malignancy algorithm (ROMA) and risk of malignancy index (RMI) as diagnostic tools of epithelial ovarian cancer in patients with a pelvic mass. *Gynecol Oncol.* 127(2):379–383.

Kim YM, Whang DH, Park J et al. 2011. Evaluation of the accuracy of serum human epididymis protein 4 in combination with CA125 for detecting ovarian cancer: A prospective case-control study in a Korean population. *Clin Chem Lab Med.* 49(3):527–534.

Kirchhoff C, Habben I, Ivell R et al. 1991. A major human epididymis-specific cDNA encodes a protein with sequence homology to extracellular proteinase inhibitors. *Biol Reprod*. 45(2):350–357.

Kong SY, Han MH, Yoo HJ et al. 2012. Serum HE4 level is an independent prognostic factor in epithelial ovarian cancer. *Ann Surg Oncol*. 19(5):1707–1712.

Lamy PJ, Roques S, Viglianti C et al. 2010. HE4, a novel marker for epithelial ovarian cancer: Evaluation of analytical performances. *Ann Biol Clin (Paris)*. 68(3):325–329.

Lenhard M, Stieber P, Hertlein L et al. 2011. The diagnostic accuracy of two human epididymis protein 4 (HE4) testing systems in combination with CA125 in the differential diagnosis of ovarian masses. *Clin Chem Lab Med*. 49(12):2081–2088.

Li F, Tie R, Chang K et al. 2012. Does risk for ovarian malignancy algorithm excel human epididymis protein 4 and ca125 in predicting epithelial ovarian cancer: A meta-analysis. *BMC Cancer*. 12:258.

Lu R, Sun X, Xiao R et al. 2012. Human epididymis protein 4 (HE4) plays a key role in ovarian cancer cell adhesion and motility. *Biochem Biophys Res Commun*. 419(2):274–280.

Macuks R, Baidekalna I, Donina S. 2012. An ovarian cancer malignancy risk index composed of HE4, CA125, ultrasonographic score, and menopausal status: Use in differentiation of ovarian cancers and benign lesions. *Tumour Biol*. 33(5):1811–1817.

Molina R, Escudero JM, Augé JM et al. 2011. HE4 a novel tumour marker for ovarian cancer: Comparison with CA 125 and ROMA algorithm in patients with gynaecological diseases. *Tumour Biol*. 32(6):1087–1095.

Montagnana M, Danese E, Giudici S et al. 2011. HE4 in ovarian cancer: From discovery to clinical application. *Adv Clin Chem*. 55:1–20.

Moore RG, Brown AK, Miller MC et al. 2008a. Utility of a novel serum tumor biomarker HE4 in patients with endometrioid adenocarcinoma of the uterus. *Gynecol Oncol*. 110(2):196–201.

Moore RG, Brown AK, Miller MC et al. 2008b. The use of multiple novel tumor biomarkers for the detection of ovarian carcinoma in patients with a pelvic mass. *Gynecol Oncol*. 108(2):402–408.

Moore RG, Jabre-Raughley M, Brown AK et al. 2010. Comparison of a novel multiple marker assay vs the Risk of Malignancy Index for the prediction of epithelial ovarian cancer in patients with a pelvic mass. *Am J Obstet Gynecol*. 203(3):228.e1–e6.

Moore RG, McMeekin DS, Brown AK et al. 2009. A novel multiple marker bioassay utilizing HE4 and CA125 for the prediction of ovarian cancer in patients with a pelvic mass. *Gynecol Oncol*. 112(1):40–46.

Moore RG, Miller MC, Eklund EE et al. 2012a. Serum levels of the ovarian cancer biomarker HE4 are decreased in pregnancy and increase with age. *Am J Obstet Gynecol*. 206(4):349.e1–e7.

Moore RG, Miller MC, Steinhoff MM et al. 2012b. Serum HE4 levels are less frequently elevated than CA125 in women with benign gynecologic disorders. *Am J Obstet Gynecol*. 206(4):351.e1–e8.

Naora H, Montell DJ. 2005. Ovarian cancer metastasis: Integrating insights from disparate model organisms. *Nat Rev Cancer*. 5(5):355–366.

Neagu M, Constantin C, Tanase C et al. 2011. Patented biomarker panels in early detection of cancer. *Recent Pat Biomark*. 1:10–24.

Nolen B, Velikokhatnaya L, Marrangoni A et al. 2010. Serum biomarker panels for the discrimination of benign from malignant cases in patients with an adnexal mass. *Gynecol Oncol*. 117(3):440–445.

Paek J, Lee SH, Yim GW et al. 2011. Prognostic significance of human epididymis protein 4 in epithelial ovarian cancer. *Eur J Obstet Gynecol Reprod Biol*. 158(2):338–342.

Ruggeri G, Bandiera E, Zanotti L et al. 2011. HE4 and epithelial ovarian cancer: Comparison and clinical evaluation of two immunoassays and a combination algorithm. *Clin Chim Acta*. 412(15–16):1447–1453.

Rustin GJ, Marples M, Nelstrop AE et al. 2001. Use of CA-125 to define progression of ovarian cancer in patients with persistently elevated levels. *J Clin Oncol*. 19:4054–4057.

Schaner ME, Ross DT, Ciaravino G et al. 2003. Gene expression patterns in ovarian carcinomas. *Mol Biol Cell*. 14(11):4376–4386.

Schummer M, Drescher C, Forrest R et al. 2012. Evaluation of ovarian cancer remission markers HE4, MMP7 and Mesothelin by comparison to the established marker CA125. *Gynecol Oncol.* 125(1):65–69.

Schummer M, Ng WV, Bumgarner RE et al. 1999. Comparative hybridization of an array of 21,500 ovarian cDNAs for the discovery of genes overexpressed in ovarian carcinomas. *Gene.* 238(2):375–385.

Schwartz DR, Kardia SL, Shedden KA et al. 2002. Gene expression in ovarian cancer reflects both morphology and biological behavior, distinguishing clear cell from other poor-prognosis ovarian carcinomas. *Cancer Res.* 62(16):4722–4729.

Siegel R, Naishadham D, Jemal A. 2012. Cancer statistics, 2012. *CA Cancer J Clin.* 62(1):10.

Solomon LA, Munkarah AR, Schimp VL et al. 2006. Maspin expression and localization impact on angiogenesis and prognosis in ovarian cancer. *Gynecol Oncol.* 101(3):385.

Steffensen KD, Waldstrom M, Brandslund I et al. 2011. Prognostic impact of prechemotherapy serum levels of HER2, CA125, and HE4 in ovarian cancer patients. *Int J Gynecol Cancer.* 21(6):1040–1047.

Trudel D, Têtu B, Grégoire J et al. 2012. Human epididymis protein 4 (HE4) and ovarian cancer prognosis. *Gynecol Oncol.* 127(3):511–515.

Van den Akker PA, Aalders AL, Snijders MP et al. 2010. Evaluation of the Risk of Malignancy Index in daily clinical management of adnexal masses. *Gynecol Oncol.* 116(3):384–388.

Van Gorp T, Cadron I, Despierre E et al. 2011. HE4 and CA125 as a diagnostic test in ovarian cancer: Prospective validation of the Risk of Ovarian Malignancy Algorithm. *Br J Cancer.* 104(5):863–870.

Veneroni R, Peracchio C, Castino R et al. 2011. Patented biomarkers for the early detection of ovarian cancer. *Recent Pat Biomark.* 1: 1–9.

Winter WE 3rd, Maxwell GL, Tian C et al. 2007. Prognostic factors for stage III epithelial ovarian cancer: A Gynecologic Oncology Group study. *J Clin Oncol.* 25(24):3621.

Wu L, Dai ZY, Qian YH et al. 2012. Diagnostic value of serum human epididymis protein 4 (HE4) in ovarian carcinoma: A systematic review and meta-analysis. *Int J Gynecol Cancer.* 22(7):1106–1112.

Yamashita S, Tokuishi K, Hashimoto T et al. 2011. Prognostic significance of HE4 expression in pulmonary adenocarcinoma. *Tumour Biol.* 32(2):265–271.

Yu S, Yang HJ, Xie SQ et al. 2012. Diagnostic value of HE4 for ovarian cancer: A meta-analysis. *Clin Chem Lab Med.* 50(8):1439–1446.

Zheng H, Gao Y. 2012. Serum HE4 as a useful biomarker in discriminating ovarian cancer from benign pelvic disease. *Int J Gynecol Cancer.* 22(6):1000–1005.

Zivanovic O, Sima CS, Iasonos A et al. 2009. Exploratory analysis of serum CA-125 response to surgery and the risk of relapse in patients with FIGO stage IIIC ovarian cancer. *Gynecol Oncol.* 115(2):209.

Section V

Uterine and Fallopian Tube Cancers

14

Biomarkers in Endometrial Cancer

Gokhan Nas, MS, Tugce Yasar, MS, Mehmet Gunduz, MD, PhD, and Esra Gunduz, DMD, PhD

CONTENTS

ABSTRACT Endometrial carcinoma (EC) is the most commonly diagnosed gynecological malignancy among western countries and fourth most common cancer in women. Most ECs are diagnosed and cured at an early stage. However, about 15%–20% of endometrial tumors exhibit an aggressive phenotype. Based on pathological and molecular characteristics, EC has been classified into two groups: type I estrogen-dependent adenocarcinoma, which has a good prognosis and an endometrioid histology, showing microsatellite instability (MSI) and mutations in PTEN, PIK3CA, K-RAS, CTNNB1 (beta-catenin) gene, etc., and type II or non-estrogen-dependent EC associated with poor prognosis and non-endometrioid histology, exhibiting p53 mutations, STK12 HER2/neu amplification, p16 overexpression, and chromosomal instability. EC develops as a result of a stepwise accumulation of alterations specific of each histological type. However, more knowledge is needed to better understand the differences in the molecular biology and the clinical outcome of EC to produce new molecular targets and better therapeutic strategies. In this chapter, we would like to highlight the present knowledge about biomarkers in EC, assessing how such markers play a role in cancer and could be applied to key clinical challenges for the treatment of this disease. Also, this chapter provides an overview of how traditional and novel molecular biomarkers used for prognosis, diagnosis as well as treatment of EC and discusses miRNAs that may influence the regulation of genes effective in EC.

14.1 Fundamentals of Endometrial Cancer

Endometrial carcinoma (EC) is the fourth most common cancer in women worldwide and is the most common gynecological malignancy in the western world. Ninety percent of the cases are sporadic, while the remaining 10% arise from a genetic background. The 5-year survival rate is around 96%, but the survival rate dramatically decreases up to 17% in cases of women diagnosed with cancer at the regional or distant stage. These patients also have an increased risk of recurrence (Society et al., 2010). Therefore, early diagnosis and treatment of the disease is crucial, and biomarkers play a major role in the process. Biomarkers are defined as a *characteristic that is objectively measured and evaluated as an indicator of normal biologic processes, pathogenic processes, or pharmacologic responses to a therapeutic intervention* (Biomarkers Definitions Working Group, 2001), and genetic, epigenetic, and molecular markers are very important when EC is classified.

There are two clinicopathologic variants of EC. The first is estrogen-dependent endometrioid endometrial carcinomas (EECs) or type I. This group represents the most majority of patients with sporadic EC, cases that arise in relatively younger pre- and postmenopausal women. A low stage, low grade, and endometrioid histology are the characteristics of good prognosis. This type of tumor expresses estrogen receptor (ER) and progesterone receptor (PR) and has a strong etiological association with estrogen exposure (Sherman et al., 1997; Lax et al., 1998). The second group consists of type II or non-endometrioid endometrial carcinomas (NEECs). It is composed of papillary serous and clear-cell carcinomas, which have been associated with a poor prognosis, higher patient age, non-endometrioid histology, and a high stage and grade. They are usually negative or weakly positive for steroid hormone receptors. These cases arise in relatively older women and are not usually preceded by a history of unopposed estrogen exposure (Oehler et al., 2003).

14.2 Molecular Genetics Associated with Endometrial Carcinoma

Type I carcinomas (EECs) are characterized by larger number of genetic alterations, including microsatellite instability (MSI) (Burks et al., 1994; Catasus et al., 1998); PTEN alterations (Tashiro et al., 1997); mutations of PIK3CA (Oda et al., 2005), K-RAS (Enomoto et al., 1991), and beta-catenin (Fukuchi et al., 1998); and DNA mismatch repair (MMR) genes. Whereas p53 mutations, STK15 and HER2/neu amplification, p16 overexpression and downregulation or loss of E-cadherin, and also loss of heterozygosity (LOH) are related to type II EC (Table 14.1). Genes overexpressed in EECs were estrogen-regulated genes, supporting the concept that EEC is a hormone-related tumor.

TABLE 14.1

Genes associated with EC Type 1 and Type 2 with Their Functions and Alterations

	Function	Alteration
K-RAS	Oncogene	Mutation
B-Raf	Oncogene	Mutation
ERBB2	Oncogene	Amplification
PIK3CA	Oncogene	Amplification, mutation
AKT	Oncogene	Mutation
FGFR2	Oncogene	Mutation
CTNNB1	Oncogene	Mutation
PTEN	Tumor suppressor	Mutation, deletion, methylation
TP53	Tumor suppressor	Mutation
ARID1A	Tumor suppressor	Mutation
CDKN2A	Tumor suppressor	Mutation, methylation
MLH1	DNA repair	Methylation
MLH2	DNA repair	Methylation
MSH3	DNA repair	Frameshift mutation
MLH6	DNA repair	Mutation
MSI	DNA repair	Methylation
ER, PR	Transcription factor	Expression
TGF-beta II	Cell growth	Frameshift mutation
IGFIIR	Cell Growth	Frameshift mutation
Bax	Apoptosis	Frameshift mutation
p16	Tumor suppressor	Expression
STK15	Oncogene	Amplification

DNA repair and the MMR system and microsatellites play a crucial role in promoting genetic stability. Microsatellites are di-, tri-, or tetranucleotide tandem repeats in DNA sequences. The number of repeats is variable in populations of DNA and within the alleles of an individual. MSI is a condition exhibited by damaged DNA, due to defects in the normal DNA repair process or during DNA replication, which are related to defects in the MMR genes. This results the microsatellites to become unstable and can shorten or lengthen them and leads to the progressive accumulation of alterations on the DNA strand (Ionov et al., 1993). MSI is found in 17%–25% of all sporadic type I ECs (Salvesen et al., 2000), but it is less frequently present in type II tumors (Tashiro et al., 1997; Catasus et al., 1998).

Telomere shortening is another important type of genomic instability observed in endometrial cancer. Only NEEC tumors were significantly associated with critical telomere shortening in the adjacent morphologically normal epithelium.

With MSI, some germline mutations of hMLH-2, MLH-1, and hMLH-6 have been described in EC (Bianchi et al., 2006; Taylor et al., 2006), and PTEN mutations were found in two short coding mononucleotide repeats (A)5 and (A)6 in 44% of EECs. On the other hand, identical PTEN mutations have been detected in MSI-negative endometrial hyperplasia with coexisting MI-positive EEC, suggesting that PTEN mutations may precede MSI (Lax et al., 2000).

The frequency of frameshift mutations has been evaluated in several genes encoding proteins critical for cell regulatory processes, such as cell growth, DNA repair, or apoptosis (TGF-betaRII, BAX, IGFIIR, MSH3, MSH6) in EECs with MSI, and frameshift mutations at one or more mononucleotide tracts were found in 73% of tumors with MSI (Catasus, 2009).

IGFIIR is also related to tumor progression in EECs with MSI, because IGFIIR frameshift mutations were detected in metastatic carcinomas (Catasus, 2000).

14.2.1 Microsatellite Instability and Methylation

In endometrial cancers, differential DNA methylation patterns are detected with MSI in EECs and NEECs, suggesting divergent epigenetic backgrounds and unique tumorigenic pathways. Genuinely, the inactivation of MLH-1 through the hypermethylation of its promoter has been described as the most common mechanism for tumor suppressor gene inactivation in endometrial cancers with MSI (Esteller et al., 1997). In the development of the MSI phenotype, MLH1 hypermethylation would be an early event in the pathogenesis of EECs. Indeed, the identification of CpG island methylation in the promoter region of some other genes such as APC, MGMT, PTEN, and CDH1 (E-cadherin) in tumors with MSI poses that epigenetic inactivation can be a common mechanism in this subset of tumors.

Hypermethylation is detected in endometrial cancer specimens, 40.4% in hMLH1, 22% in APC, 14% in E-cadherin, and 2.3% in RAR-β (Banno et al., 2006). However, no obvious DNA methylation was found in the p16 gene. Other genes inactivated by promoter hypermethylation in endometrial cancer include PgR (Ghabreau et al., 2004), the cell cycle control genes 14-3-3 sigma (Mhawech et al., 2005), homeobox gene HOXA11, thrombospondin-2 gene (THBS2) (Whitcomb et al., 2003), paternally expressed gene 3 (PEG3) (Dowdy, 2005), and the detoxifying enzyme glutathione S-transferase P1 (GSTP1) (Chan et al., 2005) (Table 14.2). The impact of methylation on these genes in endometrial cancer development has not been well identified yet.

Loss of RASSF1A function due to epigenetic gene silencing has been detected in various tumors and may contribute to the increased activity of the RAS–MAPK signaling pathway. Recent studies have demonstrated that RASSF1A inactivation by promoter hypermethylation is very common in ECs (74%), particularly in advanced-stage ECs (Pallerés, 2008).

14.2.2 Oncogenes

14.2.2.1 K-RAS

K-RAS encodes a member protein of the small GTPase superfamily and is involved in signal transduction pathways between cell surface receptors and the nucleus. K-RAS also binds

TABLE 14.2

Hypermethylated Genes in ECs
CDH1
APC
MGMT
PTEN
RAR-beta
PgR
14-3-3 sigma
HOXA11
THBS2
PEG3
GSTP1
RASSF1A

directly to PIK3CA, upregulates lipid kinase activity, and can activate the antiapoptotic AKT pathway (Enomoto et al., 1991; Lagarda et al., 2001).

K-RAS mutations are early events in endometrial carcinogenesis, and mutations of this gene have been identified in 19%–46% of ECs (Esteller et al., 1997). Alterations of K-RAS mainly involve type I tumors and have been reported in 10%–30% of the cases of EEC (Lax et al., 2000).

Different studies have shown that the frequency of K-RAS mutations rises progressively from simple to complex hyperplasia and to carcinoma and that the presence of K-RAS mutations in premalignant biopsy samples has been suggested as a marker of progression to malignancy.

14.2.2.2 B-Raf

B-Raf gene encodes a protein belonging to the raf/mil family of serine/threonine protein kinases. This protein plays a role in regulating the MAP kinase/ERKs signaling pathway, which affects cell division, differentiation, and secretion. Mutations in this gene have been associated with various cancers, including non-Hodgkin lymphoma, colorectal cancer, malignant melanoma, thyroid carcinoma, non-small-cell lung carcinoma, and adenocarcinoma of the lung.

In endometrial cancer, B-raf mutation was identified in 21% of cases, and the mutation correlated with the decreased hMLH1 expression (Feng et al., 2005). But the role of B-raf mutation in the development of endometrial cancer has not yet been clearly identified.

14.2.2.3 HER-2/neu (ERBB2)

ERBB2 gene encodes a member of the epidermal growth factor (EGF) receptor family of receptor tyrosine kinases. This protein has no ligand-binding domain of its own and therefore cannot bind growth factors. However, it does bind tightly to other ligand-bound EGF receptor family members to form a heterodimer, stabilizing ligand binding and enhancing kinase-mediated activation of downstream signaling pathways, such as those involving mitogen-activated protein kinase and phosphatidylinositol-3 kinase. Allelic variations at amino acid positions 654 and 655 of isoform (positions 624 and 625 of isoform b) have been reported, with the most common allele, Ile654/Ile655. Amplification or overexpression of this gene has been reported in numerous cancers, including breast and ovarian tumors. Overexpression of the protein product HER-2/neu is reported in 9%–30% of all ECs, being more frequent in non-endometrioid tumors, and has been associated with adverse prognostic parameters including advanced stage, high histological grade, and low overall survival (Berchuck et al., 1991; Slomovitz et al., 2004).

14.2.2.4 PIK3CA

PIK3CA is the catalytic subunit of PI3K. Mutations in this gene occur in 24%–36% of all ECs and are coexistent with PTEN mutations (Oda et al., 2005). Studies have shown that PIK3CA mutations are frequent in EECs and are associated with invasion and adverse prognostic factors, such as blood vessel invasion (Catasus et al., 2008). PIK3CA mutations described in exon 9 are associated with low-grade carcinomas. However, carcinomas with exon 20 PIK3CA mutations or PIK3CA messenger RNA (mRNA) overexpression were often high grade. PIK3CA also plays an important role in the PI3K–AKT pathway's regulation of apoptosis. This fact suggests that its alteration could represent an important step in the development and progression of EC. Activation of this pathway suppresses apoptosis that is triggered by various stimuli. Recent analysis in EC, which integrated copy number and expression data, has shown that amplifications of PIK3CA correspond to expression profiles of PI3K activation; this suggests PI3K as a potential target for new therapies (Salvesen et al., 2009).

14.2.2.5 AKT

The phosphatidylinositol 3-kinase (PI3K)–AKT pathway is activated in many human cancers and plays a key role in cell proliferation and survival. PIK3CA mutations frequently occur with other genetic alterations such as Her2/neu, K-RAS, and PTEN in several types of tumors. Endometrial cancer is known to possess various gene alterations that activate the PI3K–AKT pathway. It is reported that AKT1 (E17K) mutations were detected in 2 out of 89 tissue samples and 0 out of 12 cell lines (Shoji et al., 2009). They suggested that AKT1 mutations might be mutually exclusive from other PI3K–AKT activating alterations, although PIK3CA mutations frequently coexist with other gene aberrations. Additional mutations in AKT family members in endometrial cancers were reported in AKT2 (D399N, 426T, and 141T) and in AKT3 (E438D) (Dutt et al., 2009).

14.2.2.6 FGFR2

The FGFR2 gene provides instructions for making a protein called fibroblast growth factor receptor 2 (FGFR2). This protein is one of several fibroblast growth factor receptors, which are related proteins that are involved in important processes such as cell division, regulation of cell growth and maturation, formation of blood vessels, wound healing, and embryonic development. Alterations in the FGFR2 gene cause the receptors to become active, leading to cell proliferation. Mutations are reported in FGFR2 in 10% of primary uterine tumor samples (Byron et al., 2008). Mutations were observed in 16% of the endometrioid histology subtype tumors. In primary endometrioid endometrial cancers, FGFR2 and K-RAS mutations were mutually exclusive. Conversely, FGFR2 mutations were seen together with PTEN loss-of-function mutations. The authors also showed that endometrial cancer cell lines with activating FGFR2 mutations are selectively sensitive to the pan-FGFR inhibitor, PD173074 (Byron and Pollock, 2009). In addition, upregulation of FGF2 mRNA expression was observed in endometrial cancer specimens (Soufla et al., 2008). These data suggest that investigation of these agents may be therapeutically beneficial for endometrial cancer patients.

14.2.2.7 Beta-Catenin (CTNNB1)

The protein encoded by CTNNB1 gene is part of a complex of proteins that constitute adherens junctions (AJs). AJs are necessary for the creation and maintenance of epithelial cell layers by regulating cell growth and adhesion between cells. β-catenin also acts as a downstream transcriptional activator in the Wnt signal transduction pathway. Mutations in exon 3 of beta-catenin result in stabilization of the protein that occur in 14%–44% of all ECs and lead to cytoplasmic and nuclear accumulation, participation in signal transduction, and transcriptional activation of genes involved in the development and progression of cancer. Abnormal nuclear beta-catenin accumulation also results in transcriptional activation through the LEF/Tcf pathway of genes such as MMP-7, CCND1 (cyclin D1), Connexin 43, ITF2, c-myc, and PPAR-δ.

Nuclear accumulation of β-catenin is significantly more common in endometrioid lesions compared to non-endometrioid histologies (Moreno-Bueno et al., 2002), and it is reported that β-catenin nuclear accumulation was more frequent in endometrial hyperplasia than in EC samples, suggesting a β-catenin role in the early development of this tumor type (Nei et al., 1999).

Also, it is identified that all β-catenin mutated tumors were estrogen-receptor (ESR) positive, and most were progesterone-receptor (PgR) positive suggesting a dependence on estrogen stimulation during endometrial carcinogenesis (Koul et al., 2002).

14.2.3 Tumor Suppressor Genes

14.2.3.1 PTEN

PTEN gene was identified as a tumor suppressor that is mutated in a large number of cancers at high frequency. The protein encoded by this gene is a phosphatidylinositol-3,4,5-trisphosphate 3-phosphatase. It contains a tensin-like domain as well as a catalytic domain similar to that of the dual specificity protein tyrosine phosphatases. Unlike most of the protein tyrosine phosphatases, this protein preferentially dephosphorylates phosphoinositide substrates. It negatively regulates intracellular levels of phosphatidylinositol-3,4,5-trisphosphate in cells and functions as a tumor suppressor by negatively regulating AKT/PKB signaling pathway. PTEN has been reported to be altered in 25%–83% of tumors (Simpkins et al., 1998), and up to 83% of these cases are endometrioid carcinomas, whereas serous and clear cell carcinomas harbor mutations in this gene in just 10% of the reported cases (Mutter et al., 2000; Bansal et al., 2009). Mutations in this gene have also been observed in endometrial hyperplasia, suggesting that this could be an early event in carcinogenesis (Maxwell et al., 1998). Several groups have described a concordance between MSI status and PTEN mutations; the mutations occur in 60%–86% of MSI-positive EEC cases, but only occur in 24%–35% of MSI-negative tumors. Genetic alterations that account for PTEN protein inactivation include various mutations, an LOH, or promoter hypermethylation, with mutations occurring the most frequently (Mutter et al., 2000). PTEN promoter methylation is observed in 19% of cancers and is significantly associated with metastatic disease (Salvesen et al., 2001). Mutations in the PTEN function, along with the consequent activation of the PI3K–AKT pathway, lead to the uncontrolled function of several kinases, such as mTOR, which acts as a promoter of cellular proliferation (Salvesen et al., 2001; Boruban et al., 2008). The activation of the PI3K–AKT–mTOR signaling pathway, induced by a loss of function of the PTEN gene, suggests that mTOR inhibition may play a therapeutic role.

14.2.3.2 TP53

TP53 gene encodes tumor protein p53, which responds to diverse cellular stresses to regulate target genes that induce cell cycle arrest, apoptosis, senescence, DNA repair, or changes in metabolism. p53 is a DNA-binding protein containing transcription activation, DNA-binding, and oligomerization domains. It is postulated to bind to a p53-binding site and activate expression of downstream genes that inhibit growth and/or invasion and thus function as a tumor suppressor. Mutants of p53 that frequently occur in a number of different human cancers fail to bind the consensus DNA–binding site and hence cause the loss of tumor suppressor activity. Mutations in the p53 tumor suppressor oncogene constitute the most common genetic alterations in type II ECs (60%–85%) (Tashiro et al., 1997; Lax et al., 2000). In contrast, p53 mutations have been observed in only 17% of the cases of endometrioid EC (Lax et al., 2000). p53 alterations are frequently found with PIK3CA mutations, almost all located in exon 20, in advanced stages, and in aggressive histological types of ECs. However, concomitant PIK3CA mRNA overexpression and p53 alterations occurred exclusively in NEECs (Tashiro et al., 1997). p53 mutations are also rarely observed in ovarian clear cell adenocarcinomas in comparison to endometrioid adenocarcinoma (Okuda et al., 2003). Due to the increased incidence of p53 mutations in serous carcinomas of the uterus, it is postulated that mutation in one allele may occur during the initial stages of neoplastic transformation, while loss of the second, normal allele may occur late in the progression of carcinoma (Mountzios et al., 2011).

14.2.3.3 ARID1A

ARID1A gene encodes a member of the SWI/SNF family, whose members have helicase and ATPase activities and are thought to regulate transcription of certain genes by altering the chromatin structure around those genes. The encoded protein is part of the large ATP-dependent chromatin remodeling complex SNF/SWI, which is required for transcriptional activation of genes normally repressed by chromatin and also confers specificity to the SNF/SWI complex and may recruit the complex to its targets through either protein–DNA or protein–protein interactions.

ARID1A is mutated in approximately 50% of ovarian clear cell and 30% of ovarian endometrioid carcinomas (Wiegand et al., 2010). Uterine low-grade endometrioid carcinomas showed a relatively high-frequency loss of ARID1A expression (26% of cases, 40% of uterine endometrioid carcinomas). All mutations in endometrioid carcinomas were nonsense or insertion/deletion mutations, and tumors with ARID1A mutations showed complete loss or clonally loss of ARID1A expression. The other tumor that had a relatively high-frequency loss of ARID1A expression was gastric carcinoma (11%). Their results suggest that the molecular pathogenesis of low-grade uterine endometrioid carcinoma is similar to that of ovarian low-grade endometrioid and clear-cell carcinoma, tumors that have previously been shown to have a high-frequency loss of expression and mutation of ARID1A.

Loss of the protein ARID1A was frequent in ECs but infrequent in other types of malignancies, with loss observed in 29% of grade 1 or 2 and 39% of grade 3 endometrioid, 18% of serous, and 26% of clear-cell ECs. Loss of ARID1A expression is relatively common in high-grade carcinomas arising from the endometrium, suggesting that ARID1A mutations can trigger malignant transformation.

14.2.4 Other Genes

There are other onco- and tumor suppressor genes still under investigation for their possible involvement in ECs. Some of them are ACAA1, AP1M2, CGN, DDR1, EPS8L2, FASTKD1, GMIP, IKBKE, P2RX4, P4HB, PHKG2, PPFIBP2, PPP1R16A, RASSF7, RNF183, SIRT6, TJP3, EFEMP2, SOCS2, TFF3, CDKN2A. DCN found differentially expressed in EC, and C-myc, survivin, CCNE(Cyclin E), RUNX1, ETV5 (Ets-related protein), and human telomerase reverse transcriptase (hTERT) genes are also target genes in ECs (Table 14.3). ERM/ETV5, specifically, is upregulated in EEC and is associated with myometrial infiltration (Monge et al., 2007). In the case of EC, ETV5 has been proposed to play a role during the early events of endometrial tumorigenesis and could be associated with an initial switch to myometrial infiltration. ETV5 upregulation may participate in the process of transition from normal atrophic endometrium to simple and complex hyperplasia and EC. ETV5 has also been related to regulating the migratory and invasive properties of the tumor and to increasing protective response against the oxidative stress produced in the promotion of an EC invasion (Monge et al., 2009).

TABLE 14.3

Other Genes Over-/Underexpressed or Mutated in ECs

C-myc	ACAA1	PPF1BP2
Survivin	AP1M2	PPP1R116A
hTERT	CGN	RASSF7
ERM	DDR1	RNF183
ETV5	EPS8L2	SIRT6
RUNX	FASTKD1	TJP3
PMS-2	GMIP	EFEMP2
CYP1B1	IKBKE	SOCS2
Dkk3	P2RX4	TFF3
NF-kB	P4HB	DCN
KSR1	PHKG2	

The RUNX genes have been reported to function as both tumor suppressors and dominant oncogenes in a context-dependent manner. They are closely related and are essential for hematopoiesis, osteogenesis, and neurogenesis (Blyth et al., 2005; Planaguma et al., 2006). Chromosomal translocations involving the RUNX1 gene are well documented and have been associated with several types of leukemia. In a microarray study of invasive EC, RUNX1 was identified as one of the most highly overexpressed genes (Planaguma et al., 2004), and through immunohistochemistry analysis, it showed a strong positive correlation to p21WAF1/CIP1 (a target of p53-mediated growth arrest), especially in carcinomas that had infiltrated more than 50% of the myometrium. It has been hypothesized that in EEC p21WAF1/CIP1 and RUNX1 could interact during the initial steps of tumor dissemination. Recent studies have reported a similar codistribution of MMP-2 and MMP-9, as with ETV5, at the invasive front of EC (Planaguma et al., 2011).

HNPCC patients with endometrial cancers have an inherited germline mutation in MLH-1, MSH-2, MSH-6, or PMS-2, but endometrial cancer only develops after the instauration of a deletion or mutation in the contralateral MLH-1, MSH-2, MSH-6, or PMS-2 allele. Following this, the deficient MMR (MLH-1, MSH-2, MSH-6, or PMS-2) causes the acquisition of MSI and the development of the tumor. Inactivation of the MMR gene MLH1 by methylation of the promoter seems to be the most frequent cause of MSI in sporadic endometrioid carcinomas, followed by a loss of the expression of other two MMR genes, the MSH2 and MSH6 genes. CYP1B1 depletion in endometrial cancer cells leads to decreased cellular proliferation and induced G0–G1 cell cycle arrest, thus suggesting that CYP1B1 inhibition in endometrial cancer cells could be a useful therapeutic approach (Saini et al., 2009).

Dkk3 is a tumor suppressor gene, and Dkk3 gene expression is downregulated in endometrial cancer associated with poor prognosis affecting both proliferation and invasiveness.

14.3 Apoptosis Resistance

Recent evidence that NF-kB activation is frequent in EC may explain the presence of apoptosis resistance by activation of target genes, such as FLIP and Bcl-XL (Pallares et al., 2004; Dolcet et al., 2005; Llobet et al., 2008a,b). Also, members of the Bcl-2 family of genes are abnormal in EC. Finally, other proteins involved in apoptotic control (like survivin) have also been shown to be abnormal in EC (Pallares et al., 2005). FLIP, whose expression is frequent in ECs (Dolcet et al., 2005), is an important protein responsible for apoptosis resistance in EC. A direct evidence of the role of FLIP in TRAIL apoptosis resistance on EC cells has been provided by treatment with specific siRNA targeting FLIP (Llobet et al., 2009). The transfected cells showed a marked decrease in cell viability, after TRAIL exposition. Moreover, kinase suppressor of Ras 1 (KSR1) gene, which has been found overexpressed in EC, also regulates endometrial sensitivity to TRAIL by regulating FLIP levels (Llobet et al., 2011).

14.4 Epithelial-to-Mesenchymal Transition

Epithelial–mesenchymal transition (EMT) is a series of events during development by which epithelial cells acquire mesenchymal, fibroblast-like properties and show reduced intercellular adhesion and increased motility. Loss of expression or function of the E-cadherin, protein encoded by the CDH1 gene located at 16q21, is the hallmark of this process. The loss of epithelial characteristics, including cadherin switching and the acquisition of a mesenchymal phenotype, is achieved through repressors of E-cadherin such as the zinc finger factors Snail and Slug, the handed factors SIP-1 (Zeb-2) and EF1 (Zeb-1), and the bHLH factors E12/E47 and Twist. Reduced expression of E-cadherin results in dysfunction of the cell–cell adhesion system and promotion of tumor invasion and metastasis. In EC, partial or complete loss of E-cadherin expression correlates with adverse prognosis and shorter overall survival. Reduced E-cadherin expression has been found in 58% of ECs, being more frequent in NEECs (87%) than in EECs (22%) and in advanced-stage carcinomas. LOH of the CDH1 gene was found in 57% of NEECs but only in 22% of EECs.

14.5 miRNA Profiling of Endometrial Cancer

MicroRNAs (miRNAs) are short, 22- to 25-nucleotide noncoding sequences of RNA. These sequences control gene expression either by translational repression or by degradation of the mRNA transcript. These miRNAs may be upregulated or downregulated in various tumor types, thus displaying their roles as potential tumor suppressors or oncogenes.

Increased expression of some miRNAs is demonstrated in ECs such as mir-200, mir-183, mir-205, mir-223, and mir-425 family when compared with normal endometrial specimens. In contrast, miRNAs like mir-029a, mir-126, mir-1-2, mir-143, mir-125b, let-7a, and mir-133 had at least a twofold reduction in expression in tumors. DNMT3A, K-RAS, HMGA2 and DNA MMR genes MLH1, and MSH2 are within the possible targets of these underexpressed miRNAs. Some overexpressed miRNAs such as mir-200c and mir-183 in ECs are predicted to target PTEN. Also, mir-149, which demonstrated fourfold relative overexpression compared with early-stage cancers, is known to target TP53. You can also find miRNAs studied so far and differentially expressed in ECs (Table 14.4).

TABLE 14.4

Differentially Expressed miRNAs in ECs

mir-516	mir-033b	mir-29a	mir-125b1
let-7a	mir-425	mir-126a	mir-125b2
mir-424	mir-181c	mir-1(2)	mir-133a
mir-496	mir-19b	mir-143	mir-26a1
mir-409	mir-009	mir-125b	
mir-451	mir-205	mir-133	
mir-431	mir-423	mir-145a	
mir-516	mir-223	let-7c	
mir-503	mir-183	mir-10b	
mir-369	mir-146	mir-123	
mir-032	mir-200c	mir-26a	

14.6 Conclusion and Future Direction

EC is a common malignancy and has a relatively good prognosis when diagnosed in its early stages but is deadly in its advanced stages. The most important factors that lead EC to bad prognosis are its genetic, epigenetic, and molecular background. Epidemiology and Genetics Research Program (EGRP) at the National Cancer Institute (NCI) identified the lack of biomarkers for EC development and progression as a key challenge. Fortunately, significant progression has occurred in understanding the molecular bases for the malignant transformation of normal cells, and it is possible to take advantage of this increased understanding of tumorigenesis and develop novel therapies that target these molecular alterations. One of the comprehensive molecular characterizations of primary tumors has identified drugs targeting the PI3K/PTEN/AKT/mTOR pathway and FGFR2 as promising for further studies, also reflected currently in phase 1 and phase 2 trials in EC, that are in progress. Also, miRNA studies are important to illuminate the understanding of how endometrial carcinoma is regulated. Moreover, the appearance of novel molecular approaches such as the detection of biomarkers and tools such as the orthotopic mouse models for therapeutic trials are going to improve the diagnosis, understanding, and treatment of this disease. The findings of novel molecular markers will represent the basis for the development of a highly sensitive and specific, minimally invasive screening method for ECs. Additionally, the improvement of model organisms, which mimic the clinical behavior of EC, will also provide an advanced tool for future studies dealing with tumoral physiopathology and testing for anticancer therapies in preclinical studies.

References

ACOG, 2005. ACOG practice bulletin, clinical management guidelines for obstetrician-gynecologists, number 65, August 2005: Management of endometrial cancer. *Obstet. Gynecol.* 106, 413–425.

Banno, K., Yanokura, M., and Susumu, N., 2006. Relationship of the aberrant DNA hypermethylation of cancer-related genes with carcinogenesis of endometrial cancer. *Oncol. Rep.*, 16(6), 1189–1196.

Bansal, N., Yendluri, V., and Wenham, R.M., 2009. The molecular biology of endometrial cancers and the implications for pathogenesis, classification, and targeted therapies. *Cancer Control*, 16, 8–13.

Berchuck, A., Rodriguez, G., Kinney, R.B., Soper, J.T., Dodge, R.K., Clarke-Pearson, D.L., and Bast Jr., R.C., 1991. Overexpression of HER-2/neu in endometrial cancer is associated with advanced stage disease. *Am. J. Obstet. Gynecol.*, 164, 15–21.

Bianchi, F., Rosati, S., Belvederesi, L., Loretelli, C., Catalani, R., Mandolesi, A., Bracci, R., Bearzi, I., Porfiri, E., and Cellerino, R., 2006. MSH2 splice site mutation and endometrial cancer. *Int. J. Gynecol. Cancer*, 16, 1419–1423.

Biomarkers Definitions Working Group, 2001. Biomarkers and surrogate endpoints: Preferred definitions and conceptual framework. *Clin. Pharmacol. Ther.*, 69, 89–95.

Blyth, K., Cameron, E.R., and Neil, J.C., 2005. The RUNX genes: Gain or loss of function in cancer. *Nat. Rev. Cancer*, 5, 376–387.

Boruban, M.C., Altundag, K., Kilic, G.S., and Blankstein, J., 2008. From endometrial hyperplasia to endometrial cancer: Insight into the biology and possible medical preventive measures. *Eur. J. Cancer Prev.*, 17, 133–138.

Burks, R.T., Kessis, T.D., Cho, K.R., and Hedrick, L., 1994. Microsatellite instability in endometrial carcinoma. *Oncogene*, 9, 1163–1166.

Byron, S.A., Gartside, M.G., and Wellens, C.L., 2008. Inhibition of activated fibroblast growth factor receptor 2 in endometrial cancer cells induces cell death despite PTEN abrogation. *Cancer Res.*, 68(17), 6902–6907.

Byron, S.A. and Pollock, P.M., 2009. FGFR2 as a molecular target in endometrial cancer. *Future Oncol.*, 5(1), 27–32.

Catasus, L., Machin, P., Matias-Guiu, X., and Prat, J., 1998. Microsatellite instability in endometrial carcinomas clinicopathologic correlations in a series of 42 cases. *Hum. Pathol.*, 29, 1160–1164.

Catasus, L., Matias-Guiu, X., Machin, P. et al., 2000. Frameshift mutations at coding mononucleotide repeat microsatellites in endometrial carcinoma with microsatellite instability. *Cancer*, 88, 2290e7.

Catasus, L., Gallardo, A., Cuatrecasas, M., and Prat, J., 2008. PIK3CA mutations in the kinase domain (exon 20) of uterine endometrial adenocarcinomas are associated with adverse prognostic parameters. *Mod. Pathol.*, 21, 131–139.

Catasus, L., Gallardo, A., and Prat, J., 2009. Molecular genetics of endometrial carcinoma. *Diagn. Histopathol.*, 15(12), 554–563. doi:10.1016/j.mpdhp.2009.09.002.

Chan, Q.K.Y., Khoo, U.-S., and Chan, K.Y.K., 2005. Promoter methylation and differential expression of π-class glutathione S-transferase in endometrial carcinoma. *J. Mol. Diagn.*, 7(1), 8–16.

Dolcet, X., Llobet, D., Pallares, J., Rue, M., Comella, J.X., and Matias-Guiu, X., 2005. FLIP is frequently expressed in endometrial carcinoma and has a role in resistance to TRAIL-induced apoptosis. *Lab. Invest.* 85, 885–894.

Dowdy, S.C., Gostout, B.S., Shridhar, V., Wu, X., Smith, D.I., Podratz, K.C., and Jiang, S.-W. 2005. Biallelic methylation and silencing of paternally expressed gene 3 (PEG3) in gynecologic cancer cell lines. *Gynecol. Oncol.*, 99(1), 126–134.

Dutt, A., Salvesen, H.B., Greulich, H., Sellers, W.R., Beroukhim, R., and Meyerson, M., 2009. Somatic mutations are present in all members of the AKT family in endometrial carcinoma. *Br. J. Cancer*, 101(7), 1218–1219.

Enomoto, T., Inoue, M., Perantoni, A.O. et al., 1991. K-Ras activation in premalignant and malignant epithelial lesions of the human uterus. *Cancer Res.*, 51, 5308e14.

Esteller, M., Garcia, A., Martinez-Palones, J.M., Xercavins, J., and Reventos, J., 1997. The clinicopathological significance of K-RAS point mutation and gene amplification in endometrial cancer. *Eur. J. Cancer*, 33, 1572–1577.

Feng, Y.-Z., Shiozawa, T., and Miyamoto, T., 2005. BRAF mutation in endometrial carcinoma and hyperplasia: Correlation with KRAS and p53 mutations and mismatch repair protein expression. *Clin. Cancer Res.*, 11(17), 6133–6138.

Fukuchi, T., Sakamoto, M., Tsuda, H., Maruyama, K., Nozawa, S., and Hirohashi, S., 1998. Beta-catenin mutations in carcinoma of the uterine endometrium. *Cancer Res.*, 58, 3526e8.

Ghabreau, L., Roux, J.P., Niveleau, A., 2004. Correlation between the DNA global methylation status and progesterone receptor expression in normal endometrium, endometrioid adenocarcinoma and precursors. *Virchows Archiv.*, 445(2), 129–134.

Ionov, Y., Peinado, M.A., Malkhosyan, S., Shibata, D., and Perucho, M., 1993. Ubiquitous somatic mutations in simple repeated sequences reveal a new mechanism for colonic carcinogenesis. *Nature*, 363, 558–561.

Koul, A., Will, R., Bendahl, P.-O., Nilbert, M., and Borg, A., 2002. Distinct sets of gene alterations in endometrial carcinoma implicate alternate modes of tumorigenesis. *Cancer*, 94(9), 2369–2379.

Lagarda, H., Catasus, L., Arguelles, R., Matias-Guiu, X., and Prat, J. 2001. K-ras mutations in endometrial carcinomas with microsatellite instability. *J. Pathol.*, 193, 193–199.

Lax, S.F., Kendall, B., Tashiro, H., Slebos, R.J., and Hedrick, L. 2000. The frequency of p53, K-Ras mutations, and microsatellite instability differs in uterine endometrioid and serous carcinoma: Evidence of distinct molecular genetic pathways. *Cancer*, 88:814e24.

Lax, S.F., Pizer, E.S., Ronnett, B.M., and Kurman, R.J., 1998. Clear cell carcinoma of the endometrium is characterized by a distinctive profile of p53, Ki-67, estrogen, and progesterone receptor expression. *Hum. Pathol.*, 29, 551–558.

Llobet, D., Eritja, N., Domingo, M., Bergada, L., Mirantes, C., Santacana, M., Pallares, J. et al., 2011. KSR1 is overexpressed in endometrial carcinoma and regulates proliferation and TRAIL-induced apoptosis by modulating FLIP levels. *Am. J. Pathol.*, 178, 1529–1543.

Llobet, D., Eritja, N., Encinas, M., Llecha, N., Yeramian, A., Pallares, J., Sorolla, A., Gonzalez-Tallada, F.J., Matias-Guiu, X., and Dolcet, X., 2008a. CK2 controls TRAIL and Fas sensitivity by regulating FLIP levels in endometrial carcinoma cells. *Oncogene*, 27, 2513–2524.

Llobet, D., Eritja, N., Yeramian, A., Pallares, J., Sorolla, A., Domingo, M., Santacana, M., Gonzalez-Tallada, F.J., Matias-Guiu, X., and Dolcet, X., 2008b. The multikinase inhibitor Sorafenib induces apoptosis and sensitises endometrial cancer cells to TRAIL by different mechanisms. *Eur. J. Cancer*, 46, 836–850.

Llobet, D., Pallares, J., Yeramian, A., Santacana, M., Eritja, N., Velasco, A., Dolcet, X., and Matias-Guiu, X., 2009. Molecular pathology of endometrial carcinoma: Practical aspects from the diagnostic and therapeutic viewpoints. *J. Clin. Pathol.*, 62, 777–785.

Maxwell, G.L., Risinger, J.I., Gumbs, C., Shaw, H., Bentley, R.C., Barrett, J.C., Berchuck, A., and Futreal, P.A., 1998. Mutation of the PTEN tumor suppressor gene in endometrial hyperplasias. *Cancer Res.*, 58, 2500–2503.

Mhawech, P., Benz, A., and Cerato, C., 2005. Downregulation of 14-3-3σ in ovary, prostate and endometrial carcinomas is associated with CpG island methylation. *Mod. Pathol.*, 18(3), 340–348.

Monge, M., Colas, E., Doll, A., Gil-Moreno, A., Castellvi, J., Diaz, B., Gonzalez, M. et al. , 2009. Proteomic approach to ETV5 during endometrial carcinoma invasion reveals a link to oxidative stress. *Carcinogenesis* 30, 1288–1297.

Monge, M., Colas, E., Doll, A., Gonzalez, M., Gil-Moreno, A., Planaguma, J., Quiles, M. et al., 2007. ERM/ETV5 up-regulation plays a role during myometrial infiltration through matrix metalloproteinase-2 activation in endometrial cancer. *Cancer Res.*, 67, 6753–6759.

Moreno-Bueno, G., Hardisson, D., and Sánchez, C., 2002. Abnormalities of the APC/β-catenin pathway in endometrial cancer. *Oncogene*, 21(52), 7981–7990.

Mountzios, G., Pectasides, D., Bournakis, E., Pectasides, E., Bozas, G., Dimopoulos, M.A., and Papadimitriou, C.A., 2011. Developments in the systemic treatment of endometrial cancer. *Crit. Rev. Oncol. Hematol.*, 79(3), 278–292.

Mutter, G.L., Lin, M.C., Fitzgerald, J.T., Kum, J.B., Baak, J.P., Lees, J.A., Weng, L.P., and Eng, C., 2000. Altered PTEN expression as a diagnostic marker for the earliest endometrial precancers. *J. Natl. Cancer Inst.*, 92(11), 924–930.

Nei, H., Saito, T., Yamasaki, H., Mizumoto, H., Ito, E., and Kudo, R., 1999. Nuclear localization of β-catenin in normal and carcinogenic endometrium. *Mol. Carcinogenesis*, 25(3), 207–218.

Oda, K., Stokoe, D., Taketani, Y., and McCormick, F., 2005. High frequency of coexistent mutations of PIK3CA and PTEN genes in endometrial carcinoma. *Cancer Res.*, 65, 10669e73.

Oehler, M.K., Brand, A., and Wain, G.V., 2003. Molecular genetics and endometrial cancer. *J. Br. Menopause Soc.*, 9, 27–31.

Okuda, T., Otsuka, J., Sekizawa, A., Saito, H., Makino, R., Kushima, M., Farina, A., Kuwano, Y., Okai, T., 2003. p53 Mutations and overexpression affect prognosis of ovarian endometrioid cancer but not clear cell cancer. *Gynecol. Oncol.*, 88, 318–325.

Pallares, J., Martinez-Guitarte, J.L., Dolcet, X., Llobet, D., Rue, M., Palacios, J., Prat, J., and Matias-Guiu, X., 2004. Abnormalities in the NF-kappaB family and related proteins in endometrial carcinoma. *J. Pathol.*, 204, 569–577.

Pallares, J., Martinez-Guitarte, J.L., Dolcet, X., Llobet, D., Rue, M., Palacios, J., Prat, J., and Matias-Guiu, X., 2005. Survivin expression in endometrial carcinoma: A tissue microarray study with correlation with PTEN and STAT-3. *Int. J. Gynecol. Pathol.*, 24, 247–253.

Pallarés, J., Velasco, A., Eritja, N. et al., 2008. Promoter hypermethylation and reduced expression of RASSF1A are frequent molecular alterations of endometrial carcinoma. *Mod. Pathol.*, 21, 691e9.

Planaguma, J., Diaz-Fuertes, M., Gil-Moreno, A., Abal, M., Monge, M., Garcia, A., Baro, T. et al., 2004. A differential gene expression profile reveals overexpression of RUNX1/AML1 in invasive endometrioid carcinoma. *Cancer Res.*, 64, 8846–8853.

Planaguma, J., Gonzalez, M., Doll, A., Monge, M., Gil-Moreno, A., Baro, T., Garcia, A. et al., 2006. The up-regulation profiles of p21WAF1/CIP1 and RUNX1/AML1 correlate with myometrial infiltration in endometrioid endometrial carcinoma. *Hum. Pathol.*, 37, 1050–1057.

Planaguma, J., Liljestrom, M., Alameda, F., Butzow, R., Virtanen, I., Reventos, J., and Hukkanen, M., 2011. Matrix metalloproteinase-2 and matrix metalloproteinase-9 co-distribute with transcription factors RUNX1/AML1 and ETV5/ERM at the invasive front of endometrial and ovarian carcinoma. *Hum. Pathol.*, 42, 57–67.

Saini, S., Hirata, H., Majid, S., and Dahiya, R., 2009. Functional significance of cytochrome P450 1B1 in endometrial carcinogenesis. *Cancer Res.*, 69(17), 7038–7045.

Salvesen, H.B., Carter, S.L., Mannelqvist, M., Dutt, A., Getz, G., Stefansson, I.M., Raeder, M.B. et al., 2009. Integrated genomic profiling of endometrial carcinoma associates aggressive tumors with indicators of PI3 kinase activation. *Proc. Natl. Acad. Sci. USA*, 106, 4834–4839.

Salvesen, H.B., MacDonald, N., Ryan, A., Iversen, O.E., Jacobs, I.J., Akslen, L.A., and Das, S., 2000. Methylation of hMLH1 in a population-based series of endometrial carcinomas. *Clin. Cancer Res.*, 6, 3607–3613.

Salvesen, H.B., MacDonald, N., Ryan, A., Jacobs, I.J., Lynch, E.D., Akslen, L.A., and Das, S., 2001. PTEN methylation is associated with advanced stage and microsatellite instability in endometrial carcinoma. *Int. J. Cancer*, 91(1), 22–26.

Sherman, M.E., Sturgeon, S., Brinton, L.A., Potischman, N., Kurman, R.J., Berman, M.L., Mortel, R., Twiggs, L.B., Barrett, R.J., and Wilbanks, G.D., 1997. Risk factors and hormone levels in patients with serous and endometrioid uterine carcinomas. *Mod. Pathol.*, 10, 963–968.

Shoji, K., Oda, K., and Nakagawa S., 2009. The oncogenic mutation in the pleckstrin homology domain of AKT1 in endometrial carcinomas. *Br. J. Cancer*, 101(1), 145–148.

Simpkins, S.B., Peiffer-Schneider, S., Mutch, D.G., Gersell, D., and Goodfellow, P.J., 1998. PTEN mutations in endometrial cancers with 10q LOH: Additional evidence for the involvement of multiple tumor suppressors. *Gynecol. Oncol.*, 71, 391–395.

Slomovitz, B.M., Broaddus, R.R., Burke, T.W., Sneige, N., Soliman, P.T., Wu, W., Sun, C.C., Munsell, M.F., Gershenson, D.M., and Lu, K.H., 2004. Her-2/neu overexpression and amplification in uterine papillary serous carcinoma. *J. Clin. Oncol.*, 22, 3126–3132.

Society, A.C., 2010. *Cancer Facts and Figures 2010*. American Cancer Society, Atlanta, GA.

Soufla, G., Sifakis, S., and Spandidos, D.A., 2008. FGF2 transcript levels are positively correlated with EGF and IGF-1 in the malignant endometrium. *Cancer Lett.*, 259(2), 146–155.

Tashiro, H., Isacson, C., Levine, R., Kurman, R.J., Cho, K.R., and Hedrick, L., 1997. p53 gene mutations are common in uterine serous carcinoma and occur early in their pathogenesis. *Am. J. Pathol.*, 150, 177e85.

Taylor, N.P., Powell, M.A., Gibb, R.K., Rader, J.S., Huettner, P.C., Thibodeau, S.N., Mutch, D.G., and Goodfellow, P.J., 2006. MLH3 mutation in endometrial cancer. *Cancer Res.*, 66, 7502–7508.

Whitcomb, B.P., Mutch, D.G., Herzog, T.J., Rader, J.S., Gibb, R.K., and Goodfellow, P.J., 2003. Frequent HOXA11 and THBS2 promoter methylation, and a methylator phenotype in endometrial adenocarcinoma. *Clin Cancer Res.*, 9(6), 2277–2287.

Wiegand, K.C., Shah, S.P., Al-Agha, O.M., Zhao, Y., Tse, K., Zeng, T., Senz, J. et al., 2010. ARID1A mutations in endometriosis-associated ovarian carcinomas. *N. Engl. J. Med.*, 363, 1532–1543.

15

Biomarkers in Uterine Mesenchymal and Mixed Malignant Tumors

Rosario Rivera Buery, DMD, PhD, and Esra Gunduz, DMD, PhD

CONTENTS

ABSTRACT It is not only challenging to distinguish benign from malignant uterine tumors, but also to distinguish between malignant tumors of the same or mixed histological origin. When smooth muscle tumors of uncertain malignant potential (STUMP) are taken into consideration, it becomes more complicated to have a certain diagnosis. The use of routine hematoxylin and eosin sections assists in the diagnosis of uterine tumors. However, immunohistochemistry may further support the diagnosis distinguishing benign from malignant tumors specifically for equivocal and borderline cases. Specific markers identify critical cellular events such as differentiation, proliferation, and apoptosis to detect the tendency to malignancy. Most of the biomarkers published in scientific journals focused on differentiating benign (leiomyoma [LM]) and malignant (leiomyosarcoma [LMS]) tumors arising in the myometrium having several histological morphologies such as spindle, epithelioid, and mixed variants. Among the markers, Ki-67 is then most useful diagnostic marker separating benign from malignant uterine tumors but still not precise as to distinguish the variants of LM from LMS. Other markers include p53, p16, and p21, which are promising and may also be good targets for molecular therapies. Moreover, the cell differentiation marker CD10 may also help distinguish smooth muscle tumors from endometrial stromal sarcoma. Since the main cellular component of uterine tumors is from smooth muscles having spindle-shaped cells, precise diagnosis should be done in order to provide the best therapeutic management for the patient. Molecular studies using genetic aberrations have also been identified, which somehow may provide supporting information in the diagnosis of uterine tumors. This chapter provides an insight of the biomarkers that may be used in the diagnosis of uterine tumors based on published literatures.

15.1 Introduction

Uterine malignant tumors are a diverse group of neoplasms originating from the histological components of the uterus. These tumors are classified into smooth muscle sarcomas, stromal uterine sarcomas, and mixed uterine tumors. Leiomyosarcoma (LMS) is a rare malignant tumor with smooth muscle origin comprising about 40% of uterine sarcomas and 2%–5% of the tumors in the body of the uterus [1]. Endometrial stromal sarcoma (ESS) originated from the endometrial stroma comprising about 15% of uterine sarcomas. Carcinosarcomas although reclassified as dedifferentiated or metaplastic form of endometrial carcinoma is considered as mixed origin comprising about 40% [2].

The benign (leiomyoma [LM]) and malignant (LMS) tumors may arise in the myometrium having several histological morphologies such as spindle, epithelioid, and mixed variants [3]. The most commonly encountered is the spindle cell variant that may mimic other types of tumors. In this regard, a panel of biomarkers can be used to differentiate tumors exhibiting spindle cell formation. Although LM can be distinguished from LMS based on nuclear atypia, mitotic index, and the presence of necrosis, variants of LM like cellular LM (CLM) and bizarre LM (BLM) may exist [4]. Moreover, since both benign and malignant tumors are mostly composed of spindled-shaped cells with the same origin, distinguishing them poses a diagnostic challenge. Primarily, both benign and malignant tumors may have the same clinical presentation. In addition, histological deviation may be observed in certain smooth muscle tumors that can be classified as either benign or malignant. In 2003, certain tumors were described by the World Health Organization called *smooth muscle tumors of uncertain malignant potential* (STUMP). The incidence of those tumors creates more diagnostic challenge.

Although routine histological sections stained with hematoxylin and eosin remain the gold standard in histopathological diagnosis, the use of immunohistochemistry (IHC) with a panel of antibodies can help to distinguish equivocal and borderline cases. IHC has long been used as a tool in the diagnosis of certain diseases identifying specific proteins produced by tumor cells. Significant cellular events during tumorigenesis such as differentiation, proliferation, and apoptosis may be identified using specific markers. Moreover, molecular genetics may also give an insight on the nature of the pathogenesis of the disease. This chapter focuses on the biomarkers that may be used to distinguish benign from malignant uterine sarcomas of smooth muscle origin and uterine sarcomas originating from the endometrium as reviewed from published literatures.

15.2 Immunohistochemical Markers

15.2.1 Differentiating Leiomyosarcoma from Leiomyoma

Markers of cellular proliferation have long been implicated in the pathogenesis of malignant tumors. Among the biomarkers, expression of cell proliferation is the most numerous in distinguishing benign from malignant tumors. One of the known markers strictly associated with cellular proliferation is Ki-67 [5].

In several studies that used Ki-67 in distinguishing LM, its variants, and STUMP from LMS, the majority of the studies showed a tremendous increase in the expression of Ki-67 in LMS in comparison with STUMP, LM, and LM variants [4,6–11]. Particularly, in the studies of Mayerhofer et al. (2004) and Mittal and Demopoulos (2001), it was shown that the expression of Ki-67 in LM and STUMP was almost the same compared to the very high expression in LMS. Based on the results, both studies suggested that Ki-67 may be used as a diagnostic tool in the diagnosis of equivocal cases.

In a study by Petrovic et al. in 2010 and Chen and Yang in 2008 [4,7], it was shown that Ki-67 was not expressed in LM, but a high expression of Ki-67 was observed in STUMP and Ki-67. No statistical difference was observed between STUMP and LMS although a significant difference was observed between LM and STUMP and between LM and LMS. The lack of difference between STUMP and LMS may be brought about by the histological features of STUMP. Variations in the expression of cellular proliferation markers in STUMP have been shown in several studies. In some studies, cell proliferation markers in STUMP were similar in benign variants, while in others, the results were similar to LMS although at a lower rate [4,6–8]. This may be due to the histological features of STUMP exhibiting unusual combination of nuclear atypia, mitotic figures, and zones of necrosis but does not satisfy the criteria for the diagnosis of LMS. In a study by Vilos et al., it was mentioned that although the presence of zones of coagulative necrosis has been associated with malignant potential, the mitotic count seems to be the most significant characteristic in the progression of the tumor [12]. Thus, the variation in Ki-67 expression may be brought about by the variation in histological features. In the study by Guan et al., a close percentage in the expression of Ki-67 in CLM and LMS was presented [10]. Nevertheless, Ki-67 is a clear biomarker distinguishing benign from malignant uterine smooth muscle tumors. Various studies have also confirmed the value of Ki-67 as a reliable biomarker in uterine smooth muscle tumors [9–11,13–17].

Another proliferation marker is p53 that is a tumor suppressor protein that affects other molecules in cell cycle [18]. Studies have shown a clear difference in the expression of p53 between LM and LMS. Expression of p53 was negative even in CLM [4,8]. However, p53 expression was observed in BLM cases [4]. In two studies reviewed, expression of p53 in STUMP was almost half of the percentage with that of the LMS [4,7]. However, based on the studies reviewed, expression of p53 apparently showed that the molecule could be a potential biomarker to differentiate benign from malignant smooth muscle tumors. This observation was also evident in various studies [7–9,13–15,19].

A critical step in neoplasia is the loss of cell cycle control. p16 is a tumor suppressor acting as a negative cell cycle regulator inhibiting the catalytic activity of CDK4/cyclin D complex [20]. A number of studies showed a very low expression of p16 in LM compared to LMS. However, in the study of Chen and Yang (2008), the expression of p16 in STUMP was the same as that of LMS. In the said study, BLM showed a high percentage of p16 expression. It was suggested that p16 is a useful marker in differentiating LM from LMS but not in the case of BLM and LMS. In the study of Gannon et al. (2008), although p16 was observed in 26% of LM variants and not otherwise specified (NOS), the intensity was weak compared to a strong intensity in LMS. It was suggested that p16 would provide useful information in establishing a diagnostic criterion and parameter in the diagnosis of doubtful cases [21]. The relevance of p16 as a biomarker in differentiating benign from malignant uterine smooth muscle tumors was likewise demonstrated in previous studies [4,9,11,15,20,22].

Another cyclin-dependent molecule is p21, which inhibits the activity of CDK1 complexes. In a study by Leiser et al. in 2006, the expression of apoptotic and cell cycle regulators particularly p21, p53, and Bcl-2-associated x (bax) was investigated in LM and LMS. Results showed a significant higher expression of p21 and p53 in LMS compared to LM. However, bax was highly expressed in LM compared to LMS. It was suggested that those proteins may be involved in the pathogenesis of LMS and could be potential targets for molecular therapies. Since a clear demarcation was also shown, the markers may also differentiate benign from malignant tumors [19].

The expression of c-kit has also been investigated in uterine tumors. C-kit is a tyrosine kinase receptor of stem cell factor known in gastrointestinal stromal tumor. C-kit was observed in 53.1% cases of LMS. Direct sequencing of exon 11 was performed, but no mutation was found [23,24]. Wang observed a higher percentage of c-kit expression in LMS compared to LM suggesting that c-kit may be useful in differentiating LMS from LM [25]. Rushing also demonstrated the expression of c-kit in 100% uterine sarcomas studied, though, in one case, deletion of both exons 11 and 17 was observed [26]. On the other hand, reports about the lack of expression of c-kit have been shown [27–29].

Fascin is another marker that has been investigated in uterine smooth muscle tumor. Fascin is a major regulating factor of the cytoskeleton found in microspikes, filopodia; it is expressed by neurons and dendritic cells [30]. The expression of fascin has been observed in several carcinomas like in thymic carcinoma, endometrioid carcinoma, and hepatocellular carcinoma [31–33]. The expression of fascin was investigated in uterine smooth muscle tumors comparing the expressions in LM, LM variants, STUMP, and LMS [34]. Results showed that a high percentage of LMS expressed fascin compared to STUMP and the benign counterparts suggesting that fascin can be a reliable IHC marker in distinguishing uterine LMS from LM.

Dhingra et al. mentioned the probable role of mTORC2-PLD1 (phospholipase D) pathway in uterine LMS. This pathway functions in protein synthesis, cell cycle progression, and cell growth and proliferation [35]. In their study, an increase in the expression of p-Akt, p-mTOR, and PLD-1 was shown in LMS. It was suggested that the pathway may be used as therapeutic targets. Because of the noticeable difference in the expression of the molecules between LM and LMS, the molecules may also be potential markers in differentiating benign from malignant uterine tumors [36].

Recently, another potential biomarker was studied by Cornejo et al. in 2012 [37]. The oncofetal protein is an insulin-like growth factor mRNA-binding protein (IMP) 3 that is expressed in several malignant tumors but not in benign tumors [38–40]. Cytoplasmic staining of IMP3 was observed in 52% of cases of LMS regardless of the histological grade but was not observed in any LM case. This study was the first to describe that the expression of IMP3 is uterine smooth muscle tumors and suggested that IMP3 can be used as a biomarker enhancing the level of confidence in establishing a definitive diagnosis.

Bax protein is the first identified molecule that promotes apoptosis by competing with Bcl-2. The expression of Bax has been related in the pathogenesis of various tumors such as in melanoma, non-small-cell lung cancer, and osteosarcoma [41–43]. In the study of Leiser et al. in 2006, a significant difference in the expression of Bax was observed between LMS and LM ($p < 0.001$). It was suggested that the molecules involved in apoptotic and cell cycle regulatory pathway could be potential targets for molecular therapy. Although Bax was observed in a subset of LM, the molecule may also be used in a panel of antibodies that can be used in distinguishing benign from malignant uterine smooth muscle tumors. Expression of Bcl-2 in LMS was also mentioned in the studies of Zhai et al. and Bodner et al. [44,45].

The role of hormone receptors in the pathogenesis of uterine sarcomas has been mentioned in several studies. Particularly, the function of progesterone receptor (PR) has been investigated in various tumors. In the study of Petrovic et al. (2010), a reduction in the percentage of LMS was observed to express PR. All cases of LM and STUMP expressed PR. The reduction in the expression of PR may be one of the parameters than can be used for the diagnosis of LMS. Koivisto-Korander et al. mentioned the prognostic value of estrogen receptor and PRA in uterine LMS [46]. In addition, PR was present in LM but a marked reduction was observed in LMS [13,14]. The results of the study suggested the potential of the markers in differentiating tumors with malignant potential. Moreover, Raspollini et al. mentioned that the expressions of estrogen receptor (ER) and PR are independent predictors of the risk or recurrence and death in uterine sarcomas [47].

Interestingly, CD44 is a cell surface receptor belonging to the family of cell adhesion molecule associated with the pathogenesis of various tumors. CD44 is a transmembrane glycoprotein that interacts with hyaluronic acid, osteopontin, and matrix metalloproteinase [48,49]. The expression of the standard and isoforms of CD44 was investigated in LM and LMS. A decrease in the expression of CD44 and isoform V6 was observed in LM and LMS compared to the expression in the myometrium. However, no expression of CD44v3 was detected in LMS. The results of the study suggested that the loss of CD44v3 may be used as a diagnostic tool in differentiating LM from LMS [50].

Carbonic anhydrases have been associated with various cancers in terms of their contribution to the regulation of pH homeostasis of the tumor microenvironment [51]. This has been shown to be induced by tumor hypoxia via HIF-1a regulatory pathway. The expression of CAII and CAXII has been observed in various cancers [52–54]. Specifically, Hynninen et al. showed a statistical difference between LM and uterine sarcomas for all isozymes suggesting that the markers may be used for differential diagnosis between benign and malignant uterine tumors [55].

Another promising biomarker is LMP2. Immune-proteasome actively participates in major histocompatibility class 1–mediated tumor rejection [56]. One of the proteasome subunits induced by interferon gamma is proteasome subunit called low-molecular mass polypeptide 2 [57,58]. Hayashi and Faustman (2002) developed an animal model wherein LMP2-/- mice developed uterine LMS. Corresponding histological features characteristics of LMS were also observed in LMP2-deficient mice. LMP2 may therefore be a potential biomarker in the diagnosis of LMS. As of to date, no clinical research has been made investigating the expression of LMP2 in uterine tumors. Clinical trials have yet to be concluded [59–61]. Table 15.1 summarizes the major biomarkers differentiating LMS from LM with the corresponding references.

15.2.2 Differentiating Smooth Muscle Tumors from Endometrial Stromal Sarcoma

Smooth muscle tumors are positive to a-smooth muscle actin (SMA) and desmin [62]. Distinguishing ESS from LMS usually uses cell differentiation markers like CD10. Chu et al. mentioned that CD10 is a useful marker in differentiating ESS from uterine sarcomas of muscle in origin [63]. It was shown in their study that none of the LMS expressed CD10 while all ESS cases expressed CD10. The distinction between ESS and smooth muscle tumors is important for two reasons. Metastatic cases of ESS or primary extrauterine ESS should be recognized from other spindle cell tumors because ESS can be treated with an antiestrogen therapy [63]. McCluggage et al. in 2001 also mentioned that a positive staining for CD10 in a high-grade uterine sarcoma may be indicative of ESS differentiation rather than smooth muscle tumor [64]. However, Oliva et al. (2002) observed that CD10 expression was often seen in smooth muscle tumors, and therefore, a panel of CD10, h-caldesmon, and desmin should be used to differentiate CLM from ESS [62,65].

TABLE 15.1

Biomarkers Differentiating LMS from LM

Biomarker	LM	LM Variants	STUMP	LMS	Reference
Ki-67	8%		0%	50%	Mayerhofer et al. (2004)
	0%		67%	59%	Petrovic et al. (2010)
		0% (CLM)	0%	92%	Mittal et al. (2001)
	0%	0% (CLM) 48% (BLM)	100%	83%	Chen et al. (2008)
	0%			100%	Yanai et al. (2010)
		76.7% (CLM)		100%	Guan et al. (2012)
	0%			67%	Lee et al. (2009)
p53	0%		28%	41%	Petrovic et al. (2010)
	0%			54%	Leiser et al. (2006)
		0% (CLM)	0%	42%	Mittal et al. (2001)
	0%	0% CLM 60% BLM	50%	91%	Chen et al. (2008)
	0%			75%	Yanai et al. (2010)
	0%			29%	Cheng-han lee et al. (2009)
p16	14%	38.5% CLM 86.5% BLM	100%	100%	Chen et al. (2008)
		26% var 26% NOS		100%	Gannon et al. (2008)
	2%			87%	Cheng-han lee et al. (2009)
	12%		21%	57%	Bodner-Adler (2005)
	14%			80%	Atkins et al. (2008)
p21	0%			43%	Leiser et al. (2006)
C-kit	0%		67% high-grade ESS	75%	Wang et al. (2003)
	No comparison			100% uterine sarcomas	Rushing et al. (2003)
Fascin	4.5%	3.2%	50%	90.9%	Kefeli et al. (2009)
p-Akt	17%		65%	91%	Dhingra et al. (2010)
pmTOR	5%		59%	91%	Dhingra et al. (2010)
Phospholipase D1	0%		24%	73%	Dhingra et al. (2010)
IMP3	0%			52%	Cornejo et al. (2012)
Bax	94%			34%	Leiser et al. (2006)
PR	100%		100%	59%	Petrovic et al. (2010)
CD44v3	100%	100%		0%	Poncelet et al. (2001)

Aside from CD10, recently, the expression of oxytocin receptor (OTR) was investigated in the normal uterus, uterine smooth muscle tumors, and ESS. The study also included other proteins such as CD10. OTR has been shown to be expressed in the myometrium, mammary gland, endometrium, ovary, testes, epididymis, vas deferens, thymus, heart, and various parts of the brain [66]. OTRs have been shown in various carcinomas such as breast, endometrium, ovary, and prostate as well as in various sarcomas such as osteosarcoma and Kaposi sarcomas [67–72]. The study evaluated the use of OTR in distinguishing uterine smooth muscle tumors and ESS. Results of the study showed that OTR was more

TABLE 15.2

Biomarkers Differentiating Smooth Muscle Tumors from ESS

Biomarker	LM (%)	LM Variants (%)	ESS (%)	LMS (%)	Reference
OTR	100	100	0	100	Loddenkemper et al. (2003)
CD10	10	60	100	62	Loddenkemper et al. (2003)
		20	100	0	Chu et al. (2001)

prevalently expressed in uterine smooth muscle tumors, and none of the ESS expressed OTR. The study indicates that OTR is useful to distinguish uterine smooth muscle tumors from ESS [73] (Table 15.2).

15.3 Molecular Studies

Genetic aberration in uterine tumors has been analyzed, and distinct molecular pathways have been identified in uterine tumors [74]. Cytogenetic instability has been investigated in LMS [75–77]. Unstable genetic aberrations in 11q22 were suggested to be specific for uterine sarcomas [78]. In contrast, normal karyotype or simple aberrations were likewise found in benign tumors in which the most common is the translocation between chromosomes 12 and 14 and deletions in 7q22 [79–82]. However, Quade et al. did not find loss of heterozygosity (LOH) in the chromosomal region most frequently deleted in LM (7q), and none of the LOH markers for chromosome 10 were found in LM [74]. Since LOH in chromosome 10 was not found, it was suggested that the detection of LOH on chromosome 10 may support or may be an adjunct in distinguishing benign and malignant uterine tumor [74].

Recently in another study, mitochondrial microsatellite instability (MSI) was used to evaluate LM from LMS. A total of eight microsatellite markers were used in human samples. Results showed that no instability was found in LM cases while instability was found in 3 out of 14 patients (21.4%) with LMS with a significant p value ($p < 0.01$). The results suggest the probable use of mitochondrial MSI as a marker for the differential diagnosis of benign and malignant uterine tumors [83].

A molecular study on ESS identified alterations in 14-3-3 expression, which are ubiquitously expressed in various cellular functions. The 14-3-3 oncoprotein came from a t(10;17) genomic rearrangement, leading to the fusion of 14-3-3 (YWHAE) and any of the two identical FAM22 family members (FAM22A or FAM22B). Expression of YWHAE–FAM22 oncoprotein complex corresponded to cell growth and migration. In their study, high-grade ESS expressed the YWHAE–FAM22A/B complex that was not detected in uterine sarcomas. The results reveal diagnostically and therapeutically relevant models for characterizing aberrant 14-3-3 oncogenic functions in ESS [84].

In the course of the review of published literatures, the most commonly used markers to distinguish LM from LMS are markers of cell proliferation such as Ki-67, p53, and p16. Although histological interpretation of mitotic index, cytological atypia, and the presence of necrosis are still the standard features in differentiating LM and LMS, the biomarkers of cell proliferation are indispensable adjunct in the diagnosis of equivocal and borderline cases. On the other hand, the most frequent markers to distinguish LMS from ESS include panel of cell differentiation like a-SMA, desmin, and CD10.

15.4 Conclusion and Future Direction

To distinguish benign and malignant uterine tumors, it is necessary to use biomarkers especially for equivocal and borderline cases. As both benign and malignant tumors are mostly composed of spindled-shaped cells with the same origin, separating them poses a diagnostic challenge. To date, there are markers that are used for immunohistochemistry, like Ki-67, which can distinguish LM and LMS. But unfortunately, to separate the variants of LM and LMS remains as an unsolved problem. This problem has already raised the inspection of new biomarkers that could detect more precisely both benign and malignant tumors and the variants, as well as STUMP. Current novel biomarkers that can distinguish between uterine tumors, including p53, p16, p21, c-kit, fascin, p-Akt, pmTOR, Phospholipase D1, IMP3, Bax, PR, CD44v3, have been brought to notice (Table 15.1) in this chapter. Even though these markers are quite promising, they lack precise detection between variants of benign and malignant tumors. Another issue of uterine tumors is the difficulty to distinguish the histological origin. To separate smooth muscle tumors from endometrial sarcomas, CD10, OTR, SMA, and desmin are considered to be useful but not the accurate approach.

As a conclusion, we can state that currently there are markers for diagnosis but also new biomarkers or new evaluation methods are necessary to handle uterine tumors. New evaluation methods may be considered as the application of combination of current markers that may display more concrete results than the application of a single marker. New biomarkers are subject to innovative investigators of the field that will help both clinicians and researchers.

References

1. Lin JF, Slomovitz BM. Uterinesarcoma 2008. *Curr Oncol Rep*. November 2008;10(6):512–518.
2. D'Angelo E, Prat J. Uterine sarcomas: A review. *Gynecol Oncol*. January 2010;116(1):131–139.
3. Atkins KA. *Pathology of Uterus Smooth Muscle Tumors*, Longacre TA (ed.), 2012. http://emedicine.medscape.com/article/1611373-overview.
4. Chen L, Yang B. Immunohistochemical analysis of p16, p53, and Ki-67 expression in uterine smooth muscle tumors. *Int J Gynecol Pathol*. July 2008;27(3):326–332.
5. Scholzen T, Gerdes J. The Ki-67 protein: From the known and the unknown. *J Cell Physiol*. March 2000;182(3):311–322.
6. Mayerhofer K, Lozanov P, Bodner K, Bodner-Adler B, Obermair A, Kimberger O, Czerwenka K. Ki-67 and vascular endothelial growth factor expression in uterine leiomyosarcoma. *Gynecol Oncol*. January 2004;92(1):175–179.
7. Petrovic D, Babic D, Forko JI, Martinac I. Expression of Ki-67, P53 and progesterone receptors in uterine smooth muscle tumors. Diagnostic value. *Coll Antropol*. March 2010;34(1):93–97.
8. Mittal K, Demopoulos RI. MIB-1 (Ki-67), p53, estrogen receptor, and progesterone receptor expression in uterine smooth muscle tumors. *Hum Pathol*. September 2001;32(9):984–987.
9. Yanai H, Wani Y, Notohara K, Takada S, Yoshino T. Uterine leiomyosarcoma arising in leiomyoma: Clinicopathological study of four cases and literature review. *Pathol Int*. July 2010;60(7):506–509.
10. Guan R, Zheng W, Xu M. A retrospective analysis of the clinicopathologic characteristics of uterine cellular leiomyomas in China. *Int J Gynaecol Obstet*. July 2012;118(1):52–55.

11. Lee CH, Turbin DA, Sung YC, Espinosa I, Montgomery K, van de Rijn M, Gilks CB. A panel of antibodies to determine site of origin and malignancy in smooth muscle tumors. *Mod Pathol.* December 2009;22(12):1519–1531.
12. Vilos GA, Marks J, Ettler HC, Vilos AG, Prefontaine M, Abu-Rafea B. Uterine smooth muscle tumors of uncertain malignant potential: Diagnostic challenges and therapeutic dilemmas. Report of 2 cases and review of the literature. *J Minim Invasive Gynecol.* May–June 2012;19(3):288–295.
13. Gokaslan H, Turkeri L, Kavak ZN, Eren F, Sismanoglu A, Ilvan S, Durmusoglu F. Differential diagnosis of smooth muscle tumors utilizing p53, pTEN and Ki-67 expression with estrogen and progesterone receptors. *Gynecol Obstet Invest.* 2005;59(1):36–40.
14. Zhai YL, Kobayashi Y, Mori A, Orii A, Nikaido T, Konishi I, Fujii S. Expression of steroid receptors, Ki-67, and p53 in uterine leiomyosarcomas. *Int J Gynecol Pathol.* January 1999;18(1):20–28.
15. O'Neill CJ, McBride HA, Connolly LE, McCluggage WG. Uterine leiomyosarcomas are characterized by high p16, p53 and MIB1 expression in comparison with usual leiomyomas, leiomyoma variants and smooth muscle tumours of uncertain malignant potential. *Histopathology.* June 2007;50(7):851–858.
16. Mayerhofer K, Lozanov P, Bodner K, Bodner-Adler B, Kimberger O, Czerwenka K. Ki-67 expression in patients with uterine leiomyomas, uterine smooth muscle tumors of uncertain malignant potential (STUMP) and uterine leiomyosarcomas (LMS). *Acta Obstet Gynecol Scand.* November 2004;83(11):1085–1088.
17. D'Angelo E, Spagnoli LG, Prat J. Comparative clinicopathologic and immunohistochemical analysis of uterine sarcomas diagnosed using the World Health Organization classification system. *Hum Pathol.* November 2009;40(11):1571–1585.
18. Mirzayans R, Andrais B, Scott A, Murray D. New insights into p53 signaling and cancer cell response to DNA damage: Implications for cancer therapy. *J Biomed Biotechnol.* 2012;2012:170325.
19. Leiser AL, Anderson SE, Nonaka D, Chuai S, Olshen AB, Chi DS, Soslow RA. Apoptotic and cell cycle regulatory markers in uterine leiomyosarcoma. *Gynecol Oncol.* April 2006;101(1):86–91.
20. Bodner-Adler B, Bodner K, Czerwenka K, Kimberger O, Leodolter S, Mayerhofer K. Expression of p16 protein in patients with uterine smooth muscle tumors: An immunohistochemical analysis. *Gynecol Oncol.* January 2005;96(1):62–66.
21. Gannon BR, Manduch M, Childs TJ. Differential Immunoreactivity of p16 in leiomyosarcomas and leiomyoma variants. *Int J Gynecol Pathol.* January 2008;27(1):68–73.
22. Atkins KA, Arronte N, Darus CJ, Rice LW. The use of p16 in enhancing the histologic classification of uterine smooth muscle tumors. *Am J Surg Pathol.* January 2008;32(1):98–102.
23. Raspollini MR, Paglierani M, Taddei GL, Villanucci A, Amunni G, Taddei A. The protooncogene c-KIT is expressed in leiomyosarcomas of the uterus. *Gynecol Oncol.* June 2004;93(3):718.
24. Raspollini MR, Amunni G, Villanucci A, Pinzani P, Simi L, Paglierani M, Taddei GL. c-Kit expression in patients with uterine leiomyosarcomas: A potential alternative therapeutic treatment. *Clin Cancer Res.* May 15, 2004;10(10):3500–3503.
25. Wang L, Felix JC, Lee JL, Tan PY, Tourgeman DE, O'Meara AT, Amezcua CA. The proto-oncogene c-kit is expressed in leiomyosarcomas of the uterus. *Gynecol Oncol.* August 2003;90(2):402–406.
26. Rushing RS, Shajahan S, Chendil D, Wilder JL, Pulliam J, Lee EY, Ueland FR, van Nagell JR, Ahmed MM, Lele SM. Uterine sarcomas express KIT protein but lack mutation(s) in exon11or17ofc-KIT. *Gynecol Oncol.* October 2003;91(1):9–14.
27. Zafrakas M, Theodoridis TD, Zepiridis L, Venizelos ID, Agorastos T, Bontis J. KIT protein expression in uterine sarcomas: An immunohistochemical study and review of the literature. *Eur J Gynaecol Oncol.* 2008;29(3):264–266.
28. Raspollini MR, Pinzani P, Simi L, Amunni G, Villanucci A, Paglierani M, Taddei GL. Uterine leiomyosarcomas express KIT protein but lack mutation(s) in exon 9 of c-KIT. *Gynecol Oncol.* August 2005;98(2):334–335.
29. Klein WM, Kurman RJ. Lack of expression of c-kit protein(CD117) in mesenchymal tumors of the uterus and ovary. *Int J Gynecol Pathol.* April 2003;22(2):181–184.

30. Machesky LM, Li A. Fascin: Invasive filopodia promoting metastasis. *Commun Integr Biol.* 2010;3:263–270; Yamashiro S. Functions of fascin in dendritic cells. *Crit Rev Immunol.* 2012;32(1):11–21.
31. Sato J, Fujiwara M, Kawakami T, Sumiishi A, Sakata S, Sakamoto A, Kurata A. Fascin expression in dendritic cells and tumor epithelium in thymoma and thymic carcinoma. *Oncol Lett.* November 2011;2(6):1025–1032.
32. Gun BD, Bahadir B, Bektas S, Barut F, Yurdakan G, Kandemir NO, Ozdamar SO. Clinico pathological significance of fascin and CD44v6 expression in endometrioid carcinoma. *Diagn Pathol.* July 11, 2012;7(1):80.
33. Huang X, Ji J, Xue H, Zhang F, Han X, Cai Y, Zhang J, Ji G. Fascin and cortactin expression is correlated with a poor prognosis in hepatocellular carcinoma. *Eur J Gastroenterol Hepatol.* June 2012;24(6):633–639.
34. Kefeli M, Yildiz L, Kaya FC, Aydin O, Kandemir B. Fascin expression in uterine smooth muscle tumors. *Int J Gynecol Pathol.* July 2009;28(4):328–333.
35. Chen XG, Liu F, Song XF, Wang ZH, Dong ZQ, Hu ZQ, Lan RZ et al. Rapamycin regulates Akt and ERK phosphorylation through mTORC1and mTORC2 signaling pathways. *Mol Carcinog.* June 2010;49(6):603–610.
36. Dhingra S, Rodriguez ME, Shen Q, Duan X, Stanton ML, Chen L, Zhang R, Brown RE. Constitutive activation with overexpression of the mTORC2-phospholipase D1 pathway in uterine leiomyosarcoma and STUMP: Morphoproteomic analysis with therapeutic implications. *Int J Clin Exp Pathol.* January 28, 2010;4(2):134–146.
37. Cornejo K, Shi M, Jiang Z. Oncofetal protein IMP3: A useful diagnostic biomarker for leiomyosarcoma. *Hum Pathol.* April 2012;43(10):1567–1572.
38. Clauditz TS, Wang CJ, Gontarewicz A, Blessmann M, Tennstedt P, Borgmann K, Tribius S et al. Expression of insulin-like growth factor II mRNA-binding protein 3 in squamous cell carcinomas of the head and neck. *J Oral Pathol Med.* May 29, 2013;42(2):125–132. doi: 10.1111/j.1600-0714.2012.01178.x.
39. Wachter DL, Kristiansen G, Soll C, Hellerbrand C, Breuhahn K, Fritzsche F, Agaimy A, Hartmann A, Riener MO. Insulin-like growth factor II mRNA-binding protein 3 (IMP3) expression in hepatocellular carcinoma. A clinicopathological analysis with emphasis on diagnostic value. *Histopathology.* January 2012;60(2):278–286.
40. Wang L, Li HG, Xia ZS, Lü J, Peng TS. IMP3 is a novel biomarker to predict metastasis and prognosis of gastric adenocarcinoma: A retrospective study. *Chin Med J (Engl).* December 2010;123(24):3554–3558.
41. Fecker LF, Geilen CC, Tchernev G, Trefzer U, Assaf C, Kurbanov BM, Schwarz C, Daniel PT, Eberle J. Loss of proapoptotic Bcl-2-related multidomain proteins in primary melanomas is associated with poor prognosis. *J Invest Dermatol.* June 2006;126(6):1366–1371.
42. Sun Q, Hua J, Wang Q, Xu W, Zhang J, Zhang J, Kang J, Li M. Expressions of GRP78 and Bax associate with differentiation, metastasis, and apoptosis in non-small cell lung cancer. *Mol Biol Rep.* June 2012;39(6):6753–6761.
43. Kaseta MK, Khaldi L, Gomatos IP, Tzagarakis GP, Alevizos L, Leandros E, Papagelopoulos PJ, Soucacos PN. Prognostic value of bax, bcl-2, and p53 staining in primary osteosarcoma. *J Surg Oncol.* March 1, 2008;97(3):259–266.
44. Zhai YL, Nikaido T, Toki T, Shiozawa A, Orii A, Fujii S. Prognostic significance of bcl-2 expression in leiomyosarcoma of the uterus. *Br J Cancer.* July 1999;80(10):1658–1664.
45. Bodner K, Bodner-Adler B, Kimberger O, Czerwenka K, Mayerhofer K. Bcl-2 receptor expression in patients with uterine smooth muscle tumors: An immunohistochemical analysis comparing leiomyoma, uterine smooth muscle tumor of uncertain malignant potential, and leiomyosarcoma. *J Soc Gynecol Investig.* April 2004;11(3):187–191.
46. Koivisto-Korander R, Butzow R, Koivisto AM, Leminen A. Immunohistochemical studies on uterine carcinosarcoma, leiomyosarcoma, and endometrial stromal sarcoma: Expression and prognostic importance of ten different markers. *Tumour Biol.* June 2011;32(3):451–459.

47. Raspollini MR, Amunni G, Villanucci A, Boddi V, Simoni A, Taddei A, Taddei GL. Estrogen and progesterone receptors expression in uterine malignant smooth muscle tumors: Correlation with clinical outcome. *J Chemother*. December 2003;15(6):596–602.
48. Gotte M, Yip GW. Heparanase, hyaluronan, and CD44 in cancers: A breast carcinoma perspective. *Cancer Res*. November 1, 2006;66(21):10233–10237.
49. Kaindl T, Rieger H, Kaschel LM, Engel U, Schmaus A, Sleeman J, Tanaka M. Spatio-temporal patterns of pancreatic cancer cells expressing CD44 isoforms on supported membranes displaying hyaluronic acid oligomers arrays. *PLoS One*. 2012;7(8):e42991.
50. Poncelet C, Walker F, Madelenat P, Bringuier AF, Scoazec JY, Feldmann G, Darai E. Expression of CD44 standard and isoforms V3 and V6 in uterine smooth muscle tumors: A possible diagnostic tool for the diagnosis of leiomyosarcoma. *Hum Pathol*. November 2001;32(11):1190–1196.
51. Zavadova Z, Zavada J. Carbonic anhydrase IX (CAIX) mediates tumor cell interactions with micro environment. *Oncol Rep*. May 2005;13(5):977–982.
52. Nordfors K, Haapasalo J, Korja M, Niemela A, Laine J, Parkkila AK, Pastorekova S et al. The tumour-associated carbonic anhydrases CA II, CA IX and CA XII in a group of medulloblastomas and supratentorial primitive neuroectodermal tumours: An association of CA IX with poor prognosis. *BMC Cancer*. April 18, 2010;10:148.
53. Niemela AM, Hynninen P, Mecklin JP, Kuopio T, Kokko A, Aaltonen L, Parkkila AK et al. Carbonic anhydrase IX is highly expressed in hereditary nonpolyposis colorectal cancer. *Cancer Epidemiol Biomarkers Prev*. September 2007;16(9):1760–1766.
54. Kivela AJ, Saarnio J, Karttunen TJ, Kivela J, Parkkila AK, Pastorekova S, Pastorek J et al. Differential expression of cytoplasmic carbonic anhydrases, CA I and II, and membrane-associated isozymes, CAIX and XII, in normal mucosa of large intestine and in colorectal tumors. *Dig Dis Sci*. October 2001;46(10):2179–2186.
55. Hynninen P, Parkkila S, Huhtala H, Pastorekova S, Pastorek J, Waheed A, Sly WS, Tomas E. Carbonic anhydrase isozymes II, IX, and XII in uterine tumors. *APMIS*. February 2012;120(2):117–129.
56. Delp K, Momburg F, Hilmes C, Huber C, Seliger B. Functional deficiencies of components of the MHC class I antigen pathway in human tumors of epithelial origin. *Bone Marrow Transplant*. May 2000;25(Suppl 2):S88–S95.
57. Groettrup M, Khan S, Schwarz K, Schmidtke G. Interferon-gamma inducible exchanges of 20S proteasome active site subunits: Why? *Biochimie*. March–April 2001;83(3–4):367–372.
58. Nakajima C, Uekusa Y, Iwasaki M, Yamaguchi N, Mukai T, Gao P, Tomura M, Ono S, Tsujimura T, Fujiwara H, Hamaoka T. A role of interferon-gamma (IFN-gamma) in tumor immunity: T cells with the capacity to reject tumor cells are generated but fail to migrate to tumor sites in IFN-gamma-deficient mice. *Cancer Res*. April 15, 2001;61(8):3399–3405.
59. Hayashi T, Faustman DL. Development of spontaneous uterine tumors in low molecular mass polypeptide-2 knockout mice. *Cancer Res*. January 1, 2002;62(1):24–27.
60. Hayashi T, Horiuchi A, Sano K, Hiraoka N, Kasai M, Ichimura T, Nagase S et al. Involvement of proteasome β1i subunit, LMP2, on development of uterin leiomyosarcma. *N Am J Med Sci*. September 2011;3(9):394–399.
61. Hayashi T, Horiuchi A, Sano K, Hiraoka N, Kanai Y, Shiozawa T, Tonegawa S, Konishi I. Mice-lacking LMP2, immuno-proteasome subunit, as an animal model of spontaneous uterine leiomyosarcoma. *Protein Cell*. August 2010;1(8):711–717.
62. Oliva E, Young RH, Amin MB, Clement PB. An immunohistochemical analysis of endometrial stromal and smooth muscle tumors of the uterus: A study of 54 cases emphasizing the importance of using a panel because of overlap in immunoreactivity for individual antibodies. *Am J Surg Pathol*. April 2002;26(4):403–412.
63. Chu PG, Arber DA, Weiss LM, Chang KL. Utility of CD10 in distinguishing between endometrial stromal sarcoma and uterine smooth muscle tumors: An immunohistochemical comparison of 34 cases. *Mod Pathol*. May 2001;14(5):465–471.

64. McCluggage WG, Sumathi VP, Maxwell P. CD10 is a sensitive and diagnostically useful immunohistochemical marker of normal endometrial stroma and of endometrial stromal neoplasms. *Histopathology*. September 2001;39(3):273–278.
65. Rush DS, Tan J, Baergen RN, Soslow RA. h-Caldesmon, a novel smooth muscle-specific antibody, distinguishes between cellular leiomyoma and endometrial stromal sarcoma. *Am J Surg Pathol*. February 2001;25(2):253–258.
66. Strunecká A, Hynie S, Klenerová V. Role of oxytocin/oxytocin receptor system in regulation of cell growth and neoplastic processes. *Folia Biol (Praha)*. 2009;55(5):159–165.
67. Cassoni P, Marrocco T, Sapino A, Allia E, Bussolati G. Oxytocin synthesis within the normal and neoplastic breast: First evidence of a local peptide source. *Int J Oncol*. May 2006;28(5):1263–1268.
68. Suzuki Y, Shibata K, Kikkawa F, Kajiyama H, Ino K, Nomura S, Tsujimoto M, Mizutani S. Possible role of placental leucine aminopeptidase in the antiproliferative effect of oxytocin inhuman endometrial adenocarcinoma. *Clin Cancer Res*. April 2003;9(4):1528–1534.
69. Morita T, Shibata K, Kikkawa F, Kajiyama H, Ino K, Mizutani S. Oxytocin inhibits the progression of human ovarian carcinoma cells in vitro and in vivo. *Int J Cancer*. April 20, 2004;109(4):525–532.
70. Zhong M, Boseman ML, Millena AC, Khan SA. Oxytocin induces the migration of prostate cancer cells: Involvement of the Gi-coupled signaling pathway. *Mol Cancer Res*. August, 2010;8(8):1164–1172.
71. Petersson M. Opposite effects of oxytocin on proliferation of osteosarcoma cell lines. *Regul Pept*. October 9, 2008;150(1–3):50–54.
72. Cassoni P, Sapino A, Deaglio S, Bussolati B, Volante M, Munaron L, Albini A, Torrisi A, Bussolati G. Oxytocin is a growth factor for Kaposi's sarcoma cells: Evidence of endocrine-immunological cross-talk. *Cancer Res*. April 15, 2002;62(8):2406–2413.
73. Loddenkemper C, Mechsner S, Foss HD, Dallenbach FE, Anagnostopoulos I, Ebert AD, Stein H. Use of oxytocin receptor expression in distinguishing between uterine smooth muscle tumors and endometrial stromal sarcoma. *Am J Surg Pathol*. November 2003;27(11):1458–1462.
74. Quade BJ, Pinto AP, Howard DR, Peters WA 3rd, Crum CP. Frequent loss of heterozygosity for chromosome 10 in uterine leiomyosarcoma in contrast to leiomyoma. *Am J Pathol*. March 1999;154(3):945–950.
75. Boghosian L, Dal Cin P, Turc-Carel C, Rao U, Karakousis C, Sait SJ, Sandberg AA. Three possible cytogenetic subgroups of leiomyosarcoma. *Cancer Genet Cytogenet*. 1989, 43:39–49.
76. Nilbert M, Mandahl N, Heim S, Rydholm A, Willen H, Akerman M, Mitelman F. Chromosome abnormalities in leiomyosarcomas. *Cancer Genet Cytogenet*. 1988;34:209–218.
77. Sreekantaiah C, Davis JR, Sandberg AA. Chromosomal abnormalities in leiomyosarcomas. *Am J Pathol*. 1993;142:293–305.
78. Laxman R, Currie JL, Kurman RJ, Dudzinski M, Griffin A. Cytogenetic profile of uterine sarcomas. *Cancer*. 1993;71:1283–1288.
79. Meloni AM, Surti U, Contento AM, Davare J, Sandberg AA. Uterine leiomyomas: Cytogenetic and histologic profile. *Obstet Gynecol*. 1992;80:209–217.
80. Pandis N, Heim S, Bardi G, Flodérus U-M, Willén H, Mandahl N, Mitelman F. Chromosome analysis of 96 uterine leiomyomas. *Cancer Genet Cytogenet*. 1991;55:11–18.
81. Heim S, Nilbert M, Vanni R, Flodérus U-M, Mandahl N, Liedgren S, Lecca U, Mitelman F. A specific translocation, t(12;14)(q14–15;q23–24), characterizes a subgroup of uterine leiomyomas. *Cancer Genet Cytogenet*. 1988;32:13–17.
82. Ozisik YY, Meloni AM, Surti U, Sandberg AA. Deletion 7q22 in uterine leiomyoma: A cytogenetic review. *Cancer Genet Cytogenet*. 1993;71:1–6.
83. Lee JH, Ryu TY, Cho CH, Kim DK. Different characteristics of mitochondrial microsatellite in stability between uterine leiomyomas and leiomyosarcomas. *Pathol Oncol Res*. June 2011;17(2):201–205.
84. Lee CH, Ou WB, Mariño-Enriquez A, Zhu M, Mayeda M, Wang Y, Guo X et al. 14-3-3 fusion oncogenes in high-grade endometrial stromal sarcoma. *Proc Natl Acad Sci USA*. January 17, 2012;109(3):929–934.

16

Noninvasive Early Biomarkers in Fallopian Tube Carcinoma

Panagiotis Peitsidis, MSc, PhD

CONTENTS

ABSTRACT Primary fallopian tube carcinoma (PFTC) is an uncommon tumor accounting for approximately 0.14%–1.8% of female genital malignancies. It has been estimated, based on the data obtained from cancer registries, that the average annual incidence of PFTC is 3.6 per million women per year. The etiology of this cancer is unknown. The diagnosis of PFTC is rarely considered preoperatively and is usually first evaluated intraoperatively or by the pathology examination. Hormonal, reproductive, and genetic factors are thought to rise PFTC risk. Several pathological criteria have been used to distinguish the fallopian tube carcinoma (FTC) from epithelial ovarian carcinoma (EOC). Due to the rarity of this neoplasm, few studies exist regarding the utilization of early noninvasive biomarkers. Many of these studies have been reporting clinical experience in combination with EOC. Biomarkers involved in EOC such as cancer antigen 125 or carbohydrate antigen 125 (CA125) estimation have been used to predict and monitor PFTC and several others like vascular endothelial growth factor (VEGF) and metalloproteinases. Herein, we endeavor to perform a narrative comprehensive review on the use of several biomarkers as prognostic and predictive factors in PFTC and their application in modern therapies, obtaining material in a systematic way from the international electronic databases.

16.1 Introduction

PFTC is an uncommon tumor accounting for approximately 0.14%–1.8% of female genital malignancies (Sedlis, 1961). It is estimated, based on the data obtained from nine population-based cancer registries in the United States, that the average annual incidence of PFTC is 3.6 per million women per year. In England and Wales, 40 cases of PFTC and 4500 cases of EOC are registered annually (Woolas et al., 1997). It has been reported that the incidence of PFTC is increasing, with an age-adjusted incidence of 1.2 per million for 1953–1957 to 5.4 per million for 1993–1997 (Riska et al., 2003). About 1500 cases of PFTC have been reported in the literature until now (Ng and Lawton, 1998).

16.1.1 Etiology and Risk Factors

The etiology of this cancer is not clear and several theories that are related with EOC have been made. Several hormonal, reproductive, and genetic factors are thought to increase EOC risk and might also increase PFTC risk. High parity has been reported to be a protective (Riska et al., 2003) a previous history of pregnancy and the use of oral contraceptives has shown to decrease the PFTC risk significantly (Inal et al., 2004). It has been reported that there is no statistically significant correlation between PFTC and age, race, weight, education level, pelvic inflammatory disease, infertility, previous hysterectomy, endometriosis, lactose intolerance, or smoking (Henderson et al., 1977). Primary fallopian tube cancer has been described in high-risk breast–ovarian cancer families with germline BRCA1 and BRCA2 mutations (Meng et al., 1985). Some studies suggested that the frequency and structure of the chromosomal changes (BRCA1 or BRCA2 mutations) observed in primary fallopian tube cancer had similar characteristics with those found in breast, serous ovarian, and uterine carcinomas, and consequently, a common molecular pathogenesis was suggested (Aziz et al., 2001; Hebert et al., 2002; Jongsma et al., 2002).

16.1.2 Clinical Symptomatology of Fallopian Tube Carcinoma

The mean age of presentation is quoted as 55 years with most cases presenting in the fourth, fifth, and sixth decades. Cases have been reported in women from the ages of 17 to above 80 years (Rose et al., 1990; Baekelandt et al., 1993). In a review of 393 patients, a mean age of 55 years was described (Benedet et al., 1977), consistent with a mean age of 56.7 years in a meta-analysis of 577 patients (Ng and Lawton, 1998).

There appears to be a higher incidence in White over Black population (Rose et al., 1990). It is more common in postmenopausal women. Patients with PFTC appear to have a shorter history of symptoms than those with EOC (Ng and Lawton, 1998). The classical triad of symptoms, a serosanguinous discharge, pain and an adnexal mass, and *hydrops tubae profluens* as described by Latzko in 1916, is rarely reported nowadays (Lawson et al., 1996; Ng and Lawton, 1998). The most common clinical sign is vaginal bleeding or spotting, which is present in 50%–60% of patients; abdominal pain, colicky or dull, is present in 30%–49% of cases; abdominal or pelvic mass may appear in 60% of cases (range, 12%–84%); and ascites may be present in 15% of cases. In addition, other rare clinical presentation may occur such as acute abdominal pain, palpable inguinal node, umbilical–bone–cerebral metastases, and cerebellar degeneration (Ajithkumar et al., 2005; Pectasides et al., 2006).

16.1.3 Cytology of the Fallopian Tube Carcinoma

It has been a debate whether the cervicovaginal smear is an inadequate diagnostic tool for the diagnosis of primary fallopian tube cancer and if it should be used as a diagnostic screening tool. Positive Pap smears have been reported in only 0%–23% of cases (Takashina et al., 1985; Zreik et al., 2001). Clinicians should be aware that a discrepancy between an abnormal Pap smear and negative findings on colposcopy, cervical biopsy, and endometrial curettage could be considered as suspicious for PFTC (Pectasides et al., 2006).

16.1.4 Pathology of the Fallopian Tube Carcinoma

Primary fallopian tube cancer is usually diagnosed by a pathologist on histopathological examination. The most common histological types are shown in Table 16.1 (Alvarado-Cabrero et al., 1999; Pectasides et al., 2006). Difficulties in diagnosis exist due to the similarities shared between FTC and EOC. The diagnostic criteria to distinguish FTC from other primary tumors were established in 1950 (Hu et al., 1950). Later, the classification criteria were modified in 1978 and are the following: (a) the main tumor is in the tube and arises from the endosalpinx; (b) histologically, the pattern reproduces the epithelium of the mucosa and often shows a papillary pattern; (c) if the wall is involved, the transition between benign and malignant epithelium should be demonstrable; and (d) the ovaries and endometrium are either normal or contain less tumor than the tube (Sedlis, 1978). A significant difference between PFTC and EOC is the evidence that patients with fallopian tube cancer have a higher rate of retroperitoneal and distant metastases than those with EOC; this evidence is obtained from the international literature (McMurray et al., 1986; Gadducci et al., 2001). Metastases to the paraaortic lymph nodes have been documented in 33% of the patients with all stages of disease; this is due to the rich presence of lymphatic channels in the fallopian tube that drain into the paraaortic lymph nodes through infundibulopelvic lymphatics (Tamimi and Figge, 1981). Molecular biology studies have shown that PFTC is characterized by an extremely unstable phenotype with highly scattered DNA ploidy patterns and frequent p53 gene alterations (Lacy et al., 1995).

TABLE 16.1

Frequency of Primary Fallopian Tube Cancer Histology Types in Correlation with Frequency of Epithelial Ovarian Cancer

Type	PFTC	EOC
Serous	49.5%–83.3%	60%–80%
Endometrioid	8.3%–50%	15%–24%
Mixed	3.9%–16.7%	3%
Undifferentiated	7.8%–11.3%	1%–2%
Clear cell	1.9%	3.7%–12.1%
Transitional	11.7%	1%–2%
Mucinous	3%–7.6%	2.4%–19.9%

PFTC, primary fallopian tube cancer; EOC, epithelial ovarian cancer.

16.1.5 Staging of the Fallopian Tube Carcinoma

The surgical findings during the process of laparotomy define the staging of the primary fallopian tube cancer. Operative findings prior to debulking may be modified by histopathological as well as clinical or radiologic assessment. The current staging is provided by the International Federation of Gynecology and Obstetrics (FIGO) and has been used since 1991; the staging is exhibited on Table 16.2 (Pectasides et al., 2006). It has been found that in general, 20%–25% of patients have stage I, 20% have stage II, 45%–50% have stage III, and 5%–10% have stage IV (Ajithkumar et al., 2005).

TABLE 16.2

Staging of Primary Fallopian Tube Carcinoma (PFTC)

FIGO		TNM
0	Primary tumor cannot be assessed.	Tx
	No evidence of primary tumor.	TO
	Carcinoma in situ (preinvasive carcinoma).	Tis
I	Carcinoma confined to fallopian tubes.	T1
IA	Tumor confined to 1 tube without infiltrating the serosal surface: no ascites.	T1a
IB	Tumor confined to both tubes without infiltrating the serosal surface: no ascites.	T1b
IC	Tumor confined to 1 or both tubes with extension onto/through the tubal serosa or with positive malignant cells in the ascites or positive peritoneal washings.	T1c
II	Tumor involving both tubes with pelvic extension.	T2
IIA	Extension and/or metastases to uterus and/or ovaries.	T2a
IIB	Extension to other pelvic organs.	T2b
IIC	Stage IIA or IIB with positive malignant cells in the ascites or positive peritoneal washings.	T2c
III	Tumor involving 1 or both tubes with peritoneal implants outside the pelvis and/or positive regional lymph nodes.	T3 and/or N1
IIIA	Microscopic peritoneal metastases outside the pelvis.	T3a
IIIB	Macroscopic peritoneal metastases outside the pelvis ≤2 cm in greatest dimension.	T3b and/or N1
IIIC	Peritoneal metastases more than >2 cm in greatest dimension and/or positive regional lymph nodes.	T3c and/or N1
IV	Distant metastases beyond the peritoneal cavity.	M1
	Positive pleural cytology and/or parenchymal liver metastases.	

16.1.6 Diagnostic Procedures

Because of the rarity of the malignant neoplasms of the fallopian tube cancer and the clinical symptomatology that may mimic several pathological conditions such as salpingitis, ovarian abscess, or adnexal tumor, it is considered difficult to diagnose most of the cases prior to surgical laparotomy (Ajithkumar et al., 2005; Pectasides et al., 2006).

In many series, missing the correct diagnosis entirely in their working differential has been reported (McMurray et al., 1986).

Many different modalities for the detection of fallopian tube cancer are investigated; these include several imaging techniques such as nuclear medicine with radioactive nucleotides, magnetic resonance imaging (MRI), ultrasound, and tumor markers.

In Table 16.3 are exhibited the main diagnostic procedures and the rate of specificity and sensitivity in each method.

16.1.6.1 Hysteroscopy and Hysterosalpingography

Despite the clinical evidence that these procedures may diagnose abnormal tumor masses of the fallopian tubes, their specificity is limited; therefore, their use is limited.

In addition, it is possible to assist the dissemination of neoplastic cells and intraperitoneal seeding the fallopian tube ampulla is patent (Hinton et al., 1988).

TABLE 16.3

Overview of Different Diagnostic Studies in the Detection of Primary Fallopian Tube (PFTC)

Author Year	Country	Diagnostic Method	Diagnostic Assessment	Sensitivity (%)	Specificity (%)	Comment
Kurjak et al. (1992)	Croatia	Transvaginal Ultrasonography	Vascular resistance Indices in adnexa Color flow, Doppler	96	95	Color flow and Doppler. Indices may be used as screening method in adnexa.
Lehtovirta et al. (1990)	Finland	Radio imaging with 131I-labeled F(ab′)2 fragments of monoclonal OC-125	Detection of metastases located retroperitoneal in lymph nodes from PFTC	90	83	Metastases in lymph nodes were more frequent in patients with elevated CA125.
Hefler et al. (2000)	United States	Measuring CA125 levels in serum of patients with PFTC	Correlation of CA125 as prognostic and monitoring markers in treatment and survival of patients with PFTC	75	98	CA125 level is an independent prognostic factor of DFS and OS. CA 125 level defines response to chemotherapy.

16.1.6.2 Ultrasonography

Transvaginal and transabdominal ultrasound is an essential imaging technique in the diagnostic workup of patients with possible tubal pathology (Campbell et al., 1990).

More accurate assessment of adnexal pathology is offered with the use of transvaginal ultrasound (TVS). The sensitivity of TVS has been increased with the application of color flow and Doppler waveform measurements with possible tubal pathology demonstrated the benefits of transvaginal over transabdominal ultrasound in the imaging of fallopian tubes. The echographic appearance of fallopian tubes is nonspecific, mimicking other pelvic diseases, such as tuboovarian abscess, ovarian tumor, and ectopic pregnancy. Echogram exhibits a cystic mass with spaces and mural nodules, a sausage-shaped mass, or a multilobular mass with a cog-and-wheel appearance. Low-impedance vascular flow within the solid components has been demonstrated. In addition, it was demonstrated that transvaginal ultrasound examination with color Doppler can detect areas of neovascularization within the fallopian tube and thus may aid in the preoperative diagnosis of PFTC. Three-dimensional Doppler can show tubal wall irregularities such as papillary protrusions and pseudosepta and depictions of vascular abnormalities (arteriovenous shunts, microaneurysms, tumor lakes, blind ends, and dichotomous branching typical of malignant tumor vessels) (Timor-Trisch and Rottem, 1987; Pectasides et al., 2006).

Improved understanding of anatomical relationships may aid in distinguishing ovarian from tubal pathology. Newer studies have tried to discriminate ovarian from fallopian tube pathology; however, good experience of the operator is necessitated. Multiple sections of the tubal sausage like structures enable determination of local tumor spread and capsule infiltration. Study of the vascular architecture in cases of fallopian tube malignancy is further enhanced using 3-D power Doppler imaging (Kurjak et al., 2000).

In imaging of postmenopausal adnexal masses, the use of color flow alone has a reported specificity of only 65% assuming that flow is visible (Kurjak et al., 1992). It has been found that the differences in vessel resistance indices between benign and malignant neoplasms had a sensitivity of 96% and a specificity of 95% ($P < 0.001$). The color flow imaging during TVS is dependent from the experience of the operator, quality of instrumentation applied, and the change in imaging characteristics of tumors dependent on stage (Table 16.3) (Kurjak et al., 1992).

16.1.6.3 Computed Tomography and Magnetic Resonance Imaging

Many researchers have reported that MRI is superior to computed tomography and ultrasound in the differentiation of fallopian tube from other pelvic organs (Kawakami et al., 1993). Despite this evidence, the separation of benign neoplasms from malignant neoplasms has been considered as difficult and ultrasound has been proved to be superior to MRI and CT as a screening modality in the diagnosis of adnexal tumors in general (Kawakami et al., 1993; Kurachi et al., 1999). Several clinical imaging features may be present; the lesions may appear like small, solid, lobulated masses on CT scan or on MRI. On CT scan, the lesion obtains an attenuation equal to that of other soft tissue masses and enhances less than the myometrium. On T1-weighted MR images, the tumor is usually hypointense; on T2-weighted MR images, the tumor is often homogeneously hyperintense. Imaging can most often detect solid and cystic components having papillary projections; imaging on MRI can be remarkably enhanced by the administration of gadolinium (Kawakami et al., 1993; Kurachi et al., 1999). MRI seems to be better than CT scan or ultrasound in detecting tumor infiltration of the bladder, vagina, pelvic sidewalls, pelvic fat, and rectum (Thurnher et al., 1990).

16.1.6.4 Nuclear Scan Imaging and Metastatic Disease

The use of radio imaging with a combination of immunolymphoscintigraphy and immunoscintigraphy with ^{131}I-labeled F(ab')$_2$ fragments of monoclonal OC-125 has improved significantly the detection of retroperitoneal lymph-node metastases presenting a sensitivity of 90% and a specificity of 83% (Lehtovirta et al., 1990), Table 16.3. The results were correlated with increased levels of CA125; these findings indicate that patients having high levels of circulating CA125 are at higher risk of having metastatic disease. Another method of detecting metastatic disease is the positron emission tomography (PET) scan, which is based on the higher glucose in malignant neoplasms. Whole-body 2-deoxy-2-(18F) fluoro-D-glucose (FDG)-PET scan was used to detect sites of metastatic FTC in areas of skin nodules and bone discomfort. Chemically, FDG is a glucose analog, with the positron-emitting radioactive isotope fluorine-18 substituted for the normal hydroxyl group at the 2′ position in the glucose molecule (Lehtovirta et al., 1990; Karlan et al., 1993).

16.1.6.5 Role of CA125 as Tumor Marker in Fallopian Tube Carcinoma Diagnosis

CA125 also known as mucin 16 or MUC16 is a protein that in humans is encoded by the-*MUC16* gene. MUC16 is a member of the mucin family glycoproteins (Yin and Lloyd, 2001). CA125 is a cancer-associated antigen defined by a murine monoclonal antibody (OC125, IgG1), which was produced by immunizing mice with an ovarian serous cystadenocarcinoma cell line, OVCA433 (Bast et al., 1981).

The antigen has been detected in tissues derived from coelomic epithelium in the embryo and adult, including the pleura, pericardium, peritoneum, fallopian tube, endometrium, and endocervix. Outside this lineage, CA125 has also been detected in tracheobronchial epithelium and glands, amnion, amniotic fluid, milk, cervical mucus, and seminal fluid (DiSaia and Creasman, 2002).

CA125 is the most frequently used biomarker for ovarian cancer detection. Serum concentrations of CA125 are measured by immunoradiometric assay, introduced by Bast et al. in 1983; they suggested a 35 U/mL cutoff value for normal controls (Bast et al., 1983). Around 90% of women with advanced ovarian cancer have elevated levels of CA125 in their blood serum, making CA125 a useful tool for detecting ovarian cancer after the onset of symptoms (Suh et al., 2010). In April 2011, the UK's National Institute for Health and Care Excellence (NICE) recommended that women with symptoms that could be caused by ovarian cancer should be offered a CA125 blood test. The aim of this guideline is to help diagnose the disease at an earlier stage, when treatment is more likely to be successful. Women with higher levels of the marker in their blood would then be offered an ultrasound scan to determine whether they need further tests (NICE, 2011).

CA125 is a useful tumor marker for the diagnosis, assessment of response to treatment, and detection of tumor recurrence during follow-up (Pectasides et al., 2006). Although CA125 per se is not diagnostic for PFTC, >80% of patients have elevated pretreatment serum CA125 levels (Ajithkumar et al., 2005). Levels of CA125 greater than 65 U/mL have been defined as probable for fallopian tube malignancies with a specificity of 98% and a sensitivity of 75% (Kol et al., 1990; Hefler et al., 2000). However, serum antigen levels are found to be elevated in both benign and malignant conditions such as endometriosis pelvic inflammatory disease and early pregnancy (Zervoudis et al., 2007). Elevated serum CA125 levels have been detected more frequently in advanced or recurrent disease (Rosen et al., 1999). Some authors have reported that preoperative serum CA125 levels were >35 U/mL in 85.3% of cases (68.7% for stages I–II and 94.7% for stages III–IV of fallopian tube cancer [Gadducci et al., 2001]). Reports suggest screening with this tumor marker would be more effective if used in combination with transvaginal ultrasound (Podobnik et al., 1993). The pretreatment serum CA125 level is an independent prognostic factor of disease-free survival (DFS) and overall survival (OS) in patients with PFTC (Rosen et al., 1999; Ajithkumar et al., 2005). Serum CA125 levels after the surgical process have also been associated with response to chemotherapy (Tokunaga et al., 1990). CA125 is also a useful marker for posttreatment follow-up. It is indicated as an early and sensitive marker for tumor progression during the follow-up of the patients (Hefler et al., 2000). It has been reported that the lead time (elevated serum CA125 levels prior to clinical or radiological diagnosis of recurrence) is 3 months (range, 0.5–7 months) (Hefler et al., 2000; Ajithkumar et al., 2005).

16.1.7 Treatment of Fallopian Tube Carcinoma

The treatment of the fallopian tube cancer is based on the management of EOC. Surgery is the treatment of choice for PFTC. Surgical principles are the same as those used for ovarian cancer. In addition, chemotherapy, inhibition of angiogenesis with monoclonal antibody, radiation therapy, and hormonotherapy may be provided.

16.1.7.1 Surgical Treatment

The golden standard of the surgical management of fallopian tube cancer initiates with the staging laparotomy. There is evidence that residual disease after surgical treatment and adjuvant chemotherapy is associated with poorer prognosis (Ajithkumar et al., 2005). The residual disease is defined as the cancer cells that remain after attempts to remove the cancer have been made.

The Gynecologic Oncology Group has divided patients with advanced EOC into those with optimal residual disease, in which the maximum diameter of residual is less than or equal to 1 cm, and suboptimal residual disease, in which the residual disease is >1 cm. Similarly, these principles account for PFTC, (Hoskins et al., 1994). A careful surgical staging at presentation is paramount in the treatment of fallopian tube cancer. According to the FIGO, the following must be performed through a midline incision:

- Careful evaluation of the entire abdominopelvic cavity to delineate extent of disease
- Total abdominal hysterectomy and bilateral salpingo-oophorectomy
- Sampling of the pelvic and paraaortic lymph nodes
- Infracolic omentectomy
- Washings of the peritoneal cavity
- Biopsies of any suspicious areas including the abdominal and pelvic peritoneum

In the unlikely event that a patient is young and wishes to retain fertility, limited surgery can be considered for carcinoma in situ only after detailed evaluation and careful discussion with the patient. However, this limited approach is not encouraged in view of the high incidence of bilateral localization of the cancer. In cancer that has been established, there is no role for conservative surgery or cytoreduction, which is the medical term used in surgical oncology (FIGO, 1998).

16.1.7.2 Adjuvant Chemotherapy in Fallopian Tube Carcinoma

Based on the propensity for microscopic distant spread and the relatively high risk for recurrence despite complete surgical resection, chemotherapy seems to have a strong rationale as adjuvant treatment for patients with early-stage disease.

Single-agent chemotherapy does not seem to be effective, while platinum-based combination chemotherapy is the most commonly used adjuvant therapy for these patients, identical to EOC patients (Pectasides et al., 2006). Patients with stage IA and IB may not require adjuvant therapy, as for patients with EOC (Ajithkumar et al., 2005; Pectasides et al., 2006). The current gold-standard chemotherapy for EOC in North America is a platinum (carboplatin)–taxane (paclitaxel) combination, and in Britain, it is platinum followed on relapse by a taxane (Pectasides et al., 2006).

Paclitaxel is a mitotic inhibitor, which was a drug isolated from the bark of the Pacific yew tree, *Taxus brevifolia,* and was originally named taxol. Paclitaxel is one of several cytoskeletal drugs that target tubulin. Paclitaxel-treated cells have defects in mitotic spindle assembly, chromosome segregation, and cell division. Unlike other tubulin-targeting drugs such as colchicine that inhibit microtubule assembly, paclitaxel stabilizes the microtubule polymer and protects it from disassembly. Chromosomes are thus unable to achieve a metaphase spindle configuration. This blocks progression of mitosis, and prolonged activation of the mitotic checkpoint triggers apoptosis or reversion to the G-phase of the cell cycle without cell division (Bharadwaj and Yu, 2004).

In a large study with 41 patients treated with combination of paclitaxel and carboplatin, the authors concluded that adjuvant platinum- and paclitaxel-based chemotherapy should be regarded as the standard treatment in patients with PFTC. Early-stage disease and optimal debulking are associated with improved time to progression (TTP) of disease and OS (Papadimitriou et al., 2008).

16.1.7.3 Inhibition of Angiogenesis in Fallopian Tube Cancer with Bevacizumab

Bevacizumab (trade name Avastin, Genentech/Roche) is a humanized monoclonal antibody that inhibits VEGF and especially (VEGF-A). VEGF-A is a growth factor, a natural protein that stimulates angiogenesis in physiological processes and in cancer.

Bevacizumab binds directly to VEGF to form a protein complex that is incapable of further binding to VEGF receptor sites thus effectively reducing available VEGF. The bevacizumab/VEGF complex is both metabolized and excreted directly (Los et al., 2007).

Bevacizumab was approved by the U.S. Food and Drug Administration (FDA) for certain metastatic cancers. It received its first approval in 2004, for combination use with standard chemotherapy for metastatic colon cancer (Los et al., 2007).

Bevacizumab is administered intravenously for the treatment of colon, breast, and lung cancer. The main side effects are hypertension and heightened risk of bleeding. Bowel perforation as well as nasal septum perforation and renal thrombotic microangiopathy and ovarian failure has been reported (Muggia, 2012).

A systematic electronic search in the PubMed/MEDLINE database using the keywords bevacizumab and fallopian tube cancer revealed 16 articles dating from 2007 to 2012. Of the 16 studies, 7 studies reporting the use of bevacizumab in PFTC were selected from inclusion. The design of the studies was the following: three were phase II trials (trials that aim to assess the therapeutic efficacy and toxicity of new treatment regimens), one observational study, one randomized trial, and one case report. The main characteristics of the selected studies are exhibited on Table 16.4. In general, it was noted that bevacizumab may be combined

TABLE 16.4

List of the Selected Studies Reporting the Use of Bevacizumab in Patients with Fallopian Tube Cancer, Ovarian Cancer, and Peritoneal Cancer

Author Year	Country	Study Design	Purpose	Regiments Used	Patient Population	Results	Adverse Effects	Comment
Micha et al. (2007)	United States	Phase II trial	To assess response rate and toxicity	Bevacizumab Paclitaxel Carboplatin	$n = 20$ with EOC, peritoneal, and PFTC	CR ($n = 3$) PR ($n = 10$) SD ($n = 1$) DP ($n = 1$)	Hypertension ($n = 2$) Polyneuritis ($n = 1$)	Bevacizumab can be safely administered.
Arora et al. (2008)	United States	Case Report	Efficacy of bevacizumab in refractory metastatic PFTC	Bevacizumab	$n = 1$ with PFTC	CR	NS	Significance of antiangiogenesis treatment in PFTC.
Nimeiri et al. (2008)	United States	Phase II trial	To assess the activity and tolerability of bevacizumab and erlotinib	Bevacizumab Erlotinib	$n = 13$ with EOC, peritoneal, and PFTC	CR ($n = 1$) PR ($n = 1$) SD ($n = 7$)	Anemia ($n = 1$) Nausea ($n = 2$) Vomiting ($n = 1$) Hypertension ($n = 1$) Diarrhea ($n = 2$)	No strong suggestion that this combination was superior to single agent.
Cheng et al. (2009)	United States	Retrospective analysis	To assess the efficacy and tolerability of bevacizumab combined with other agents in nonprotocol patients	Bevacizumab Paclitaxel Cyclophosphamide	$n = 64$ with EOC, peritoneal, and PFTC	CR ($n = 25$) SD ($n = 23$)	GI perforations ($n = 2$) GI mild adverse effects ($n = 15$)	Promising clinical benefits with bevacizumab.

McGonigle et al. (2011)	United States	Phase II trial	To assess the efficacy and toxicity of bevacizumab combined with topotecan in platinum-resistant patients	Bevacizumab topotecan	$n = 40$ with EOC, peritoneal, and PFTC	PR ($n = 10$) SD ($n = 14$) PD ($n = 16$)	Neutropenia (18%) Hypertension (20%) Gastrointestinal toxicity (18%) Pain (13%) Metabolic toxicity (15%) Bowel obstruction (10%) Cardiotoxicity (8%)	Acceptable toxicity and efficacy in platinum-resistant patients.
Aghajanian et al. (2012)	United States	Randomized blinded	To compare the efficacy of gemcitabine+bevacizumab versus gemcitabine+carboplatin	Bevacizumab Gemcitabine Carboplatin	$n = 484$ with EOC, peritoneal, and PFTC	Response rate (78.5% vs. 57.4%); $P < 0.0001$	Hypertension (17.4% vs. < 1%) Proteinuria (8.5% vs. < 1%)	Combination of bevacizumab+ gemcitabine is more effective
Del Carmen et al. (2012)	United States	Phase II trial	To assess the safety and efficacy of doxorubicin plus carboplatin, plus bevacizumab	Bevacizumab Carboplatin Doxorubicin	$n = 54$ with EOC, peritoneal, and PFTC	Response rate 72.2% (95% CI: 58.4, 83.5)	Severe gastrointestinal effects ($n = 3$) Mild general effects ($n = 50$)	Effective combination adverse effects were usual in frequency.

CR, complete response; PR, partial response; SD, stable disease; DP, disease progression; PFTC, primary fallopian tube cancer, EOC, epithelial ovarian cancer; CI, confidence interval; GI, gastrointestinal.

with several chemotherapeutic agents in the treatment of PFTC, EOC, and peritoneal cancer. Several adverse effects have been reported of which hypertension was the most common, gastrointestinal toxicities and perforations, anemia, metabolic disorders, polyneuritis, etc. (Micha et al., 2007; Arora et al., 2008; Nimeiri et al., 2008; Cheng et al., 2009; McGonigle et al., 2011; Aghajanian et al., 2012; Del Carmen et al., 2012).

Bevacizumab has been criticized by the international media for its high cost and the fact that only it contributes to prolongation of life in cancer patients; this evidence is without doubt its greatest disadvantage in the management of malignant tumors. In an article published in one of the most prestigious medical journals, it has been reported that bevacizumab extended life by 4.7 months (20.3 months vs. 15.6 months) in the initial study, at a cost of $42,800–$55,000 (Mayer, 2004). Larger studies with randomized design and multicentric participation are necessitated to reach to new conclusions for the future of bevacizumab.

16.1.7.4 Radiotherapy in Fallopian Tube Carcinoma

Although radiotherapy has been used traditionally in the past as an adjuvant therapy for PFTC, its role in the era of effective chemotherapy is less well defined and controversial (Pectasides et al., 2006). Radiotherapy has been given in the form of external beam pelvic and abdominal radiotherapy while brachytherapy has also been used. It has been felt that radiotherapy did not improve survival rates when given adjuvant treatment and was associated with severe side effects. This may be because most patients receiving radiotherapy may already have had abdominal disease that would have conferred a poorer prognosis. Although the current consensus is that radiotherapy should not be used as adjuvant treatment, these results suggest that there may still be a role of postoperative pelvic radiotherapy in patients who are staged accurately (Ng and Lawton, 1998; Ajithkumar et al., 2005; Pectasides et al., 2006).

16.1.7.5 Hormonotherapy in Fallopian Tube Carcinoma

Hormonal agents have been used in the treatment of fallopian tube cancer. The fallopian tube is hormone dependent due to the histology characteristics of the tubal epithelium, which is derived from the same source as the endometrial epithelium.

Usually, progestational agents have been used in combination with chemotherapeutic agents; however, no studies have been reported with randomized design that could reach to safer and more conclusive results regarding their administration (Baekelandt et al., 1993; Pectasides et al., 2006).

16.1.7.6 Prognostic and Predictive Factors in Fallopian Tube Carcinoma

Prior to reporting the prognostic and preventive factors in fallopian tube cancer, it is necessary to explain these two essential definitions in oncology in general. It is extremely essential to analyze these elements because the experimental studies with various tumor markers have been correlated with prognostic factors.

As prognostic factors are defined, the clinical and histological findings in patients diagnosed with cancer or the molecular markers expressed in the neoplasms define their biological activity and are related statistically with the recurrence and the survival of the patients (Allred, 1997).

As predictive factors are defined, these factors are related with the response of adjuvant treatment in special protocols of management. The assessment of prognostic and predictive factors follows the initial surgical management and must be performed prior to initiation of adjuvant treatment.

Prognostic factors reflect the metastatic potential and/or growth rate of the tumor and are used to select patient outcomes without consideration of treatment given; predictive factors, on the other hand, reflect the sensitivity or resistance of a tumor to a therapeutic agent and therefore are used to predict which patients are likely to respond to a specific treatment (Henry and Hayes, 2006).

After 20 years of continuous disease, few factors may be used securely in order to evaluate two important parameters, the DFS and the OS, which are used as indicators for the management of disease. DFS measures the proportion of people among those treated for a cancer who will remain free of disease at a specified time after treatment. Overall, survival is an indication of the proportion of people within a group who are expected to be alive after a specified time. It takes into account death due to any cause—both related and unrelated to the cancer in question (Allred, 1997).

The percentage of OS in PFTC has been estimated to be 30%–50% whereas in patients with EOC it has been estimated to be 40%; this is related with the fact that many patients are diagnosed in more advanced stages of disease (Baekelandt et al., 1993; Ajithkumar et al., 2005). The prognostic factors in PFTC are similar to those applied in patients with EOC. These are the following in order of importance:

- *The stage of disease*: The stage of the disease is the most important prognostic factor for many neoplastic diseases. It has been estimated that 5-year survival in patients with PFTC may reach 65% and more (Baekelandt et al., 1993). A meta-analysis of six large studies enrolling 278 patients with PFTC has exhibited a 5-year survival of 62% for stage I; 36% for stage II; 17% for stage III; and 0% for stage IV. In addition, in another study enrolling 115 patients, the following results regarding 5-year survival were reported: for stages I and II of disease, 50.8% and for stages III and IV, 13.6% (Rosen et al., 1993). Furthermore, in a more recent study enrolling 416 patients, it was reported that a 5-year survival for stage I is (n = 102) 95%; for stage II, (n = 29) 75%; for stage III, (n = 52) 69%; and for stage IV, (n = 151) 45% (Kosary and Trimble, 2002).
- *The residual disease*: It is considered of great importance; this factor is assessed after the initial cytoreductive surgery and it is reported by the surgeon. As it was aforementioned, the larger the residual disease, the worse the prognosis. It was reported that patients with residual disease <1 cm had a 5-year survival of 55% in contrast to patients with residual disease who had residual disease >1 cm and exhibited a 22% percentage of 5-year survival (Gadducci et al., 2001).
- *The depth of invasion*: The depth of invasion is a prognostic factor that is defined through microscopy in the histological examination of the extracted surgical specimen. The depth of invasion was reported for the first time in 1970 by the American pathologist Breslow in a study about melanoma (Breslow, 1970). Since then, it has been studied as a prognostic factor in various malignancies. It has been shown that the larger depth of tumor invasion in the organ wall is related with more common failure of adjuvant treatment thus worsening the prognosis (Peters et al., 1988).
- *The histological grading*: The histological grading of the malignant tumors is related with the survival of patients with PFTC in a study with univariate design analysis

(Gadducci et al., 2001). The grade of tumor has been associated with the spread of the cancer in the lymph vessels, and the existence of lymph vessel tumor emboli might present prognostic importance (Klein et al., 1994).

- *The age of the patient*: Increased age at diagnosis is associated with increased risk for recurrence and deterioration of prognosis (Pectasides et al., 2006).
- *The histological type*: Some histological types of PFTC develop worse prognosis, for instance, serous versus endometrioid type of PFTC (Ng and Lawton, 1998; Ajithkumar et al., 2005).

16.1.8 General Aspects in Early Noninvasive Fallopian Tube Carcinoma Markers

Tumor markers or biomarkers are chemical substances that can be detected and identified in body fluids (serum and urine) and tissues and are used for diagnosis, follow-up, and as prognostic markers among patients with cancer. They can be classified into three categories: (1) *oncodevelopmental antigens*, (2) *cancer-associated antigens*, and (3) *tumor markers* representing biochemical and metabolic alterations, usually as a reaction of the host against the tumor. Tumor markers may also be classified as *tumor-specific markers*, *organ-specific markers*, and reaction products against cancer or cancer-associated metabolic changes (Riska and Leminen, 2007).

Tumor markers may have prognostic and predictive value; three key issues in tumor marker evaluation are essential and these are utility, magnitude, and reliability (Henry and Hayes, 2006).

FTC is the rarest gynecological carcinoma; there is obviously lack of studies in contrast to ovarian cancer; usually, tumor markers that have been applied in ovarian carcinoma have also been tested on FTC.

The most common tumor marker/biomarker studied is the CA125 antigen; its role in FTC has been analyzed and explained in details in the previous chapter. Herein, we endeavor to review the most essential biomarkers that have been used in clinical practice in patients with PFTC.

16.1.8.1 Serum Markers

16.1.8.1.1 Role of Human Chorionic Gonadotropin in Fallopian Tube Carcinoma

Human chorionic gonadotropin (hCG) is a glycoprotein consisting of two subunits, that is, the α- and β-subunit hCG is a very useful marker for monitoring pregnancy, pregnancy-related disorders, and trophoblastic disease, but it is very rarely useful in nontrophoblastic malignancies (Marcillac et al., 1992).

In these, the free β-subunit of hCG (hCGβ) in serum is fairly often elevated, for example, in ovarian carcinoma, elevated serum hCGβ levels have been observed in 30%–40% of the patients. Furthermore, hCGβ is an independent prognostic factor in ovarian, colorectal, and renal cell carcinoma (Vartiainen et al., 2001).

In an experimental study, hCG was collected preoperatively from the serum of 61 patients with PFTC and quantified with an in-house time-resolved immunofluorometric assay; the detection limit was 0.5 pmol/L. The patients were followed up for recurrence and survival; the prognostic value of the serum markers was compared with those of stage, grade, and histological type; overall, 5-year survival was 38% when serum hCGβ was below 3.5 pmol/L, while it was 18% when the level was higher. Clearly elevated serum concentrations of hCGβ predict survival in FTC, but in multivariate analyses, only hCG β is a prognostic factor independent of stage and histology (Riska et al., 2006).

The strong correlation between serum hCGβ and prognosis is intriguing and the true role in cancer pathophysiology is not clear. Some mechanisms through which hCG could affect tumor aggressiveness have recently been elucidated. hCGβ may exert antiapoptotic activity, and suppression of hCGβ expression reduces tumor growth of hCGβ expressing tumors (Devi et al., 2002). However, so far, a limitation in the use of hCGβ is the paucity of sufficiently sensitive commercially available assays (Riska et al., 2006). Among patients with high serum hCGβ levels, more aggressive treatments could be used and maybe in the future, they could benefit from antitumor vaccines and therapy (Riska et al., 2006). More studies with larger population and randomized design are required to reach to safer conclusions regarding the use of hCG as biomarker in PFTC.

16.1.9 Immunohistochemical Markers

16.1.9.1 Significance of HER2 as Prognostic Factor

Human epidermal growth factor receptor 2 (HER2) also known as Neu, ErbB-2, cluster of differentiation 340 (CD340), or p185 is a protein that is encoded in humans by the ERBB2 gene. HER2 is a member of the epidermal growth factor receptor (EGFR/ErbB) family. HER2 is encoded by ERBB2, a known proto-oncogene located at the long arm of human chromosome 17 (17q12). HER2 is named because it has a similar structure to human EGFR, or HER1. Neu is so named because it was derived from a rodent glioblastoma cell line, a type of neural tumor. ErbB-2 was named for its similarity to ERBB (avian erythroblastosis oncogene B), the oncogene later found to code for EGFR. Gene cloning showed that HER2, Neu, and ErbB-2 are all encoded by the same gene (Coussens et al., 1985).

The ErbB family is composed of four plasma-membrane-bound receptor tyrosine kinases. All four contain an extracellular ligand-binding domain, a transmembrane domain, and an intracellular domain that can interact with a multitude of signaling molecules and exhibit both ligand-dependent and ligand-independent activity. HER2 can heterodimerize with any of the other three receptors and is considered to be the preferred dimerization partner of the other ErbB receptors (Olayioye, 2001).

The HER2/neu proto-oncogene encodes a 185 kDa transmembrane glycoprotein with intrinsic tyrosine-kinase activity that resembles the receptor for epidermal growth factor. Aberrant HER2/neu protein overexpression occurs in human gynecologic adenocarcinomas, including those of the ovary, endometrium, breast, fallopian tube, and cervix, and is secondary to gene amplification and/or overexpression of the p185HER2 protein. Overexpression of HER2/neu was found to be a poor prognostic factor for survival from advanced-stage ovarian cancer, node-positive breast cancer, and endometrial cancer (Cirisano and Karlan, 1996).

New agent such as EGFR tyrosine-kinase inhibitors and especially an agent called pertuzumab are used relatively as adjuvant treatment of ovarian cancer in combination with paclitaxel (Haldar et al., 2011).

A Cochrane systematic review and meta-analysis in 2011 has reported that EGFR inhibitors, including pertuzumab, may add activity to conventional chemotherapy for the treatment of platinum-resistant ovarian cancer. Further RCTs are necessary before EGFR inhibitors are introduced as first- or second-line treatment of ovarian cancer (Haldar et al., 2011).

Electronic search of PubMed medical database using the keywords *HER2/neu* and *fallopian tube cancer* yielded several studies regarding the expression of HER2 in

TABLE 16.5

Summary of Studies with HER2 Expression in Patients with Primary Fallopian Tube Carcinoma

Author Year	Country	Population (Specimen)	Methods	Results	Comment
Lacy et al. (1995)	United States	N = 43	ABPC	N = 11/43 positive	No prognostic significance
Stuhlinger et al. (1995)	Austria	N = 73	PCR	N = 65/73	No amplification of HER2
Chung et al. (2000)	Hong Kong	N = 18	ABPC	N = 16/18	May exist a role in tumorigenesis
Nowee et al. (2007)	The Netherlands	N = 28	CGH-ARRAY	N = 12/28	May exist a role in tumorigenesis
Papadimitriou et al. (2009)	Greece	N = 26	ABPC	N = 2/26	No prognostic significance

ABPC, avidin–biotidin–peroxidase complex; PCR, polymerase chain reaction; CHG-ARRAY, color genome hybridization array.

specimen of patients with PFTC that have been published; the results are exhibited on Table 16.5. All of them were related with immunohistochemical expression of HER2 in tissue specimen of patients with PFTC.

In their study, Lacy et al. (1995) investigated the immunohistochemical expression of HER2 in 43 patients with PFTC via avidin–biotin–peroxidase complex method; the results were correlated with clinical characteristics like survival and stage. HER2 overexpression was found in 11 cases (25.6%). The authors could not demonstrate that these molecular markers had prognostic relevance in this disease, but the size of their cohort was limited. However, the potential prognostic relevance of HER2 expression in tubal cancers should be pursued in a larger cohort (Lacy et al., 1995).

Another study from Austria examined tissue specimen from 73 patients with PFTC (Stühlinger et al., 1995). The tissue was embedded in paraffin and investigated for HER2 oncogene amplification with a quantitative polymerase chain reaction method. The authors stated that DNA could be extracted and successfully prepared in 65/73 samples. However, none of the tissue samples exhibited amplified the HER2 oncogene. These findings suggested that the HER2 oncogene does not play a role in tumor transformation and progression in FTCs. This contrasts with observations in ovarian carcinomas, with which FTCs share many clinical, histological, and biochemical similarities (Stühlinger et al., 1995).

The expression of HER2 in PFTC specimen was investigated in a study from Hong Kong; the authors included specimen from 18 patients with PFTC. They correlated the expression of HER2 with the expression of oncogene p53 and clinicopathological features were examined. HER2 was detected in 16 cases (89%) but no significant correlation was found. The authors reported that the high incidence of p53 and HER2 overexpression in fallopian tube adenocarcinoma suggests that these genes may play a role in its tumorigenesis (Chung et al., 2000).

In a more recent study from the Netherlands, the authors aimed to determine the expression of p53, HER2/neu, and p27(Kip1) in serous FTC in relation to stage and grade and to investigate DNA copy number changes in HER2 and P27KIP1 as a potential mechanism of altered expression status (Nowee et al., 2007).

Immunohistochemistry was performed on 28 serous FTCs and 10 normal fallopian tubes. p53 protein accumulated and p27(Kip1) was downregulated significantly in early-stage FTCs compared with normal fallopian tubes. HER2/neu overexpression was absent in normal fallopian tubes and in all stage I FTCs (n = 6) but present in 57% (12/21) of advanced-stage FTCs. No differences in expression between grade 2 and 3 tumors were detected. HER2 gain/amplification was found by array comparative genomic hybridization in 23% (3/13) of analyzed FTCs and all showed overexpression. HER2/neu overexpression also occurred without DNA copy number changes in three other cases. For p27(Kip1), expression and DNA copy number were unrelated. HER2 showed overexpression, caused by gain/amplification in 50%, and may be involved in progression of FTC. These data contribute to a better understanding of the molecular carcinogenesis of FTC and to possible new therapeutic approaches (Nowee et al., 2007).

In a research study from Greece, the authors retrospectively analyzed the specimen of 26 patients with PFTC. Tissue blocks were reviewed and sections were stained for HER2 with the use of the avidin–biotin–peroxidase complex method (Papadimitriou et al., 2009). There were 2 (8%) positive stains for HER2; the results were correlated with survival and stage; no statistical significance was observed from the correlation; therefore, it was concluded that early-stage disease and optimal debulking are associated with improved outcome and HER2 could not be established as prognostic factor due to the fact that the study population was low (Papadimitriou et al., 2009).

Larger series with PFTC are necessitated to reach to more conclusive and solid understandings about the role of HER2 as prognostic factor.

16.1.9.2 Laminin as Prognostic Factor in Fallopian Tube Carcinoma

Laminins are major proteins in the basal lamina (one of the layers of the basement membrane), a protein network foundation for most cells and organs. The laminins are an important and biologically active part of the basal lamina, influencing cell differentiation, migration, adhesion, as well as phenotype and survival.

Laminins are trimeric proteins that contain an α-chain, a β-chain, and a γ-chain, found in five, four, and three genetic variants, respectively. The laminin molecules are named according to their chain composition. Thus, laminin-511 contains α5, β1, and γ1 chains (Aumailley et al., 2005).

Fifteen laminin trimers have been identified. The laminins are combinations of different α-, β-, and γ-chains. There are five forms of α-chains, LAMA1, LAMA2, LAMA3, LAMA4, and LAMA5; four of β-chains, LAMB1, LAMB2, LAMB3, and LAMB4; and three of γ-chains, LAMC1, LAMC2, and LAMC3 (Colognato and Yurchenco, 2000).

There were two prospective studies studying the role of laminin as prognostic factor as the electronic search of database PubMed yielded: one study from Poland by Halon et al. (2003) and one study from the United States by Kuhn et al. (2012).

In their study, Halon et al. (2003) used formalin fixed, paraffin-embedded tissue samples from 70 patients diagnosed with PFTC. The tissues were cut into 4 μm sections and were immunohistochemically stained for laminin using the avidin–biotin–peroxidase complex method. Primary laminin and lyophilized monoclonal NCL-LAMININ clone LAM-89 were used also. The expression of laminin in the tissues was correlated with clinicopathological features such as FIGO stage, histological type, grade, and survival. Intracellular expression of laminin was found in 46 cases and extracellular in 28 cases; no statistical significance was found in correlation with clinicopathological features; therefore, laminin could not be applied as prognostic factor.

Recently, in the study by Kuhn et al. (2012), a reappraisal was reported. The authors performed RNA sequencing to compare transcriptomes between high-grade serous carcinomas (HGSCs) and normal fallopian tube epithelium (FTE). They performed immunohistochemical analysis for laminin γ1, TP53 mutations, p53, and Ki-67 in 32 cases of concurrent HGSC and serous tubal intraepithelial carcinoma (STIC). Laminin γ1 immunostaining intensity was found to be significantly higher in STIC and HGSC compared with adjacent FTE in all cases ($P < 0.001$). What is essential is that laminin γ1 staining was identified in all 13 STICs that lacked p53 immunoreactivity because of null mutations. These findings suggested that the overexpression of laminin γ1 immunoreactivity and alteration of its staining pattern in STICs can serve as a useful tissue biomarker, especially for those STICs that are negative for p53 and have a low Ki-67 labeling index (Kuhn et al., 2012). This study indicated that laminin γ1 may be provided in the future as immunochemical biomarker in FTC. Further studies are necessitated to establish this role.

16.1.9.3 Vascular Endothelial Growth Factor and Fallopian Tube Carcinoma

VEGF is a highly specific mitogen for vascular endothelial cells. Five VEGF isoforms are generated as a result of alternative splicing from a single VEGF gene. The most important member is VEGF-A; other members are placenta growth factor (PGF), VEGF-B, VEGF-C, and VEGF-D. The latter ones were discovered later than VEGF-A, and, before their discovery, VEGF-A was called just VEGF. These isoforms differ in their molecular mass and in biological functions such as their ability to bind to cell-surface heparan-sulfate proteoglycans. The expression of VEGF is potentiated in response to hypoxia, by activated oncogenes and by a variety of cytokines. VEGF induces endothelial cell proliferation, promotes cell migration, and inhibits apoptosis. In vivo VEGF induces angiogenesis as well as permeabilization of blood vessels and plays a central role in the regulation of vasculogenesis. Deregulated VEGF expression contributes to the development of solid tumors by promoting tumor angiogenesis and to the etiology of several additional diseases that are characterized by abnormal angiogenesis. Consequently, inhibition of VEGF signaling abrogates the development of a wide variety of tumors. The various VEGF forms bind to two tyrosine-kinase receptors, VEGFR-1 (*flt-1*) and VEGFR-2 (*KDR/flk-1*), which are expressed almost exclusively in endothelial cells (Neufeld et al., 1999).

VEGF expression in specimen of 26 women with PFTC was retrospectively analyzed with the avidin–biotin–peroxidase complex technique. The results were correlated with the clinical and pathological characteristics of these patients in order to investigate if VEGF expression may be considered as prognostic factor. Positive immunostaining was observed in 22 patients (85%); however, statistical analysis did not confirm any prognostic significance (Papadimitriou et al., 2009). VEGF could not be considered as prognostic factor due to low cohort of patients.

16.1.9.4 Genomic Sequencing for Inherited Cancer

Inherited mutations in BRCA1 and BRCA2 create a lifetime risk of ovarian carcinoma of between 20% (for BRCA2) and 50% or even higher (for BRCA1) (King et al., 2003). It has been estimated that 13%–15% of patients with ovarian carcinoma in North America carry germline mutations in BRCA1 or BRCA2 (Zhang et al., 2011).

Hereditary ovarian carcinoma also occurs in the context of Lynch syndrome (hereditary nonpolyposis colorectal cancer [HNPCC]), but the proportion of ovarian carcinoma explained by germline mutations in the mismatch repair genes has not been determined. Inherited mutations in RAD51C, RAD51D, and PALB2 have also been reported in patients with familial ovarian carcinoma (Walsh et al., 2011).

Women with early-stage ovarian carcinoma have far better survival than women whose carcinomas are diagnosed at later stages, but current methods of early detection have not proven effective. In contrast, risk-reducing salpingo-oophorectomy in women with BRCA1 or BRCA2 mutations dramatically reduces the risk of ovarian carcinoma and significantly decreases overall mortality (Walsh et al., 2011).

In order to detect the genes related with hereditary cancer, breast, ovary, and adnexa, a massively parallel sequencing approach has been validated, named BROCA, in honor of Paul Broca, the nineteenth-century neurosurgeon, oncologist, anatomist, and evolutionist, who elegantly described inherited breast and ovarian cancer (Walsh et al., 2011).

The test analyzes blood samples from patients and this assay sequences all exons and flanking intronic sequences of the following genes: *APC, ATM, ATR, BABAM1, BAP1, BARD1, BMPR1A, BRCC36, BRIP1, CDH1, CDK4, CDKN2A, CHEK1, CHEK2, FAM175A* (Abraxas), *MLH1, MRE11A, MSH2* (+*EPCAM*), *MSH6, MUTYH, NBN, PALB2, PMS2, PRSS1, PTEN, RAD50, RAD51, RAD51B, RAD51C, RAD51D, RBBP8, RET, SMAD4, STK11, TP53, TP53BP1, UIMC1, VHL, XRCC2,* and *XRCC3*. A total of 1.1 Mb (1.1 million base pairs) are sequenced and the average coverage ranges from 320 to >1000 sequencing reads per bp. Genomic regions are captured using biotinylated RNA oligonucleotides (SureSelect), prepared in paired-end libraries with ~200 bp insert size, and sequenced on an Illumina HiSeq2000 instrument with 100 bp read lengths, in a modification of a procedure described by Walsh et al. (2011). Large deletions and duplications are detected using methods described by Nord et al. (2011).

The BROCA panel was used in a large study that enrolled 360 women, of those, 273 women with ovarian carcinomas, 48 with peritoneal carcinomas, 31 with FTCs, and 8 with synchronous endometrial and ovarian carcinomas. Targeted capture by BROCA baits and genomic sequencing yielded median 449-fold coverage; 98.4% of bases had >50-fold coverage, our threshold for variant detection (Walsh et al., 2011).

From the 31 patients with fallopian tube cancer, a proportion of 0.93 germline loss-of-function mutations was found in BRCA1; BRCA2; BARD1, BRIP1, CHEK2, MRE11, NBN, PALB2, RAD50; or RAD51C; MSH6; or p53 (Walsh et al., 2011).

For the BROCA test, the reagent cost is ~$200 per sample and decreases as more samples are multiplexed per lane. Sensitivity is high, demonstrated by the detection of a mosaic germline TP53 mutation present in only 20% of sequenced alleles (Walsh et al., 2011).

The authors concluded that one-fifth of ovarian carcinoma appears to be associated with inherited risk, and the speed and cost of BROCA will allow immediate translation into clinical laboratories, and throughput is sufficient for larger epidemiological studies. The BROCA test is not patented and the design of capture baits is freely available (Walsh et al., 2011). More information can be obtained in the following website address: http://web.labmed.washington.edu/tests/genetics/BROCA.

16.1.10 Future Perspectives

Fallopian tube cancer is an extremely rare clinical entity, as it has been mentioned. Therefore, there is not a plethora of studies, and there is limited screening appliance. Its diagnosis is usually confirmed postoperatively in pathology specimen. FIGO guidelines suggest that fallopian tube should be treated as EOC, in all aspects of surgery chemotherapy and radiotherapy.

References

Ajithkumar TV, Minimole AL, John MM et al. 2005. Primary fallopian tube carcinoma. *Obstet Gynecol Surv* 60:247–252.

Aghajanian C, Blank SV, Goff BA, Judson PL, Teneriello MG, Husain A, Sovak MA, Yi J, Nycum LR. 2012. OCEANS: A randomized, double-blind, placebo-controlled phase III trial of chemotherapy with or without bevacizumab in patients with platinum-sensitive recurrent epithelial ovarian, primary peritoneal, or fallopian tube cancer. *J Clin Oncol* 30(17):2039–2045.

Allred C. 1997. Prognostic and predictive factors in breast cancer assessed by immunohistochemi try. United States and Canadian Academy of Pathology. *Long Course, Breast Pathology*, March 5. Orlando, FL: Marriott's Orlando World Center, pp. 77–97.

Alvarado-Cabrero I, Young RH, Vamvakas EC et al. 1999. Carcinoma of the fallopian tube: A clinicopathological study of 105 cases with observations on staging and prognostic factors. *Gynecol Oncol* 72:367–379.

Arora N, Tewari D, Cowan C, Saffari B, Monk BJ, Burger RA. 2008. Bevacizumab demonstrates activity in advanced refractory fallopian tube carcinoma. *Int J Gynecol Cancer* 18(2):369–372.

Aumailley M, Bruckner-Tuderman L, Carter WG, Deutzmann R, Edgar D, Ekblom P, Engel J et al. 2005. A simplified laminin nomenclature. *Matrix Biol* 24(5):326–332.

Aziz S, Kuperstein G, Rosen B et al. 2001. A genetic epidemiological study of carcinoma of the fallopian tube. *Gynecol Oncol* 80:341–345.

Baekelandt M, Kockx M, Wesling F et al. 1993. Primary adenocarcinoma of the fallopian tube. Review of the literature. *Int J Gynecol Cancer* 3:65–71.

Bast RC Jr, Feeney M, Lazarus H, Nadler LM, Colvin RB, Knapp RC. 1981. Reactivity of a monoclonal antibody with human ovarian carcinoma. *J Clin Invest* 68:1331–1337.

Bast RC Jr, Klug TL, St John E, Jenison E, Niloff JM, Lazarus H, Berkowitz RS, Leavitt T, Griffiths CT, Parker L. 1983. A radioimmunoassay using a monoclonal antibody to monitor the course of epithelial ovarian cancer. *N Engl J Med* 309:883–887.

Benedet JL, Miller DM. 1992. Tumors of fallopian tube: Clinical features, staging and management. In: Coppleson M, Monoghan JM, Morrow CP et al., eds. *Gynecologic Oncology: Fundamental Principles and Clinical Practice*. Edinburgh, U.K.: Churchill Livingstone, pp. 853–860.

Benedet JL, White GW, Fairey RN, Boyes DA. 1977. Adenocarcinoma of the fallopian tube. Experience with 41 patients. *Obstet Gynecol* 50(6):654–657.

Bharadwaj R, Yu H. 2004. The spindle checkpoint, aneuploidy, and cancer. *Oncogene* 23(11):2016–2027.

Breslow A. 1970. Thickness, cross-sectional areas and depth of invasion in the prognosis of cutaneous melanoma. *Ann Surg* 172(5):902–908.

Campbell S, Royston P, Bhan V et al. 1990. Novel screening strategies for early ovarian cancer by transabdominal ultrasonography. *Br J Obstet Gynaecol* 97:304–311.

Cheng X, Moroney JW, Levenback CF, Fu S, Jaishuen A, Kavanagh JJ. 2009. What is the benefit of bevacizumab combined with chemotherapy in patients with recurrent ovarian, fallopian tube or primary peritoneal malignancies? *J Chemother* 21(5):566–572.

Chung TK, Cheung TH, To KF, Wong YF. 2000. Overexpression of p53 and HER-2/neu and c-myc in primary fallopian tube carcinoma. *Gynecol Obstet Invest* 49(1):47–51.

Cirisano FD, Karlan BY. 1996. The role of the HER-2/neu oncogene in gynecologic cancers. *J Soc Gynecol Investig* 3(3):99–105.

Colognato H, Yurchenco PD. 2000. Form and function: The laminin family of heterotrimers. *Dev Dyn* 218(2):213–234.

Coussens L, Yang-Feng TL, Liao YC, Chen E, Gray A, McGrath J, Seeburg PH, Libermann TA, Schlessinger J, Francke U. 1985. Tyrosine kinase receptor with extensive homology to EGF receptor shares chromosomal location with neu oncogene. *Science* 230(4730):1132–1139.

Del Carmen MG, Micha J, Small L, Street DG, Londhe A, McGowan T. 2012. A phase II clinical trial of pegylated liposomal doxorubicin and carboplatin plus bevacizumab in patients with platinum-sensitive recurrent ovarian, fallopian tube, or primary peritoneal cancer. *Gynecol Oncol* 126(3):369–374.

Devi GR, Oldenkamp JR, London CA, Iversen PL. 2002. Inhibition of human chorionic gonadotropin beta-subunit modulates the mitogenic effect of c-myc in human prostate cancer cells. *Prostate* 53:200–210.

DiSaia PJ, Creasman WT, eds. 2002. *Clinical Gynecologic Oncology*. 6th ed. St. Louis, MO: Mosby, p. 675.

FIGO Report. 1998. Carcinoma of the fallopian tube: Patients treated in 1990–1992. Distribution by age groups. *J Epidemiol Biostat* 3:93.

Gadducci A, Landoni F, Sartori E et al. 2001. Analysis of treatment failures and survival of patients with fallopian tube carcinoma: A cooperation task force (CTF) study. *Gynecol Oncol* 81:150–159.

Haldar K, Gaitskell K, Bryant A, Nicum S, Kehoe S, Morrison J. 2011. Epidermal growth factor receptor blockers for the treatment of ovarian cancer. *Cochrane Database Syst Rev* (10):CD007927.

Hałoń A, Rabczyński J. 2003. PCNA and laminin as prognostic factors in primary fallopian tube carcinoma. *Folia Morphol (Warsz)* 62(4):475–478.

Hebert-Blouin MN, Koufogianis V, Gillett P et al. 2002. Fallopian tube cancer in a BRCA1 mutation carrier: Rapid development and failure of screening. *Am J Obstet Gynecol* 186:53–54.

Hefler LA, Rosen AC, Graf AH et al. 2000. The clinical value of serum concentrations of cancer antigen 125 in patients with primary fallopian tube carcinoma: A multicenter study. *Cancer* 89:1555–1560.

Henderson SR, Harper RC, Salazar OM. 1977. Primary carcinoma of the fallopian tube: Difficulties of diagnosis and treatment. *Gynecol Oncol* 5:168–179.

Henry NL, Hayes DF. 2006. Uses and abuses of tumor markers in the diagnosis, monitoring, and treatment of primary and metastatic breast cancer. *Oncologist* 11(6):541–552.

Hinton A, Bea C, Winfield AC, Entman SS. 1988. Carcinoma of the fallopian tube. *Urol Radiol* 10(2):113–115.

Hoskins WJ, McGuire WP, Brady MF, Homesley HD, Creasman WT, Berman M, Ball H, Berek JS. 1994. The effect of diameter of largest residual disease on survival after primary cytoreductive surgery in patients with suboptimal residual epithelial ovarian carcinoma. *Am J Obstet Gynecol* 170(4):974–979; 979–980.

Hu CY, Taymour ML, Hertig AT. 1950. Primary carcinoma of the fallopian tube. *Am J Obstet Gynaecol* 59:58–67.

Inal MM, Hanhan M, Pilanci B et al. 2004. Fallopian tube malignancies: Experience of Social Security Agency Aegean Maternity Hospital. *Int J Gynecol Cancer* 14:595–599.

Jongsma AP, Piek JM, Zweemer RP et al. 2002. Molecular evidence for putative tumour suppressor genes on chromosome 13q specific to BRCA1 related ovarian and fallopian tube cancer. *Mol Pathol* 55:305–309.

Karlan BY, Hoh C, Tse N, Futoran R, Hawkins R, Glaspy J. 1993. Whole-body positron emission tomography with (fluorine-18)-2-deoxyglucose can detect metastatic carcinoma of the fallopian tube. *Gynecol Oncol* 49(3):383–388.

Kawakami S, Togashi K, Kimura I, Nakano Y, Koshiyama M, Takakura K, Konishi I, Mori T, Konishi J. 1993. Primary malignant tumor of the fallopian tube: Appearance at CT and MR imaging. *Radiology* 186(2):503–508.

King MC, Marks JH, Mandell JB, New York Breast Cancer Study Group. 2003. Breast and ovarian cancer risks due to inherited mutations in BRCA1 and BRCA2. *Science* 302:643–646.

Klein M, Rosen A, Lahousen M et al. 1994. Lymphogenous metastasis in the primary carcinoma of the fallopian tube. *Gynecol Oncol* 55:336–338.

Kol S, Gal D, Friedman M, Paldi E. 1990. Preoperative diagnosis of fallopian tube carcinoma by transvaginal sonography and CA-125. *Gynecol Oncol* 37(1):129–131.

Kosary C, Trimble EL. 2002. Treatment and survival for women with Fallopian tube carcinoma: A population-based study. *Gynecol Oncol* 86:190–191.

Kuhn E, Kurman RJ, Soslow RA, Han G, Sehdev AS, Morin PJ, Wang TL, Shih IM. 2012. The diagnostic and biological implications of Laminin Expression in serous tubal intraepithelial carcinoma. *Am J Surg Pathol* Sept 18 [Epub ahead of print] 36(12):1826–1834.

Kurachi H, Maeda T, Murakami T et al. 1999. A case of fallopian tube carcinoma: Successful preoperative diagnosis with MR imaging. *Radiat Med* 17:63–66.

Kurjak A, Kupesic S, Jacobs I. 2000. Preoperative diagnosis of the primary fallopian tube carcinoma by three-dimensional static and power Doppler sonography. *Ultrasound Obstet Gynecol* 15(3):246–251.

Kurjak A, Schulman H, Sosic A, Zalud I, Shalan H. 1992. Transvaginal ultrasound, color flow, and Doppler waveform of the postmenopausal adnexal mass. *Obstet Gynecol* 80(6):917–921.

Lacy MQ, Hartmann LC, Keeney GL et al. 1995. C-erbB-2 and p53 expression in fallopian tube carcinoma. *Cancer* 75:2891–2896.

Lawson F, Lees C, Kelleher C. 1996. Primary cancer of the fallopian tube. In: Studd J, ed. *Progress in Obstetrics and Gynaecology*. New York: Churchill Livingstone, 12(22):393–401.

Lehtovirta P, Kairemo KJ, Liewendahl K, Seppälä M. 1990. Immunolymphoscintigraphy and immunoscintigraphy of ovarian and fallopian tube cancer using F(ab')2 fragments of monoclonal antibody OC 125. *Cancer Res* 50(3 Suppl):937s–940s.

Los M, Roodhart JML, Voest E. 2007. Target practice: Lessons from phase III trials with Bevacizumab and Vatalanib in the treatment of advanced colorectal cancer. *Oncology* 12(4):443–450.

Marcillac I, Troalen FF, Bidart JM, Ghillani P, Ribrag V, Escudier B, Malassagne B, Droz JP, Lhomme C, Rougier P et al. 1992. Free human chorionic gonadotropin beta subunit in gonadal and nongonadal neoplasms. *Cancer Res* 52:3901–3907.

Mayer, RJ. 2004. Two steps forward in the treatment of colorectal cancer. *N Engl J Med* 350(23):2406–2408.

McGonigle KF, Muntz HG, Vuky J, Paley PJ, Veljovich DS, Greer BE, Goff BA, Gray HJ, Malpass TW. 2011. Combined weekly topotecan and biweekly bevacizumab in women with platinum-resistant ovarian, peritoneal, or fallopian tube cancer: results of a phase 2 study. *Cancer* 117(16):3731–3740.

McMurray EH, Jacobs AJ, Perez CA et al. 1986. Carcinoma of the fallopian tube. Management and sites of failure. *Cancer* 58:2070–2075.

Meng ML, Gan-Gao, Scheng-Sun et al. 1985. Diagnosis of primary adenocarcinoma of the fallopian tube. *J Cancer Res Clin Oncol* 110:136–140.

Micha JP, Goldstein BH, Rettenmaier MA, Genesen M, Graham C, Bader K, Lopez KL, Nickle M, Brown JV 3rd. 2007. A phase II study of outpatient first-line paclitaxel, carboplatin, and bevacizumab for advanced-stage epithelial ovarian, peritoneal, and fallopian tube cancer. *Int J Gynecol Cancer* 17(4):771–776.

Muggia F. 2012. Bevacizumab in ovarian cancer: Unanswered questions. *Drugs* 72(7):931–936.

Neufeld G, Cohen T, Gengrinovitch S, Poltorak Z. 1999. Vascular endothelial growth factor (VEGF) and its receptors. *FASEB J* 13(1):9–22.

Ng P, Lawton F. 1998. Fallopian tube carcinoma—A review. *Ann Acad Med Singapore* 27(5):693–697.

Nimeiri HS, Oza AM, Morgan RJ, Friberg G, Kasza K, Faoro L, Salgia R, Stadler WM, Vokes EE, Fleming GF; Chicago Phase II Consortium; PMH Phase II Consortium; California Phase II Consortium. 2008. Efficacy and safety of bevacizumab plus erlotinib for patients with recurrent ovarian, primary peritoneal, and fallopian tube cancer: A trial of the Chicago, PMH, and California Phase II Consortia. *Gynecol Oncol* 110(1):49–55.

NICE Guidance. Women should be offered a blood test for ovarian cancer. United Kingdom National Institute for Health and Clinical Excellence. 2011-04-27.

Nord AS, Lee M, King MC, Walsh T. 2011. Accurate and exact CNV identification from targeted high-throughput sequence data. *BMC Genomics* 12:184.

Nowee ME, Dorsman JC, Piek JM, Kosma VM, Hämäläinen K, Verheijen RH, van Diest PJ. 2007. HER-2/neu and p27Kip1 in progression of Fallopian tube carcinoma: an immunohistochemical and array comparative genomic hybridization study. *Histopathology* 51(5):666–673.

Olayioye MA. 2001. Update on HER-2 as a target for cancer therapy: Intracellular signaling pathways of ErbB2/HER-2 and family members. *Breast Cancer Res* 3(6):385–389.

Papadimitriou CA, Markaki S, Lianos E, Peitsidis P, Vourli G, Nikitas N, Vlachos G, Rodolakis A, Antsaklis A, Dimopoulos MA. 2009. Clinicopathological features of primary fallopian tube carcinoma: A single institution experience. *Eur J Gynaecol Oncol* 30(4):389–395.

Papadimitriou CA, Peitsidis P, Bozas G, Grimani I, Vlahos G, Rodolakis A, Lianos E, Bamias A, Lainakis G, Dimopoulos MA. 2008. Paclitaxel- and platinum-based postoperative chemotherapy for primary fallopian tube carcinoma: A single institution experience. *Oncology* 75(1–2):42–48.

Pectasides D, Pectasides E, Economopoulos T. 2006. Fallopian tube carcinoma: A review. *Oncologist* 11(8):902–912.

Peters WA, Andersen WA, Hopkins MP, Kumar NB, Morley GW. 1988. Prognostic features of carcinoma of the fallopian tube. *Obstet Gynecol* 71:757.

Podobnik M, Singer Z, Ciglar S, Bulic M. 1993. Preoperative diagnosis of primary fallopian tube carcinoma by transvaginal ultrasound, cytological finding and CA-125. *Ultrasound Med Biol* 19(7):587–591.

Riska A, Alfthan H, Finne P, Jalkanen J, Sorvari T, Stenman UH, Leminen A. 2006. Preoperative serum hCGbeta as a prognostic marker in primary fallopian tube carcinoma. *Tumour Biol* 27(1):43–49.

Riska A, Leminen A. 2007. Updating on primary fallopian tube carcinoma. *Acta Obstet Gynecol Scand* 86(12):1419–1426.

Riska A, Leminen A, Pukkala E. 2003. Sociodemographic determinants of incidence of primary fallopian tube carcinoma, Finland 1953–97. *Int J Cancer* 104:643–645.

Rose P, Piver MS, Tsukada Y. 1990. Fallopian tube cancer—The Roswell Park experience. *Cancer* 66:2661–2667.

Rosen A, Klein M, Lahousen M et al. 1993. Primary carcinoma of the fallopian tube a retrospective analysis of 115 patients. Austrian Cooperative Study Group for Fallopian Tube Carcinoma. *Br J Cancer* 68:605–609.

Rosen AC, Klein M, Hafner E et al. 1999. Management and prognosis of primary fallopian tube carcinoma. Austrian Cooperative Study Group for Fallopian Tube Carcinoma. *Gynecol Obstet Invest* 47:45–51.

Sedlis A. 1961. Primary carcinoma of the fallopian tube. *Obstet Gynecol Surv* 16:209–226.

Sedlis A. 1978. Carcinoma of the fallopian tube. *Surg Clin North Am* 58:121–129.

Stühlinger M, Rosen AC, Dobianer K, Hruza C, Helmer H, Kein M, Koukal T, ReinerA, Klein M, Spona J. 1995. HER-2 oncogene is not amplified in primary carcinoma of the fallopian tube. Austrian Cooperative Study Group for Fallopian Tube Carcinoma. *Oncology* 52(5):397–399.

Suh KS, Park SW, Castro A, Patel H, Blake P, Liang M, Goy A. 2010. Ovarian cancer biomarkers for molecular biosensors and translational medicine. *Expert Rev Mol Diagn* 10(8):1069–1083.

Takashina T, Ito E, Kudo R. 1985. Cytologic diagnosis of primary tubal cancer. *Acta Cytol* 29:367–372.

Tamimi HK, Figge DC. 1981. Adenocarcinoma of the uterine tube: Potential for lymph node metastases. *Am J Obstet Gynecol* 141:132–137.

Thurnher S, Hodler J, Baer S, Marincek B, von Schulthess GK. 1990. Gadolinium-DOTA enhanced MR imaging of adnexal tumors. *J Comput Assist Tomogr* 14(6):939–949.

Timor-Tritsch IE, Rottem S. 1987. Transvaginal ultrasonographic study of the fallopian tube. *Obstet Gynecol* 70:424–428.

Tokunaga T, Miyazaki K, Matsuyama S et al. 1990. Serial measurement of CA 125 in patients with primary carcinoma of the fallopian tube. *Gynecol Oncol* 36:335–337.

Vartiainen J, Lehtovirta P, Finne P, Stenman UH, Alfthan H. 2001. Preoperative serum concentration of hCG beta as a prognostic factor in ovarian cancer. *Int J Cancer* 95:313–316.

Walsh T, Casadei S, Lee MK et al. 2011. Mutations in 12 genes for inherited ovarian, fallopian tube, and peritoneal carcinoma identified by massively parallel sequencing. *Proc Natl Acad Sci USA* 108(44):18032–18037.

Woolas RP, Smith JHF, Sarharnis P et al. 1997. Fallopian tube carcinoma: An under-recognized primary neoplasm. *Int J Gynecol Cancer* 7:284–288.

Yin BW, Lloyd KO. 2001. Molecular cloning of the CA125 ovarian cancer antigen: Identification as a new mucin, MUC16. *J Biol Chem* 276(29):27371–27375.

Zervoudis S, Peitsidis P, Iatrakis G, Panourgias E, Koureas A, Navrozoglou I, Dubois JB. 2007. Increased levels of tumor markers in the follow-up of 400 patients with breast cancer without recurrence or metastasis: Interpretation of false-positive results. *J BUON* 12(4):487–492.

Zhang S, Royer R, Li S et al. 2011. Frequencies of BRCA1 and BRCA2 mutations among 1,342 un selected patients with invasive ovarian cancer. *Gynecol Oncol* 121:353–357.

Zreik TG, Rutherford TJ. 2001. Psammoma bodies in cervico vaginal smears. *Obstet Gynecol* 97:693–695.

Section VI

Vaginal and Vulvar Cancers

17

Biomarkers for Early Detection of Vaginal Cancers

Zeynep Ocak, MD, Muradiye Acar, PhD, Mehmet Gunduz, MD, PhD, and Esra Gunduz, DMD, PhD

CONTENTS

ABSTRACT Primary carcinoma of the vagina (PCV) is a rare cancer that develops when malignant cells are formed in the vagina. The main risk factors are gynecological, reproductive, environmental, and age. Approximately 65%–95% of vaginal cancers are squamous cell carcinoma (SCC), which forms in the tissues lining the vagina. As PCV is rare, little is known about its etiology, symptoms, prognostic factors, or biological markers, and it is often detected at advanced stages. In recent years, a few studies have investigated gene and protein expression in PCV. The most recent genomic studies reported that PCV has a highly aneuploid distribution of nuclear DNA and that aggressive tumors have high proliferative activity. Proteomic studies have identified alterations and interactions of several proteins from different pathways. For example, the expression levels of some biological markers are related to tumor location, which might indicate different origins of the disease, but none of these markers can explain the variations in survival. Biological markers may also be used to diagnose vaginal cancer that has spread within the vagina and metastasized to other parts of the body or to determine whether a particular treatment is effective. This chapter focuses on recent developments in the early detection of noninvasive and invasive biomarkers related to vaginal cancer.

17.1 Introduction

The vagina is a part of the female genital system that extends from the vulva to the uterine cervix. It is lined by squamous epithelium; glandular structures are very rare (Yavagal et al., 2011). Primary carcinoma of the vagina (PCV) constitutes approximately 1%–2% of all gynecological malignancies and affects primarily postmenopausal women. Despite continuous therapeutic advances, the prognosis for PCV is still poor, with a 78% survival rate at stage I and an overall 5-year survival rate of ~53% (Hellman et al., 2012). Early detection is vital for prognosis and choice of appropriate therapy. Routine Pap smear screening can aid in the detection of PCV because vaginal and cervical cancers share similar risk factors, and it is generally accepted that these carcinomas share the same etiology, that is, HPV infection. Therefore, any suspicious area identified during a physical examination should undergo biopsy for pathological examination and diagnosis (Beller et al., 2003).

An increased biological knowledge of PCV is necessary to understand the molecular mechanisms of carcinogenesis and to identify tumor-associated markers that will facilitate definitive diagnosis, prognosis, and treatment (Hellman et al., 2012). Investigations of molecular markers of PCV are uncommon since there are few study samples and assessments lack the statistical significance necessary for use as a prognostic indicator. This chapter will focus on the biomarkers that are used or proposed for the early detection of PCV to decrease the risk and support the management of the disease at early stages.

17.1.1 Importance

Vaginal cancers remain a serious health problem. The American Cancer Society estimates that only 2680 women are diagnosed with vaginal cancer each year in the United States (Table 17.1). About 840 women will succumb, since many vaginal cancers do not cause symptoms until they reach an advanced stage (Table 17.2). Most vaginal squamous cell cancers begin as precancerous changes, called vaginal intraepithelial neoplasia (VAIN), which do not usually produce any symptoms and may not be detected during a routine

TABLE 17.1

Vaginal Cancer (C52), Number of New Cases, and Crude and European Age-Standardized (AS) Incidence Rates per 100,000 Population, United Kingdom, 2008

	England	Wales	Scotland	Northern Ireland	United Kingdom
Cases	194	19	33	12	258
Crude rate	0.7	1.2	1.2	1.3	0.8
AS rate	0.5	0.8	0.8	0.9	0.6
AS rate—95% LCL*	0.5	0.4	0.5	0.4	0.5
AS rate—95% UCL*	0.6	1.2	1.1	1.4	0.7

Source: Welsh Cancer Intelligence and Surveillance Unit, http://www.wcisu.wales.nhs.uk.
*The European age-standardised incidence rates (AS rates) do not differ significantly between the constituent countries of the UK.

TABLE 17.2

Numbers and Rates of Deaths, Cancer of the Vagina, United Kingdom, by Country, 5-Year Average, 2004–2008

	England		Wales		Scotland		Northern Ireland		United Kingdom[a]	
Number of deaths										
Females	77		7		8		2		93	
Crude rate per 100,000 population										
Females	0.30		0.43		0.30		0.20		0.30	
Age-standardized (European) rate per 100,000 female population										
Females	0.19		0.26		0.20		0.12		0.19	
95% CI[b]	0.17	0.21	0.17	0.35	0.14	0.26	0.04	0.20	0.18	0.21

Source: Welsh Cancer Intelligence and Surveillance Unit, http://www.wcisu.wales.nhs.uk.
[a] Totals may not add due to rounding.
[b] Squamous cell carcinoma in situ of the vagina is a lesion that falls within the more general category known as vaginal intraepithelial neoplasia (VAIN).

examination of the vagina. However, routine Pap testing can find some cases of VAIN and early invasive vaginal cancer (Michalas, 2000). Still, the primary goal of a Pap test is to find not vaginal cancer or VAIN but cervical precancers and early cervical cancers. Routine cytology screening is less sensitive and specific for vaginal cancers. The development of high-throughput technologies has improved the identification of molecular targets related to carcinogenesis, and these advancements will facilitate screening, early detection, management, and personalization of targeted therapy. Thus far, the use of biomarkers has not significantly increased the specificity and the sensitivity of early detection of vaginal cancer. Thus, biomarker discovery is a current challenge in clinical medicine and cytopathology.

17.1.2 Epidemiology

Squamous cell cancer of the vagina is seen mostly among older women, with almost half of cases detected in women aged 70 years or older. Only 15% of the cases are seen among women younger than 40 years of age, and the incidence of vaginal cancer increases with age (Figure 17.1). Similar to cervical cancer, the majority of vaginal cancer cases (68%) occur in developing countries but are reported primarily in developed countries (Figure 17.2).

17.1.3 Types of the Cancer

Approximately 80%–90% of PCV cases are associated with metastasis (Creasman, 2005) and 30% of PCV cases have a history of *in situ* or invasive cervical cancer. The various types of vaginal cancer detected worldwide are summarized in Table 17.3.

17.1.3.1 Squamous Cell Carcinoma

Squamous cell carcinoma (SCC) is the most common histological type of PCV (Hellman et al., 2012) and often develops slowly over many years. These cancers begin as the

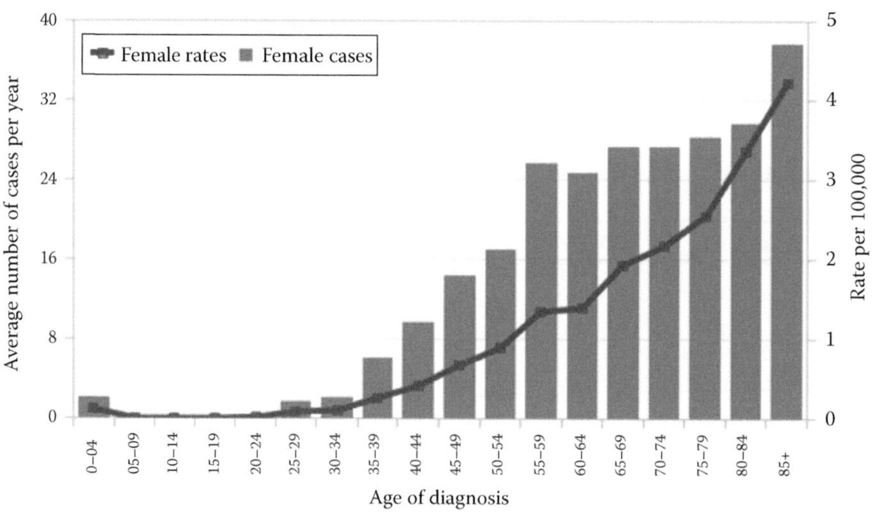

FIGURE 17.1
Vaginal cancer (C52), age-specific incidence rates, and average number of new cases per year, 2006–2008, United Kingdom.

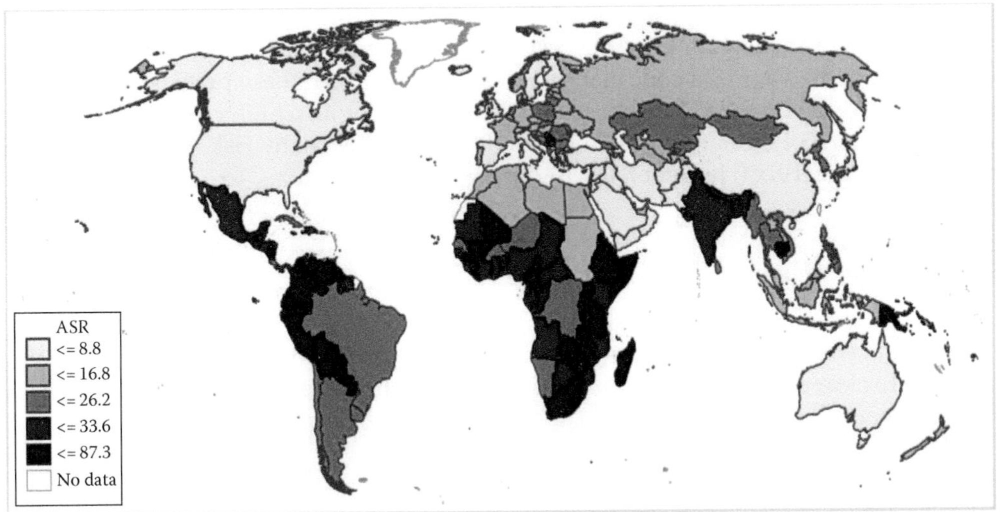

FIGURE 17.2
Age-standardized incidence rates of vaginal cancer in year 2008. ASR, age-standardized incidence rate; rates per 100,000 women per year. (From Office for National Statistics. Cancer Statistics: Registrations Series MB1, http://www.ons.gov.uk/ons/search/index.html?newquery=series+mb1.)

TABLE 17.3

Cancer of Vagina: Number and Distribution of Cases and 5-Year Relative Survival by Histology, Age 20+, 12 SEER Areas, 1988–2001

Histology	ICD-O Code	Cases	Percent	Five Year Relative Survival Rate (%)
Total	8000–9989	1041	100.0	49.4
Squamous	8050–8130	705	67.7	53.6
Squamous, NOS[a]	8070	530	50.9	52.4
All other squamous	8050–8069, 8071–8130	175	16.8	56.8
Adenocarcinoma	8140–8147, 8160–8162, 8180–8221, 8250–8506, 8520–8550, 8560, 8570–8573, 8940–8941	172	16.5	59.0
Clear cell	8310	20	1.9	b
All other adenocarcinomas	8140–8147, 8160–8162, 8180–8221, 8250–8309, 8311–8506, 8520–8550, 8560, 8570–8573, 8940–8941	152	14.6	58.5
Other specified carcinomas	8030–8045, 8150–8155, 8170–8171, 8230–8248, 8510–8512, 8561–8562, 8580–8671	13	1.2	b
Carcinoma, NOS[a]	8010–8022	40	3.8	32.9
Other specified types	8720–8790, 8935, 8950–8979, 8982, 9000–9030, 9060–9110, 9350–9364, 9380–9512, 9530–9539	106	10.2	16.9
Melanoma	8720–8790	92	8.8	13.3
All other specified types	8935, 8950–8979, 8982, 9000–9030, 9060–9110, 9350–9364, 9380–9512, 9530–9539	14	1.3	b
Unspecified	8000–8004	5	0.5	b

Source: Ries, L.A.G. et al., SEER Survival Monograph: *Cancer Survival Among Adults: U.S. SEER Program, 1988–2001, Patient and Tumor Characteristics*. National Cancer Institute, SEER Program, NIH Pub. No. 07-6215, Bethesda, MD, 2007.

[a] NOS, not otherwise specified.

[b] Statistic not displayed due to less than 25 cases.

squamous cells that form the epithelial lining of the vagina and are commonly seen in the upper part of the vagina near the cervix. Precancerous changes occur in some of the normal cells of the vagina, a condition known as VAIN. Later, these precancer cells transform into cancerous cells. SCC of the vagina is associated with a high rate of infection with oncogenic strains of human papillomavirus (HPV) and has many risk factors in common with SCC of the cervix (Hacker et al., 2012).

17.1.3.2 Adenocarcinoma

Adenocarcinomas account for ~10% of vaginal cancers in women over 50 years of age, with a 5-year survival rate of 60%. Young women exposed to diethylstilbestrol (DES) *in utero* are prone to clear cell adenocarcinoma. HPV infection has also been described in a case of vaginal adenocarcinoma (Hacker et al., 2012).

17.1.3.3 Melanoma

Melanomas account for ~10% of vaginal cancers and tend to affect the lower or outer portion of the vagina. The tumors vary in size, color, and growth patterns and are often deeply invasive. Radical surgery, often involving some type of pelvic exenteration, is the primary treatment; however, the overall 5-year survival rate is only 10% (Hacker et al., 2012).

17.1.3.4 Sarcoma

Sarcomas account for ~4% of vaginal cancers. These cancers do not form on the surface of the vagina but deep in the vaginal wall. The most common type of vaginal sarcoma is rhabdomyosarcoma, which is hardly ever seen in adults and is more common among children. Leiomyosarcoma is more often seen in adults and tends to occur in women older than 50 years of age. Survival rates of these types of vaginal cancers are significantly improved by conservative surgery in conjunction with preoperative or postoperative chemotherapy and radiotherapy (Hacker et al., 2012).

17.1.4 Current Methods for Early Diagnosis, Prognosis, and Therapy with Specificity, Sensitivity, Advantages, and Disadvantages

17.1.4.1 Early Diagnosis

The vagina should be examined during routine cervical screening for precancerous conditions such as VAIN. Either conventional cytology or liquid-based cytology can then be used for analysis (Hacker et al., 2012). With conventional cytology, the sample is smeared directly onto a glass microscope slide and sent to the laboratory. Despite the drawbacks, this method is efficient and relatively inexpensive. With liquid-based cytology, a cell sample is added directly into a special preservative liquid for analysis. When abnormalities are observed on a Pap test, the cervix, vagina, and vulva can be examined with a specialized instrument known as a colposcope (Wentzensen et al., 2009). A biopsy is necessary if an area of abnormality is seen on the cervix or vagina.

17.1.4.2 Prognosis

Patient prognosis depends primarily on the stage of the disease. Women older than 60 years of age who are symptomatic at the time of diagnosis with lesions of the middle and lower third of the vagina or who have poorly differentiated tumors have a lower chance of survival (Figure 17.3). In addition, the extent of vaginal wall involvement and the stage of the disease in vaginal SCC patients are associated with survival (Hacker et al., 2012).

As soon as it is diagnosed, vaginal cancer can be staged by clinical examination of the patient. Guidelines from the International Federation of Gynecology and Obstetrics (FIGO) form the basis for the current system of vaginal cancer staging combined with the American Joint Committee on Cancer (AJCC) TNM system (Table 17.4).

Combination strategies that include surgery, chemotherapy, and radiation treatment can prolong survival but is often too late to prevent death. A detailed description of vaginal cancer stages is provided in Table 17.5.

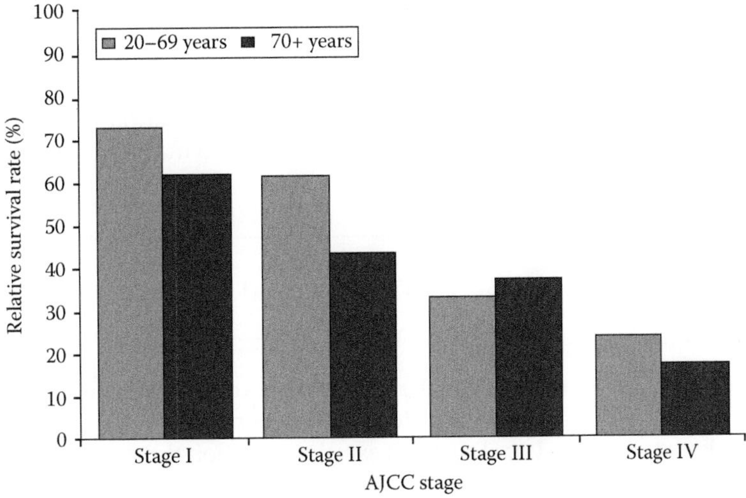

FIGURE 17.3
Cancer of vagina: 5-year relative survival rate (%) by age (20+) and stage (SEER modified AJCC, 3rd edition), 12 SEER areas, 1998–2001.

TABLE 17.4
Carcinoma of the Vagina: FIGO Nomenclature

Stage 0	Carcinoma *in situ*; intraepithelial neoplasia Grade III.
Stage I	The carcinoma is limited to the vaginal wall and if detected.
Stage II	The carcinoma has involved the subvaginal tissue but has not extended to the pelvic wall.
Stage III	The carcinoma has extended to the pelvic wall.
Stage IV	The carcinoma has extended beyond the true pelvis or has involved the mucosa of the bladder or rectum; bullous edema as such does not permit a case to be allotted to stage IV. IVa tumor invades bladder and/or rectal mucosa and/or direct extension beyond the true pelvis. IVb Spread to distant organs.

Sources: Hacker, N. et al., *Int. J. Gynecol. Obstet.*, 119, S97, 2012; Kosary, C.L., Cancer of the vagina, in *SEER Survival Monograph*, Chapter 19.

TABLE 17.5

Clinical Stages of Vaginal Carcinoma according to American Joint Committee on Cancer (AJCC) with 5-year Survival Rate

Stage	Description	Five Years Survival Rate (%)
I	Vaginal cancer is defined as tumor confined to vagina with no lymph node metastases.	85
II	Vaginal cancer is defined as tumor that invades paravaginal tissues but not to pelvic wall with no lymph node metastases.	78
III	Vaginal cancer is defined as tumor extending to pelvic wall or either tumor confined to the vagina or tumor with lymph node metastases invading paravaginal tissues.	58
IV	Vaginal cancer is defined as either tumor invasion of the mucosa of the bladder or rectum or extension beyond the true pelvis.	58

Source: Kosary, C.L., Cancer of the vagina, in *SEER Survival Monograph*, Chapter 19.

17.1.4.3 Therapies

All treatment must be individualized and will vary depending on the stage of disease and the site of vaginal involvement. Invasive vaginal cancer is treated primarily with radiation therapy and surgery. Chemotherapy in combination with radiation may be used to treat advanced disease. For most patients, it is important to try to maintain vaginal function.

17.2 Treatment Strategy, Targeted Therapy, and Pharmacogenomics

17.2.1 Treatment Strategy

There are several treatment options for the preinvasive and invasive lesions of the vagina. Different treatment methods can be used for VAIN depending on individual patient characteristics (Hacker et al., 2012). Local surgical excision, ablation through intracavitary radiotherapy, and laser vaporization with carbon dioxide laser can be used. 5-fluorouracil (5-FU) can be used in patients with a widespread multifocal disease (Krebs, 1986). Alternatively, multifocal VAIN 2/3 in HPV-positive young women can be treated by imiquimod 5% cream. Total vaginectomy with split-thickness skin grafting may be necessary in extensive lesions of the vagina (Haidopoulos et al., 2005).

In invasive cancer of the vagina, treatment varies according to the stage of the disease and site of vaginal involvement. Surgery has a role in only a certain group of patients. In invasive stage I carcinoma of the upper posterior vagina, radical hysterectomy, upper vaginectomy, and pelvic lymphadenectomy may be performed. In hysterectomized patients, radical upper vaginectomy and pelvic lymphadenectomy may be performed. Surgery may also be used in young patients with the aim of ovarian transposition before radiotherapy, for primary pelvic exenteration in advanced stage disease (IVA), and for bilateral groin dissection in such patients if the lesion involves the lower third of the vagina and for exenteration in patients with central recurrence after radiotherapy (Dalrymple et al., 2004; Hacker et al., 2012). Most of the patients with vaginal cancer is a candidate for radiation therapy that is performed as teletherapy and intracavitary/interstitial brachytherapy. Concurrent use of cisplatin-based chemoradiation may be thought in locally advanced cases, but there is limited experience with this mode of treatment in the management of PCV (Hacker et al., 2012).

17.2.2 Targeted Therapy and Pharmacogenomics

Personalized medicine tailors a patient's treatment strategy to their unique genetic makeup. In oncology, personalized medicine is being used in combination with pharmacogenomics, which is the study of how interindividual genetic variation determines drug response or toxicity (Gossage and Madhusudan, 2007). Pharmacogenomic attempts to facilitate physician decision making regarding optimal drug selection, dose, and treatment duration on a patient-by-patient basis. Recent advances in genome-wide genotyping and sequencing technologies have identified a number of pharmacogenetic markers that can predict the response to chemotherapy. However, effectively implementing these pharmacogenetic markers in the clinic remains a major challenge.

So far, pharmacogenetic tests have not been routinely performed for drugs used in the treatment of vaginal cancer.

17.3 Invasive and Noninvasive Markers: Advantages and Disadvantages

Molecular biomarkers are distinct biochemical indicators of normal biological or pathogenic processes or pharmacological responses to a therapeutic intervention. A biomarker might be a molecule secreted by a tumor or may also be a specific response of the body to the presence of cancer. It is possible to categorize biomarkers as invasive or noninvasive based on the sampling technique. Noninvasive biomarkers can easily be obtained from bodily fluids such as serum, urine, or saliva, while invasive biomarkers require sophisticated invasive interventions. The specificity and sensitivity of invasive biomarkers are high, but invasive intervention in the body may result in side effects such as anxiety and discomfort, prolonged recovery time, and high follow-up costs (Schönhofer, 2006; Schönhofer et al., 2008). In contrast, noninvasive biomarkers reduce anxiety and discomfort and increase accessibility for clinical tests. But so far, specific noninvasive technique has not been identified that can be used routinely for the diagnosis of vaginal cancer.

17.4 Noninvasive Molecular Biomarkers

Proteins or enzymes produced and released either by tumor cells or by host cells and whose presence may be detected in the serum or other biological fluids (Sharma, 2009) are termed noninvasive tumor biomarkers. A number of such markers have recently been assayed noninvasively in collected biofluids. However, biomarkers are not highly sensitive and specific for vaginal cancer detection and identifying a reliable marker remains a major challenge. Thus, attempts to identify new prognostic indicators and tumor markers for vaginal cancer are ongoing. Platforms for the discovery of novel biomarkers using integrated genomic, transcriptomic, proteomic, and epigenomic approaches are now available. These techniques will contribute to the early detection and diagnosis of vaginal cancer and allow oncologists to delineate patients who need aggressive adjuvant, neoadjuvant, or combination therapy.

17.4.1 Serum Biomarkers

Synthesis of free βhCG and its subunits has also been reported in some pelvic carcinomas such as colon, urinary tract, prostate, uterus, and vulvovaginal carcinomas.

17.4.2 Genetic Biomarkers

Alterations in genes, such as oncogenes and tumor suppressors genes that regulate cell proliferation, survival, and other homeostasis functions, initiate a specific disease called carcinogenesis. Genetic gain and loss, for example, change in gene dosage, is predominantly responsible for oncogenic transformation. Early diagnosis and improved therapeutics may be possible by identifying these defects.

17.4.2.1 Cytogenetic Biomarkers (DNA, RNA, miRNA, Antibody, Autoantigen, etc.)

Newer cytogenetic techniques have the potential to provide improved diagnostic and prognostic means. In several tumors, cytogenetic evidence is critical for understanding the neoplasia process and for the development of new therapeutic modalities. Based on chromosome banding techniques, only a few karyotypes with nonrecurrent chromosome abnormalities have been reported in PCV. Although chromosomal rearrangements and different DNA aneuploidies such as trisomy of chromosome 8 and duplication of the long arm of chromosome 1 can be observed in PCV, the association of these abnormalities with the clinicopathological variables is not known (Jens et al., 2004; Manor et al., 2009).

17.4.2.2 Copy Number Variations

The most frequent copy number changes in vaginal carcinomas were mapped to chromosome arms 3q and 5p. In a study, the pattern of genomic alterations in PCV was analyzed using comparative genomic hybridization, and it was found that 70% of vaginal carcinomas carry relative copy number increases that map to chromosome arm 3q (Habermann et al., 2004). This pattern of genomic alteration in PCV was salient similar to the one observed in cervical carcinomas (Heselmeyer et al., 1996), which further strengthened the hypothesis of related etiological pathways.

17.5 Invasive Molecular Biomarkers

17.5.1 Proteomic Biomarkers

In recent years, a few studies have been carried out to investigate gene and protein expressions in vaginal carcinoma. The first study investigated protein expression profiles using 2D polyacrylamide gel electrophoresis (2-DE) in PCV compared with cervical carcinoma. Correlation analysis revealed highly correlated similarities between the tissue specimens. Vaginal and cervical carcinomas demonstrated a few constitutional similarities in their protein expression patterns, which could indicate a similarity of the etiology of the two conditions (Hellman et al., 2004).

The second study examined expression profiles of three proteins (DEAD box, erbB3-binding protein, and biliverdin reductase [BVR]) using 2-DE and matrix-assisted laser desorption/ionization-time of flight mass spectrometry (MALDI-TOF-MS) in PCV compared with cervical carcinoma (Hellman et al., 2009). These proteins were uniquely altered in PCV (Hartwell et al., 2006; Kim et al., 2010).

Another study investigated the prognostic value of DNA content and biological markers for cell cycle regulation and invasion in PCV. According to the study, most of the PCV patients showed no overexpression of p53 and high expression of p21, cyclin A, and Ki67. Loss or underexpression of E-cadherin was found in 94% (68/72) of PCV patients, and all patients showed immunopositivity for the laminin-5F2 chain (Hellman et al., 2012). The expression level of some markers was related to tumor location, which might be indicative of different genesis. Overexpression of p53 was associated with short-term survival, but the only independent predictors of survival were age at diagnosis and tumor size (Hellman et al., 2012).

17.5.1.1 DEAD-Box Protein

DEAD-box proteins are the major family of superfamily 2 (SF2) helicases, which covers all aspects of RNA metabolism, including translation, transcription, and splicing (Abdelhaleem, 2004; Cordin et al., 2006). DEAD-box proteins are accepted to take part in the overlapping of RNA by destabilizing RNA secondary or tertiary structures. Members of this family are believed to be involved in different biological activities such as cellular growth and division depending on their distribution patterns. Furthermore, p21waf1/cip1 transcription independent from p53 may be regulated by these proteins, and based on this effect, it may be a tumor suppressor gene (Chao et al., 2006). The DEAD-box protein 48 was identified on a duty in vaginal carcinoma. On the other hand, it was also discovered in pancreatic cancer and has been proposed as a potential serum marker with a comprehensive study (Xia et al., 2005).

17.5.1.2 ErbB3-Binding Protein

The ErbB3-binding protein 1 (Ebp1) has been implicated in a number of human cancers. Ebp1 is an important member of the family of proliferation-associated 2G4 proteins (PA2G4s) and has a significant role in proliferation, cellular growth, and differentiation. It triggers activation of the transmembrane receptor erbB3 (Kowalinski et al., 2007), which initiates the Ras pathway. The Ras–Raf–MEK pathway is the major downstream signaling pathway that emanates from all EGFR complexes. The EGFR signaling system incorporates the four transmembrane proteins erbB1–erbB4, with intracellular tyrosine domains and extracellular ligand-binding domains. In vaginal cancer, the erbB3-binding protein was found to be modified, demonstrating involvement of the Ras pathway (Hellman et al., 2009). In another study, it was found that ebp1 expression was decreased in clinical prostate cancer and that increased expression of EBP1 in hormone-refractory cells led to an amelioration of the androgen-independent phenotype because ebp1 overexpression resulted in downregulation of the androgen receptor (Zhang et al., 2005).

17.5.1.3 Biliverdin Reductase

Biliverdin (BV) has emerged as a cytoprotective and important anti-inflammatory molecule. BVR is a serine/threonine/tyrosine kinase that catalyzes reduction of BV to bilirubin (Wegiel and Otterbein, 2012). There are two isoforms of BVR. The first one is BVR-A, which catalyzes conversion of BV-a specifically. It is expressed in the majority of adult tissues and is inducible with stress. The second one is BVR-B, which is present during embryogenesis and is an isoform specific for the BV-d and b isomers. In BVR-A and BVR-B, entirely BVR has been shown to preclude cellular agedness (Kim et al., 2011) and apoptosis (Jansen and Daiber, 2012). BVR consists of zinc metalloprotein and variables that are responsible from protecting the cell from oxidative damages (Baranano et al., 2002; Lerner- Marmarosh et al., 2005). Moreover, increases in BVR expression have been detected in renal cell carcinoma (Maines et al., 1999) and hepatocellular carcinoma (Melle et al., 2007).

17.5.1.4 p53

The p53 protein is an important tumor suppressor because of its ability to produce apoptosis in the tumor cells. This protein can arrest the cell cycle, and it allows cell repair before the beginning of replication. The p53 protein also has an important role in the embryonic development of vertebrates by maintaining the proliferation and apoptosis of the cells (Levine et al., 2004; Pintusa et al., 2007). The expression of p53 in PCV has been investigated in only a few studies, and overexpression was found in 12%–50% of PCV. However, no significant association between the p53 alteration and survival has so far been observed in PCV. Overexpression of p53 was related to short-term survival rates, but the only independent predictors of survival were age at diagnosis and tumor size (Hellman et al., 2012).

17.5.1.5 p21

The p21 protein is a potential cyclin-dependent kinase inhibitor; it is also known as p21WAF1/Cip1 and responsible for controlling the response of cell cycle to various stimuli both by p53-dependent and p53-independent mechanisms. The location of p53-activated fragment (WAF1) gene is on human chromosome 6p21 and encodes a 21 kDa protein (p21) that helped to identify through reductive hybridization screening for transcriptional targets of the p53 tumor suppressor protein. The WAF1 gene contains several p53 response elements in its body. So, the activation of p53 induces p21 protein expression and affects the G1 in response to DNA damage (Warfel and El-Deiry, 2013). Besides, to its regulation by the classical p53 pathway, p21 expression is also adjusted at the transcriptional level of oncogenes and tumor suppressor proteins that induce p21 expression by binding of different transcription factors to specific elements placed in the p21 promoter. Thus, p21 might also act as an oncogene and promote cell proliferation. p21 is overexpressed in PCV, prostate, breast, and cervical cancers, among others, and in many instances, it has also been associated with poor prognosis. High p21 expression can cause antiapoptotic and mitogenic activity that may contribute to the pathogenesis of cancer (Hellman et al., 2012).

17.5.1.6 Cyclin A and Ki67

Cyclin A is normally expressed from late G1 to late G2 phases. Cyclin A complex has substrates in both the nucleus and the cytoplasm. These substrates shuttle between the two compartments. The Ki67 antibody was originally identified as a reliable marker for a nuclear antigen present in proliferating cells, from late G1 to M phase, and is therefore approved as a ubiquitous proliferation marker (He et al., 2011). The roles of cyclin A and Ki67 in the proliferative activity of PCV have been studied in two reports. High expressions of cyclin A and Ki67 were detected in most of PCV patients (71% and 83%, respectively). In a study, a high expression of cyclin A and Ki67 was found in PCV, but no association with survival was observed (Hellman et al., 2012). On the contrary, according to other studies, the expressions of cyclin A and Ki67 have repeatedly been proven to be of prognostic value for survival and recurrence in several other tumors (e.g., breast, colon, rectal, and anal cancer) (Aamodt et al., 2009; Nilsson et al., 2006).

17.5.1.7 E-Cadherin

In several studies, PCV showed loss of E-cadherin expression, suggesting that it is an aggressive malignancy with poor prognosis. The suppression of E-cadherin is central in epithelial–mesenchymal transition and is regulated by various intracellular signaling pathways activated by multiple extracellular signals as well as some other factors (Beavon, 2000). Growth factors, Wnt, and estrogens are the most known multiple extracellular signals. There is also growing evidence of a strong connection between estrogen signaling and E-cadherin expression (Hellman et al., 2012). In this study, a remarkable downregulation was observed in E-cadherin expression in all PCV cases. Disturbances in the E-cadherin-mediated signaling pathways and in the control of E-cadherin-mediated cell adhesion also seem to be important in vaginal tumorigenesis.

17.5.1.8 Laminin-5F2 Chain

The laminin-5F2 chain, an important component of the epithelial basement membranes, plays an important role in the adhesion of cells to the basement membrane and in cell migration (Lundgren et al., 2003). The laminin-5F2 chain has seen by expressing on cytoplasm of migrating keratinocytes and metalloproteinase-2, which is a specific cleavage of laminin-5F2 responsible for cell migration during tumor invasion and tissue remodelling. Depending upon these reasons, lots of cancer types such as pancreatic, gastric, colorectal, and gallbladder cancers arose (Masuda et al., 2012). Its increased expression has been correlated with a more aggressive tumor behavior and with a worse prognosis. But, in another study, the expression level of laminin-5F2 chain was found to have no correlation with survival (Hellman et al., 2012).

17.5.2 Human Papillomavirus

HPV is a very common cause of genital infection, of which at least 40 types are known (Figure 17.4). HPV infects the mucosal areas of the vulva, vagina, cervix, and anus. While HPV is necessary for the development of genital cancer, it is not in itself sufficient; other cofactors are necessary for progression from cervical HPV infection to cancer. Tobacco smoking, parity, oral contraceptive use, and coinfection with HIV have been identified as established cofactors. HPV DNA is detected among 91% of invasive vaginal carcinomas and 82% of high-grade vaginal neoplasias (VAIN3) (Table 17.6). HPV 16 and 18 account for >70% of vaginal cancers (De Vuyst et al., 2009). A few studies have investigated the role of HPV in the prognosis of patients treated for PCV (Ikenberg et al., 1994) (Table 17.7). All of these studies suggest that women with HPV-positive tumors have increased overall survival. Thus, HPV detection might be considered a valuable prognostic biomarker in patients with PCV. HPV-positive early-stage (FIGO I and II) PCV has a better prognosis than early HPV-negative tumors (Immaculada et al., 2012). The introduction of HPV vaccination may also reduce the burden of vaginal and cervical cancers in the coming decades. HPV vaccination has been widely used all over the world (Brunner et al., 2011; Ikenberg et al., 1994) (Figure 17.5).

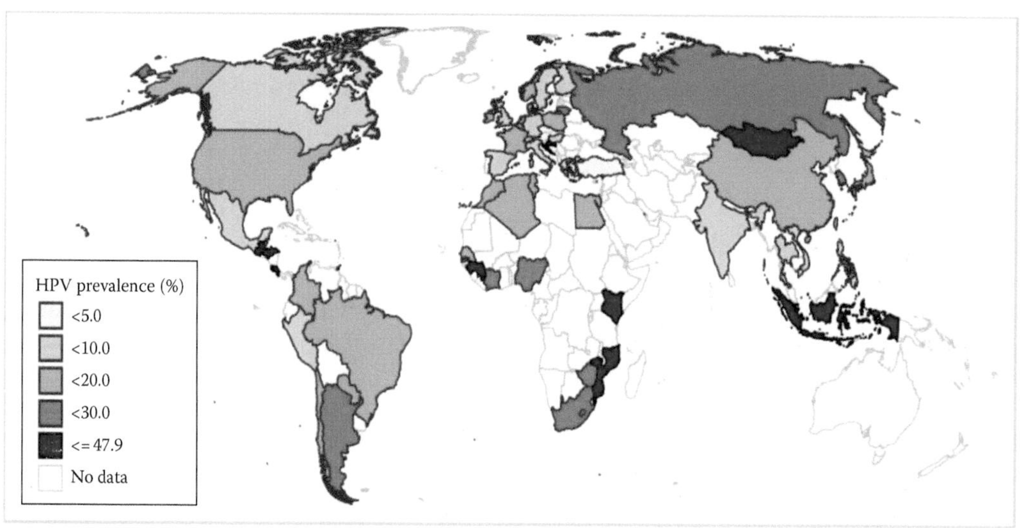

FIGURE 17.4
World prevalence of HPV among women with normal cytology.

TABLE 17.6
Proteomic Markers Studied in Vaginal Cancer

Gene Symbol	Gene Name	Function	Chromosome Location	Detection	Reference
DDX53	DEAD (Asp-Glu-Ala-Asp) box polypeptide 53	Cell-cycle arrest	Xp22.13	2-DE	Cordin et al. (2006)
TP53	Tumor protein p53	Tumor suppressor	17p13.1	Immunostaining	Levine et al. (2004)
CDKN1A	Cyclin-dependent kinase inhibitor, p21	Promotes cell cycle arrest	6p21.2	Immunostaining	Warfel and El-Deiry (2013)
CCNA2	Cyclin A	Cellular proliferation	4q27	Immunostaining	Nilsson et al. (2006)
MKI67	Antigen identified by monoclonal antibody Ki-67	Cellular proliferation	10q26.2	Immunostaining	Scholzen et al. (2000)
LAMA5	Laminin, alpha 5, laminin-5F2 chain	Adhesion of cells to the basement membrane	20q13.2–q13.3	Immunostaining	Masuda et al. (2012)
PA2G4	Proliferation-associated 2G4, 38kDa, erbB3-binding protein	Cellular growth and differentiation	12q13.2	Immunostaining 2-DE	Kowalinski et al. (2007)
BLVRA	Biliverdin reductase	Catalyze the conversion of biliverdin to bilirubin	7p13	2-DE	Wegiel and Otterbein (2012)
CDH1	Cadherin 1, type 1, E-cadherin (epithelial)	Cell–cell signaling	16q22.1	Immunostaining	Abudukadeer et al. (2012)

Sources: Hellman, K. et al., *Int. J. Gynecol. Cancer,* 2012.

TABLE 17.7

Studies on HPV Prevalence among Cases of Vaginal Cancer in the World

Study	HPV Detection Method	Histology	No Tested	HPV Prevalence % (95% CI)
Ferreira (2008, Portugal)	INNO-LiPA	SCC	21	80.9 (58.1–94.6)
Madsen (2008, Denmark)	GP5+/6+ PCR-EIA assay and type specific for HPV 16, 18, 31,33, 35, 39, 45, 51, 52, 56, 58, 59, 66, and 68 and other 23 low-risk HPV	SCC	27	88.9 (70.9–97.7)
Habermann et al. (2004, Sweden)	PGMY09/11.	SCC	8	25.0 (3.2–65.1)
Koyamatsu (2003, Japan)	E7 (115–158 bp) for HPV 16, HPV 18, L1 (250 bp) for HPV 6,11,16,18,31,33,42,52,58	SCC	16	43.8 (19.8–70.1)
Daling (2002, United States of America)	MY09/11 for 6/11, 16, 18/45, 31	SCC	25	64.0 (42.5–82.0)
Carter (2001, United States of America)	MY09/11 and RFLP; type specific for 16, 18.	SCC	54	90.7 (79.7–96.9)
Waggoner (1994, United States of America)	L1 primers and E6/E/7	Adenocarcinoma	7	28.6 (3.7–71.0)
Kiyabu (1989, United States of America)	E6 for HPV 16 and HPV 18.	SCC	14	64.3 (35.1–87.2)

Source: IARC, Globocan 2002 | WHO GBD 2004 (for WHO region estimates only).

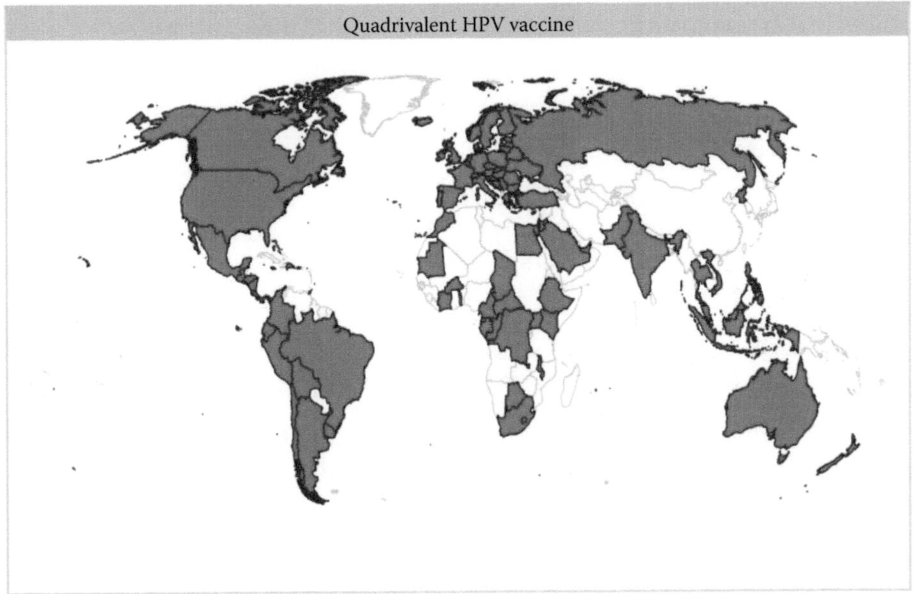

FIGURE 17.5
Global HPV vaccine licensure as of March 2009.

Two vaccines against the most common type of HPV infection that causes vaginal and cervical cancers are available. Gardasil is recommended for use in females 9–26 years of age, and Cervarix is recommended in females 9–25 years of age. Gardasil is also approved for use in males 9–26 years of age to prevent anal cancer and associated precancerous lesions since ~90% of anal cancers are linked to HPV infection. These vaccines cannot protect against established infections, nor do they protect against all HPV types.

17.6 Imaging Biomarkers

Imaging makers are being routinely utilized for the diagnosis of vaginal cancer of various stages. Several types of imaging markers are available.

17.6.1 Computed Tomography

The size, shape, and position of a tumor, along with the area to which the cancer has spread, can be determined by a computed tomography (CT) scan. It is also possible to identify enlarged lymph nodes that might contain cancer cells (American Cancer Society, 2012).

17.6.2 Magnetic Resonance Imaging

Magnetic resonance imaging (MRI) images are especially effective for examination of pelvic tumors. This technique allows detection of enlarged lymph nodes in the groin and cancer that has spread to the brain or spinal cord (American Cancer Society, 2012). However, in vaginal cancer, the situation is different for it rarely occurs in this case.

17.6.3 Positron Emission Tomography

Positron emission tomography (PET) uses radiolabeled glucose, which tends to concentrate more in cancerous cells than in normal tissues. Although PET scans can be used to identify areas to which the cancer has spread, they are often not helpful in vaginal cancer cases (American Cancer Society, 2012).

17.6.4 Endoscopic Tests

These tests are commonly used for the evaluation of vaginal cancer (American Cancer Society, 2012).

17.6.5 Proctosigmoidoscopy

Proctosigmoidoscopy focuses on the rectum and part of the colon. This procedure might be advisable for patients whose vaginal cancers are large and/or located in the part of the vagina next to the rectum and colon (American Cancer Society, 2012).

17.6.6 Cystoscopy

A cystoscopy is used to check for the spread of vaginal cancer to the bladder when a vaginal cancer is large and/or located in the front wall of the vagina near the bladder (American Cancer Society, 2012).

17.6.7 Lymphangiogram

A lymphangiogram is used to x-ray the lymph system and determine whether the cancer has spread to the lymph nodes. With this procedure, a dye is injected into the lymph vessels in the feet and travels upward through the lymph nodes and lymph vessels. X-rays are taken to identify blockages (American Cancer Society, 2012, Vaginal cancer).

17.7 Integrative Omics-Based Molecular Markers for Early Diagnosis

Omics techniques, like MS and arrays, have aided in the identification, measurement and quantification of DNA, messenger RNAs, and proteins derived from the body (Morel et al., 2004). Laboratory-based, high-throughput omics studies are generating promising results and translational application of these could benefit cancer patients by facilitating early diagnosis and appropriate therapies. However, the cost per sample for commercial use is still not economically feasible. The next-generation sequencing alone or coupled with other techniques has been beneficial in defining the genetic signatures of specific cancers and discovering specific biomarkers that could be used for early cancer diagnosis and target-based therapies (Bhati et al., 2012).

17.8 Recommended Tests for Early Diagnosis

There is currently no sufficiently accurate screening test proven to be effective for the early detection of vaginal cancer because it is such a rare condition. However, during routine cervical screening, the vagina should be examined. These tests can detect precancerous conditions such as VAIN. Women with a history of cervical intraepithelial or invasive neoplasia are at increased risk, but regular cytological screening gives a low yield. The incorporation of newer testing modalities, including HPV testing, may allow the screening interval to be increased, and cost-effective screening, in this group of patients (Hacker et al., 2012). Three 2D electrophoresis studies of vaginal carcinoma reported over 120 proteins that were *different* in squamous cervical cancer tissues (Alonso et al., 2012; Bae et al., 2005; Hellman et al., 2004; Zhu et al., 2009). However, no biomarker panels emerged from these data sets. Many of the proteomic techniques are still not sufficiently sensitive and specific to identify all proteins from a complex biological sample, like serum or plasma. Thus, clinical proteomics technology must focus on increasing the sensitivity, reproducibility, and specificity of novel biomarker detection (Tacu et al., 2010). Vaginal cancer and cervical cancer are relatively homogeneous in terms of their protein expression and so the biomarkers indicative of their presence may be similar or identical.

17.9 Advantages and Challenges in Developing Molecular Biomarkers for Early Detection

Biomarkers are increasingly commonly used during routine patient management as part of appropriate diagnostic tests. The aims of diagnostic tests are to identify patients at the earliest cancer stage possible; to avoid false positives, psychological stress, and unnecessary treatments; and finally, to minimize the cost. The use of biomarker-based diagnostics for cancer includes risk assessment, disease stratification and prognosis, noninvasive screening for early-stage disease, detection and localization, response to therapy, and for those in remission, screening for disease recurrence. No test is perfect, and sensitivity, specificity, and cost become trade-offs when applying diagnostics to disease management. Combining multiple biomarkers can minimize the risks. For instance, one might combine a biomarker with high sensitivity and low specificity, which would determine potentially lethal cancers but could result in many false positives, with a second biomarker with lower sensitivity but higher specificity. When defining and targeting a population with an increased cancer incidence, screening tests will result in a higher positive predictive value and result in a higher pretest rate. Improving the sensitivity of a screening test to >90%–95% will reduce diagnostic time and provide a sharp decrease in the cost per case detected by $230,000 when screening women aged 50–54 years for diseases such as ovarian cancer (~30 cases/100,000).

17.10 Commercially Available Molecular Biomarkers for Early Diagnosis, Prognosis, and Therapy

Early detection and appropriate therapeutic measures have decreased the vaginal cancer mortality rate. The conventional Pap test is widely used globally, and a variety of liquid-based cytology techniques have increased its sensitivity and specificity and decreased the false-positive rate. ThinPrep® and SurePath™ are approved by the FDA for use in the United States and are the most widely used methods worldwide. The manufacturer of ThinPrep (Cytyc Corporation, Boxborough, MA) and Becton Dickinson and Company have now acquired SurePath from TriPath Imaging Inc.

Current tests for HPV are DNA based, detecting the viral genome in vaginal cells. AMPLICOR HPV, the LINEAR ARRAY HPV Genotyping, the PapilloCheck, and the INNO-LiPA HPV are commercially available elsewhere in the world but have not been approved in the United States. The FDA has approved three HPV tests. These are the APTIMA® HPV assay (Gen-Probe, San Diego, Calif, United States), the Cervista HPV HR (high risk) (Hologic, Bedford, Mass, United States), and the Hybrid Capture 2 (hc2) test (Qiagen, Valencia, Calif, United States). Abbott and Roche Laboratories Inc., among others, have invested in the development of a nucleic-acid-based HPV test. The Cervista HPV 16/18 test (Hologic, Bedford, Mass, United States) and cobas 4800 HPV tests (Roche Molecular Systems) are approved by the FDA for HPV genotyping. NorChip AS (Klokkarstua Norway) has developed an mRNA-based HPV test known as PreTect HPV-Proofer (Ratner, 2011). Quest Diagnostics (NYSE: DGX), the leading provider of diagnostic testing, has introduced a new laboratory assay, the telomerase RNA component (*TERC*) test (Andersson et al., 2009). In younger women, HPV infection is often transient and overtreatment of these women is a serious problem. *TERC* is a powerful marker that discerns histologically confirmed low-grade from high-grade cervical disease. In the future, one could envision a screening strategy in which

HPV-positive Pap smears are triaged with the help of the *TERC* marker to contribute to greater evidence-based individualized clinical management (Andersson et al., 2009).

Recently, Guided Therapeutics, Inc. developed the LightTouch™ noninvasive diagnostic device for SCC cancer detection. Unlike the Pap test and HPV testing, which require a tissue sample, LightTouch is a fast, painless test that significantly improves early detection of cervical precancerous and cancers, independent of the sample type (Vlaicu, 2009).

Proteomics technology, such as MS, 2DGE protein array, and MS imagery, has been recently used for biomarker discovery in cancer. MS, such as by surface-enhanced laser desorption/ionization-TOF (SELDI-TOF) and MALDI-TOF, represents an advantageous high-throughput approach (Conrads et al., 2003).

In the basic approach, *integral* protein complexes from tissue or body fluids may be resolved by TOF-MS with high reproducibility and accuracy. In several patents, the ProteinChip® high-throughput protein expression technology coupled with SELDI-TOF-MS is described as being able to determine the protein profiles of biological samples known to be extremely complex.

17.11 Conclusion

In the last 5 years, over 200 papers describing cancer biomarker panels have been published; 20% of these claim that the identified biomarkers can be used for early diagnosis. In 2010, 30% of the published literature focused on early diagnosis of cancer, which emphasizes the importance of biomarker discovery to cancer research. The biomolecular pathways of HPV-induced carcinogenesis are well understood and are proving beneficial for the early detection of vaginal cancer. Despite this, advances in screening methods are urgently needed to provide an efficient, cost-effective screening tool to identify women at risk of HPV-associated malignancies. The recent introduction of FDA-approved prophylactic HPV vaccines will eventually reduce the incidence of gynecological cancers; however, it will be a few years before this benefit is realized.

Genome-wide scanning will assist in identifying a novel panel of candidate genes for cancer screening in the near future. The use of noninvasive imaging techniques for the early detection of precancerous conditions is also a rapidly developing area. Additionally, a number of new proteomics technologies and strategies exist that have not yet been widely applied to reproductive disease research. Nevertheless, good progress is being made, and rapidly emerging technologies for protein detection, coupled with prefractionation techniques and developments in bioinformatics, are now enabling a deeper understanding of the proteome of tissues and biological fluids.

The combination of Pap tests, HPV detection, noninvasive imaging, genomics, proteomics, and identification of more robust biomarkers could be used in clinical practice to identify asymptomatic individuals at risk of vaginal and cervical cancer, facilitating early diagnosis.

References

Aamodt R, Jonsdottir K, Andersen SN et al. 2009. Differences in protein expression and gene amplification of cyclins between colon and rectal adenocarcinomas. *Gastroenterol Res Pract* 285830.

Abdelhaleem M. 2004. Over-expression of RNA helicases in cancer. *Anticancer Res* 24:3951–3953.

Abudukadeer A, Bakry R, Goebel G, Mutz-Dehbalaie I, Widschwendter A, Bonn GK, Fiegl H. 2012. Clinical relevance of CDH1 and CDH13 DNA-methylation in serum of cervical cancer patients. *Int J Mol Sci* 13(7):8353–8363.

Alonso I, Felix A, Torné A, Fusté V, del Pino M, Castillo P, Balasch J, Pahisa J, Rios J, Ordi J. 2012. Human papillomavirus as a favorable prognostic biomarker in squamous cell carcinomas of the vagina. *Gynecol Oncol* 125:194–199.

American Cancer Society guidelines for the early detection of cancer. *American Cancer Society*. 2012. Retrieved from http://www.cancer.org/Healthy/FindCancerEarly/CancerScreeningGuidelines/american-cancer-society-guidelines-for-the-early-detection-of-cancer.

Andersson S, Sowjanya P, Wangsa D et al. 2009. Detection of genomic amplification of the human telomerase gene TERC, a potential marker for triage of women with HPV-positive, abnormal Pap smears. *Am J Pathol* 175(5):1831–1847.

Baranano DE, Rao M, Ferris CD, Snyder SH. 2002. Biliverdin reductase: A major physiologic cytoprotectant. *Proc Natl Acad Sci USA* 99:16093–16098.

Bae SM, Lee CH, Cho YL, Nam KH, Kim YW, Kim CK, Han BD, Lee YJ, Chun HJ, Ahn WS. 2005. Two-dimensional gel analysis of protein xpression profile in squamous cervical cancer patients. *Gynecol Oncol* 99:26–35.

Beavon IR. 2000. The E-cadherin-catenin complex in tumour metastasis: Structure, function and regulation. *Eur J Cancer* 36:1607–1620.

Beller U, Maısonneuve P, Benedet JI, Heıntz A, Ngan H, Pecorellı S, Odıcıno F, Creasman. W. 2003. Carcinoma of the vagina. *Int J Gynaecol Obstet* 83(1):27–39.

Bhati A, Gupta H, Chhabra H, Kumari A, Patel T. Omics of cancer. 2012. *Asian Pacific J Cancer Prev* 13(9):4229–4233.

Bruni L, Barrionuevo-Rosas L, Serrano B, Brotons M, Albero G, Cosano R, Muñoz J, Bosch FX, de Sanjosé S, Castellsagué X. 2014. ICO Information Centre on HPV and Cancer (HPV Information Centre). Human Papillomavirus and Related Diseases in the World. Summary Report 2014-08-22.

Brunner AH, Grimm C, Polterauer S et al. 2011. The prognostic role of human papillomavirus in patients with vaginal cancer. *Int J Gynecol Cancer* 21:923–929.

Chao CH, Chen CM, Cheng PL, Shih JW, Tsou AP, Lee YH. 2006. DDX3, a DEAD box RNA helicase with tumor growth-suppressive property and transcriptional regulation activity of the p21waf1/cip1 promoter, is a candidate tumor suppressor. *Cancer Res* 66:6579–6588.

Cole LA. 1997. Immunoassay of human chorionic gonadotropin, its free subunits, and metabolites. *Clin Chem* 43:2233–2243.

Conrads TP, Zhou M, Petricoin EF 3rd, Liotta L, Veenstra TD. 2003. Cancer diagnosis using proteomic patterns. *Expert Rev Mol Diagn* 3(4):411–420.

Cordin O, Banroques J, Tanner NK, Linder P. 2006. The DEAD-box protein family of RNA helicases. *Gene* 367:17–37.

Creasman WT. 2005. Vaginal cancers. *Curr Opin Obstet Gynecol* 17:71–76.

De Vuyst H, Clifford GM, Nascimento MC et al. 2009. Prevalence and type distribution of human papillomavirus in carcinoma and intraepithelial neoplasia of the vulva, vagina and anus: A meta-analysis. *Int J Cancer* 124:1626–1636.

Dalrymple JL, Russell AH, Lee SW et al. 2004. Chemoradiation for primary invasive squamous carcinoma of the vagina. *Int J Gynecol Cancer* 14(1):110–117.

Desai AA, Innocenti F, Ratain MJ. 2003. Pharmacogenomics: Road to anticancer therapeutics nirvana? *Oncogene* 22:6621–6628.

Gossage L, Madhusudan S. 2007. Cancer pharmacogenomics: Role of DNA repair genetic polymorphisms in individualizing cancer therapy. *Mol Diagn Ther* 11(6):361–380.

Habermann JK, Hellman K, Freitag S, Heselmeyer-Haddad K, Hellström AC, Shah K, Auer G, Ried T. 2004. A recurrent gain of chromosome arm 3q in primary squamous carcinoma of the vagina. *Cancer Genet Cytogenet* 148(1):7–13.

Hacker N, Eifel P, Velden J. 2012. Cancer of the vagina. *Int J Gynecol Obstet* 119(Suppl 2):S97–S99.

Haidopoulos D, Diakomanolis E, Rodolakis A, Voulgaris Z, Vlachos G, Intsaklis A. 2005. Can local application of imiquimod cream be an alternative mode of therapy for patients with high-grade intraepithelial lesions of the vagina. *Int J Gynecol Cancer* 15(5):898–902.

Hartwell L, Mankoff D, Paulovich A, Ramsey S, Swisher E. 2006. Cancer biomarkers: A systems approach. *Nat Biotechnol* 24:8.

He Z, Campolmi N, Ha Thi BM, Dumollard JM, Peoc'h M, Garraud O, Piselli S, Gain P, Thuret G. 2011. Optimization of immunolocalization of cell cycle proteins in human corneal endothelial cells. *Mol Vis* 17:3494–3511.

Hellman K, Alaiya AA, Becker S, Lomnytska M, Schedvins K, Steinberg W, Hellstro AC, Andersson S, Hellman U, Auer G. 2009. Differential tissue-specific protein markers of vaginal carcinoma. *Br J Cancer* 100:1303–1314.

Hellman K, Alaiya AA, Schedvins K, Steinberg W, Hellstro AC, Auer G. 2004. Protein expression patterns in primary carcinoma of the vagina. *Br J Cancer* 91:319–326.

Hellman K, Johansson H, Andersson S, Pettersson F, Auer G. 2012. Prognostic significance of cell cycle- and invasion-related molecular markers and genomic instability in primary carcinoma of the vagina. *Int J Gynecol Cancer* 23(1):41–51.

Heselmeyer K, Schröck E, du Manoir S, Blegen H, Shah K, Steinbeck R, Auer G, Ried T. 1996. Gain of chromosome 3q defines the transition from severe dysplasia to invasive carcinoma of the uterine cervix. *Proc Natl Acad Sci USA* 93(1):479–484.

Ikenberg H, Runge M, Goppinger A et al. 1990. Human papillomavirus DNA in invasive carcinoma of the vagina. *Obstet Gynecol* 76:432–438.

Ikenberg H, Sauerbrei W, Schottmüller U, Spitz C, Pfleiderer A. 1994. Human papillomavirus DNA in cervical carcinoma—Correlation with clinical data and influence on prognosis. *Int J Cancer* 59(3):322–326.

Immaculada A, Felix A, Torné A, Aureli A, Fusté V. 2012. Human papillomavirus as a favorable prognostic biomarker in squamous cell carcinomas of the vagina. *Gynecologic Oncology* 125(1):194–199.

Jansen T, Daiber A. 2012. Direct antioxidant properties of bilirubin and biliverdin. Is there a role for biliverdin reductase? *Front Pharmacol* 16(3):30.

Jens KH, Hellmanc K, Freitagd S, Heselmeyer-Haddada K, Hellstro AC, Shahe K, Auerb G, Rieda T. 2004. A recurrent gain of chromosome arm 3q in primary squamous carcinoma of the vagina. *Cancer Genet Cytogenet* 148:7–13.

Kim CK, Truong LX. Nguyen Joo KM, Nam DH, Park J, Lee KH, Cho SW, Ahn JY. 2010. Binding protein Ebp1 in brain tumors 3. *Cancer Res* 70:23.

Kim HP, Wang X, Galbiati F, Ryter SW, Choi AM. 2004. Caveolae compartmentalization of heme oxygenase-1 in endothelial cells. *FASEB J* 18:1080.

Kim SY, Kang HT, Choi HR, Park SC. 2011. Biliverdin reductase A in the prevention of cellular senescence against oxidative stress. *Exp Mol Med* 431:15–23.

Kowalinski E, Bange G, Wild K, Sinning I. 2007. Expression, purification, crystallization and preliminary crystallographic analysis of the proliferation-associated protein Ebp1. *Acta Crystallogr Sect F Struct Biol Cryst Commun* 63:768–770.

Krebs HB. 1986. Prophylactic topical 5-fluorouracil following treatment of human papillomavirus-associated lesions of the vulva and vagina. *Obstet Gynecol* 68(6):837–841.

Lerner-Marmarosh N, Shen J, Torno MD, Kravets A, Hu Z, Maines MD. 2005. Human biliverdin reductase: A member of the insulin receptor substrate family with serine/threonine/tyrosine kinase activity. *Proc Natl Acad Sci USA* 102:7109–7114.

Levine AJ, Finlay CA, Hinds PW. 2004. P53 is a tumor suppressor gene. *Cell* 116:S67–S69.

Lundgren C, Frankendal B, Silfversward C et al. 2003. Laminin-5 gamma2-chain expression and DNA ploidy as predictors of prognosis in endometrial carcinoma. *Med Oncol* 20:147–156.

Maines MD, Mayer RD, Erturk E, Huang TJ, Disantagnese A. 1999. The oxidoreductase, biliverdin reductase, is induced in human renal carcinoma pH and cofactor-specific increase in activity. *J Urol* 162:1467–1472.

Manor E, Bodner L, Kachko P, Kapelushnik J. 2009. Trisomy 8 as a sole aberration in embryonal rhabdomyosarcoma (sarcoma botryoides) of the vagina. *Cancer Genet Cytogenet* 195:172–174.

Masuda R, Kijima H, Imamura N et al. 2012. Laminin-5γ2 chain expression is associated with tumor cell invasiveness and prognosis of lung squamous cell carcinoma. *Biomed Res* 33(5):309–317.

Melle C, Ernst G, Scheibner O, Kaufmann R, Schimmel B, Bleul A, Settmacher U, Hommann M, Claussen U, Eggeling FV. 2007. Identification of specific protein markers in microdissected hepatocellular carcinoma. *J Proteome Res* 6:306–315.

Michalas SP. 2000. The Pap test: George N. Papanicolaou (1883–1962) A screening test for the prevention of cancer of uterine cervix. *Eur J Obstet Gynecol Reprod Biol* 90:135–138.

Morel NM, Holland JM, van der Greef J, Marple EW, Clish C, Loscalzo J, Naylor S. 2004. Primer on medical genomics. Part XIV: Introduction to systems biology—A new approach to understanding disease and treatment. *Mayo Clin Proc* 79(5):651–658.

Nilsson PJ, Lenander C, Rubio C et al. 2006. Prognostic significance of Cyclin A in epidermoid anal cancer. *Oncol Rep* 16:443–449.

Pintusa SS, Fomina ES, Oshurkovb IS, Ivanisenkoa VA. 2007. Phylogenetic analysis of the p53 and p63/p73 gene families. *In Silico Biology* 7:319–332.

Ratner ML. 2011. Can E6E7 alter the competitive balance in the crowded HPV test market? *In Vivo: The Business & Medicine report*, 2011.

Ries LAG, Young JL, Keel GE, et al. 2007. *SEER Survival Monograph: Cancer Survival Among Adults: U.S. SEER Program, 1988–2001, Patient and Tumor Characteristics*. National Cancer Institute, SEER Program, NIH Pub. No. 07-6215, Bethesda, MD.

Sharma S. 2009. Tumor markers in clinical practice: General principles and guidelines. *Indian J Med Paediatr Oncol* 30(1):1–8.

Scholzen TE, Kalden DH, Brzoska T et al. 2000. Expression of proopiomelanocortin peptides in human dermal microvascular endothelial cells: Evidence for a regulation by ultraviolet light and interleukin-1. *J Invest Dermatol* 115(6):1021–1028.

Schönhofer B. 2006. Nicht-invasive Beatmung – Grundlagen und moderne Praxis, UNI-MED, Bremen.

Schönhofer B et al. 2008. Nicht-invasive Beatmung bei akuter respiratorischer Insuffizienz. *Deutsches Ärzteblatt* 105(24):424–433.

Tacu C, Neagu M, Constantin C, Sajin M. 2010. Biomarkers discovery in cancer—Up-dates in methodology. *Roum Arch Microbiol Immunol* 69:48–55.

Vaissière T, Sawan C, Herceg Z. 2008. Epigenetic interplay between histone modifications and DNA methylation in gene silencing. *Mutat Res* 659:40–48.

Vlaicu M. 2009. *FDA Medical Device: Non-Invasive Cervical Cancer Detection (OTC:GTHP)*. Guided Therapeutics Inc.

Warfel NA, El-Deiry WS. 2013. p21WAF1 and tumourigenesis: 20 years after. *Curr Opin Oncol* 25(1):52–58.

Wegiel B, Otterbein LE. 2012. Go green: The anti-inflammatory effects of biliverdin reductase. *Front Pharmacol* 3:47.

Wentzensen N, Sherman ME, Schiffman M, Wang SS. 2009. Utility of methylation markers in cervical cancer early detection: Appraisal of the state-of-the-science. *Gynecol Oncol* 112:293–299.

Xia Q, Kong XT, Zhang GA, Hou XJ, Qiang H, Zhong RQ. 2005. Proteomics-based identification of DEAD-box protein 48 as a novel autoantigen, a prospective serum marker for pancreatic cancer. *Biochem Biophys Res Commun* 330:526–532.

Yavagal S, de Farias TF, Medina CA, Takacs P. 2011. Normal vulvovaginal, perineal, and pelvic anatomy with reconstructive considerations. *Semin Plast Surg* 25(2):121–129.

Zhang Y, Wang XW, Jelovac D, Nakanishi T, Yu MH, Akinmade D, Goloubeva O, Ross DD, Brodie A, Hamburger AW. 2005. The ErbB3-binding protein Ebp1 suppresses androgen receptor-mediated gene transcription and tumorigenesis of prostate cancer cells. *Proc Natl Acad Sci USA* 102(28):9890–9895.

Zhu X, Lv J, Yu L, Zhu X, Wu J, Zou S, Jiang S. 2009. Proteomic identification of differentially-expressed proteins in squamous cervical cancer. *Gynecol Oncol* 112:248–256.

18

Noninvasive Early Biomarkers for Vulvar Cancer

Sara Iacoponi, MD, PhD, Marcos Cuerva, MD, PhD, Mar Gil, MD, Elisa Moreno-Palacios, MD, Alicia Hernández, MD, PhD, Javier De Santiago, MD, PhD, and Ignacio Zapardiel, MD, PhD

CONTENTS

ABSTRACT Vulvar carcinoma represents 5% of all female genital cancers (1–2 in 100,000 person/year). Squamous cell carcinoma is the most common histological type of vulvar cancer and represents 80%–90% of the cases. Nowadays, there is a big concern about the postoperative sequela and mutilation associated with radical surgery, which is the most common treatment for this disease. Due to this, there are high expectations in new tumor markers that could serve as prognostic indicators to guide treatment decisions. Several molecular pathological markers have been investigated in vulvar squamous cell carcinoma, such as p16, p21, p14, p27, cyclin A, cyclin D1, p53, VEGF, TGFa, HER-2, EGFR, HPV, CD44v3, CD44v6, MMP-12, caspase 3, Bcl-2, and nm23-H1. But not every vulvar carcinoma has the same behavior and origin. Only among the vulvar squamous cell carcinomas, there are four histological subtypes: basaloid, warty, verrucoid, and keratinizing or non-keratinizing squamous cell carcinomas. This means that there are many possible specific markers that may be useful in only some of the subtypes. This chapter summarizes the biomarkers that are in actual use and others that are in study in the diagnoses and treatment of vulvar cancer. Unfortunately, all the conclusions regarding the prognostic value of the markers for vulvar cancer are based on small trials, with a lack of multivariate analyses. Therefore, these markers should not modify the medical practice due to their lack of evidence.

18.1 Introduction

18.1.1 Epidemiology

Vulvar cancer represents 5% of all gynecological cancers and 1% of all cancers in women, with an incidence of 1–2/100,000 women (Hacker, 2005). It classically affects older women, with an average age of 65–70 years (Beller et al., 2006), although lastly an increase in the incidence has been detected among women younger than 50 years old (Joura, 2002).

From 1985 to 1997, the incidence has rose from 5% to 16% in young women. There are two groups with high incidence of vulvar cancer, the highest being in women 70–80 years old in the first group and in women under 50 years old in the second group (Joura, 2002). An increase of 2.4% from 1992 to 1998 has been reported, above all in women under 65 years old (Howe et al., 2001). In a country like Spain (42 million habitants), there are around 500 deaths per year because of this pathology (SEGO, 2010).

18.1.2 Types of Vulvar Cancer

Ninety percent of vulvar carcinomas are squamous cell carcinomas (SCCs) and the remaining 10% includes a wide variety of tumors such as melanoma, adenocarcinoma of Bartholin's gland, or Paget's disease (Finan and Barre, 2003).

The vulva, as an anatomic structure, is formed by the dermis; mucous components like the clitoris, hymen, and urethra; and glandular structures like the Bartholin's gland and Skene's gland. Due to these different tissues, different types of tumors may appear, such as glandular tumors and epithelial tumors (Table 18.1) (SEGO, 2010).

18.1.3 Vulvar Squamous Carcinoma

Among the vulvar SCCs, there are three different kinds, depending on their aspect and etiology: the condylomatous type, the basaloid type, and the keratinizing type.

The condylomatous and basaloid tumors share the same risk factors of cervical cancer (e.g., high number of sexual partners, starting sexual activity at an early age, genital condylomas, and tobacco). The main etiological factor is the human papillomavirus (HPV).

TABLE 18.1

Histological Classification of the Vulva Epithelial Tumors (OMS 2003)

Squamous and related tumors and precursors	Squamous cell carcinoma, not otherwise specified	Keratinizing
		Nonkeratinizing
		Basaloid
		Warty
		Verrucous
		Keratoacanthoma-like
		Variant with tumor giant cell
		Others
	Basal cell carcinoma	
	Squamous intraepithelial neoplasia	Vulvar intraepithelial neoplasia (VIN 3)/squamous cell carcinoma in situ
	Benign squamous lesions	Condyloma acuminatum
		Vestibular papilloma
		Fibroepithelial polyp
		Seborrheic and inverted follicular keratosis
		Keratoacanthoma
Glandular tumors	Paget's disease	
	Bartholin's gland tumors	Adenocarcinoma
		Squamous cell carcinoma
		Adenoid cystic carcinoma
		Adenosquamous carcinoma
		Transitional cell carcinoma
		Small-cell carcinoma
		Adenoma
		Adenomyoma
		Others
	Tumors arising from specialized anogenital mammary-like glands	Adenocarcinoma of mammary gland type
		Papillary hidradenoma
		Others
	Adenocarcinoma of Skene's gland origin	
	Adenocarcinoma of other types	
	Adenoma of minor vestibular glands	
	Mixed tumor of the vulva	
Tumors of skin appendage origin	Malignant sweat gland tumors	
	Sebaceous carcinoma	
	Syringoma	
	Nodular hidradenoma	
	Trichoepithelioma	
	Trichilemmoma	
	Others	

The most important risk factors for vulvar cancer are immunosuppression, HPV infection, and old age (Sillman et al., 1984).

In immunosuppressed patients, there is an increase in the incidence of cervical and vulvar carcinomas, which suggests that the immune deficiency could be a factor in the oncogenesis, possibly due to an inefficient status of the oncosuppressor genes in the cells infected by HPV (Tyring, 2003).

These risk factors (high number of sexual partners, starting sexual activity at an early age, genital condylomas, and tobacco) are not associated with the keratinizing type, which have risk factors such as old age and other unknown factors.

A relation between cardiovascular disease and gynecological cancer has also been suggested, although there is no known cause. Forty percent of patients with gynecological cancer have a high blood pressure. Other chronic vascular and metabolic diseases, including diabetes and obesity, are common in patients with vulvar carcinomas (Edwards and Balat, 1996). In two case–control studies published by Mabuchi et al. (1985) and Brinton et al. (1990), they did not find an increase in cardiovascular disease in these patients, but tobacco was identified as a risk factor in young patients, mostly associated with genital condylomas. In these studies, the nulliparity, early menopause, and the use of oral contraceptive were not related to an increase in the disease incidence. Only the vulvar intraepithelial neoplasm (VIN) and the vulvar dystrophy were statistically related to these factors (Ansink and Heintz, 1993).

There are many studies that have reported an association between herpes simplex virus (HSV) and the VIN; and due to this relation, it has been reported as a possible factor together with HPV in the pathogenesis of VIN (Kaufman, 1995).

Well-differentiated squamous cell carcinoma generally affects old women (70–80 years old) and its incidence has remained stable in time. It has not been related to HPV infection. It is associated with vulvar dystrophy, squamous cell hyperplasia, and lichen sclerosus (LS) (SEGO, 2010).

The condylomatous and basaloid SCC types are more frequent in younger women (under 55 years old). They are associated with HPV infection, particularly type 16 and VIN. Their incidence is increasing and frequently, there is simultaneously a vaginal and cervical damage.

18.1.3.1 Vulvar Intraepithelial Neoplasm

The VIN is the lesion that affects the vulva previously to a vulvar SCC and it is characterized by a loss of the differentiation of the epithelial cells that appear hyperchromatic, with pleomorphic nucleus and abnormal mitosis. The abnormal cells can appear with dyskeratosis, hyperkeratosis, parakeratosis and pigment incontinence (Puig-Tintoré, 2011).

IN 1986 VIN was classified into three stages, VIN 1 (mild dysplasia), VIN 2 (moderate dysplasia), and VIN 3 (severe dysplasia) according to the thickness of the epithelium affected by the nuclear mimetism with the same classification as the CIN (Lai and Mercurio, 2010).

As we know, most of the VIN appear due to a viral cause and the progression to cancer is similar in the three stages of VIN. A new classification of the International Society for the study of vulvovaginal disease was established in 2004; the new classification divides VIN into two groups, common VIN associated with HPV with the condylomatous and basaloid pattern and the well-differentiated VIN, nonrelated to HPV, that is related to squamous cell hyperplasia or to LS (Sideri et al., 2005).

In the new classification, the term VIN is used only for high-grade lesions (VIN 2, VIN 3). The term VIN 1 has been erased because usually it represents reactive changes as a consequence of the HPV infection that should be described only as atypia (Bergeron, 2008; Puig-Tintoré, 2011).

A broad meta-analysis with 3322 patients found, after 33 months follow-up, that 9% of nontreated VIN and 3% of treated VIN ended in a vulvar carcinoma.

In the well-differentiated VIN, the behavior is more aggressive than in the common type, with a shorter intraepithelial phase and a higher risk of progression (up to 32.8%) (van Seters et al., 2005).

The VIN related with vulvar carcinoma could be considered as an independent prognostic factor for recurrence. Rarzier et al. analyzed 108 patients with vulvar cancer recurrence; out of these patients, 23% had an association to a common VIN. The author observed that the existence of tumor-related VIN was an independent factor for survival (Rarzier et al., 2001).

In vulvar tissue of patients affected by carcinoma, precursor lesions such as VIN, or LS, it is common to find an aneusomy of chromosome 17, but not in the vulvar tissue of patients without a tumoral lesion. In relation to chromosome 17, there is a study that reports that normal chromosome 17 of vulvar carcinomas associated with LS and the loss of chromosome 17 material in tissues of vulvar carcinomas associated with HPV support the division in two different kinds of vulvar cancer (Carlson et al., 2000).

There is a small study of 17 cases of VIN and 26 cases of vulvar carcinoma that showed the presence of endothelial growth factor in 92% of cases of cancer and in 6% of cases of VIN, but it was not observed in ordinary vulvar tissue. This would indicate a role of angiogenesis in VIN progression to invasive cancer (Mc Lean et al., 2000).

Yang and Hart investigated the clinicopathological features of 12 cases of differentiated VIN. Squamous hyperplasia (SH) was present in the epidermis adjacent to the lesion in 10 patients and LS in 4 patients. Four patients subsequently developed an invasive vulvar cancer. Ten of the twelve patients were p53 positive. In only one differentiated VIN, there was a lesion that was p53 negative, and HPV was identified. These results suggested that differentiated VIN has a strong association with HPV-negative vulvar SCC and p53 gene alteration appears to be involved in the development of differentiated VIN (Yang and Hart, 2000).

Survival rates are related to inguinal nodal status at the time of diagnosis. In patients with an operable disease without nodal involvement, the OS is 90%; however, in patients with nodal involvement, the 5-year OS rate is approximately 50%–60% (Homesley et al., 1991).

The most important risk factors for node metastasis are the clinical node status, age, differentiation grade, tumor stage, tumor size, depth of stromal invasion, and presence of lymphovascular space invasion (Homesley et al., 1993).

The survival rate of vulvar cancer has increased in the last decades due to the introduction of radical vulvectomy *en bloc* with inguinofemoral and pelvic lymphadenectomy, replacing the simple excision of the lesion. However, due to the high morbidity of this surgery, in the last 20 years, the treatment of vulvar cancer has moved to a more conservative and tailored treatment (De Hullu and van der Zee, 2006).

The first step in reducing morbidity was performed by Byron, who introduced the triple incision technique, which showed the same oncological outcomes, with a recurrence of the skin bridge at only 2.4%, but a greater morbidity reduction (Woelber et al., 2011). Posteriorly, the implementation of tumor-wide excision and the sentinel node (SN) biopsy has achieved a great reduction in morbidity. The current standard of pathological margin of at least 8 mm in patients with early-stage disease has added benefits to this aspect (Heaps et al., 1990; De Hullu et al., 2002; De Hullu and van der Zee, 2006; Chan et al., 2007).

18.1.3.2 Lichen Sclerosus and Hyperplasia

LS, classified as a nonneoplastic epithelial disorder of the vulva, is the most common dermatologic disease in this specialized area of the skin, accounting for as much as 23% of new patients seen in vulvar clinic (Mc Lean et al., 1998). LS is an inflammatory dermatosis whose etiology remains unknown, though there have been several theories proposed, like immunological, hormonal, enzymatic, and infectious (Bamberger and Perrett, 2002). Vulvar LS has a 3%–5% reported prospective risk of malignant transformation, but histological analysis of vulvar SCC demonstrates LS in the adjacent skin in more than 75% of cases (Mc Lean, 1993).

Like LS, SH is a pruritic disorder often seen in postmenopausal women. The clinical appearance is of raised white plaques on the vulva. Histological features are of epithelial hyperplasia with acanthosis, hyperkeratosis, parakeratosis, and irregular prolongation of the rete ridges (Bamberger and Perrett, 2002).

18.1.3.3 Paget's Disease of the Vulva

Paget's disease of the vulva (PDV) is a rare intraepithelial carcinoma in situ disease accounting for 1% of all vulvar neoplasm. It usually occurs in postmenopausal women with presenting symptoms of pruritus and soreness appearing as erythematous scaly patches with island of hyperkeratosis. Paget's cell can be distinguished by their pronounced nuclear atypia and pleomorphism (Ordonez et al., 1987). Unlike Paget's disease of the breast where almost all cases are associated with an underlying ductal carcinoma in situ or an invasive carcinoma of the breast, the number of associated carcinoma present in extramammary Paget's disease is thought to be much less (Bamberger and Perrett, 2002). In one study of PDV cases (Boehm and Morris, 1971) had an underlying cancer and in a later study, 24% of extramammary Paget's disease cases had an underlying cancer (Chanda, 1985).

18.2 Noninvasive Markers

The development of noninvasive tests for cancer detection is of high importance. It could bring the possibility of detecting vulvar carcinomas at its earliest stages decreasing the mortality and the morbidity, improving the survival rate, and screening the high-risk patients. Although many molecular markers have been identified, there is still minor evidence and low clinical use regarding vulvar carcinomas. On one hand, the vulvar cancer biomarkers that have been studied are found in the vulvar tissue, which means that at least a biopsy is required (unfortunately, no useful biomarkers have been found so far in urine or serum). On the other hand, the different types of vulvar carcinomas have different etiologies, which mean that different biomarkers are needed depending on the subtype of vulvar carcinoma that we want to study.

There is still not an official classification of vulvar cancer biomarkers, but several different ones have been used in different publications. We are going to use one based on the one used by Knopp in his review about vulvar cancer biomarkers (Knopp et al., 2009).

18.2.1 HPV

HPV is a double-stranded DNA virus. Most of the HPV subtypes cause benign proliferative lesions or warts, but some subtypes are oncogenic. It has been longer discussed if the detection of HPV is useful for the prognosis as a biomarker in vulvar cancer. The vulvar carcinomas, when HPV is involved, have a better prognosis according to some studies and no influence in the prognosis according to others, which results in a lack of evidence in order to set a prognosis (Ansink et al., 1994; Monk et al., 1995; Pinto et al., 2004).

Usually, vulvar carcinomas are divided into the ones related to HPV or not related. The patients with vulvar carcinoma positive for HPV are younger and smokers and show a high rate of multifocal disease (Rouzier et al., 2001). For detecting the HPV virus, polymerase chain reaction (PCR) is the most sensitive method and also a high expression of p16 has been suggested as a marker for HPV activity and vulvar lesions, because of the high expression found in vulvar SCCs.

The infection by HPV can be considered as an early step in the carcinogenesis of the vulvar cancers related to this infection (the viral integration leads to the disruption of the E2 region and to an increased expression of E6 and E7 interacting and inactivating the p53 and pRb among others). But one of the biggest and more important difficulties if HPV is used as a biomarker for vulvar cancer is that its detection results in an overestimation, because there are many infections that do not lead to a neoplasm. For example, van de Nieuwenhof found an association between HPV and vulvar SCCs in 26.9%; but only in 19.6% HPV could be considered as the cause (van de Nieuwenhof et al., 2009). In order to elucidate the reason why some patients develop neoplasms and cancer due to the HPV infection and others do not, the immune response to the HPV virus is being studied. CD83 glycoprotein as a marker of dendritic cells maturation seemed a promising marker, but unfortunately, a recent study did not observe associations between genetic variations of the CD83 and the risk of vulvar cancer (Bodelon et al., 2012).

It is maybe more interesting considering the immune response that is caused by the HPV infection. It is well known that immunosuppressed patients are in higher risk of developing a malignancy because of HPV. The immune response to HPV is caused by cells of the innate and adaptive immune system. It has been observed that there are less CD1a and CD207 dendritic cells in HPV-positive VIN than in women without HPV infection, and the amount of these cells has been inversely correlated to the stage of VIN (Singh et al., 2006; van Seters et al., 2008).

The study of the immune response is also promising, because there must be biomarkers in serum correlated with this response. HPV16-specific CD4 T-cells and CD8 T-cells reactive to HPV16 oncopeptides E6 and E7 have been detected in serum determinations of patients with vulvar neoplasms, and they may be related to the disease prognosis (Todd et al., 2004; van Poelgeest et al., 2005).

18.2.2 Cell Cycle

The cell cycle in eukaryotic cells and therefore in human cells is divided into four phases: G1, S, G2, and M (and G0 as separate phase).

G1 is the phase during which the cell gets prepared for the DNA replication process. During the G1 phase, the cell integrates mitogenic and growth inhibitory signals, and depending on them, the cell can enter into three different paths: to progress to the next stage, pause, or exit the cell cycle.

The S phase is defined as the phase in which DNA synthesis occurs.

G2 is the phase during which the cell prepares for the division process, after the phase S.

The M phase means mitosis. It is the phase when the replicated chromosomes are segregated into separate cores and cytokinesis occurs to form two daughter cells.

The transitions in the cell cycle are controlled by cyclin-dependent kinases that are regulated by cyclins sequentially.

To keep the cell in the cycle, cyclin-dependent kinase complexes and cyclin-independent kinase complexes will phosphorylate the retinoblastoma protein (pRb). Depending on the phosphorylation of the pRb, transcription factors like E2F are released, which activate the transcription of genes responsible for the progression to the S phase. An overexpression of kinases and cyclins can cause a failure in the stop signals of cells in G1 phase, causing an uncontrolled proliferation and tumor growth. Therefore, inhibitors of cyclin-dependent kinases are important in controlling the cell cycle.

Among the inhibitors of cyclin-dependent kinases, there are two families of inhibitors, depending on the kinases they inhibit:

1. One of the families is the INK4 family, consisting of p15INK4b, p16INK4a (p16), p19INK4d, and p18INK4c proteins.
2. The other family is known as Cip/Kip and consists of p21WAF1/CIP1 protein (p21), p27Kip1 (p27), and p57KIP2 proteins (Sherr and Roberts, 1999).

The literature suggests that lesions or disturbances of these cyclin-dependent kinases inhibitor proteins play an important role in the tumorigenesis; however, it is still not clear how its detection alters the prognosis for vulvar cancers.

In the cell cycle, the proteins that have been more studied are the alterations that occur at the level of expression of cyclin D1, p16, and pRb and are believed to be important events in the beginning and development of vulvar carcinogenesis.

18.2.2.1 pRb

The pRb belongs to the pocket proteins family. The members of this pocket proteins family have a pocket for functional binding to other proteins. In this family, there are also p107 and p130 proteins that are structurally and functionally similar to pRb.

Related to vulvar cancer, it has been found that there is an increase in the frequency of loss of expression of the pRb/p130 depending on the nature of the lesion: benign lesions or invasive SCCs (Zamparelli et al., 2001). A previous study showed that the loss of expression of the protein of retinoblastoma increased from stage I to stage IV of 16.7%–50% (Chan et al., 1998).

18.2.2.2 Cyclin D1

Cyclins are cell cycle modulators, and they act, as mentioned, through the cyclin-dependent kinases. Some cyclins are related to the retinoblastoma gene and act by inhibiting the expression of the pRb. Cyclins are metabolized by the ubiquitin and destroyed in the cytoplasm during the S phase.

Cyclin D1 is the most widely studied cyclin in relation to the vulvar carcinogenesis. Its aberrant expression has been found in precursor lesions adjacent to malignant vulvar tumors (Rolfe et al., 2001). The increase in expression of cyclin D1 has been observed in 26% of cases of squamous cell tumors of the vulva according to Knopp et al.; although they refer that cyclin D1 is not a relevant prognostic, they consider cyclin A1 more relevant (Knopp et al., 2005). Other authors have observed an increase in the expression of cyclin D1 in squamous cell tumors of the vulva, although always in relation to the p16 protein expression.

18.2.2.3 Ki-67

The expression of cyclin D1 is comparable to that of Ki-67. As occurs with cyclin D1, there is a greater expression of Ki-67 when cell proliferation is increased.

Ki-67 is a well-known and reliable marker of growth of a cell population. It is expressed in the core of proliferating cells during G1, S, G2, and M, but not in G0. The cytoplasmic staining complexes are only expressed during the M phase (Brown and Gatter, 1990).

In normal vulvar epithelium, Ki-67 shows a localized pattern of expression in the parabasal cells. Ki-67 is not expressed in the basal epithelial layer of normal vulvar epithelium, but it does appear in the basal epithelial layers in VIN neoplasms (van der Avoort et al., 2007). In cases of VIN 3, there is a diffuse expression of Ki-67, while in vulvar carcinomas, the Ki-67 is expressed in either a localized or diffuse staining pattern (Modesitt et al., 2000).

Ki-67 has been related to lymph node metastases prediction. Some studies found an association between its expression and lymph node metastases, but a study of Emanuels et al. (1996) demonstrated that there is no association between lymph node metastases and the expression of Ki-67. Afterward, another study did find a significant relation between the type of expression of Ki-67 and the frequency of lymph node metastases. This study differs between three types of Ki-67 expression, diffuse, localized, and infiltrating, and found that the diffuse expression and infiltrating expression are associated with a higher rate of lymph node involvement and shorter disease-free survival after treatment (Hantschmann et al., 2000).

18.2.2.4 p16INK4a

p16INK4a is an inhibitor of cyclin-dependent kinase 4. The activity of p16 in normal cells is related to proliferation inhibition. The p16 protein is a key element in the path, in that it shares with the cyclin D, cyclin-dependent kinase 4, and retinoblastoma gene, so they are often studied together (Funk et al., 1997).

Thus, in regard to vulvar carcinogenesis, an INK4a-promoter hypermethylation with a simultaneous loss of expression of p16 has been detected in squamous vulvar cancers and VIN 3 lesions (Gasco et al., 2002). On the other hand, in VIN 3 lesions associated with HPV, there is an alteration in the expression of p16, but in this case, there is an overexpression.

Knopp et al. (2004) found that the p16 expression is significantly correlated with clinical outcome. Other studies have not shown a statistically significant association, probably because larger numbers of patients are required in the studies (Tringler et al., 2007).

18.2.2.5 p14

The p14 protein is encoded in the same locus as the INK4a family. The p14 protein is capable of inhibiting the destruction of the p53 by the ubiquitin protein. Thereby, p14 stabilizes p53 and allows the action of this tumor suppressor protein.

Studies on p14 and vulvar carcinomas show an overexpression of p14 in 36% of vulvar carcinomas (Knopp et al., 2006). This overexpression is more in relation with tumors with HPV-positive infection, and therefore, the action of p14 is not effective.

These studies express a correlation between the expression of p14 and the specific survival at 5 years. The expression of p14 is associated with a better prognosis in vulvar cancers when they are not associated with HPV; this association has not been demonstrated in vulvar cancers related to HPV infection (Knopp et al., 2006).

18.2.2.6 p27

The p27 protein belongs to the family Cip/Kip and has a regulatory function that responds to extracellular signals. The oncogene E7 of HPV-16 can join it without degrading it, although its inactivation is not yet clearly related to oncogenesis.

p27Kip1 gene is a negative regulator of the G1 phase of the cell cycle and is considered a tumor suppressor gene. Loss of p27 protein expression seems to be associated with the development of vulvar carcinomas (Sgambato et al., 2000; Knopp et al., 2004). The p27 protein as inhibitor of cyclins and therefore of cyclin-dependent kinases has been implicated in the regulation of cellular proliferation in response to extracellular signals.

The progressive loss of p27 protein expression has been linked to the progression of benign and malignant tumors, and its subsequent decrease is related to the acquisition of metastatic potential and poor prognosis (Sgambato et al., 2000; Lee and Yang, 2001). In relation to vulvar cancer, the study of Zannoni et al. (2006) shows that a reduction in the expression of the p27 protein may be associated with the development of vulvar cancer and may play an important role in the early phase of vulvar tumorigenesis. In the same study, there were no differences in p27 protein expression related to advanced tumor grades and stages in vulvar carcinomas.

18.2.2.7 p21

The p21 protein is considered as the p53 executor. The p21 gene is under the transcriptional control of p53 (el-Deiry et al., 1994). Expression of p21 is diminished or absent in resting cells and is involved in the activity of cyclin-dependent kinases. Its activity seems to have no prognostic value, although some studies have linked its activity with survival. Knopp et al. (2004) found a relationship between the high expression of the p21 and a worse prognosis, while low expression was present in well-differentiated cases. This relationship with the survival demonstrated mainly in stages 1 and 2 of the International Federation of Gynecology and Obstetrics (FIGO) is paradoxical, because as a protein that activates the p53, high activity would be expected to be associated with a higher tumor suppression.

18.2.2.8 p53

The p53 protein is considered an oncosuppressor protein. p53 allows the cell cycle to progress after checking that the genome is intact. The p53 protein is expressed if the DNA is damaged, stopping the cell cycle through p21.

The p53 tumor suppressor gene is located on chromosome 17p. An overexpression of wild-type p53 protein induces a growth arrest.

Mutations of the p53 and p53 protein overexpression are found in about 50% of vulvar carcinomas and in a high percentage of VIN lesions (Scheistrøen et al., 1999). However, reports about the correlation between the expression of p53 and prognosis in patients with vulvar carcinomas are contradictory.

Scheistrøen et al. (1999) reported a significantly shorter disease-related survival at 5 years for patients with p53 overexpression compared with patients with p53 negative tumors in a cohort of 160 patients. In another study, conducted by Salmaso et al. (2000), it was observed that the high expression of p53 was strongly associated with increased grade and progression of the tumor. Together, these studies indicate that p53 may be an important prognostic marker in the future.

18.2.2.9 BCL-2

There is a scarce expression of bcl-2 in normal vulva, but there is an increase in vulvar carcinomas and VIN lesions.

BCL-2 gene is one of the central control genes in the regulation of apoptosis. It encodes an antiapoptotic protein family: Bcl-2 and Bcl-X and proapoptotic proteins, for example, Bax and Bcl-xs.

However, the expression of bcl-2 does not influence the prognosis of patients; there is no difference in disease-free survival and OS depending on its expression (Hefler et al., 1999).

18.2.3 Angiogenesis

Angiogenesis is the stimulation of growth of new vascular endothelial cells and development of new blood vessels. Angiogenesis is therefore a critical factor in the progression and metastasis of solid tumors (Folkman, 1971). The onset of angiogenesis marks a phase of rapid proliferation, local invasion, and ultimately metastasis, although angiogenesis can also have a role to play in premalignant lesions (Folkman et al., 1989). Vascular endothelial growth factor (VEGF) is a multifunctional cytokine with potent angiogenic activity. It acts selectively on endothelial cells by binding to specific class III receptor tyrosine kinases. VEGF stimulates angiogenesis through its action as an endothelial mitogen and its ability to increase vascular permeability (Ellis et al., 2002). VEGF is widely distributed and has been shown to play a coordinated role in endothelial cell proliferation and assembly of the vessel wall in a variety of normal and abnormal circumstances (Ferrara, 1999).

Several studies have demonstrated its overexpression in a variety of tumors including those of breast, ovary, bladder, and vulva (Ellis et al., 2002).

Another factor that has been shown to stimulate angiogenesis is platelet-derived endothelial cell growth factor (PD-ECGF). This protein promotes cell growth and chemotaxis in endothelial cell in vivo and angiogenesis in vitro (Ishikawa et al., 1989).

Angiopoietin 1 (Ang-1) and angiopoietin 2 (Ang-2) are growth factors that are ligands for the *ties*, a family of receptor tyrosine kinases that are as selectively expressed within the vascular endothelium as are the VEGF receptors (Dumont et al., 1993).

Numerous ephrin ligands (e.g., ephrins A1, B1, B2) bind to the Eph receptor tyrosine kinases; these comprise the largest known family of growth factor receptors and include EphA2, EphB2, EphB3, and EphB4. In the settings of angiogenesis, as in tumor or in the female reproductive system, the endothelium of new vessels strongly reexpresses ephrin B2, suggesting that ephrin B2 may also be important in this angiogenic setting (Yancopoulos et al., 2000).

Many studies have used measurements of microvessel density (MVD) in regions of high vessel density (HVD), also termed vascular *hot spots*, to assess the role of tumor angiogenesis in prognosis. Elevated MVD was associated with both low relapse-free survival and OS (Bamberger and Perrett, 2002). Angiogenesis and angiogenic factors are now available in the search for new targets for the improvement of prognosis in patients with vulvar cancer.

Bancher-Todescha et al. (1997), using immunohistochemistry, examined the expression of VEGF and MVD in vulvar intraepithelial neoplasia. They demonstrated that, for both VEGF expression and MVD, the differences between VIN 1 and VIN 3 and between VIN 2 and VIN 3 were statistically significant and the highest values were found in VIN 3. In contrast, Doldi et al. (1996) detected by dot blot VEGF mRNA analysis/expression in both SCC benign and premalignant lesion of 15 human vulvar tissue specimens. VEGF mRNA was detected in all tissues studied. It was highly expressed in both VIN and VIN associated with HPV infection, but minimally expressed in SCC. Such data suggest that VEGF in both invasive and potentially invasive (VIN) lesions of the vulva may be involved in malignant progression and may be a valuable marker of vulvar lesions that go on to become invasive.

Wong Te Fong et al. (2000) evaluated the expression of VEGF and PD-ECGF/TP in different types of vulvar tissue. VEGF was expressed in 86% of the SCC and 7% of VIN samples. However, VEGF was not expressed in normal vulva, LS alone, or in LS adjacent to SCC. PD-ECGF/TP was expressed in 73%–100% of pathological samples and in 20% of the normal vulvar samples.

VEGF expression may be a predictive factor in identifying which VIN lesions are more likely to become invasive. The fact that LS adjacent to carcinoma did not express VEGF indicates that VEGF is not a predictive marker of cases of LS likely to progress to carcinoma. The presence of PD-ECGF/TP in the majority of sections tested hinders its use as a prognostic tool, unlike VEGF, but may indicate its involvement in early angiogenic events (Bamberger et al., 2002).

Ellis et al. (2002) studied the role of VEGF and PD-ECGF/TP in PDV and suggest that PD-ECGF/TP may have a role to play in the pathogenesis of PDV, but not its malignant progression. However, VEGF is not involved in PDV pathogenesis, since it was not expressed in any case, including those associated with invasive disease.

Hefler et al. (1999) evaluated serum concentrations of VEGF in patients with vulvar cancer and in healthy female controls with respect to correlation of VEGF with clinicopathological parameters and impact on the patient's prognosis.

Hefler found serum concentrations of VEGF to be markedly elevated in patients with vulvar cancer compared with healthy female controls. Furthermore, serum concentrations VEGF were shown to be associated with tumor stage but not with tumor dedifferentiation. Patients with vulvar cancer had significantly higher serum concentrations of VEGF compared with healthy female controls, and serum concentrations of VEGF were associated with advanced tumor stage and had a significantly shorter disease-free survival and OS. Although associated with impaired disease-free survival and OS, pretreatment serum concentrations of VEGF are not an independent predictor of outcome in patients with vulvar cancer.

Concluding, tissue VEGF expression and MVD are predictive factors for identifying which VIN lesions are more likely to become invasive, but VEGF is not a predictive marker of cases of LS likely to progress to carcinoma.

18.2.4 Epidermal Growth Factor Receptor's Family

The EGFR family of receptor tyrosine kinases consists of four members: HER-1 (EGFR), HER-2, HER-3, and HER-4. They play a crucial role in growth, differentiation, and morbidity of normal as well as cancer cells (Knopp et al., 2009).

The EGFR (also HER-1) is a 170kd transmembrane tyrosine kinase. Its main ligands are epidermal growth factor (EGF) and transforming growth factor (TGF) (Brustmann, 2007). The EGFR plays a critical role in cancer development and progression for autocrine stimulation of cell proliferation, apoptosis, angiogenesis, and metastatic spread. After ligand binding, the dimerization of EGFR with itself or with other member of its tyrosine kinase receptors leads to high-affinity binding, activation of the intrinsic protein tyrosine kinase activity, and tyrosine autophosphorylation, thereby eliciting a cascade of biochemical and physiological responses involved in receptor-mediated signal transduction. As a consequence of its biological roles, EGFR has been subject to investigation for targeted therapies, with monoclonal antibodies and small-molecule tyrosine kinase inhibitors as anticancer modalities (Alvarez et al., 2006).

Different studies have shown that EGFR is expressed in many types of healthy tissues and is overexpressed in epithelial neoplasms of different origins and tumor-derived cell lines. Brustmann (2007) observed that the EGFR immunoexpression increased significantly from healthy epithelia to vulvar condyloma, high-grade vulvar intraepithelial neoplasia, and keratinizing SCC of vulva (6% in high VIN vs. 41% in SCC), but was not related to stage, grade, or recurrence in SCC.

Woelber found an EGFR copy number increase in 39.3% of the vulvar carcinomas; 17% of vulvar carcinoma showed EGFR high polysomy including 9% with an amplification of the EGFR gene. Genomic EGFR alterations showed a clear association with high-tumor stages, tumors with high depth of invasion, and higher number of positive locoregional lymph nodes. All of these features underline the influence of EGFR on local tumor progression as well as the development of metastases (Woelber et al., 2011). Johnson et al. (1997) found that in a patients with lymph node metastasis, the mean EGFR level in the primary tumor was 65% versus 88% in the metastatic lesion ($p < 0.001$). It is possible that in the future, the levels of EGFR expression could be used for detecting in which group of low-risk tumors an inguinal lymphadenectomy could be avoided (Oonk et al., 2007).

The HER-2 gene, located on chromosome 17q21, encodes for a transmembrane glycoprotein growth factor receptor processing a tyrosine kinase domain. The HER-2 protein recognizes growth stimuli and acts by two principal pathways, phosphatidylinositol 3 kinase (PI3K) and extracellular signal–regulated kinase (ERK). Activation of both pathways is intimately correlated with aggressiveness in various human cancers, like breast, ovarian, vulvar, and gastric adenocarcinoma (Masuguchi et al., 2011).

In addition, a high level of HER-2 in primary vulvar cancer was significantly correlated with high-grade tumors and high count of mitotic figure and lymph node metastasis (Gordinier et al., 1997).

The high number of vulvar carcinoma with an increased expression of HER-2 and EGFR indicates that monoclonal antibodies to HER-2 and EGFR may be used for the therapy of metastatic vulvar carcinoma (Knopp et al., 2009).

Kim characterized EGFR signal transduction and cellular response to treatment with EGFR inhibitor alone or in combination with cisplatin in vulvar cancer cell. He demonstrated that EGFR inhibitor abrogates proliferative signals in vulvar cancer cell expressing EGFR. Given the poor response of vulvar cancer to conventional chemotherapy, the results are encouraging and they support the idea that EGFR inhibition could be plausible strategy in vulvar cancer (Kim et al., 2009).

18.2.5 CAIX

Carbonic anhydrase IX (CAIX) is a transmembrane zinc metalloenzyme that catalyzes the reversible hydration of CO_2 to HCO_3 and plays an important role in tissue pH homeostasis. Apart from its role in pH regulation, CAIX has a function in cell adhesion and is important for growth and survival of tumor cells under normoxia and hypoxia (Robertson et al., 2004).

CAIX shows a very limited expression pattern in nonneoplastic tissue, but it is overexpressed in a wide variety of malignant cell lines and tumors. High levels of CAIX were found to be associated with unfavorable patient outcome in breast carcinomas, bladder cancer, advanced cervical carcinomas, and lung cancer (Choschzick et al., 2010).

The CAIX expression in vulvar cancer is not yet determined. Choschzick found that an increased level of CAIX was significantly associated with advanced pT stage, tumor size, depth of invasion, and lymph node metastases. All of these features are well known to be related with unfavorable clinical outcome. The exclusive expression of CAIX in cancerous tissues makes the enzyme a possible target for therapy. Currently developed CAIX-targeting antibodies (G250) achieved antitumor activity in mouse xenograft tumor models and phase II clinical trials (Bauer et al., 2009).

18.2.6 Cyclooxygenase-2 and Caspase 3

Cyclooxygenase is the enzyme that catalyzes the conversion of arachidonic acid to prostaglandin H2, the rate-limiting step in the synthesis of prostaglandins, and other eicosanoids from membrane phospholipids. Two isoforms of COX are expressed in human tissue. COX-1 is constitutively expressed in most mammalian cell and generates prostaglandins necessary for normal physiological function. COX-2 is normally undetectable but is rapidly inducible in response to a variety of stimuli. COX has been shown to be selectively overexpressed in head and neck, bronchial, pancreatic, breast, gastric, colon, and vulvar cancer (Chang et al., 2004).

In a study of Fons et al., COX-2 overexpression has been significantly associated with poor disease-specific survival (HR, 4.01; 95% CI, 1.10–14.64; $p = 0.035$) (Fons et al., 2007). COX-2 expression was independently associated with disease-free and disease-specific survival (Fons et al., 2009). In other study of Ferrandina et al., COX-2 overexpression was significantly associated with lymph node metastases. In this study, the authors, analyzing the role of COX-2 expression in nonneoplastic and neoplastic vulvar epithelial lesions, suggested that its overexpression may contribute to vulvar tumorigenesis. However, the authors reported a strong COX-2 expression in high-grade VIN, with respect to low-grade VIN, suggesting that upregulation of COX-2 can play a role in tumor onset and progression, but not in LS case (Ferrandina et al., 2004).

In addition, COX-2 was expressed in an increasing degree in the evolution of LS of the vulva into squamous cell cancer (Raspollini et al., 2007).

Caspase 3 belongs to the protease family, which has probably the best correlation with apoptosis. In Fons's study, caspase 3 expression has been a significant prognostic factor in predicting disease-specific survival. Cumulative 5-year survival in patients with caspase-3-positive tumors was 86% compared with a 64% 5-year survival in patients with caspase-3-negative tumors. Until now, there are no data available with regard to the prognostic significance of caspase 3 expression in vulvar cancer (Fons et al., 2007).

This means that although caspase 3 and COX-2 are promising, their prognostic value has to be determined in relation to clinical and pathological variables in a validation study.

18.2.7 CD44v3 and v6

The transmembrane receptor protein CD44 belongs to the family of cell-surface adhesion molecules mediating cell–cell and cell–matrix interactions (Underhill, 1992). CD44 is involved in lymphocyte functions such as cell activation, motility, division, adhesion to extracellular matrix, and adhesion to stromal cells (Mackay et al., 1994). Alternative splicing of the CD44 gene located on chromosome 11 produces various isoforms of the CD44 protein (Screaton et al., 1992). Aberrant expression of isoforms, such as CD44v3 and CD44v6, is indicative of a loss of splice control in malignant cells and increases the affinity of malignant cells to extracellular matrix ligands such as hyaluronan (Salles et al., 1993). It has been shown that the expression of CD44 isoforms is associated with metastasis and poor prognosis in human malignancies such as breast cancer, colorectal cancer, and gastrointestinal lymphoma (Tempfer et al., 1998). Data with respect to the immunohistochemically detected expression of CD44v3 and CDDv6 in gynecologic malignancies are inconsistent. In vulvar carcinoma, these isoforms, CD44v63 and Cd44v6, were shown to predict lymph node involvement and poor prognosis. Furthermore, a possible clinical role for CD44v3 antibodies in detecting occult lymph node metastases in patients with vulvar carcinoma has been proposed (Rodriguez-Rodriguez et al., 2000).

In Tempfer's study, CD44 isoforms CD44v5, CD44v6, and CD44v7-8 were detected in 83% (25/30), 63% (19/30), and 27% (8/30) of the tumor samples, respectively. Patients with tumors overexpressing CD44v6 showed a significantly shorter relapse-free survival ($p = 0.002$) and OS ($p = 0.003$) compared with patients with tumors lacking CD44v6 overexpression. They found no correlation between the expression of CD44 isoforms and clinical stage and histological grade (Tempfer et al., 1996). Overexpression of CD44v6, but not CD44v3, was associated with an impaired prognosis with respect to both disease-free survival and OS. A clinical use of CD44v6 as an additional stratification marker in prospective studies involving patients with vulvar carcinoma remains to be determined (Hefler et al., 2002).

18.2.8 Estrogen Receptors

Vulvar SCC in elderly women develops following a HPV-negative pathway. Zannoni et al. studied if there were differences in the expression of estrogen receptors (ERs) between the tumoral vulvar tissue and the nontumoral one; they found out that there are changes in both ERα and ERβ expression: ERα is lost in tumoral vulvar tissue while ERβ is decreased (Zannoni et al., 2011a). The same author also studied if the expression of ER was related with tumor dimension, histological grading, depth of stromal invasion, epithelial disorders, and number of lymph nodes removed; and an association between the expression of ER and the histological grading was found (Zannoni et al., 2011b). Due to these publications, the expression of ERs seems to be a possible useful biomarker for vulvar cancer in the future.

18.3 Patented Biomarker Panels

There are several biomarkers being used for the early diagnosis and prognosis of different kinds of carcinomas. And every biomarker has a different meaning for the prognosis and future development of the disease. Due to this, several patented biomarker panels have appeared in order to help with the diagnosis, prognosis, and therapy monitoring, using the information of different markers in the same analysis.

Unfortunately, in vulvar cancer, due to the lack of known serum or urine biomarkers and due to the still few evidence in the use of the biomarkers found in vulvar biopsies, there are still no specific patented biomarker panels, such as the ones for ovarian or endometrial cancer.

Nowadays, there are some studies on gynecological cancers that also study possible future vulvar biomarkers such as the *Northwestern Ovarian Cancer Early Detection & Prevention Program: A Specimen and Data Study* that also includes patients with vulvar cancer. So, we hope and expect that new biomarkers will be discovered and evidence will grow with already known ones, so that in a short future, there will be panels useful for clinical practice.

18.4 Conclusion and Future Direction

Vulvar cancer includes a wide variety of histological types implying different etiologies and therefore different possible early biomarkers. Many molecular markers have been identified and studied in different types of vulvar carcinomas, some of them with prognostic implications.

HPV DNA is a marker of vulvar carcinoma that can be helpful for the basaloid and warty carcinomas.

To the cyclin-dependent kinase inhibitors belong p27, p16, and p21. A low level of p16 protein and a high level of p21 protein have been correlated to shorter disease-related survival in patients with vulvar carcinomas. The loss of expression of p27 has been related to the acquisition of metastatic potential and poor prognosis. Another marker is p53 protein. p53 protein overexpression has been found in 35%–68% of vulvar carcinomas and has been associated with shorter disease-related survival at 5 years.

Related to the angiogenesis process is VEGF and MVD. An increased in the expression of VEGF has been associated with tumor progression and poor prognosis in many vulvar cancer types.

Growth factors such as EGFR and HER-2 have been associated with high-grade tumors and lymph node metastasis. EGFR and HER-2 may be used as therapeutic targets in the future, by developing monoclonal antibodies against them.

The transmembrane receptor protein CD44 also appears as a possibly useful marker. An increased expression of CD44 is correlated with reduced disease-free survival and overall survival.

Although many markers have been studied, there is still minor evidence and little clinical use regarding vulvar carcinomas. Nowadays, biomarkers should not change our current medical practice in vulvar cancer. Further multivariable studies with higher number of cases are needed.

References

Alvarez G et al. 2006. Expression of epidermal growth factor receptor in squamous cell carcinomas of the anal canal is independent of gene amplification. *Mod Pathol*, 19, 942–949.

Ansink AC and Heintz AP. 1993. Epidemiology and etiology of squamous cell carcinoma of the vulva. *Eur J Obstet Gynecol Reprod Biol*, 48, 111–115.

Ansink AC et al. 1994. Human papillomavirus, lichen sclerosus, and squamous cell carcinoma of the vulva: Detection and prognostic significance. *Gynecol Oncol*, 52(2), 180–184. doi:10.1006/gyno.1994.1028.

Bamberger ES and Perrett CW. 2002. Angiogenesis in benign, pre-malignant and malignant vulvar lesions. *Anticancer Res*, 22, 3853–3866.

Bancher-Todesca D, Obermair A, Bilgi S, Kohlberger P, Kainz C, Breitenecker G, Leodlter S, and Gitsch G. 1997. Angiogenesis in vulvar intraepithelial neoplasia. *Gynecol Oncol*, 64, 496–500.

Bauer S et al. 2009. Targeted therapy of renal cell carcinoma: Synergic activity of cG250-TNF and IFNg. *Int J Cancer*, 125, 115–123.

Beller U et al. 2006. Carcinoma of the vulva. *Int J Gynecol Obstet*, 95(suppl. 1), S7–S27.

Bergeron C. 2008. Nouvelle terminologie histologique des neoplasies intraepitheliales de la vulve. *Gynecol Obstet Fertil*, 36, 74–78.

Bodelon C, Madeleine MM, Johnson LG, Du Q, Malkki M, Petersdorf EW, and Schwartz SM. 2012. Genetic variation in CD83 and risks of cervical and vulvar cancers: A population-based case-control study. *Gynecol Oncol*, 124(3), 525–528.

Boehm F and Morris JMCL. 1971. Paget's disease and apocrine gland carcinoma of the vulva. *Obstet Gynecol*, 38, 185–192.

Brinton LA, Nasca PC, Mallin K, Baptiste MS, Wilbanks GD, and Richart RM. 1990. Case-control study of cancer of the vulva. *Obset Gynecol*, 75, 859–866.

Brown DC and Gatter KC. 1990. Monoclonal antibody Ki-67: Its use in histopathology. *Histopathology*, 17(6), 489–503.

Brustmann H. 2007. Epidermal growth factor receptor is involved in the development of an invasive phenotype in vulvar squamous lesions, but is not related to MIB-1 immunoreactivity. *Int J Gynecol Pathol*, 26, 481–489.

Carlson JA et al. 2000. Chromosome 17 aneusomy detected by fluorescence in situ hybridization in vulvar squamous cell carcinomas and synchronous vulvar skin. *Am J Pathol*, 157, 973–983.

Chan JK et al. 2007. Margin distance and other clinic-pathologic prognostics factors in vulvar carcinoma: A multivariate analysis. *Gynecol Oncol*, 104, 636–641.

Chan MK et al. 1998. Expression of p16INK4 and retinoblastoma protein Rb in vulvar lesions of Chinese women. *Gynecol Oncol*, 68(2), 156–161.

Chanda JJ. 1985. Extramammary Paget's disease: Prognosis and relationship to internal malignancy. *J Am Acad Dermatol*, 113, 1009–1018.

Chang BW et al. 2004. Prognostic significance of cyclooxygenase-2 in oropharyngeal cell carcinoma. *Clin Cancer Res*, 10, 1678–1684.

Choschzick M, Woelber L, Hess S, zu Eulenburg C, Schwarz, Simon R, Mahner S, Jaenicke F, and Muller V. 2010. Overexpression of carbonic anhydrase IX (CAIX) in vulvar cancer is associated with tumor progression and development of locoregional lymph node metastases. *Virchows Arch*, 45, 483–490.

De Hullu JA et al. 2002. Vulvar carcinoma, the Price of less radical surgery. *Cancer*, 95, 2331–2338.

De Hullu JA and van der Zee AG. 2006. Surgery and radiotherapy in vulvar cancer. *Crit Rev Oncol Hemat*, 60, 38–58.

Doldi N, Origoni M, Bassan M, Ferrari D, Rossi M, and Ferrari A. 1996. Vascular endothelial growth factor expression in human vulvar neoplastic and no neoplastic tissue. *J Reprod Med*, 41, 844–848.

Dumont DJ, Gradwohl GJ, Fong GH, Auerbach R, and Breitman ML. 1993. The endothelial- specific receptor tyrosine kinase, tek, is a member of a new subfamily of receptors. *Oncogene*, 8, 1293–1301.

Edwards CL and Balat O. 1996. Characteristics of patients with vulvar cancer: An analysis of 94 patients. *Eur J Gynaecol Oncol*, 17, 351–353.

el-Deiry WS, Harper JW, O'Connor PM, Velculescu VE, Canman CE, et al. 1994. WAF1/CIP1 is induced in p53-mediated G1 arrest and apoptosis. *Cancer Res*, 54(5), 1169–1174.

Ellis PE et al. 2002. The role of vascular endothelial growth factor—A (VEGF-A) and Platelet-derived Endothelial cell growth factor/Thymidine phosphorylase (PD-ECGF/TP) in Paget`s disease of the vulva and breast. *Anticancer Res*, 22, 857–862.

Emanuels AG et al. 1996. Quantitation of proliferation-associated markers Ag-NOR and Ki-67 does not contribute to the prediction of lymph node metastases in squamous cell carcinoma of the vulva. *Human Pathol*, 27(8), 807–811.

Ferrandina G et al. 2004. Expression of cyclooxygenase-2 (COX-2) in non –neoplastic and neoplastic vulvar epithelial lesions. *Gynecol Oncol*, 92, 537–544.

Ferrara N. 1999. Vascular endothelial growth factor: Molecular and biological aspects. *Curr Top Microbiol Immunol*, 237, 1–30.

Finan MA and Barre G. 2003. Bartholin's gland carcinoma, malignant melanoma and other rare tumors of the vulva. *Best Pract Res Clin Obstet Gynaecol*, 17, 609–633.

Folkman J. 1971. Tumor angiogenesis: Therapeutic implications. *N Engl J Med*, 285, 1182–1186.

Folkman J, Watson K, Ingher D, and Hanahan D. 1989. Induction of angiogenesis during the transition from hyperplasia to neoplasia. *Nature*, 339, 58–61.

Fons G, Burger M, ten Kate F, and van der Velden J. 2007. Identification of potential prognostic markers for vulvar cancer using immunohistochemical staining of tissue microarrays. *Int J Gynecol Pathol*, 26(2), 188–193.

Fons G, Burger M, ten Kate F, and van der Velden J. 2009. Assessment of promising protein markers for vulvar cancer. *Int J Gynecol Cancer*, 19(4), 756–760.

Funk JO et al. 1997. Inhibition of CDK activity and PCNA-dependent DNA replication by p21 is blocked by interaction with the HPV-16 E7 oncoprotein. *Genes Dev*, 11(16), 2090–2100.

Gasco M et al. 2002. Coincident inactivation of 14-3-3sigma and p16INK4a is an early event in vulval squamous neoplasia. *Oncogene*, 21(12), 1876–1881.

Gordinier ME, Steinhoff MM, Hogan JW, Peipert JF, Gajewski WH, Falkenberry SS, and Granai CO. 1997. S-Phase fraction, p53, and HER-2/neu status as predictors of nodal metastasis in early vulvar cancer. *Gynecol Oncol*, 67(2), 200–202.

Hacker NF. 2005. Vulvar cancer. In: Berek JS and Hacker NF, (eds.), *Practical Gynecologic Oncology*, 4th edn. Philadelphia, PA: Williams & Wilkins, pp. 585–602.

Hantschmann P et al. 2000. Tumor proliferation in squamous cell carcinoma of the vulva. *Int J Gynecol Pathol*, 19(4), 361–368.

Heaps JM et al. 1990. Surgical-pathologic variables predictive of local recurrence in squamous cell carcinoma of the vulva. *Gynecology*, 38, 309–301.

Hefler L et al. 2002. The prognostic value of inmunohistochemically detected CD44v3 and CD44v6 expression in patients with surgically staged vulvar carcinoma. *Cancer*, 94(1), 125–130.

Hefler L, Tempfer C, and Kainz C. 1999. Expression of Bcl-2 in vulvar cancer tissue. *Gynecol Oncol*, 73(2), 338–339.

Hefler L, Tempfer C, Obermair A, Frischmuth K, Sliutz G, Reinthaller A, Leodolter S, and Kainz C. 1999. Serum concentrations of vascular endothelial growth factor in vulvar cancer. *Clin Cancer Res*, 5, 2806–2809.

Homesley HD et al. 1991. Assessment of current International Federation of Gynecology and Obstetrics staging of vulvar carcinoma relative to prognostic factors for survival (a Gynecologic Oncology Group study). *Am J Obstet Gynecol*, 164(4), 997–1003; discussion 1003–1004.

Homesley HD et al. 1993. Prognostic factors for groin node metastasis in squamous cell carcinoma of the vulva (a Gynecologic Oncology Group study). *Gynecol Oncol*, 49(3), 279–283.

Howe HL et al. 2001. Annual report to the nation on the status of cancer (1973 through 1998), featuring cancers with recent increasing trends. *J Natl Cancer Inst*, 93, 824–842.

Ishikawa F et al. 1989. Identification of angiogenic activity and the cloning expression of platelet-derived endothelial cell growth factor. *Nature*, 338, 557–561.

Johnson GA, Mannel R, Khalifa M, Walker JL, Wren M, Min KW, and Benbrook DM. 1997. Epidermal growth factor receptor in vulvar malignancies and its relationship to metastasis and patient survival. *Gynecol Oncol*, 65(3), 425–429.

Joura EA. 2002. Epidemiology, diagnosis and treatment of vulvar intraepithelial neoplasia. *Curr Opin Obstet Gynecol*, 14, 39–43.

Kaufman RH. 1995. Distinguished professor series. Intraepithelial neoplasia of the vulva. *Gynecol Oncol*, 56(1), 8–21.

Kim SH, Song YC, Kim SH, Jo H, and Song YS. 2009. Effect of epidermal growth factor receptor inhibitor alone and in combination with cisplatin on growth of vulvar cancer cell. *Acad Sci*, 1171, 642–648.

Knopp S et al. 2004. p16INK4a and p21Waf1/Cip1 expression correlates with clinical outcome in vulvar carcinomas. *Gynecol Oncol*, 95(1), 37–45.

Knopp S et al. 2005. Cyclins D1, D3, E, and A in vulvar carcinoma patients. *Gynecol Oncol*, 97(3), 733–739.

Knopp S et al. 2006. p14ARF, a prognostic predictor in HPV-negative vulvar carcinoma. *Am J Clin Pathol*, 126(2), 266–276.

Knopp S, Tropé C, Nesland JM, and Holm R. 2009. A review of molecular pathological markers in vulvar carcinoma: Lack of application in clinical practice. *J Clin Pathol*, 62, 212–218.

Lai KM and Mercurio G. 2010. Medical and surgical approaches to vulvar intraepithelial neoplasia. *Dermatol Ther*, 23, 477–484.

Lee MH and Yang HY. 2001. Negative regulators of cyclin-dependent kinases and their roles in cancers. *Cell Mol Life Sci*, 58(12–13), 1907–1922.

Mabuchi K, Bross DS, and Kessler II. 1985. Epidemiology of cancer de vulva. A case-control study. *Cancer*, 55, 1843–1848.

Mackay CR, Terpe H, Stauder R, Marston W, Stark H, and Guenthert U. 1994. expression and modulation of CD44 variant isoforms in humans. *J Cell Biol*, 124, 71–82.

Masuguchi S, Jinnin M, Fukushima S, Makino T, sakai K, Inoue Y, Igata T, and Ihn H. 2011. The expression of HER-2 in extramammary Paget's disease. *Biosci Trends*, 5(4), 151–155.

Mc Lean AB. 1993. Precursors of vulval cancers. *Curr Obstet Gynaecol*, 3, 149–156.

Mc Lean AB et al. 2000. Role of angiogenesis in benign, premalignant and malignant vulvar lesions. *J Reprod Med*, 45, 609–612.

Mc Lean AB, Roberts DT, and Reid WMN. 1998. Review of 1000 women seen at two specially designated vulval clinics. *Curr Obster Gynaecol*, 8, 159–162.

Modesitt SC et al. 2000. Expression of Ki-67 in vulvar carcinoma and vulvar intraepithelial neoplasia III: Correlation with clinical prognostic factors. *Gynecol Oncol*, 76(1), 51–55.

Monk BJ, Burger RA, Lin F, Parham G, Vasilev SA, and Wilczynski SP. 1995. Prognostic significance of human papillomavirus DNA in vulvar carcinoma. *Obstet Gynecol*, 85(5 Pt 1), 709–715.

Oonk MHM, Bock GH, van der Veen DJ, ten Hoor KA, de Hullu JA, Hollema H, and van der Zee AGJ. 2007. EGFR expression is associated with groin node metastases in vulvar cancer, but does not improve their prediction. *Gynecol Oncol*, 104, 109–113.

Ordonez NG, Awalt H, and Mackay B. 1987. Mammary and extramammary Paget's disease. An immunocytochemical and ultrastructural study. *Cancer*, 59, 1173–1183.

Pinto AP, Schlecht NF, Pintos J, Kaiano J, Franco EL, Crum CP, and Villa LL. 2004. Prognostic significance of lymph node variables and human papillomavirus DNA in invasive vulvar carcinoma. *Gynecol Oncol*, 92(3), 856–865.

Puig-Tintoré M. 2011. Curso formación continuada de prevención del cáncer cervical: Prevención secundaria. Madrid, Spain: Editores médicos. Modulo 4.

Raspollini MR, Asirelli G, and Taddei GL. 2007. The role of angiogenesis and COX-2 expression in the evolution of vulvar lichen sclerosus to squamous cell carcinoma of the vulva. *Gynecol Oncol*, 106, 567–571.

Robertson N, Potter C, and Harris AL. 2004. Role of carbonic anhydrase IX in human tumor cell growth, survival, and invasion. *Cancer Res*, 64, 6160–6165.

Rodriguez-Rodriguez L, Sancho-Torres I, Gibbon DG, Watelet LF, and Mesonero C. 2000. CD44v9 and CD44v10 are potential molecular markers for squamous cell carcinoma of the vulva. *J Soc Gynecol Invest*, 7, 70–75.

Rolfe KJ et al. 2001. Cyclin D1 and retinoblastoma protein in vulvar cancer and adjacent lesions. *Int J Gynecol Cancer*, 11(5), 381–386.

Rouzier R et al. 2001. Prognostic significance of epithelial disorders adjacent to invasive vulvar carcinomas. *Gynecol Oncol*, 81, 414–419.

Salles G, Zain M, Jiang W, Boussiotis V, and Shipp M. 1993. Alternatively spliced CD44 transcripts in diffuse large cell lymphomas: Characterization and comparison with normal activated B cells and epithelial malignancies. *Blood*, 82, 3539–3547.

Salmaso R et al. 2000. Prognostic value of protein p53 and ki-67 in invasive vulvar squamous cell carcinoma. *Eur J Gynaecol Oncol*, 21(5), 479–483.

Scheistrøen M et al. 1999. p53 protein expression in squamous cell carcinoma of the vulva. *Cancer*, 85(5), 1133–1138.

Screaton GR, Bell MV, Jackson DG, Cornelis FB, Gerth U, and Bell JI. 1992. Genomic structure of DNA encoding the lymphocyte homing receptor CD44 reveals at least 12 alternatively spliced exons. *Proc Natl Acad Sci USA*, 89, 12160–12164.

SEGO (Spanish Society of Gynecology and Obstetrics). 2010. Cancer escamoso invasor de vulva. Oncoguia.

Sgambato A et al. 2000. Multiple functions of p27(Kip1) and its alterations in tumor cells: A review. *J Cell Physiol*, 183(1), 18–27.

Sherr CJ and Roberts JM. 1999. CDK inhibitors: Positive and negative regulators of G1-phase progression. *Genes Dev*, 13(12), 1501–1512.

Sideri M et al. 2005. Squamous vulvar intraepithelial neoplasia: 2004 modified terminology, ISSVD vulvar oncology subcommittee. *J Reprod Med*, 50 (11), 807–810.

Sillman F et al. 1984. The relationship between papillomavirus and lower genital intraepithelial neoplasia in immunosuppressed women. *Am J Obstet Gynecol*, 150, 300–308.

Singh K, Yeo Y, Honest H, Ganesan R, and Luesley D. 2006. Antigen processing and correlation with immunological response in vulval intraepithelial neoplasia—A study of CD1a, CD54 and LN3 expression. *Gynecol Oncol*, 102(3), 489–492.

Tempfer C, Gitsch G, Haeusler G, Reinthaller A, Koelbl H, and Kainz C. 1996. Prognostic value of immunohistochemically detected CD44 expression in patients with carcinoma of the vulva. *Cancer*, 78(2), 273–277.

Tempfer C, Sliutz G, Haeusler G, Speiser P, Reinthaller A, Breitenecker G, Vavra N, and Kainz C. 1998. CD44v3 and v6 variant isoform expression correlates with poor prognosis in early-stage vulvar cancer. *Br J Cancer*, 78(8), 1091–1094.

Todd RW, Steele JC, Etherington I, and Luesley DM. 2004. Detection of CD8+ T cell responses to human papillomavirus type 16 antigens in women using imiquimod as a treatment for high-grade vulval intraepithelial neoplasia. *Gynecol Oncol*, 92(1), 167–174.

Tringler B, Grimm C, Dudek G, Zeillinger R, Tempfer C, Speiser P, Joura E, Reinthaller A, and Hefler LA. 2007. p16INK4a expression in invasive vulvar squamous cell carcinoma. *Appl Immunohistochem Mol Morphol*, 15(3), 279–283.

Tyring SK. 2003. Vulvar squamous cell carcinoma: Guidelines for early diagnosis and treatment. *Am J Obstet Gynecol*, 189(3 Suppl), S17–S23.

Underhill C. 1992. CD44: The hyaluronan receptor. *J Cell Sci*, 103, 293–298.

Van De Nieuwenhof HP, Van Kempen LCLT, De Hullu JA, Bekkers RLM, Bulten J, Melchers WJG, and Massuger LFAG. 2009. The etiologic role of HPV in vulvar squamous cell carcinoma fine tuned. *Cancer Epidemiol Biomarkers Prev*, 18(7), 2061–2067.

van der Avoort IAM et al. 2007. MIB1 expression in basal cell layer: A diagnostic tool to identify premalignancies of the vulva. *Mod Pathol*, 20(7), 770–778.

van Poelgeest MIE et al. 2005. Detection of human papillomavirus (HPV) 16-specific CD4+ T-cell immunity in patients with persistent HPV16-induced vulvar intraepithelial neoplasia in relation to clinical impact of imiquimod treatment. *Clin Cancer Res*, 11(14), 5273–5280. doi:10.1158/1078-0432.CCR-05-0616.

van Seters M et al. 2008. Disturbed patterns of immunocompetent cells in usual-type vulvar intraepithelial neoplasia. *Cancer Res*, 68(16), 6617–6622.

van Seters M, Beurden M, and Craen A. 2005. Is the assumed natural history of vulvar intraepithelial neoplasia III base don enough evidence? A systematic review of 3322 published patients. *Gynecol Oncol*, 97, 645–651.

Woelber L et al. 2011. Prognostic value of pathological resection margin distance in squamous cell cáncer of the vulva. *Ann Surg Oncol*, 18(13), 3811–3818.

Wong Te Fong LF, Rolfe KJ, Crow JC, Reid WMN, MacLean AB, and Perrett CW. 2000. Vascular endothelial growth factor (VEGF) and platelet derived endothelial cell growth factor/thymidine phosphorylase (PD_ECGF/TP) as potential markers in malignant progression of vulvar intraepithelial neoplasia (VIN) and lichen sclerosus to vulvar cancer. *J Obstet Gynaecol*, 20, 559.

Yancopoulos GD et al. 2000. Vascular specific growth factors and blood vessel formation. *Nature*, 407, 242–248.

Yang B and Hart WR. 2000. Vulvar intraepithelial neoplasia of the simplex (differentiated)type: A clinicopathologic study including analysis of HPV and p53 expression. *Am J Surg Pathol*, 24, 429–441.

Zamparelli A et al. 2001. Expression of cell-cycle-associated proteins pRB2/p130 and p27kip in vulvar squamous cell carcinomas. *Hum Pathol*, 32(1), 4–9.
Zannoni GF et al. 2006. Expression of the CDK inhibitor p27kip1 and oxidative DNA damage in non-neoplastic and neoplastic vulvar epithelial lesions. *Mod Pathol*, 19(4), 504–513.
Zannoni GF et al. 2011a. Changes in the expression of oestrogen receptors and E-cadherin as molecular markers of progression from normal epithelium to invasive cancer in elderly patients with vulvar squamous cell carcinoma. *Histopathology*, 58(2), 265–275.
Zannoni GF et al. 2011b. Cytoplasmic expression of oestrogen receptor beta (ERβ) as a prognostic factor in vulvar squamous cell carcinoma in elderly women. *Histopathology*, 59(5), 909–917.

Index

C

D

E

H

I

J

K

L

P

R

S

T

W

Y

Z